VOLUME

5

Bipolar Disorder

WPA Series
Evidence and Experience in Psychiatry

Other Titles in the *WPA Series* Evidence and Experience in Psychiatry

Volume 1—Depressive Disorders
Mario Maj and Norman Sartorius

Volume 2—Schizophrenia
Mario Maj and Norman Sartorius

Volume 3—Dementia
Mario Maj and Norman Sartorius

Volume 4—Obsessive-Compulsive Disorder
*Mario Maj, Norman Sartorius,
Ahmed Okasha and Joseph Zohar*

Bipolar Disorder

Edited by

Mario Maj
University of Naples, Italy

Hagop S. Akiskal
University of California, San Diego, USA

Juan José López-Ibor
Complutense University of Madrid, Spain

Norman Sartorius
University of Geneva, Switzerland

WPA Series
Evidence and Experience in Psychiatry

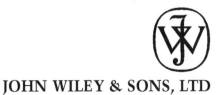

JOHN WILEY & SONS, LTD

Reprinted October 2002 , July 2003

Other Wiley Editorial Offices

John Wiley & Sons Inc., 111 River Street, Hoboken, NJ 07030, USA

Jossey-Bass, 989 Market Street, San Francisco, CA 94103-1741, USA

Wiley-VCH Verlag GmbH, Boschstr. 12, D-69469 Weinheim, Germany

John Wiley & Sons Australia Ltd, 33 Park Road, Milton, Queensland 4064, Australia

John Wiley & Sons (Asia) Pte Ltd, 2 Clementi Loop #02-01, Jin Xing Distripark, Singapore
129809

John Wiley & Sons Canada Ltd, 22 Worcester Road, Etobicoke, Ontario, Canada M9W 1L1

British Library Cataloguing in Publication Data

A catalogue record for this book is available from the British Library

ISBN 0-471-56037-5

Typeset in 10/12 Palatino from author's disks by Kolam Information Services Private Ltd,
Pondicherry
Printed and bound in Great Britain by TJ International Ltd, Padstow, Cornwall
This book is printed on acid-free paper responsibly manufactured from sustainable forestry
in which at least two trees are planted for each one used for paper production.

Contents

Review Contributors

Professor Hagop S. Akiskal VA Psychiatry Service (116A), University of California at San Diego, 3350 La Jolla Village Dr., San Diego, CA 92161, USA

Professor Mark S. Bauer Veterans Affairs Medical Center, Brown University Department of Psychiatry and Human Behavior, 830 Chalkstone Avenue, Providence, RI 02908–4799, USA

Professor Charles L. Bowden Department of Psychiatry, Mail Code 7792, University of Texas Health Science Center, 7703 Floyd Curl Drive, San Antonio, TX 78229–3900, USA

Dr Peter Brieger Department of Psychiatry and Psychotherapy, Martin-Luther-University, Halle-Wittenberg, 06097 Halle, Germany

Dr Carrie L. Ernst Departments of Medicine and Psychiatry, Harvard Medical School, Boston, MA, USA

Professor Joseph Goldberg New York Presbyterian Hospital, Payne Whitney Clinic, Box 140, 525 E 68th Street, New York, NY 10021, USA

Dr Nathan Herrmann Department of Psychiatry, University of Toronto, Sunnybrook and Women's College Health Sciences Centre, 2075 Bayview Ave. Toronto, Ontario M5P 3C6, Canada

Dr Anthony Levitt Department of Psychiatry, University of Toronto, Sunnybrook and Women's College Health Sciences Centre, 2075 Bayview Ave. Toronto, Ontario M5P 3C6, Canada

Professor Andreas Marneros Department of Psychiatry and Psychotherapy, Martin-Luther University, Halle-Wittenberg, 06097 Halle, Germany

Dr Ayal Schaffer Department of Psychiatry, University of Toronto, Sunnybrook and Women's College Health Sciences Centre, 2075 Bayview Ave. Toronto, Ontario M5P 3C6, Canada

Professor Kenneth I. Shulman Department of Psychiatry, University of Toronto, Sunnybrook and Women's College Health Sciences Centre, 2075 Bayview Ave. Toronto, Ontario M5P 3C6, Canada

Preface

Until recently, bipolar disorder was predominantly viewed as a relatively rare condition characterized by periods of euphoric excitement and depressive retardation, which was easy to diagnose and to treat, whose treatment was exclusively pharmacological, and whose outcome was usually favourable.

This perception has changed dramatically in the last decade or so. It has become clear that the rubric "bipolar disorder" actually encompasses a variety of conditions, whose overall lifetime prevalence in the general population may be as high as 5%. The concept of bipolarity extended to bipolar type II has been validated by new research; mixed and psychotic forms of bipolar disorder have turned out to be much more frequent than previously thought; the concomitance of alcohol or drug abuse and of anxiety disorders has been found to be common in bipolar patients and to mask in many cases the disorder of mood. The foregoing developments have made the diagnosis of bipolar disorder a complex clinical endeavour in those cases involving variations on the classical picture. Moreover, the onset of the disorder in childhood or adolescence has been reported to be not so rare, and to generate further diagnostic uncertainties.

The impact of long-term lithium monotherapy on the course of bipolar disorder has been found to be often less than satisfactory. Several alternative drugs have been introduced in clinical practice, and the choice of the most appropriate drug or combination of drugs in the individual patient has become much more complex. The specific problems posed by the treatment of the depressive phase of bipolar disorder have been recognized. Research has documented that some psychosocial interventions may be a useful addition to pharmacotherapy in bipolar patients. The outcome of bipolar disorder has been proved to be frequently sub-optimal, and sometimes chronically deteriorating from both psychopathological and psychosocial perspectives, and the economic burden of the disorder has been reported to be huge.

The debate about some of the above issues, however, remains open. Although for clinical purposes the broadening of the boundaries of bipolar disorder may bring the benefit of new treatments to the less than manic spectrum of the disorder, the concept of a bipolar spectrum has been criticized by some authorities on methodological grounds. It has been argued that the dilution of the concept could lead to decreased reliability in research studies and that the very concept of bipolar spectrum may lack an organizing principle. However, recent familial-genetic studies are beginning to provide a theoretical framework whereby pedigrees of probands with mania include a significant excess of a broad spectrum of affective psychopathology beyond classic mania. Paralleling some of these clinical and theoretical issues, the definition of "mood stabilizer" has emerged as a new controversy; research studies on the increasingly rich variety of agents used in bipolar disorder have not yet provided a consistent answer to this important psychopharmacological question.

It would appear that the foregoing developments and debate have had a relatively limited impact on clinical practice worldwide. Although bipolar II disorder appears in ICD-10, it is not an official diagnostic rubric, which may in part explain why it is not used in clinical practice in many countries; even in North America, where bipolar II disorder is an official diagnosis, such patients with depression, mood instability, and mild brief hypomania are likely to receive the diagnosis of a personality disorder or "unipolar" depression. Of greater concern is the fact that bipolar patients with psychotic symptoms and a deteriorating course are still likely to receive a diagnosis of schizophrenia in many clinical centres around the globe. Thus, long-term treatment of bipolar patients with conventional neuroleptics remains a common problematic practice. New mood stabilizers remain underused in many countries (while they are possibly overused in some others in the absence of adequate data), and the popularity of the individual compounds varies considerably from one country to another (which is not necessarily based on available evidence either). Furthermore, recently introduced psychosocial interventions for bipolar disorder are virtually unknown in many parts of the world.

The WPA series "Evidence and Experience in Psychiatry" has been launched as part of the effort of the World Psychiatric Association to bridge the gap between research data and clinical practice concerning the most prevalent mental disorders. The present volume aims to review the above-mentioned developments and controversies concerning the diagnosis and management of bipolar disorder, and to provide psychiatrists of all countries of the world with a balanced state-of-the-art update of the emerging scientific evidence and accumulated clinical wisdom. We are offering this book to enhance clinical awareness of this prevalent, underdiagnosed, undertreated, and often socially disabling disorder.

Mario Maj
Hagop S. Akiskal
Juan José López-Ibor
Norman Sartorius

1

Classification, Diagnosis and Boundaries of Bipolar Disorders: A Review

Hagop S. Akiskal

International Mood Center, University of California at San Diego, VA Psychiatry Service (116A), 3350 La Jolla Village Drive, San Diego, CA 92161, USA

INTRODUCTION

The New Bipolar Era

After relative neglect in the age of melancholy during the 1970s and 1980s, there has been a renaissance of bipolar disorder during the last decade of the 20th century. Major monographs which cover the psychopathology of the illness have been published, beginning with the Goodwin–Jamison encyclopaedic coverage of *Manic Depressive Illness* [1], the Marneros and Angst's book on *Bipolar Disorders: 100 Years After Manic Depressive Insanity* [2] and the present author's monograph entitled *Bipolarity: Beyond Classic Mania* [3]. Several volumes deal primarily with biological aspects [4–6]. Two poignant autobiographical accounts [7, 8] have helped in the cause of destigmatizing the illness. Other books have been written to address the needs of patients and their families, while at the same time maintaining a scholarly base [7, 9].

The new bipolar era has also witnessed the development of innovative pharmacological and psychosocial interventions specifically geared for this disorder. Despite these advances, bipolar disorder continues to be a disabling disorder for many of its sufferers. One recent monograph on its course and outcome [10] opened with a chapter on "Poor outcome bipolar disorders". A large recent survey [11] of the members of the Depressive and Manic-Depressive Association in the United States found that early misdiagnosis was common, and often a decade elapsed before the correct diagnosis. The signs and symptoms of the classical cyclical illness are

Bipolar Disorder. Edited by Mario Maj, Hagop S. Akiskal, Juan José López-Ibor and Norman Sartorius.
© 2002 John Wiley & Sons Ltd.

unmistakable. However, the illness may begin insidiously with manifestations of a subthreshold or disturbances of a temperamental nature buried in early childhood or adolescence [12]. The course may be irregular or "chaotic" [13], or mixed/cycling [14]. In as many as 50%, psychotic symptoms dominate the clinical picture [15, 16]. Alcohol and substance abuse may mask or complicate underlying mood swings [17, 18]. Other comorbidities include anxiety states, singly or in combination, giving rise to atypical clinical presentations [19, 20]. As the primary aim of this chapter is to review the current body of research evidence and clinical experience in the diagnosis and classification of bipolar disorder, there will be no attempt to exhaustively review comorbidity. The latter will be limited to the most disputed clinical boundaries of bipolar disorder.

The spectrum of psychopathology under the rubric of "bipolar disorder" has been expanded to include bipolar II (major depression plus hypomania) [21], bipolar III (pharmacologically occasioned hypomania during treatment of depression) and beyond [22]. These broader or "softer" phenotypes [23] have enriched bipolar disorder phenotypes, while at the same time inviting criticism on methodological grounds [24]. As juvenile and late-life bipolarity is covered in Chapter 5 of this volume, the main focus of the present chapter will be on the expression of the disorder in adults.

What emerges from the foregoing developments in bipolar illness is a group of overlapping clinical subtypes. Certainly the core classical euphoric disorder responding to lithium is recognized as a valid clinical entity [25, 26]. But bipolarity encountered in contemporary clinical practice extends much beyond this core category [27]. The title of this chapter refers to "bipolar disorders" in the plural, but for the sake of convenience, throughout this chapter, the singular noun will be used. This terminologic convention notwithstanding, the present chapter will offer arguments for and against pluralistic versus unitary concepts of bipolarity.

US vs. International Concepts

The extension of the boundaries of bipolarity is reflected in the American Psychiatric Association's *Diagnostic and Statistical Manual of Mental Disorders* in its 4th edition (DSM-IV) [28]. In this manual, bipolar disorders include bipolar disorder proper (also known as bipolar I), followed by bipolar II, cyclothymia, and bipolar not otherwise specified. This is implicit acceptance of the concept of some sort of a bipolar severity spectrum, contrasted with a depressive disorder spectrum consisting of major depressive disorder, dysthymia, and depression not otherwise specified. The rubric "unipolar disorder", however, is wisely avoided because of the risk for bipolar transformation of major depressive disorder even after many episodes [29–34]. The World Health Organization Classification in its 10th revision (ICD-10) [35] is less committed to the concept of spectrum. Depressive disorders are extensively documented, but again, the term "unipolar" is avoided. While bipolar disorder is recognized along with cyclothymia, the latter is classified with dysthymia under persistent affective disorders. ICD-10 does not formally recognize bipolar II disorder as a specific nosologic category; it is merely given as an example of the nondescript "other" category on the edge of bipolar affective disorders. After providing a superb description of hypomania, ICD-10 makes the surprising statement—and in a spirit contrary to Kraepelin [36]—that recurrent depressive disorder is the diagnosis to be given even if there is evidence of "brief episodes of mild mood elevations and over-activity which fulfil the criteria for hypomania" during the recovery process. Where the US and international manuals agree is in rejecting hypomania—as well as mania!—occurring in response to anti-depressants from inclusion in the "bipolar" rubric. Finally, both manuals accept the concept of bipolar mixed states, consisting of simultaneous admixtures of both poles of the illness. However, there does not appear to be a formal provision for rapid cycling in the international classification.

It is noteworthy that the modern US concept of bipolar or manic-depressive illness—imported almost entirely from classical European psychiatry—today seems to encompass a broader conglomeration of affective conditions than its present counterpart in the European or international classification. Only two decades before the publication of DSM-IV, the US–UK diagnostic project [37] had demonstrated that the US concept of affective disorder was rather narrow, whereas the UK concept included a good chunk of what in the US was classified as schizophrenia, neurosis, or personality disorder. Before embarking on detailed descriptions of contemporary classification and diagnostic practice, this chapter will briefly allude to the historical origins of these reversals in conceptual and nosological systems across the two continents. These differences in part reflect the conservative European tradition versus the greater tendency to experiment with new ideas in the United States. The United States has, of course, benefited from psychiatric talent emigrating from different parts of the world who have brought their diverse psychiatric heritage.

In closing these introductory remarks on bipolar disorder, it would be relevant to point out that, as is the case for other sections of the classification, the ICD-10 definitions of bipolar phases and subtypes pay greater attention to their phenomenology, and less to arbitrary cutoffs on the number of symptoms and their duration, with which DSM-IV is burdened. The latter permits greater operationalization for DSM-IV categories, rendering them more reliable, without assuring clinical validity. As an illustration of the ICD-10 vs. DSM-IV contrast in this regard, I have reproduced excerpts from the

ICD-10 (Table 1.1a) and DSM-IV (Table 1.1b) definitions of hypomania. In ICD-10, the hypomanic patient is presented in all of his liveliness, and the essence of the aroused hyperactive affective state is thereby captured. The DSM-IV criteria merely identify submanic signs and symptoms without capturing the qualitative attributes of hypomania. With the former, we understand the way of being of the hypomanic patient; with the latter we know the precise range of his signs and symptoms. The two approaches are complementary: both are necessary for the diagnostic process.

TABLE 1.1 Hypomania according to ICD-10 and DSM-IV

(a) Excerpts from ICD-10 description of hypomania

Persistent mild elevation of mood, increased energy and activity, and usually marked feelings of well-being and both physical and mental efficiency. Increased sociability, talkativeness, overfamiliarity, increased sexual energy, and a decreased need for sleep are often present but not to the extent that they lead to severe disruption of work or result in social rejection. Irritability, conceit, and boorish behavior may take the place of the more euphoric sociability. Concentration and attention may be impaired, thus diminishing the ability to settle down to work or to relaxation and leisure, but this may not prevent the appearance of interests in quite new ventures and activities, or mild over-spending. Several of [these] features . . . consistent with elevated or changed mood and increased activity, should be present for at least several days on end . . .

(b) DSM-IV criteria for hypomanic episode

A. A distinct period of persistently elevated, expansive, or irritable mood, lasting throughout at least 4 days, that is clearly different from the usual nondepressed mood.

B. During the period of mood disturbance, three (or more) of the following symptoms have persisted (four if the mood is only irritable) and have been present to a significant degree:
   1. Inflated self-esteem or grandiosity
   2. Decreased need for sleep
   3. More talkative than usual or pressure to keep talking
   4. Flight of ideas or subjective experience that thoughts are racing
   5. Distractibility
   6. Increase in goal-directed activity (either socially, at work or school, or sexually) or psychomotor agitation
   7. Excessive involvement in pleasurable activities that have a high potential for painful consequences (e.g., the person engages in unrestrained buying sprees, sexual indiscretions, or foolish business investments)

C. The episode is associated with an unequivocal change in functioning that is uncharacteristic of the person when not symptomatic.

D. The disturbance in mood and the change in functioning are observable by others.

E. The episode is not severe enough to cause marked impairment in social or occupational functioning, or to necessitate hospitalization, and there are no psychotic features.

HISTORICAL ORIGINS

Aretaeus

A state of raving madness with exalted mood was recognized by the ancient Greeks [2]. Its relation to melancholia was probably noted as early as the first century BC by Soranus, who described mania as a remitting illness which, in some patients, had admixtures with melancholia: continual wakefulness and fluctuating states of anger and merriment, sometimes of sadness and futility during the same episode (this description foreshadowed contemporary mixed states).

Aretaeus of Cappadocia (circa AD 150) [38] is usually credited with more explicitly stating the connection between the two major mood states: "It appears to me that melancholy is the commencement and a part of mania." He proceeded to describe euphoric mania as we know it in contemporary psychiatry: "There are infinite forms of mania but the disease is one. If mania is associated with joy, the patient may laugh, play, dance night and day, and go to the market crowned as if victor in some contest or skill. The ideas the patients have are infinite. They believe they are experts in astronomy, philosophy, or poetry."

Aretaeus also described the more severe excitements that develop from this base (end stage mania according to Carlson and Goodwin [39]): "The patient may become excitable, suspicious, and irritable; hearing may become sharp; get noises and buzzing in the ears; or may have visual hallucinations; bad dreams and his sexual desires may get uncontrollable; aroused to anger, he may become wholly mad and run unrestrainedly, roar aloud; kill his keepers, and lay violent hands upon himself."

In another magnificent passage reproduced below, Aretaeus further commented on *secondary* personality changes (of what today some might mistakenly attribute to personality disorder): "They are prone to change their mind readily; to become base, mean-spirited, illiberal, and in a little time extravagant, munificent, not from any virtue of the soul, but from the changeableness of the disease."

Aretaeus also described mania as a disease of adolescent and young men given intermittently to "active habits, drunkenness, lechery" and an immoderate life-style (what today might be called hyperthymic and cyclothymic temperaments). Exacerbations were more frequent in the spring. A modern concept of mania indeed!

Falret and Baillarger

The connection of mania to melancholia was rediscovered 17 centuries later in Falret's "folie circulaire" [40] and Baillarger's "folie à double forme" [41].

That accomplishment was made possible by the humane treatment of the mentally ill in Paris around the turn of the 18th century, which emphasized systematic longitudinal clinical observations of patients, detailed in case records. Bourgeois and Marneros [42] have noted that Falret's concept of circular insanity identified a disorder with highly regular cyclicity and lucid intervals, but that the ultimate prognosis for recovery was often grave, especially in cases with short free intervals (Falret thereby foreshadowed the modern concepts of rapid- and continuous-cycling forms). Baillarger's description of insanity with two phases was less concerned with the free interval and, therefore, the prognosis of the disorder was variable.

The humanitarian reforms introduced in the 19th century may have eventually played a role in changing the prognosis of these disorders: they ensured that standards of general health and nutrition would improve the outlook of patients with mania and melancholia who—unlike those with insanity that evolved into "dementia"—could be discharged from the asylum. In his brilliant historical review on the "two manias", Hare [43] has noted that mania, which in European asylums was once considered to be an incurable illness, thereby became transformed into a disorder with better prognosis.

Kraepelin

The foregoing developments, among others, paved the way to Kraepelin's synthesis at the turn of the 19th century [36]. His unique contribution was not so much in the grouping together of melancholia and mania, but his compelling methodologic rationale based on rigorous observation. His work established manic-depressive illness as a nosological and, he hoped, a disease entity. It was based on the following validating principles: a) the various forms had a common "heredity" measured as a function of familial aggregation, i.e., depression could occur in the families of manic patients and vice versa; b) frequent transitions from depression to mania or the reverse occurred during longitudinal follow-up; c) the superimposed epi-sodes were sometimes opposite to the patient's habitual temperament, i.e., mania could arise from a depressive temperament and depression from a "manic" temperament; d) depressive and manic features could intermix during the same episode (this concept of mixed states was considerably enriched by Weygandt [44], a Kraepelin disciple); e) a recurrent course with illness-free intervals characterized most cases.

Prognosis played such a central role in Kraepelin's formulation of manic-depressive insanity that he may have excluded many patients who failed to make adequate recovery from affective episodes. What was perhaps more objectionable to his contemporaries was his inclusion of clinical depressions without the opposite pole in the enlarged manic-depressive group. The following two passages, reproduced from Kraepelin, explain his rationale for such inclusion: as mania is often followed by depressive states and even minor depressive dips without clinical significance, the reverse could be true for depressive attacks: "When the depression disappears with remarkable rapidity, one must be prepared for a manic attack—an increased feeling of well-being may take the place of depression; this we must perhaps regard as a manic indication, even when it acquires no real morbid extent."

" . . . In association with the states of depression . . . slighter indications of manic symptoms can be demonstrated with extreme frequency, as temporary exalted mood, laughing, singing, dancing, feelings of happiness at time of recovery." (Kraepelin remarked that patients, and sometimes physicians, considered these brief hypomanic excursions as expressions of pleasure at recovery, and thereby missed the manic-depressive nature of the disorder. In the quoted passages Kraepelin was actually describing what today will certainly be considered bipolar II disorder or variants thereof.)

Kraepelin's grouping of states of manic and depressive disorders into a unitary disorder was developed as early as the sixth (1899) edition of his *Lehrbuch der Psychiatrie*. Its opening passage on manic-depressive insanity reads: "Manic-depressive insanity includes on the one hand the whole domain of so-called periodic and circular insanity, on the other hand simple mania, the greater part of the morbid states termed melancholia and also a not inconsiderable number of cases of amentia [confusional insanity]. Lastly, we include here certain slight and slightest colorings of mood, some of them periodic, some of them continuously morbid, which on the one hand are to be regarded as the rudiment of more severe disorders, on the other hand, pass over without boundary into the domain of personal predisposition."

For Kraepelin, the core pathology of clinical depression was expressed in three related domains: lowering of mood, and slowed or retarded physical and mental activity. In mania the opposite dominated the clinical picture: mood was elated and both physical and mental activity accelerated. Mixed states occurred when in either state at least one domain was replaced by its opposite. Table 1.2 summarizes three of Kraepelin's six mixed state prototypes, still commonly observed in contemporary clinical practice. Patients with "involutional melancholia" (referring to 40- to 55-year-old patients with extreme anxiety, irritability, agitation, and delusions) were originally excluded from the larger manic-depressive rubric; he believed the etiology of the former to be vascular or degenerative. However, in the eighth edition of the *Lehrbuch*, he classified involutional melancholia within the manic-depressive group as a special form of mixed state; follow-up conducted by his pupil Dreyfus [45] had shown the occurrence of unmistakable excited phases. This historical note contradicts the myth that Kraepelin was "rigid";

TABLE 1.2 Kraepelin's concept of mixed states in contemporary practice

Type of mixed state	Mood	Thinking	Activity
Anxious-depressive mania	⇓	⇑	⇑
Excited depression	⇓	⇓	⇑
Depression with flight of ideas	⇓	⇑	⇓

indeed he did change his mind when evidence pointed to the contrary. (Curiously, the question of depressive mixed state is still a controversial issue, as further discussed in Koukopoulos and Koukopoulos' superb paper on "agitated depression as a mixed state" [46].)

Kraepelin's concept of manic-depressive insanity was not just unitary. In suggesting that the range of illness manifestations spanned from temperament—"personal disposition" in his formulation in German—all the way to depressive, mixed, manic and psychotic states, Kraepelin was formulating what today we consider a spectrum concept of manic-depressive illness [27].

CONTEMPORARY CLASSIFICATORY APPROACHES

The Unipolar-Bipolar Distinction

In the short span of 12 years, Karl Leonhard [47] in 1957, Jules Angst [48] in 1966, Carlo Perris [49] in 1966, and George Winokur, Paula Clayton, and Theodore Reich [50] in 1969—working independently on two continents in four different countries—proposed that depressive disorders without manic or hypomanic episodes (unipolar depression) are distinct from depressive episodes that begin at earlier ages and alternate with manic or hypomanic episodes (bipolar disorder). The main difference between the two affective subtypes is the greater familial loading for mood disorder—especially for bipolar disorder—among bipolar probands. This polarity-based distinction has proven to be of great heuristic research and clinical benefit [1, 2]. The most documented differentiating features between unipolar and bipolar depressions (most data based on bipolar I disorder) are summarized in Table 1.3.

Although, in the extreme, bipolar and unipolar disorders are discriminable clinically, familially, and therapeutically, observations during the past two decades have shown areas of overlap between those extremes that might be considered "pseudo-unipolar".

Firstly, there are those depressive patients who experience very brief hypomanic episodes, as described by Angst [51]. Despite the fact that the

TABLE 1.3 Differentiating characteristics of bipolar and unipolar depressions

	Bipolar	Unipolar
History of mania or hypomania (definitional)	Yes	No
Sex ratio	Equal	Women > men
Age at onset	Teens, 20s, and 30s	30s, 40s, 50s
Postpartum episodes	More common	Less common
Onset of episode	Often abrupt	More insidious
Number of episodes	Numerous	Fewer
Duration of episodes	3 to 6 months	3 to 12 months
Psychomotor activity	Retardation > agitation	Agitation > retardation
Sleep	Hypersomnia > insomnia	Insomnia > hypersomnia
Family history		
Bipolar disorder	High	Low
Unipolar disorder	High	High
Pharmacological response		
Antidepressants	Induce hypomania/ mania	Induction of hypomania/mania is rare
Lithium carbonate	Acute antidepressant effect	Generally ineffective

Research Diagnostic Criteria (RDC) [52] set the lowest threshold to two days for probable hypomania (seven days for definite), DSM-IV—which is derived from it—arbitrarily settled down with a threshold of four days.

Secondly, 10–20% of patients with major depressive disorder subsequently develop hypomanic or manic episodes and so should be reclassified as having bipolar I or II disorder [29–33]. This occurs with an average latency of six years from first depressive attack. A disciple of Kraepelin would argue that some, though not all, such patients must have been "cryptic" bipolar at the temperamental level, possibly indicated by trait mood lability or mild cyclothymic tendencies; others may have displayed "manic" or hyperthymic traits—upbeat, driven, overenergetic and overconfident individuals—without having ever reached the threshold of a discrete episode of hypomania.

Thirdly, there exist "unipolar" patients in bipolar pedigrees, or clinically depressed patients who have a bipolar first-degree relative [53–5]. Indeed Winokur [56], the US proponent of the unipolar-bipolar distinction, wondered whether a common genetic factor linked the two disorders.

The foregoing observations may, in part, explain why some apparently "unipolar" patients respond to lithium monotherapy or lithium augmentation [57–60]. A practitioner—or a researcher for that matter—who systematically follows up his or her patients will often encounter primarily depressed patients who display rudimentary or muted manifestations of hypomania. As Kraepelin demonstrated in his monograph—and Post's group [61] has systematically endorsed—course captured graphically is one of the best ways to identify these less-than-manic expressions of the illness. Kraepelin, after diagramming 18 illustrative patterns for the entire spectrum of manic-depressive illness, declared that the illness pursued an indefinite number of courses. He was naturally sceptical of any subdivisions, for that would have undermined his unitary concept of manic-depressive illness! The question for the contemporary practitioner is whether there are validated clinical subtypes in the interface of depressive and manic extremes of affective illness.

The Bipolar Spectrum

The unipolar-bipolar distinction left undefined many affective conditions lying in between [62]. We encounter such patients in the pedigrees of bipolar probands: indeed, relatives of bipolar patients suffer predominantly of illnesses that are depressive in nature (by a factor of 3 or 4) [54]. Based on such data and clinical intuition, we argued that these phenotypically "unipolar" relatives of bipolar probands are "genotypically" bipolar [23]: we thereby estimated that 4–5% of the general population belongs to a broad bipolar spectrum with predominantly depressive phenomenology and muted bipolar features. This prediction has now been confirmed in the new wave of epidemiologic studies [63–65], which have documented that the classical figure of 1–1.6% for bipolar disorder [66–68] is too conservative, and that at least 5% of the community manifests bipolarity, much of it depressive in form, but coupled with less-than-manic, brief excitements. The most compelling data derive from the Zurich epidemiological study by Angst [65]. This work, conducted by one of the original researchers who was highly influential in promoting the concept of bipolar disorder, persuasively argues for the need to enlarge bipolarity at the subthreshold (brief hypomania) end of the spectrum. These seemingly "subclinical" manifestations from a symptomatological point of view have proven—in association with depressive features—to have significant adverse psychosocial consequences.

In a pioneering contribution, Dunner et al [21] had identified these less-than-manic patients as bipolar II on the basis of hospitalization for depression, and hypomanic periods that did not require hospitalization. Fieve and Dunner [69] had reserved the diagnosis of bipolar I disorder for bipolar patients who had required hospitalization for mania. Although one may question whether hospitalization is an adequate criterion for defining the diagnostic threshold for mania, the work of these investigators nonetheless represented an important advance—for both research methodology and clinical practice—in paving the way for the recognition of the large universe of bipolar patients whose excited periods remained ambulatory. Subsequently, Angst et al [70] introduced the concept of "Dm" for these genetic variants of the more classic "MD" and "Md" subtypes. The Akiskal and Mallya [23] proposal for a "soft bipolar spectrum" is a more inclusive term for bipolar conditions beyond classic mania, and extends the foregoing definitions by incorporating depressions with hypomanic episodes (core bipolar II), cyclothymic and hyperthymic traits, as well as those with familial bipolarity; the spectrum also includes hypomanic periods which occur during pharmacotherapy or other somatic treatments (bipolar III). A related proposal based on extensive clinical observations has been made by Noble Endicott [71], who further expanded the spectrum to include, among others, cyclic depressions without hypomania, but abrupt onset and offset. Klerman [72], too, had earlier written in favour of a "spectrum of mania", based on nosological considerations. More recently, Cassano et al [73] have described yet another variant of the bipolar spectrum concept based on a symtomatologic continuum between subthreshold and full-blown clinical expressions of bipolarity.

Just a few years after the publication of DSM-III—and in response to a request by the American Psychiatric Association as to whether the new diagnostic manual provided adequate coverage for all affective diagnoses—we reported that the foregoing bipolar spectrum conditions were as prevalent as their unipolar counterparts (Table 1.4) in a consecutive case series of personally examined affective states [23]. A major validation of the concept of a bipolar spectrum that ranges from levels of mania through hypomania and hyperthymia has come from the Pisa–Memphis collaborative study [74]: it demonstrated that bipolar I and II disorders and depressions arising from the hyperthymic temperament could be distinguished from major depressive disorder (without manic spectrum features) on the basis of bipolar family history. The French national collaborative study (EPIDEP) [75] has the largest data in support for the inclusion of hypomania associated with pharmacotherapy within the bipolar spectrum, based on familial bipolarity essentially indistinguishable from that of spontaneous hypomania.

The genetic investigation of Bertelsen et al [76] is one of the strongest lines of evidence for the broad bipolar concept: monozygotic twins discordant for strictly defined mood disorders were broadly concordant for such conditions as mood-labile temperaments at the (untreated) end of the spectrum, and schizophreniform disorders beyond the boundaries of classic affective disorders at the psychotic end of the spectrum. One could therefore argue that the same putative bipolar genotype expressed itself in phenotypes which range from the very mild near normal to the extremely ill.

TABLE 1.4 Primary affective diagnoses in 102 patients in a community mental health centre (summarized from Akiskal and Mallya [23])

Diagnosis*	%
Bipolar I	18
Bipolar II	18
Bipolar III	9
Cyclothymia**	5
Unipolar (major depression)	44
Dysthymia**	6

*Sampling involved taking every 50th patient over a 10-year period and eliminating those with non-affective diagnoses.
**In the absence of major mood disorders.

Like the unipolar-bipolar distinction, the bipolar spectrum is a heuristic clinical classification. Bipolar II disorder, which is the most common expression of the spectrum, in some pedigrees seems to "breed true" [77–80]. It is therefore likely that genetic heterogeneity underlies the proposed clinical spectrum of bipolarity. However, it is not clear at this time how to subdivide the broad clinical terrain of bipolarity on genetic grounds. Alda *et al* [81] have proposed that lithium-responsive bipolar patients, typified by euphoric mania, might constitute the core genetic subtype within the spectrum. However, this would exclude at least 50% of bipolar I patients, who do not respond to lithium. Also, judging from the fact that bipolar II disorder is common in bipolar pedigrees, at least some bipolar II patients (presumably a "sunny" or stable phenotype) must represent muted expressions of the core genotype. Other bipolar II patients might represent an autonomous or "dark" phenotype in association with cyclothymic instability; this temperament has emerged as distinct from other more stable temperaments in an epidemiologic study [82]. Much work lies ahead of us in terms of defining putative phenotypes to guide the search for genotypes within the clinical spectrum of bipolar disorders.

Two recent critical reviews represent contrasting views on the boundaries of bipolar disorder. Cassano *et al* [73] argue that the bipolar spectrum is a "clinical reality" but in search of diagnostic and assessment methodology. The other critique by Baldessarini [24] argues for a more cautious approach which would restrict any broadening of the presently accepted official boundaries of DSM-IV. Paradoxically, Baldessarini's historical overview of bipolarity—from Aretaeus [38] to Goodwin and Jamison [1]—includes largely authors or investigators whose work supports a broad concept (Table 1.5). This is because the thrust of historical development in bipolar disorder has been *for* a broad spectrum! Where Baldessarini and Cassano converge is in their requirement of methodological purity, which may be

TABLE 1.5 Historical evolution of the concept of bipolar disorder (according to Baldessarini [24])

150 AD	Aretaeus	Melancholia → mania
1854	Falret & Baillarger	Circular and double insanity
1867	Griesinger	Unitary mental disorder
1882	Kahlbaum	Cyclothymia
1899	Kraepelin	Manic depressive psychosis
1960s	Angst, Perris, Winokur	Unipolar-bipolar distinction
1976	Dunner et al	Bipolar II
1976	Mendels	Pseudo-unipolar depression
1978	Pope and Lipinski	"Schizophrenic" symptoms in manic depressive psychosis
1983	Akiskal	Bipolar spectrum
1990	Goodwin and Jamison	Manic-depressive illness

necessary for certain research operations, versus practice considerations that, we would contend, do not require pristine methodological designs, nor unwieldy assessment instruments which are unrealistic in a clinical setting. A recently published instrument by Hirschfeld et al [83] to screen for the bipolar spectrum appears to be relatively straightforward, with acceptable sensitivity and good specificity, though it has not yet been used extensively in clinical practice. The same is true for several other instruments developed primarily for use in epidemiologic or high risk studies [84, 85].

The compelling clinical rationale for the spectrum concept is that practitioners with preventive focus in most fields of medicine have historically diagnosed illnesses in their earlier and milder expressions. Those described in textbooks—as well as ICD-10 or DSM-IV—as "typical" cases, are actually relatively uncommon in clinical experience. In other words, what those manuals describe as "atypical" (or not otherwise specified) are, in reality, quite typical!

To recapitulate, candidates proposed for inclusion in a broadly conceived bipolar spectrum are mania; recurrent depressions with hypomania (irrespective of duration), pharmacologically mobilized hypomania, as well as those in association with cyclothymic and hyperthymic temperaments; and finally recurrent (pseudo-unipolar) depressions with bipolar family history, or cyclic depressions responsive to lithium. An International Exchange on Bipolar Disorder (IEBD) [86] among 30 clinician-researchers from both sides of the Atlantic took place in Barcelona in the spring of 1998 to consider, among others, the current status of clinically validated bipolar subtypes. Table 1.6 summarizes the deliberations of this group.

Neither the unipolar-bipolar distinction, nor the competing bipolar spectrum concept have received unqualified support. Indeed, both have

TABLE 1.6 Barcelona international "consensus" on bipolar subtypes *beyond DSM-IV and ICD-10** (summarized from Akiskal *et al* [86])

- Mood incongruent bipolar psychosis
- Bipolar I (mania)
- Mixed mania (≥ 2 *depressive symptoms*)
- Bipolar II (*hypomania ≥ 2 days*)
- *Somatic treatment-induced hypomania*
- Rapid cycling
- Cyclothymia
- *Recurrent brief hypomania*

*Italic entries represent recommended revisions to these manuals.

been criticized [24, 87]. Even since before Kraepelin, the pendulum in international classification has moved back and forth between unitary (spectrum) and discontinuity (unipolar-bipolar) positions. Circa 2001, the pendulum seems to be moving towards the spectrum position [1, 3], even though its ultimate range remains undefined.

MANIA, HYPOMANIA, CYCLOTHYMIA AND HYPERTHYMIA

Mania

Classic *euphoric mania* is unmistakable: the elated mood is accompanied by grandiosity, psychomotor acceleration, a rush of ideas, distractibility, and decreased need for sleep [36]. The manic patient is witty, his behaviour expansive, jesting, and dramatic. The patient lifts the clinician's spirits, but can be irritating as well. Although this mode of emotional communication is highly characteristic of mania [88], as contrasted with schizophrenia, it is not specifically mentioned in the diagnostic guidelines of ICD-10 and DSM-IV. Perhaps it is deemed to be unreliable, in that manic mood is changeable. Bursting into tears is common, but not necessarily lasting. Also, for many patients the high is so excessive that it is experienced as intense nervousness. Moreover, when crossed, the patient can become extremely hostile. Thus, lability and irritable hostility are as much features of the manic mood as is elation, and appear as such in both ICD-10 and DSM-IV.

Accelerated psychomotor activity, which for some investigators [89] constitutes the hallmark of mania, is characterized by an overabundance of energy and activity and by rapid and pressured speech. Subjectively, the patient experiences an unusual sense of physical vitality (eutonia), not specifically mentioned in DSM-IV and ICD-10 manuals. Thinking processes are accelerated, subjectively experienced as flight of ideas. The patient may speak with such pressure that it is difficult to follow his associations, often based on rhyming or chance perceptions, which may therefore appear "loose". The pressure to speak may continue despite the development of hoarseness—this, too, is neither in DSM-IV, nor ICD-10. The psychomotor disinhibition in mania is often associated with risk-taking behaviour in many domains [88]. They are distractible and move quickly, not only from one thought to another, but from one person to another, showing heightened interest in every new activity that strikes their fancy. They are indefatigable and engage in various activities in which they usually display poor judgement. Examples include preaching or dancing in the street; abuse of long distance calling; buying new cars, hundreds of records, expensive jewellery, or other unnecessary items; paying the bills of total strangers in bars; giving away one's furniture; engaging in questionable business ventures; gambling; unplanned trips; and sudden marriages. Such pursuits can lead to personal and financial ruin. The sexual appetite is typically increased and often leads to sexual misadventures, resulting in marital disasters— hence the multiple separations or divorces that are so characteristic of the disorder. Sexual indiscretion is even more problematic now, in view of the spectre of HIV infection. Although both ICD-10 and DSM-IV consider such behavioural excesses as cardinal signs of mania, neither manual makes specific reference to the meddlesome behaviour of manic patients [90]: they are intrusive in their increased involvement with others, leading to marked—and often lifelong—friction with family members, friends, and colleagues. A corollary of psychomotor activation, and another cardinal sign of mania, is decreased need for sleep, whereby the patient sleeps for only a few hours but feels energetic on awakening. Some may actually go sleepless for several days, which could lead to a dangerous escalation of manic activity, and sometimes, to physical exhaustion. Weight loss may occur because of such hyperactivity and neglect of nutritional needs. Delirious mania, an extremely severe, yet rare, expression of mania (also known as "Bell's mania") [91] involves frenzied physical activity that continues unabated, leading to a medical emergency that is life threatening. Pseudodementia, a confused manic state, has also been reported [92].

Manic thinking is overly positive, optimistic, and expansive. The patient presents an inflated self-esteem, a grandiose sense of confidence and boasts about his achievements [36]. Behind that façade, however, there may be a vague and painful recognition that the positive self-concepts do not represent reality [88]. Such insight, if present at all, is transient; indeed, manic patients are notoriously refractory to self-examination. Denial, lack of insight, and impaired judgement [93, 94]—cardinal cognitive derangements of mania—are not listed in the DSM-IV criteria for manic episode or bipolar disorders. This is a serious omission: poor judgement plays an important role in the way manic patients manage their personal life, harming themselves and their loved ones. Their proverbial poor adherence to pharmacotherapy is due to their denial that there is anything wrong with their exalted mental state. Finally, their lack of insight makes their delusions less amenable to challenge.

According to Kurt Schneider [95], manic *psychosis* is characterized by delusions of exceptional mental and physical fitness and talent; delusions of wealth, aristocratic ancestry, or other grandiose identity; delusions of assistance; or delusions of reference and persecution, based on the belief that enemies are observing or following them out of jealousy at their special abilities. At the height of mania patients may even see visions or hear voices congruent with their euphoric mood and grandiose self-image. Psychosis in the setting of mania is thus typically mood-congruent. The sense of physical well-being and mental alacrity is so extraordinary that manic patients believe that they possess superior powers or that they are great healers, inventors or famous reformers. Their senses are so vivid that colours and textures are richer, and reality more exotic, both of which can be easily transformed into a vision. Such enhanced perceptions [88], briefly mentioned in ICD-10, are nowhere to be found in DSM-IV. The thoughts of manic patients are so rapid and vibrant that they feel they can hear them. Mental processes in mania are so powerful, that some patients feel their brains have special communication channels with a deity or the cosmos. Thus, certain first-rank Schneiderian-type symptoms, which have been traditionally considered mood-incongruent, can be understood phenomenologically to arise from the powerful mental experiences of mania. A high proportion of manic patients abuse alcohol and stimulants [96, 97]— as well as other substances—ostensibly to enhance or modulate their moods and, therefore, mood-incongruence can sometimes be explained on the basis of intoxication or withdrawal [17]. However, not all mood-incongruent psychotic experiences in mania are understandable on phenomenologic grounds, nor on the basis of cerebral pathology. At the height of mania, severely ill manic patients may experience or display most signs and symptoms deemed "schizophrenic" in form [15, 16, 39, 98]. Major exceptions are poverty of content of thought and lasting flattening of affect [99]. Caution should be exercised to avoid over-diagnosing schizophrenia in certain ethnic groups, as African-American and UK Caribbean manic patients are more likely to present clinically with severe illness and psychotic symptoms [100–103].

Neither ICD-10 nor DSM-IV specifically address the diagnostic questions posed by the 5–10% of bipolar patients who pursue a chronic manic course [104]. These cases represent deterioration of bipolar disorder dominated by recurrent manic episodes arising from a hyperthymic baseline. The psychomotor excitement in these cases is gradually replaced by chronic grandiose delusions; the mood is one of near constant elation; with minimal subjective distress and insight totally lacking, the patient sees no reason to adhere to any treatment regimen. Because of their social deterioration, Kraepelin had subsumed such patients under the category of "manic dementia". Organic factors such as head trauma and chronic alcohol abuse may contribute to the deteriorative course. A persistent cheerful disposition, non-schizoid premorbid adjustment, prior manic episodes, and a family history of bipolar disorder—as well as the absence of flagrant formal thought disorder—can be marshalled in validating the affective nature of these poor-prognosis manic states [88].

The descriptive and phenomenologic features of mania reviewed suggest the need to enrich DSM-IV by at least three domains presently absent from its formal diagnostic criteria: 1) social disinhibition leading to meddlesome and intrusive behaviour; 2) enhanced perceptions; 3) impaired insight and judgement. A new ordering of the symptomatologic criteria of mania which incorporate these three domains is summarized in Table 1.7.

It is relevant to end this section on mania by noting that its clinical diagnosis has very high reliability among trained clinicians (kappa= .93) [105], making the use of mania rating scales unnecessary in routine clinical practice. Such scales [106–108] are primarily for research purposes. Psychopharmaceutical trials, in particular, have benefited from the use of such scales.

Hypomania

The signs and symptoms of hypomanic episodes as described in DSM-IV are insufficiently discriminatory from those for mania. The distinction is based on severity: psychotic symptoms are absent, duration is shorter, and

TABLE 1.7 Proposed enrichment of the DSM-IV symptomatologic criteria for mania

- Euphoria—which can easily shift to irritability and hostility
- Psychomotor activation
- Boundless energy
- Grandiose self-esteem
- Pressure of speech—flight of ideas
- Heightened perceptions
- Marked distractibility of attention
- Little need for sleep
- Increased risk-taking—squandering money
- Social disinhibition
- Lechery
- Denial—loss of insight—impaired judgement

major life disruptions are uncharacteristic—indeed, hypomania can be adaptive [62, 109]. Thus, hypomania is a non-psychotic, milder or sub-threshold manic state of short duration and without marked impairment. Although hypomanic episodes represent a departure from the person's habitual baseline, they are typically experienced as ego-syntonic. Hence, family and significant others generally provide more reliable reports.

Brief hypomanic episodes among Memphis cyclothymic outpatients [110] revealed features which are deceptively adaptive when taken singly and without regard to long-term course: carefree and cheerful; high energy, eutonia and vitality; could get by with less sleep than usual for the person; sharper senses and creative thinking; overconfident and overly optimistic; talkative; overly gregarious and people-seeking; heightened sexual drive and behaviour; spending sprees; and over-involvement in new projects and activities. More often than not, hypomania is recurrent and part of cyclothymia and, therefore, considerable impairment invariably occurs as a result of repeated mood swings. The Zurich epidemiologic project [111] reported a broader range of hypomanic manifestations in the community: less sleep; more energy and strength; more self-confidence; increased activities; enjoying work more than usual; more social activities; spending too much money; more ideas and plans; less shy and less inhibited; more talkative than usual; increased sex drive; increased consumption of coffee, cigarettes, and alcohol; overly optimistic with euphoria; increased laughter, joking and puns; and sharp thinking with new ideas. The psychometric properties of the Zurich hypomania scale are under investigation [112]. Suffice it to say that the "sunny" or positive features of hypomania are observed primarily among those with sporadic hypomania. Both the Memphis and Zurich observations are based on individuals who had never been hospitalized for mania, and thus capture the rich phenomenology for hypomania beyond the narrow band criteria in DSM-IV. Also, both studies stipulated a modal duration of two days. This threshold has been recently validated in an Italian study [113]: indeed, nearly all patients in a large consecutive series of private outpatients had hypomania less than four days, and nearly all were recurrent. An earlier Italian study [74] on bipolar II patients which used a definition of hypomania duration of two days—whether it was in association with episodes of major depression or part of cyclothymia—found the rate of bipolar family history in these patients to be similar to that of bipolar I patients, and significantly higher than that of pure major depressive disorder. Manning *et al* [114], reporting on a consecutive case series of depressive and anxious patients in general medical practice, have also presented data in favour of the two-day threshold for hypomania.

In conclusion, the four-day threshold of DSM-IV hypomania is unjustified [86] and unnecessarily narrows down the range of bipolar spectrum disorders diagnosable in clinical, epidemiologic, and genetic studies. The IEBD

[86] recommended four days in sporadic cases, and two days for the more prevalent recurrent forms.

Cyclothymia

Both Kraepelin [36] and Kretschmer [115] described cyclothymic individuals in whom low-grade affective manifestations of a subdepressive and mild hypomanic nature oscillated over long periods of the life span. While in the classical, and especially German, literature [116] cyclothymia refers to the entire range of manic-depressive manifestations, in its current usage [117] the term cyclothymic disorder is restricted to a subthreshold bipolar trait or temperament.

In most cyclothymes presenting clinically [118], depressive or irritable moodiness predominates; in a minority of cases, intermittent hypomanic features are more characteristic. Cyclothymic mood swings could occur throughout life without progression to major affective episodes, or represent the prodromal phases of more severe episodic mood disorders; upon recovery from these episodes, patients tend to return to their cyclothymic baseline. Relatively neglected by the contemporary psychiatric establishment and clinical psychology, several large-scale studies have nonetheless examined cyclothymic disorder and its variants in juvenile and young adult subjects.

The earliest of these studies was carried out at the University of Tennessee, Memphis [110] in the late 1970s: 10% of a mental health clinic population met criteria for subsyndromal mood swings over long periods of teenage and young adult years. They presented clinically because of social disruptions in their lives, such as romantic failure, financial extravagance, repeated change of line of work or college studies, frequent geographic moves, and polysubstance abuse. The underlying bipolar diathesis was validated on the basis of biphasic subsyndromal changes in energy, activity, mood, and cognition, each phase typically lasting from two days to a week; family history for bipolar disorder was obtained from cyclothymes at rates comparable to that from full-blown bipolar disorder; during prospective follow-up, one out of three cyclothymes progressed to full-blown clinical depression or hypomania (some of which were during antidepressant use for depression), and rarely to manic states. This observation suggests that cyclothymia and bipolar II disorder form a continuum [118]. The same finding emerged in the French EPIDEP study [119], where 88% of cyclothymes in a national cohort of major depressives were independently diagnosed as bipolar II.

In collaboration with a team of clinical researchers from Pisa [82], we studied 1010, 14–25-year-old students: high internal consistency and diagnostic specificity was found for six of the eight criteria for cyclothymic temperament according to Akiskal and Mallya [23]: lethargy alternating with eutonia; shaky self-esteem alternating between low self-confidence and overconfidence; decreased verbal output alternating with talkativeness; mental confusion alternating with sharpened and creative thinking; unexplained tearfulness alternating with excessive punning and jocularity; and introverted self-absorption alternating with uninhibited people-seeking. This *subthreshold* oscillation of hypomanic and depressive periods, with infrequent euthymia, identified 6.3% of the student population as cyclothymic [120]. These biphasic shifts, lasting typically no more than a few days at a time in each direction, represent the *habitual* long-term functioning of the individual. Both the Memphis and Pisa studies of cyclothymia utilized a semi-structured interview format. An auto-questionnaire version of this cyclothymia scale called TEMPS-A (Temperament Evaluation of Memphis, Pisa, Paris and San Diego) [121] found excellent internal consistency for the set of 21 items of cyclothymia, of which those with the highest factorial loading are listed in Table 1.8. Translated into 12 languages, TEMPS-A is presently being investigated in different countries. The French national EPIDEP study [119] has reported high (positive) correlation between patient self-rating vs. clinician interview, and a conservative cutoff of 10 or more items for a provisional identification of the cyclothymic temperament in clinical populations.

Another large study [122] examining cyclothymia was conducted in college students in Albany, New York, in the early 1980s. Constructing a self-rated inventory based in part on the University of Tennessee descriptions of cyclothymia—and modifying them on the basis of the classical psychiatric literature and psychometric considerations—these authors reported that 4–6% of students could be described as cyclothymic. Many of these cyclothymic students developed depressive and/or suicidal crises—often in association with substance abuse—during prospective observation, underscoring the public health importance of cyclothymia as a putative bipolar diathesis. The General Behavior Inventory (GBI), which has derived from this body of work, has not proven to be particularly useful for clinical practice. Its research applications have been more promising. For instance, high GBI cyclothymia scores have been reported in the offspring of bipolar probands [123].

A consistent finding in the foregoing studies is the strong familial association of cyclothymia with bipolar disorder. However, it phenotypically appears more linked to bipolar II rather than bipolar I disorder. Cyclothymia is emerging as a bipolar trait of great public health significance: occurring in up to 6% of individuals in the general population, it may serve as the reservoir of bipolar genes, and perhaps of greatness in human societies. The stormy temperament of cyclothymic people, which often causes much suffering to themselves and their loved ones, nonetheless appears to be an important ingredient in creative pursuits in a variety of domains of life and art [117, 124–127].

TABLE 1.8 Self-rated items loading heavily on the cyclothymic temperament in affectively ill outpatients (summarized from Akiskal *et al* [121])

.601 I constantly switch between being lively and sluggish
.578 My mood often changes for no reason
.564 My ability to think varies greatly from sharp to dull for no apparent reason
.538 My mood and energy are either high or low, rarely in between
.532 The way I see things is sometimes vivid, but at other times lifeless
.514 I often feel tired for no reason
.506 I get sudden shifts in mood and energy
.504 I often start things and lose interest before finishing them
.484 I often have a strong urge to do outrageous things
.445 I feel all emotions intensely

Hyperthymia

Little attention has been paid in the contemporary psychiatric literature to long-term adaptive traits of yet another temperament representing sub-threshold expression of the manic/hypomanic spectrum, i.e. hyperthymia [127]. Hyperthymic individuals are distinguished from patients with chronic mania, which is a psychotic disorder. They are distinguished from hypomanics because the latter typically manifest short-lived episodes distinct from the patient's baseline. By contrast, hyperthymia is characterized by lifelong *traits* of upbeat, energy-driven, and overconfident disposition. This is in contrast to the constant mood swings of the cyclothymic. Our criteria for this trait hypomanic disposition, currently under investigation in an expanded version as part of TEMPS-A [121], are shown in Table 1.9.

Hyperthymia received a brilliant description by Kurt Schneider, though he subsumed it under *psychopathic personalities* [128]. Most modern authors, e.g. Akiskal [127], Possl and von Zerssen [129], following Kraepelin, have defined it as a "manic" temperament. In effect, the defining attributes of hyperthymia represent a muted, highly adaptive, version of mania at the trait level. The contemporary literature (since 1966) is sparse on hyperthymia—barely 15 papers! Empirical studies among these are even more sparse. This might be due to the fact that these attributes represent the signature temperament of leaders and famous people and hence are not easily accessible for investigation. However, hyperthymic traits do precede manic episodes, and can be retrospectively examined. An excellent description of the biographical features of this temperament—based on systematic chart review of manic patients in Munich—is provided by Possl and von Zerssen [129]: vivid, active, extraverted; verbally aggressive, self-assured; strong-willed; self-employed; risk-taking; sensation-seeking; breaking social norms; generous and spendthrift.

TABLE 1.9   The hyperthymic temperament (expanded from Akiskal and Mallya [23])

Four or more of the following attributes, which are *not episode-bound* and constitute part of the *habitual long-term* functioning of the individual:
- Upbeat and exuberant
- Articulate and jocular
- Self-reliant, confident, optimistic
- Versatile with broad interests
- Energetic—thrives on action
- Full of plans
- Habitual short sleeper
- High level of libido
- Uninhibited and novelty-seeking
- Over-involved and meddlesome

Eckblad and Chapman [130] studied college students at the University of Wisconsin: 6% met lifetime criteria for hypomanic tendencies that, interestingly, were associated with occasional mini-depressive dips. Two other studies using the same instrument reported depressive states both in cross-section [131] and upon prospective follow-up [132]. In brief, despite its trait hyperthymic characteristics, this temperament does appear to predispose to depression as well. In the Pisa–San Diego collaborative study [120], also conducted among students, 8% could be categorized as hyperthymic on the basis of the entire complement of seven persistent hypomanic traits from the original Akiskal–Mallya operational criteria [23].

The main evidence linking hyperthymia to the bipolar spectrum has come from the use of family history as an external validator [74]: major depressive patients who met at least five of seven of the hyperthymic attributes had rates of familial bipolarity significantly higher than strictly unipolar patients without these temperamental attributes, and from a familial perspective were indistinguishable from bipolar II patients. This study needs to be replicated with "blind" methodology. The possible inclusion of these "hyperthymic depressions" within the bipolar spectrum [22]—depending on the clinical sample and the number of hyperthymic items used for diagnosis—could shrink the unipolar depressive universe by 10–20% [74]. However, current data are uncertain about the boundary of hyperthymic temperament and normality. This temperament then, as currently measured, may be considered clinically relevant only in association with major depression [22, 23, 82]. Further psychometric characterization of hyperthymia will be important for both clinical and genetic research.

Hyperthymia also appears relevant to the course of manic and depressive states [133–135]. When this temperament occurs in association with mania, the latter would often pursue a recurrent course. However, as further discussed in the next section, when hyperthymic traits precede depressive states, they tend to colour the depression with "mixed" (hypomanic) features.

BIPOLAR DEPRESSIVE PHASE AND MIXED STATES

Depressive Phase

Like mania, bipolar depression may manifest psychotic symptoms of usually mood-congruent nature [16]. However, delusional and hallucinatory experiences are less common. Stupor, uncommonly observed today, represents the most severe expression of the depressive phase of bipolar disorder. In the elderly, bipolar depression may present as a pseudodementia. "Neurastheniform" symptoms [32] with reverse vegetative signs (i.e., "atypical depression" in the sense of DSM-IV) are more characteristic of juvenile bipolar depressives, particularly adolescents and young adult women.

Psychomotor retardation, with or without hypersomnia, is generally considered the hallmark of the uncomplicated depressive phase of bipolar disorder [136]. Onset and offset are often abrupt, though gradual onset over several weeks can also occur. Patients may recover into a free interval or switch directly into mania [137, 138]: switching into an excited phase is not infrequently associated with somatotherapy (e.g., ECT, sleep deprivation, and antidepressants).

The characteristics which distinguish the depressive phase of bipolars from unipolars have been the subject of several prospective studies [31, 32]. Table 1.10 lists the most useful predictors of bipolar I outcome. The composite profile of such a depressive is that of a young person (< 25 years old), with "loaded" affective family history—or at least one definite bipolar first-degree kin—who is psychomotor retarded, or psychotically depressed; in a woman the depressive psychosis can be purperal. Bipolar II switching is more complex, as it involves temperamental factors (and is to be discussed later in this chapter under the heading of bipolar II disorder).

Depressive Mixed State

5–10% of depressed patients switch to the opposite pole upon antidepressant treatment [139–141]. Other destabilizing factors, uncovered in pioneering studies conducted by Himmelhoch et al [142], include cerebral factors and alcohol and drug abuse or withdrawal. The process can be acute or subacute and many patients develop a driven depression with psychomotor restlessness; they may be "stuck" for many months in a depressive phase with severe anxiety and "hypomanic" admixtures such as marked irritability, tension, crowded thoughts and sexual arousal.

Although neither DSM-IV nor ICD-10 specifically recognize a mixed depressive phase with few hypomanic and/or excitatory symptoms occurring during a full-blown depression—what Kraepelin had described as excited depression and depression with racing thoughts—these cases have been reported by several contemporary clinical observers [23, 46, 143–145]. Berner and colleagues from the Vienna school [146] have drawn attention to mixed states where a drive state opposite to that of the prevailing emotional disturbance develops, for instance sexual impulses in the setting of a clinical depression. Severe agitated depression with associated hypomania was described by Himmelhoch et al [143] as a variant of bipolar mixed states. Koukopoulos and Koukopoulos [46] have described intensely agitated depressions which they consider as forms of not unipolar, but bipolar depressive mixed states. Perugi et al [144] also identified such a mixed depressive syndrome. However, Swann et al [147] could not find sufficient evidence to classify agitated depression as a mixed state. The work of the present author [23] has revealed the existence of ambulatory depressive mixed states related to bipolar II disorder. These patients meet minimum criteria for a major depressive episode, plus intense activation in a variety of symptom domains brought about by overzealous prescription of antidepressants: dramatic expressions of suffering; unrelenting dysphoria, irritability, and lability; psychomotor agitation against a background of retardation; extreme fatigue with racing thoughts; intense sexual excitement; free-floating anxiety, and panic attacks; as well as suicidal obsessions in a significant minority of cases. Finally, milder mixed states have been described by Benazzi [145] among bipolar II patients, involving irritability, distractability and racing thoughts.

It has been suggested [148], in confirmation of Kraepelin's conceptualization, that psychomotor retardation is the "signature" of bipolar depression.

TABLE 1.10 Diagnostic performance of variables significantly associated with bipolar outcome in patients with major depression (summarized from Akiskal et al [32])

Variable	Sensitivity (%)	Specificity (%)
Pharmacologic hypomania	32	100
Bipolar family history	56	98
Loaded pedigrees	32	95
Hypersomnic-retarded depression	59	88
Psychotic depression	42	85
Postpartum onset	58	84
Onset of depression before age 26	71	68

However, the foregoing considerations suggest that bipolar depression is not always of the retarded type; indeed, some degree of psychomotor restlessness or agitation is often present. Whether the latter should be taken as evidence of "mixity" is not universally agreed upon. In the clinical judgement of the present author, the nonrecognition of such a depressive mixed state as bipolar is tantamount to clinical disaster, as antidepressants are likely to aggravate it.

Mixed Mania

Mixed mania—commonly referred to as "dysphoric mania" [149]—is characterized by dysphorically excited moods, irritability, anger, panic attacks, pressured speech, agitation, suicidal crises, severe insomnia, grandiosity, hypersexuality, persecutory delusions and confusion. Severely psychotic mixed states are at risk for being misdiagnosed as schizoaffective. Defined as the simultaneous presence of depressive and hypo/manic symptoms, mixed states represented a major line of evidence for Kraepelin's concept linking mania and depression. As reviewed earlier in the historical section of this chapter, for him the diagnosis of mixed episodes was justified if *any elements* from affective, psychomotor and cognitive domains were incongruent with the other two: for instance, anxious and depressive cognitions occurring during a manic episode. Kraepelin's broad definition of mixed states is only partially reflected in ICD-10; DSM-IV, which requires full-fledged manic and syndromal depressive manifestations, is even more conservative.

Unlike the relative paucity of research on the depressive phase of bipolar disorder, there has been a true renaissance [14, 86] during the past decade in characterizing bipolar mixed states in bipolar I disorder. It has been reported that an average of 40% of bipolar I patients develop a mixed state at some point during their illness course [86]. However, this mean rate reflects a great deal of inter-centre variability (14–67%), as data derive from diverse clinical and research settings. Moreover, there is no terminological uniformity in the literature, with a regrettable tendency to use such terms as "mixed state", "mixed mania", "depression during mania", and "dysphoric mania" interchangeably.

Despite the foregoing uncertainties, several consistent findings have emerged. Alcohol abuse and neuropsychiatric conditions are prevalent in mixed states [142]. Mixed states have been best characterized in female inpatients [133, 150, 151], often arising from a prior course of illness with more depressive than manic episodes and with a tendency to repeat over time, though this is based on retrospective examination. Family history is more often depressive than manic [150], and suicidal behaviour is a distinct risk [152–154]. Confusion and psychotic features, including mood incongruence, are also common clinical presentations [144, 150, 151].

From a diagnostic standpoint, the most important consideration is the emerging international consensus that the DSM-IV threshold for syndromal depression during mania is too restrictive in the diagnosis of mixed mania [14, 133, 144, 155, 156]. Overall, the most compelling data comes from the French national EPIMAN study [133], which was conducted in four centres in France, involving over 105 patients. Semi-structured diagnostic interviews were conducted based on the DSM-IV schema for mixed state, but with suspension of the arbitrary threshold of full syndromal depression, as recommended by McElroy et al [14]. Patients were extensively tested psychometrically, including the French version of the TEMPS-A [157]. They entered the study on the basis of meeting full criteria for index manic episodes. The rates for strictly defined DSM-IV mixed states were low, 6.7%. But using a cutoff of two or more depressive symptoms, 37% could be characterized as dysphoric manic. As expected, these patients scored more than 10 on the modified Hamilton Rating Scale for Depression (HAM-D). Depressed mood and suicidal thoughts had the best predictive value for the diagnosis of mixed mania. Another important finding was that mixed manic patients, compared with those with pure mania, had a higher percentage of depressive temperamental traits. Such data suggest that mixed mania can be defined categorically by two or more depressive symptoms, psychometrically on the basis of HAM-D > 10, or dimensionally on the basis of depressive temperamental traits (similar to long-standing dysthymia). The latter had also been observed in our collaboration with Perugi's clinical research team [144], supporting the present author's hypothesis that mixed states are best conceived as a reversal of temperament to its episode of opposite polarity [158]. In other words, dysphoric mania arises from the intrusion of a depressive temperament into a manic episode—stated differently, when mania is superimposed on a depressive temperament.

There are no long-term studies of mixed mania examining prospectively the list of discriminatory depressive symptoms developed by McElroy [14]. Cassidy et al [159] have proposed a list which coheres with an emerging world literature [88] on a constellation of largely emotional-cognitive symptoms as the most discriminatory (Table 1.11) and worthy of further investigation. McElroy et al [14] proposed a cut-off of ≥ 3, Akiskal et al [133] ≥ 2, and Swann et al [160] ≥ 1 depressive symptoms in the midst of mania for the diagnosis of dysphoric mania. These are not mere nosologic exercises, because even one depressive symptom during mania has been reported to predict low response to lithium and good response to divalproex [160]. Mixed mania also appears to respond well to atypical antipsychotics such as olanzapine [161].

TABLE 1.11 Discriminatory depressive signs and symptoms in the diagnosis of dysphoric mania (based on McElroy *et al* [14]; Bauer *et al* [155]; Cassidy *et al* [159]; Akiskal *et al* [133])

- Depressed mood
- Irritability/hostility
- Mood lability
- Anhedonia
- Hopelessness/helplessness
- Suicidal ideation and/or attempt
- Guilt
- Fatigue

BIPOLAR SUBTYPES AND THEIR VARIANTS

Bipolar I Disorder

Typically beginning in the teenage years, the 20s, or the 30s, the first episode of bipolar I disorder could be manic, depressive, or mixed [1, 88]. One common mode of onset is mild retarded depression, or hypersomnia, for a few weeks or months, which then often switches into a manic episode. In others, several depressive episodes occur before the first mania. It is not uncommon for the illness to be ushered with a severely psychotic manic episode that might present schizophreniform features. In a special subgroup the illness pursues a recurrent manic course [162, 163]. Lastly, Keller *et al* [164] have brought attention to patients whose course includes mixed/cycling features which take longer to remit.

Although the sex ratio is 1:1, men experience more manic episodes, and women more depressive and mixed episodes [1]. On average, manic episodes predominate in youth and depressive episodes in later years [48]. A partial exception is the group of "secondary manias", which usually occur in association with various cerebral, endocrine, and other systemic medical conditions later in life [165]. Irritable mood tends to prevail in secondary manias [166]. Family history for bipolar disorder, and recurrence or depressive switches, are unusual in these maniform states [165]. The latter features suggest that many such cases do not belong to bipolar I disorder. However, postpartum mania—often mixed or schizophreniform in nature—should, on the basis of family history and course, be probably classified under bipolar I disorder [167].

Dilsaver *et al* [168] and Cassidy *et al* [169] have recently described different cross-sectional subtypes within the larger manic population. We will not attempt to review this fascinating literature, which is still inconclusive, in part because there is virtually no data on the prospectively defined longitudinal stability of these subtypes.

Bipolar II Disorder

These patients typically present with a major depressive episode, and upon further inquiry, history for hypomanic episodes is elicited [21]. Accurate diagnosis then depends on the vagaries of the patient's memory and how rigorously the clinician pursues queries about hypomania—and, most importantly, whether relatives are available to respond to such queries. Otherwise, unless noted in the patient's past psychiatric record, the examining psychiatrist may have little clue from the patient's current depressive presentation about the bipolar elements in the patient's history. Accordingly, rates of bipolar II disorder were, until recently, underestimated.

The under-diagnosis of bipolar II disorder due to failure to detect hypomania is of critical importance for both clinical practice and genetic investigations. There have been two signal methodological developments with respect to this question. The first is by Rice *et al* [170], who reported that although the reliability of the bipolar II disorder diagnosis was low, all such diagnoses occurred in pedigrees with bipolar disorder, suggesting that once hypomania was identified in association with major depressive disorder, it did carry major diagnostic weight. The other important methodological observation was made by Dunner and Tay [171], who found that clinicians specifically trained to recognize bipolar II disorder, far outperformed structured instruments such as the Schedule for Affective Disorders and Schizophrenia (SADS) or the Structured Clinical Interview for DSM-III-R (SCID). Both methodologic points cohere with recommendations made earlier by the present author: documenting hypomania among subjects suspected of cyclothymia requires repeated expert interview at several points in time. Although these considerations go against the general tenets in the literature on structured interviewing, they are consistent in suggesting that the proper identification of bipolar II disorder requires a more sophisticated approach in diagnostic interviewing. Stated differently, because many bipolar II patients have an underlying cyclothymic temperamental dysregulation [33, 118, 119], their clinical presentations are varied and inconsistent and often prove confusing in cross-section. That is, they could present with cross-sectional features of atypical depression, and lifelong history of anxiety states, bulimia, substance abuse, and cluster B personality disorders [172]. Atypical depressive features are perhaps the most important clinical markers for bipolar II disorder [173]. Indeed, a prospective study found that atypical depression often progressed to bipolar spectrum disorders [174].

Faced with patients with atypical depressive features as defined in DSM-IV, the clinician's task is to identify a pattern of cyclic depressions with discrete hypomanic periods as the core underlying diagnosis behind varied comorbid manifestations. The affective dysregulation of bipolar II disorder extends beyond elation and depression, to include, among others, such negative affective arousal states as panic, irritability, and mood lability [19, 20, 33]. Although counterintuitive, such complex anxious bipolar cases appear to have a stronger genetic basis than bipolar II disorder without panic attacks [175].

Vieta et al [176] have succintly summarized the complexity of bipolar II disorder as follows: less severe in symptom intensity, but more severe in course. This would suggest that trait factors might underlie its special features. Analyses from the National Institute of Mental Health (NIMH) Collaborative Depression Study [33] on "unipolar" patients who switched to bipolar II disorder may shed further light on its defining trait characteristics. Of 559 patients with major depressive disorder at entry, 48 converted to bipolar II disorder during a prospective observation period of 11 years. At entry into the study, what characterized these "unipolar" converters to bipolar II disorder was early age at onset of first depression, recurrent depression, high rates of divorce or separation, high rates of scholastic and/or job maladjustment, isolated "antisocial acts", drug abuse—in brief, a tempestuous biography. In addition, the index depressive episode was further characterized by such features as phobic anxiety, interpersonal sensitivity, obsessive-compulsive symptoms, somatization (with subpanic symptoms), worse in evening, self-pity, demandingness, subjective or overt anger, jealousy, suspiciousness, and ideas of reference—again testifying to a broad mélange of "atypical" depressive symptoms with "borderline" taint. Temperamental attributes obtained at index interview proved decisive (sensitivity = 91%) in identifying those who switched from depression to hypomania: these attributes consisted of trait "mood lability", "energy-activity", and "daydreaming" (all characteristic of Kretschmer's description of the cyclothymic temperament). Mood lability was the most specific predictor (specificity = 86%) of which depressions will prospectively switch to bipolar II disorder. This study testifies to the fact that bipolar II disorder is a complex affective disorder with biographical instability deriving from an intense temperamental dysregulation. *Mood lability—with rapid shifts, often in a depressive polarity—was the hallmark of "unipolar" patients who switched to bipolar II disorder.* The foregoing characteristics revealed in a prospective study on a large clinical sample in five university centres provide a pattern recognition which clinicians can use in their diagnostic evaluation for ascertaining bipolar II disorder diagnosis and its variants. It is noteworthy that conversion to bipolar I disorder was *not* predicted by any of the foregoing features, and supports the separation of bipolar II from bipolar I disorder within the clinical spectrum of bipolarity.

The diagnosis of bipolar II disorder is crucial, not only because of its therapeutic implications, but also for prognostic reasons. Since the Dunner et al original report [21], the literature has supported the risk for high suicidality in this group of patients [177]. Some, perhaps many, "unipolar" suicides are hidden bipolar II cases. It is of great public health significance not to miss the diagnosis of bipolar II disorder in patients presenting with major depression. During the past decade, a great deal of research has been conducted on the clinical prevalence of bipolar II disorder among patients presenting with major depression to various medical centres and clinics worldwide. What emerges is that from 27 to 65% of all patients with major depression conform to bipolar II disorder or its variants [22, 23, 71, 74, 86, 114, 119, 125, 172, 178–180]. I wish to emphasize that the data are not limited to academic centres that specialize in mood disorders, but include at least two large outpatient psychiatric private practice settings [179,180]. Nor are these high rates limited to psychiatric settings; at least one such report has come from a family practice clinic [114]. Moreover, according to Simpson *et al* [80], bipolar II disorder may represent the most common phenotype of bipolar disorder.

The French National EPIDEP study [119], based on a sample from a variety of clinical settings—private and public, inpatient and outpatient, academic and general psychiatric sector—have provided the most compelling data on the high prevalence of bipolar II disorder among patients with major depression. The main objective of this study was to assist practising psychiatrists in recognizing bipolarity in all of its varieties. The major finding was that at index interview 22% of patients with major depression could be diagnosed as bipolar II (based primarily on past history of hypomania in the records); a month later, upon re-interview, 40% of patients were diagnosed within the bipolar II spectrum on the basis of more in-depth evaluation and collateral information from significant others, as well as *observed* hypomania by the clinician. These data indicate that clinicians in diverse practice settings can be trained to recognize bipolar II disorder and its variants, leading to changes in diagnostic practice at the national, and by extension, international level.

Bipolar III Disorder

What about the diagnostic status of hypomania that becomes first manifest upon pharmacological challenge with antidepressants? Based in part on the contributions by Lewis and Winokur [181], Angst [182], and Kupfer *et al* [183], both DSM-IV and ICD-10 have denied bipolar legitimacy to these patients. This decision regrettably did not consider a more extensive literature which existed before the publication of these manuals [31, 32, 184–187], and which favoured annexing this realm to the bipolar terrain. New reports [188–190] have been published since then. Mood stabilizers do not seem to fully prevent antidepressant-associated switches [191], though an adequate level of a mood stabilizer might be protective [192]. Antidepressant-mobilized hypomanic episodes tend to be somewhat milder, less likely to occur with selective serotonin reuptake inhibitors (SSRIs) compared with tricyclics [140], and more euphoric with monoamine oxidase inhibitors than tricyclics, which are likely to induce more dysphoric hypomania [193]. However, during prospective observation, nearly all adult patients with antidepressant-associated hypomanic episodes progress months or years later to bipolar episodes with spontaneous hypomania or mania [32]; this is also true for adolescent depressives [31]. A return to Table 1.10, where the most sensitive and specific parameters in the prospective prediction of bipolar outcome are summarized, reveals that pharmacologically occasioned hypomania is the most specific. The data in the table further indicate that depressions with bipolar family history should be closely observed for eventual bipolar transformation. Systematic probing may also reveal spontaneous hypomanic excursions buried in the past history, which had been considered "normal" mood fluctuation.

Antidepressant-associated hypomania is not limited to major depressions. It occurs in as many as a third of dysthymic patients [194,195], as well as in 10–30% of social phobic, obsessive-compulsive, and panic disorders [20, 136]. This would suggest that soft bipolarity, in a significant minority of cases, may be ushered by panic attacks as well as socially anxious or obsessive inhibitions: switching on antidepressants may provide the first suggestive evidence for bipolarity in these patients. These clinical considerations, which require more extensive research validation, are of great significance in clinical practice. But the general principle that antidepressant-associated hypomania is indicative of a bipolar diathesis should no longer be in doubt.

Rapid Cycling

Rapid cycling bipolar patients, as defined in DSM-IV, experience a minimum of four episodes (mania/hypomania and major depression) per year [196, 197]. They most frequently arise from a bipolar II terrain [198], and thus present with at least four alternating depressive-hypomanic cycles per year. As a result, these patients rarely have freedom from affective episodes during the rapid-cycling phase of their illness, which is usually dominated by depression.

Rapid cycling lies along a continuum based on the duration of episodes which, by definition, must meet the symptom severity thresholds for mania/hypomania and depression. Rapid (≥ 4/year), ultra-rapid (≥ 4/month), and ultradian (within a day) cycling patterns can be recognized clinically; they are distinguished from cyclothymic disorder which pursues a *subthreshold* course as far as symptoms are concerned. However, cyclothymia often precedes, and probably predisposes to, bipolar II rapid cycling.

In rapid cycling, the illness takes on a roller coaster course for both patient, family, and the physician. Such cycling appears to be on the rise [199]. Fortunately, it is a transient phase in the course of bipolar disorder: in 2–4 years, most rapid cycling observed during naturalistic follow-up tends to return to a less cycling pattern [198]. Nonetheless, some authorities believe that rapid cycling may continue indefinitely [200]. Rapid cycling has been reported to occur in 13–56% of bipolar patients (see [201] for a review). The higher rates come from research institutions which specialize in refractory bipolar disorders; its prevalence is less than 20% in most studies. Risk factors discussed in the literature—but without unanimous agreement—include cyclothymic temperament, borderline hypothyroidism, and possibly excessive use of antidepressants. Although few doubt the role of female sex, a meta-analysis by Tondo and Baldessarini [202] found only modest association to female sex. Such discrepancies are likely due to methodologic differences in case definition and inclusion criteria.

Rapid cycling is ordinarily a *post hoc* diagnosis. This may be another explanation for some of the discrepancies in the literature regarding risk factors. However, retrospective systematic analysis of large samples may minimize biased observations. Thus, Perugi *et al* [203], reporting on 320 bipolar patients, have shown that bipolar illness with depression as the episode at onset is significantly more likely than manic and mixed state onsets to have developed rapid cycling, suicidal behaviour, and psychotic symptoms; mixed onsets, too, had high rates of suicide attempts, but differed from depressive onsets in having significantly more chronicity, yet negligible rates of rapid cycling. Because those with depressive onset had received significantly higher rates of antidepressant treatment, the findings lend indirect support to the hypothesis that antidepressants may have played a role in the induction of rapid cycling. It is impossible, however, to entirely rule out the alternative explanation that bipolar II disorder, which often forms the basis of rapid cycling, presented such difficulty in clinical management due to the complex anxious-depressive elements, that psychiatrists may have been "forced" out of desperation to overuse antidepressants! It is noteworthy that the Perugi study confirmed Himmelhoch's [142] observation that rapid cycling was distinct from mixed states. However, in ultra-rapid cycling there may be considerable overlap with mixity.

Bipolar Disorder Not Otherwise Classified

This is a residual category in which ICD-10 places bipolar II disorder, and DSM-IV places what is *beyond* bipolar II disorder. Neither manual considers the existence of hyperthymic traits which could precede (or follow) depressive episodes [23, 24]. It is also curious that hypomania/mania in association with antidepressant treatment is not even mentioned as a candidate for bipolar disorder not otherwise classified—it is simply voted out of existence! The intention of these august manuals is apparently to dump them among major depressive disorders.

Other possible candidates on the edges of bipolarity include seasonal depressions without discernible hypomanic episodes, as well as other recurrent depressions of abrupt onset and offset [71]. There also exist patients— about whom clinicians write [22]—with episodic obsessive-compulsive symptoms, periodic states of irritability, or acute suicidal crises in the absence of clear-cut affective symptoms; still others who experience cyclic neurasthenic or sleep complaints or severe brief recurrent depressions [22]. Lastly, McElroy et al [204] have drawn attention to the possible bipolar nature of some impulse-ridden behaviours such as those in the realm of aggression control, gambling and paraphilias. The foregoing conditions require further extensive studies before any link to bipolarity can be claimed.

DISPUTED BOUNDARIES OF BIPOLARITY

Until recently, compared to the UK, bipolar disorder was often misdiagnosed as schizophrenia in the US [15, 16, 37]. We are aware of at least one data-based paper on this subject from another country [205]. Current data from the US [206] indicate that schizophrenia no longer tops the list in missed bipolar diagnoses. A national survey of the US Depressive and Manic-Depressive Association [207] recently revealed that disorders within the broader affective range—major depressive and comorbid anxiety disorders, and borderline personality with its affective tempests—precede for a decade bipolar diagnoses. This change may have occurred because schizophrenia in the US classification is now limited to a deteriorating disorder. On the other hand, the concept of depressive disorders in DSM-IV (as well as in ICD-10) appears over-inclusive, in part reflecting the contemporaneous revolution in antidepressant development. By contrast, bipolar II variants with brief ($\leq$ 4 days) hypomanic episodes and depressive mixed states (isolated hypomanic symptoms intruding into depressive states) are not officially recognized; also the boundaries between cyclothymic mood swings and borderline mood lability have not been clarified in these manuals.

The overinclusive boundaries of bipolar disorder discussed in this chapter in part reflect the clinical judgement of investigators that depressed patients with soft pre-bipolar indicators will be spared the risk of antidepressant treatment with its attendant cycle acceleration and possible chronicization [22, 208]. Such clinical logic is also predicated on the premise that the increasing availability of mood stabilizers beyond lithium might be beneficial for bipolar patients beyond classic mania. This is not a new phenomenon: the introduction of chlorpromazine in 1952 [209] and lithium salts in the 1960s [210] were considered major factors in changing diagnostic practice in North America.

Although biological markers such as the dexamethasone suppression test and the thyrotropin-releasing hormone (TRH)/thyroid-stimulating hormone (TSH) test have been reported to distinguish bipolar from unipolar disorder [211–213], they have not been shown to be useful in routine practice. Faced with subthreshold, unusual or confusing bipolar and comorbid presentations, a systematic clinical approach is still the only valid method in differential diagnosis: a) to characterize in great detail all the clinical features of the current episode; b) to elicit a history of more typical manic/hypomanic episodes in the past; c) to assess whether the presenting complaints recur in a periodic or cyclical fashion; d) to substantiate the adequacy of social functioning between periods of illness; e) to construct a family pedigree; f) to document switching on an antidepressant, and to obtain history of unequivocal therapeutic response to mood-stabilizing medication or electroconvulsive therapy in either the patient or the family.

Using the foregoing validating approach, it is possible to examine the bipolar links of many DSM-IV disorders, such as schizophrenic and schizoaffective psychoses, borderline personality disorder, impulse-control disorders (e.g., kleptomania, gambling), polysubstance abuse, dipsomania, circadian rhythm sleep disorder (delayed sleep phase type), and bulimia nervosa. Notably, those conditions exhibit selected bipolar features, such as cyclicity, circadian patterns, disinhibited behaviour, temperamentality, mood lability, and impulsive behaviour. However, solid evidence linking the foregoing to the bipolar spectrum is presently lacking. The relationship of depressive disorders to the bipolar spectrum has been documented throughout this chapter. Our thesis has been that the depressive pole of bipolarity—and its varied expressions—have been relatively neglected in both the official diagnostic system and in the research literature. In this section we briefly examine the differential diagnosis of bipolar disorder from its closest three neighbours, which present the greatest challenge in clinical practice.

Schizoaffective Disorder

Although current molecular genetic data have revealed intriguing links between some forms of schizophrenia and bipolar disorder [214], circa 2001, their clinical differentiation does not seem to pose as much trouble as in the past. Clinical differentiation of bipolar disorder from schizoaffective disorder is another matter.

According to ICD-10, the concept of schizoaffective disorder should be restricted to recurrent psychoses with full affective and schizophrenic symptoms occurring nearly simultaneously during each episode. Research by the present author [16] has shown that such a diagnosis should not be considered in a bipolar psychosis where mood-incongruent psychotic features can be explained on the basis of one of the following: a) affective psychosis superimposed on mental retardation, giving rise to extremely hyperactive and bizarre manic behaviour; b) affective psychosis complicated by concurrent cerebral disease, substance abuse, or substance withdrawal, all of which are known to give rise to numerous Schneiderian symptoms; c) mixed episodes of bipolar disorder, which are notorious for signs and symptoms of protracted psychotic disorganization.

In DSM-IV, the rubric of "schizoaffective disorder" is used more broadly than that in ICD-10. Thus, patients with manic episodes will receive a schizoaffective diagnosis if delusions or hallucinations occur in the interepisodic period in the absence of prominent affective symptoms. As discussed earlier, many psychotic symptoms in bipolar disorders are of an explanatory nature, whereby the patient tries to make sense of the core experiences of the manic excitement. Such explanatory delusional process can be carried over into the interepisodic period. These patients would thereby be delusional in the absence of prominent mood symptoms and, technically (that is, by DSM-IV criteria), might be considered schizoaffective. Taylor and Amir [215] have suggested that greater emphasis be placed on Bleulerian signs—formal thought disorder and affective blunting—rather than the mood-incongruent positive features in the interepisodic period emphasized in DSM-IV. The more serious problem with the DSM-IV schizoaffective construct is that it has very low reliability [216]. Full discussion of this subject [217] is beyond the scope of this chapter. Suffice it to say that while schizodepressive patients are heterogeneous (many of them are more allied with schizophrenia), schizobipolar patients [218, 219] can more confidently be assigned to the psychotic end of the bipolar spectrum.

Borderline Personality Disorder

There is a great deal of confusion in clinical psychiatry today concerning the boundaries between bipolar II disorder, cyclothymic disorder and borderline personality disorder. Such individuals also often use various substances, which further complicates their diagnostic status. Although much has been written from either personality disorder [220] or mood disorder perspectives [221], definitive studies to convince the opposite groups are lacking or what has been published is conflicting. In the present author's clinical judgement, conceptualizing borderline conditions as belonging to the bipolar spectrum has the advantage that it opens therapeutic opportunities for them.

The diagnosis of borderline personality disorder is usually applied to teenage and young adult females with labile emotionality of particularly hostile nature. Indeed the DSM-IV diagnostic criteria for the disorder indicate a liberal mélange of low-grade affective symptoms and behaviour. The overlap between borderline personality and bipolar II disorder is extensive, e.g., affective instability and impulsivity, disinhibition on antidepressants, familial bipolarity [221], such that giving a "borderline" diagnosis to a person with mood disorder is often redundant. Mood lability is not unique to borderline personality disorder: it is also a prospectively validated trait characteristic of bipolar II disorder [33]. When personality disorder diagnoses are used, they may lead to neglect of the bipolar disorder, resulting in half-hearted treatment of the affective component; failure to respond would then be blamed on the patient's "self-defeating character" and/or "resistance" to get well, thereby blaming the patient and exculpating the clinician.

Although more systematic research needs to be done on the complex interface of borderline and soft bipolar disorders, clinically they are often inseparable. It is generally preferable to diagnose mood disorders at the expense of personality disorders, which should not be difficult to justify in most cases where the validating strategies outlined earlier are satisfied. When features of both borderline and bipolar spectrum disorders coexist, it is good practice to defer the axis II diagnosis, and embark upon competent treatment of the presenting bipolar disorder. Although not all personality disturbances recede with the competent treatment of the affective disorder, so many experienced clinicians have seen such disturbances improve [222] or even melt away [223] with the successful resolution of the bipolar disorder that erring in favor of bipolar spectrum diagnoses is justified on clinical grounds.

Alcohol and Substance Use Disorders

The very high comorbidity of these disorders with the bipolar spectrum cannot be explained away as the chance occurrence of two prevalent disorders [96, 224, 225]. This is particularly true for the high lifetime co-occurrence of bipolarity and alcohol abuse. Self-medication for subthreshold bipolar symptoms is insufficiently appreciated by both psychiatrists and substance use disorder experts. Whereas stimulants can be used to enhance hypomania [110, 226–228], alcohol can both enhance or calm down excited mood states. The present author believes that a modest amount of daily alcohol may have some therapeutic value in a subgroup of bipolar patients. This can perhaps be inferred from the fact that bipolar disorder following alcohol abuse usually manifests a decade later than bipolar disorder without such abuse [97]; however, one cannot rule out the possibility that the protracted use of alcohol may have played a formative influence on the bipolar disorder in such cases. Given the clinical dangers of missing an otherwise treatable disorder, bipolar disorder should be given serious consideration as the primary diagnosis if marked bipolar manifestations continue one month after the period of detoxification. According to Winokur *et al* [97], family history of mania can further buttress a bipolar diagnosis in such situations: indeed, alcohol, stimulant abuse and mania are often unilineal in such families.

The DSM-IV category of alcohol or substance-induced mood disorder is difficult to validate clinically because, in the absence of an affective diathesis, detoxification should, in principle, rapidly clear affective disturbances occurring in persons who abuse substances. Erring in favour of underlying bipolar spectrum diagnoses opens the door for the potential therapeutic benefit of mood-stabilizing anticonvulsants. This is not to say that the scientific literature provides stronger endorsement to the self-medication hypothesis [17] over competing hypotheses. Actually, the hypothesis that the two sets of disorders might share a common diathesis is perhaps more appealing from a scientific perspective. The present author submits that, in practice, certain classes of anticonvulsants represent rational choices in addressing drug withdrawal, destabilization due to kindling, and the destabilization inherent to bipolar mood swings [229]. This clinical opinion, though perhaps not fully defensible on the merits of the available evidence, is pragmatic in routine clinical practice.

SUMMARY

Consistent Evidence

The weight of the reviewed evidence indicates that bipolar disorder is broader than what is included in DSM-IV and ICD-10. It ranges from psychotic extremes to attenuated forms that manifest at the level of disordered temperament. It includes:

- *Bipolar I disorder.* Manic episodes with or without major depression can escalate to extremely psychotic expressions, including mood-incongruent and/or schizobipolar forms.
- *Bipolar II disorder.* Recurrent major depressions associated with spontaneous hypomania may represent the most common phenotype

of bipolar disorder. Current data indicate that the modal duration of hypomanic episodes is two days.

- *Cyclothymic depression.* These are major depressive episodes superimposed on cyclothymic and/or trait mood lability, representing a common variant of bipolar II disorder with tempestuous course.
- *Bipolar III disorder.* As for clinically depressed patients who experience hypomania during antidepressant treatment (sometimes referred to as *bipolar III*), the evidence from US studies as well as those conducted in Europe is nearly unanimous in supporting bipolar spectrum status for these patients.
- *Rapid cycling.* This represents a transient phase in the course of bipolar, especially bipolar II, disorder which occurs in up to 20% of patients.
- *Mixed states.* These states, the most extensively studied of which are the *dysphoric manias*, occur in the course of an average of 40% of bipolar patients. Current international consensus indicates that they do not need to have the full constellation of depressive symptoms. Two or more depressive symptoms appear sufficient in imparting mixed state status to mania.

Incomplete Evidence

- *Depressive mixed states.* Although Kraepelin had included slight hypomanic intrusions into depressive episodes in his rubric of mixed states, they have commanded insufficient research interest. Nonetheless, there is increasing evidence that depressions with several excitatory phenomena (such as intense panic, mood lability, hostility, agitation, crowded thoughts, sexual arousal and restlessness) represent an excited or agitated depression that conforms to Kraepelin's concept of mixed state. Alcohol, stimulants, and antidepressants are implicated in their genesis. Their bipolar status should be further clarified, because they may be mistakenly regarded as anxious or resistant depressions, thereby exposing them to the risk of even greater destabilization by one antidepressant trial after another.
- *Hyperthymic depression.* This rubric too has received insufficient clinical attention. Nonetheless, it has been suggested that clinically depressed patients with lifelong traits of cheerful disposition, high drive and energy, and overconfidence do belong to the soft bipolar spectrum based on family history for bipolar disorder. Also, such depressions are likely to be destabilized by antidepressants.
- *Recurrent brief hypomania.* This prevalent condition, often "comorbid" with recurrent brief depression and major depression, seems to represent the subthreshold terrain of cyclothymic and bipolar II disorders. Hence

its public health significance and the consequent need for wider recognition and research in this epidemiologic terrain.

- *Driven dysthymia.* It would be also relevant to mention that, among dysthymic subjects characterized by brooding and low confidence, there exist some driven individuals who might be mobilized by antidepressants, particularly SSRIs, into short-lived hypomanic states and sometimes protracted hyperthymia. Family history is often bipolar in these individuals. They might be considered a putative sub-bipolar dysthymic subtype within the soft bipolar spectrum.

Areas Still Open to Research

- *Borderline personality disorder.* Patients within the soft bipolar spectrum, especially when recurrence rate is high and the interepisodic period is not free of affective manifestations, often meet criteria for Axis II cluster B personality disorders. This is particularly true for bipolar II disorder arising from a cyclothymic baseline. In view of their extreme mood lability—especially when pursuing subacute or chronic course—these patients are often misclassified as borderline personality disorder. Treatment considerations suggest that, in the presence of prominent affective symptoms of bipolar nature, a bipolar spectrum diagnosis should perhaps have precedence over Axis II disorders. Actually, subthreshold mood lability has been prospectively validated as a sensitive and specific predictor of bipolar II outcome. More work along these lines is necessary to sway the personality disorder-centric view of this interphase.
- *Prominent mood swings associated with alcohol and substance abuse.* Substance—and especially alcohol—abuse is highly comorbid across the entire spectrum of bipolar disorders. In DSM-IV, so-called alcohol and/or substance-induced mood disorders have been given an exaggerated preferential status over bipolar spectrum diagnoses. It is not uncommon at all for mood swings to persist following detoxification, suggesting that these disorders may have much in common with bipolar spectrum conditions such as recurrent brief hypomania, cyclothymia, or hyperthymia. This is a fertile clinical area in search of investigators with the requisite will to measure bipolarity broadly across different patterns of alcohol and substance use, abuse, and addiction. The author hypothesizes that molecular genetics may ultimately reveal genes common to these disorders—bridging them via some temperamental dimensions along novelty-seeking, impulsivity or cyclothymic lines.
- *The future.* Table 1.12 provides a summary of all conventional and putative diagnostic subtypes for which plausible data exists for inclusion within a broadly conceived bipolar spectrum proposal by myself and

TABLE 1.12 A proposed broad spectrum of bipolar disorders (modified from Akiskal and Pinto [22])

- **Bipolar $\frac{1}{2}$:** Schizobipolar disorder
- **Bipolar I:** Manic-depressive illness
- **Bipolar I $\frac{1}{2}$:** Depression with protracted hypomania
- **Bipolar II:** Depression with spontaneous discrete hypomanic episodes
- **Bipolar II $\frac{1}{2}$:** Depression superimposed on cyclothymia
- **Bipolar III:** Depression plus hypomania occurring in association with antidepressant or other somatic treatment
- **Bipolar III $\frac{1}{2}$:** Prominent mood swings in association with substance and/or alcohol (ab)use
- **Bipolar IV:** Depression superimposed on hyperthymia

Olavo Pinto [22]. The classification is offered for its heuristic value in that it combines both categorical (prototypical) and dimensional (spectrum) conceptualizations. To avoid burdening the diagnostic schema with undue complexity, considerations of comorbidity, mixity and rapid cycling have been left out of this proposed classification. However, it is easy to see that rapid cycling pertains primarily to bipolar II, II $\frac{1}{2}$, and III $\frac{1}{2}$, while mixity in its broadest sense applies to the entire spectrum. Obviously the proposed expansion of the bipolar spectrum will require a great deal of more systematic research during the coming decade. Shared oligogenic inheritance might ultimately provide answers to boundary problems within and on the boundaries of the bipolar spectrum.

The justification for such subthreshold expansions of bipolarity for defining "dilute" yet complex phenotypes is for future genetic investigation, as well as in the service of public health. Such lowering of illness boundaries is happening in diabetes mellitus type II as well as in hypertension. However, in psychiatry, we have just begun to develop instruments to detect bipolar spectrum disorders. The search for genetic markers needs to somehow consider the broader phenotypes discussed herein. The pursuit of such work—whether diagnostic, psychometric or molecular genetic—is also of paramount importance in early detection of bipolar disorder in juvenile subjects and in the offspring of bipolar parents.

REFERENCES

1. Goodwin F.K., Jamison K.R. (1990) *Manic-Depressive Illness*. Oxford University Press, New York.
2. Marneros A., Angst J. (Eds) (2000) *Bipolar Disorders: 100 Years after Manic Depressive Insanity*. Kluwer, Dordrecht.

3. Akiskal H.S. (Ed.) (1999) *Bipolarity: Beyond Classic Mania.* Saunders, Philadelphia.
4. Goodnick P.J. (Ed.) (1998) *Mania: Clinical and Research Perspectives.* American Psychiatric Press, Washington.
5. Young L.T., Joffe R.T. (Eds) (1997) *Bipolar Disorder: Biological Models and their Clinical Application.* Dekker, New York.
6. Soares J.C., Gershon S. (Eds) (2000) *Bipolar Disorders: Basic Mechanisms and Therapeutic Implications.* Dekker, New York.
7. Duke P., Hochman G. (1992) *A Brilliant Madness: Living with Manic Depressive Illness.* Bantam, New York.
8. Jamison K. (1996) *An Unquiet Mind.* Random House, New York.
9. Whybrow P.C. (1997) *A Mood Apart.* HarperCollins, New York.
10. Goldberg J.F., Harrow M. (Eds) (1999) *Bipolar Disorders: Clinical Course and Outcome.* American Psychiatric Press, Washington.
11. Lish J.D., Dime-Meenan S., Whybrow P.C., Price R.A., Hirschfeld R.M. (1994) The National Depressive and Manic-Depressive Association (DMDA) survey of bipolar members. *J. Affect. Disord.*, **31**: 281–294.
12. Akiskal H.S., Downs J., Jordan P., Watson S., Daugherty D., Pruitt D.B. (1985) Affective disorders in referred children and younger siblings of manic depressives: mode of onset and prospective course. *Arch. Gen. Psychiatry*, **42**: 996–1003.
13. Gottschalk A., Bauer M.S., Whybrow P.C. (1995) Evidence of chaotic mood variation in bipolar disorder. *Arch. Gen. Psychiatry*, **52**: 947–959.
14. McElroy S.L., Keck P.E., Pope H.G.J., Hudson J.I., Faedda G.L., Swann A.C. (1992) Clinical and research implications of the diagnosis of dysphoric or mixed mania or hypomania. *Am. J. Psychiatry*, **149**: 1633–1644.
15. Pope H.G., Lipinski J.F. (1978) Diagnosis in schizophrenia and manic-depressive illness: a reassessment of the specificity of "schizophrenic" symptoms in the light of current research. *Arch. Gen. Psychiatry*, **35**: 811–828.
16. Akiskal H.S., Puzantian V.R. (1979) Psychotic forms of depression and mania. *Psychiatr. Clin. North Am.*, **2**: 419–439.
17. Khantzian E.J. (1997) The self-medication hypothesis of substance use disorders: a reconsideration and recent applications. *Harvard Rev. Psychiatry*, **4**: 231–244.
18. Salloum I.M., Thase M.E. (2000) Impact of substance abuse on the course and treatment of bipolar disorder. *Bipolar Disord.*, **2**: 269–280.
19. Young L.T., Cooke R.G., Robb J.C., Levitt A.J., Joffe R.T. (1993) Anxious and nonanxious bipolar disorder. *J. Affect. Disord.*, **29**: 49–52.
20. Perugi G., Akiskal H.S., Ramacciotti S., Nassini S., Toni C., Milanfranchi A., Musetti L. (1999) Depressive comorbidity of panic, social phobic, and obsessive-compulsive disorders re-examined: is there a bipolar II connection? *J. Psychiatr. Res.*, **33**: 53–61.
21. Dunner D.L., Gershon E.S., Goodwin F.K. (1976) Heritable factors in the severity of affective illness. *Biol. Psychiatry*, **11**: 31–42.
22. Akiskal H.S., Pinto O. (1999) The evolving bipolar spectrum. Prototypes I, II, III, and IV. *Psychiatr. Clin. North Am.*, **22**: 517–534.
23. Akiskal H.S., Mallya G. (1987) Criteria for the "soft" bipolar spectrum: treatment implications. *Psychopharmacol. Bull.*, **23**: 68–73.
24. Baldessarini R.J. (2000) A plea for integrity of the bipolar disorder concept. *Bipolar Disord.*, **2**: 3–7.
25. Gershon S., Yuwiler A. (1960) Lithium ion: a specific psychopharmacological approach to the treatment of mania. *J. Neuropsychiatry*, **1**: 229–241.

26. Grof P., Alda M., Grof E., Zvolsky P., Walsh M. (1994)   Lithium response and genetics of affective disorders. *J. Affect. Disord.*, **32**: 85–95.
27. Akiskal H.S. (1996)   The prevalent clinical spectrum of bipolar disorders: beyond DSM-IV. *J. Clin. Psychopharmacology*, **16** (Suppl. 1): 4s–14s.
28. American Psychiatric Association (1994)   *Diagnostic and Statistical Manual of Mental Disorders*, 4th ed., American Psychiatric Association, Washington.
29. Dunner D.L., Fleiss J.L., Fieve R.R. (1976)   The course of development of mania in patients with recurrent depression. *Am. J. Psychiatry*, **133**: 905–908.
30. Rao A.V., Nammalvar J. (1977)   The course and outcome in depressive illness—A follow-up study of 122 cases in Madurai, India. *Br. J. Psychiatry*, **130**: 392–396.
31. Strober M., Carlson G. (1982)   Bipolar illness in adolescents with major depression: clinical, genetic, and psychopharmacologic predictors in a three- to four-year prospective follow-up investigation. *Arch. Gen. Psychiatry*, **39**: 549–555.
32. Akiskal H.S., Walker P., Puzantian V.R., King D., Rosenthal T.L., Dranon M. (1983)   Bipolar outcome in the course of depressive illness: phenomenologic, familial, and pharmacologic predictors. *J. Affect. Disord.*, **5**: 115–128.
33. Akiskal H.S., Maser J.D., Zeller P.J., Endicott J., Coryell W., Keller M., Warshaw M., Clayton P., Goodwin F.K. (1995)   Switching from "unipolar" to bipolar II: an 11-year prospective study of clinical and temperamental predictors in 559 patients. *Arch. Gen. Psychiatry*, **52**: 114–123.
34. Coryell E., Endicott J., Maser J.D., Keller M.B., Leon A.C., Akiskal H.S. (1995)   Long-term stability of polarity distinctions in the affective disorders. *Am. J. Psychiatry*, **152**: 365–372.
35. World Health Organization (1992)   *The ICD-10 Classification of Mental and Behavioural Disorders. Clinical Descriptions and Diagnostic Guidelines*. World Health Organization, Geneva.
36. Kraepelin E. (1921)   *Manic-depressive Insanity and Paranoia*. Livingstone, Edinburgh.
37. Cooper J.E., Kendell R.E., Gurland B.J., Sharpe L., Copeland J.R.M., Simon R. (1972)   *Psychiatric Diagnosis in New York and London*. Oxford University Press, London.
38. Adams F. (Ed.) (1856)   *The Extant Works of Aretaeus, the Cappadocian*. Sydenham Society, London.
39. Carlson G.A., Goodwin F.K. (1973)   The stages of mania: a longitudinal analysis of the manic episode. *Arch. Gen. Psychiatry*, **28**: 221–228.
40. Falret J.P. (1854)   Mémoire sur la folie circulaire. *Bulletin de l'Académie de Médicine*, **19**: 382–415.
41. Baillarger J. (1854)   De la folie à double forme. *Ann. Med. Psychol.* (Paris), **6**: 367–391.
42. Bourgeois M.L., Marneros A. (2000)   The prognosis of bipolar disorders: course and outcome. In *Bipolar Disorders: 100 Years after Manic Depressive Insanity* (Eds A. Marneros, J. Angst), pp. 405–436, Kluwer, Dordrecht.
43. Hare E. (1981)   The two manias: a study of the evolution of the modern concept of mania. *Br. J. Psychiatry*, **138**: 89–99.
44. Weygandt W. (1899)   *Über die Mischzustände des Manisch-Depressiven Irreseins*. Lehmann, Munich.
45. Dreyfus G.L. (1907)   *Die Melancholie, ein Zustandsbild des Manisch-Depressiven Irreseins*. Fisher, Jena.
46. Koukopoulos A., Koukopoulos A. (1999)   Agitated depression as a mixed state and the problem of melancholia. *Psychiatr. Clin. North Am.*, **22**: 547–564.

47. Leonhard K. (1979) *The Classification of Endogenous Psychoses*. Irvington, New York.
48. Angst J. (1973) The etiology and nosology of endogenous depressive psychoses. *Foreign Psychiatry*, **2**: 1–108.
49. Perris C. (1966) A study of bipolar (manic-depressive) and unipolar recurrent depressive psychoses. *Acta Psychiatr. Scand.*, **194** (Suppl.).
50. Winokur G., Clayton P.J., Reich T. (1969) *Manic-Depressive Illness*. Mosby, St. Louis.
51. Angst J. (1995) Epidémiologie du spectre bipolaire. *Encéphale*, **21**: 37–42.
52. Spitzer R.L., Endicott J., Robins E. (1978) Research Diagnostic Criteria: rationale and reliability. *Arch. Gen. Psychiatry*, **35**: 773–782.
53. Smeraldi E., Negri E., Melica M. (1977) A genetic study of affective disorders. *Acta Psychiatr. Scand.*, **56**: 382–398.
54. Gershon E.S., Hamovit J., Guroff J.J., Dibble E., Leckman J.F., Sceery W., Targum S.D., Nurnberger J.I. Jr., Goldin L.R., Bunney W.E., Jr (1982) A family study of schizoaffective, bipolar I, bipolar II, unipolar and control probands. *Arch. Gen. Psychiatry*, **39**: 1157–1167.
55. Tsuang M.T., Faraone S.V., Fleming J.A. (1985) Familial transmission of major affective disorders. Is there evidence supporting the distinction between unipolar and bipolar disorders? *Br. J. Psychiatry*, **146**: 268–271.
56. Winokur G. (1980) Is there a common genetic factor in bipolar and unipolar affective disorder? *Compr. Psychiatry*, **21**: 460–468.
57. Kupfer D.J., Pickar D., Himmelhoch J.M., Detre T.P. (1975) Are there two types of unipolar depression? *Arch. Gen. Psychiatry*, **32**: 866–871.
58. Mendels J. (1976) Lithium in the treatment of depression. *Am. J. Psychiatry*, **133**: 373–378.
59. Bowden C. (1978) Lithium-responsive depression. *Compr. Psychiatry*, **19**: 227–231.
60. De Montigny C., Grunberg F., Mayer A., Deschenes J.P. (1981) Lithium induces rapid relief of depression in tricyclic antidepressant drug non-responders. *Br. J. Psychiatry*, **138**: 252–256.
61. Leverich G.S., Post R.M. (1998) Life charting of affective disorders. *CNS Spectrums*, **3**: 21–37.
62. Akiskal H.S. (1983) The bipolar spectrum: new concepts in classification and diagnosis. In *Psychiatry Update: The American Psychiatric Association Annual Review*, Vol. 2 (Ed. L. Grinspoon), pp. 271–292, American Psychiatric Press, Washington.
63. Lewinsohn P.M., Klein D.L., Seeley J.R. (1995) Bipolar disorders in a community sample of older adolescents: prevalence, phenomenology, comorbidity, and course. *J. Am. Acad. Child Adolesc. Psychiatry*, **34**: 454–463.
64. Szádóczky E., Papp Z., Vitrai J., Rihmer Z., Füredi J. (1998) The prevalence of major depressive and bipolar disorder in Hungary. *J. Affect. Disord.*, **50**: 155–162.
65. Angst J. (1998) The emerging epidemiology of hypomania and bipolar II disorder. *J. Affect. Disord.*, **50**: 143–151.
66. Regier D.A., Boyd J.H., Burke J.D. Jr., Rae D.S., Myers J.K., Kramer M., Robins L.N., George L.K., Karno M., Locke B.Z. (1988) One-month prevalence of mental disorders in the United States. *Arch. Gen. Psychiatry*, **45**: 977–986.
67. Kessler R.C., McGonagle K.A., Zhao S., Nelson C.B., Hughes M., Eshleman S., Wittchen H.U., Kendler K.S. (1994) Lifetime and 12-month prevalence of DSM-III-R psychiatric disorders in the United States: results from the national comorbidity survey. *Arch. Gen. Psychiatry*, **51**: 8–19.

68. Weissman M.M., Bland R.C., Canino G.J., Faravelli C., Greenwald S., Hwu H.-G., Joyce P.R., Karam E.G., Lee C.-K., Lellouch J. *et al* (1996) Cross-national epidemiology of major depression and bipolar disorder. *JAMA*, **276**: 293–299.

69. Fieve R.R., Dunner D.L. (1975) Unipolar and bipolar affective states. In *The Nature and Treatment of Depression* (Eds F.F. Flach, S.S. Draghi), pp. 145–160, Wiley, New York.

70. Angst J., Frey R., Lohmeyer B., Zerbin-Rüdin E. (1980) Bipolar manic-depressive psychoses: results of a genetic investigation. *Hum. Genet.*, **55**: 237–254.

71. Endicott N.A. (1989) Psychophysiological correlates of "bipolarity". *J. Affect. Disord.*, **17**: 47–56.

72. Klerman G.L. (1981) The spectrum of mania. *Compr. Psychiatry*, **22**: 11–20.

73. Cassano G.B., Dell'Osso L., Frank E., Miniati M., Fagiolini A., Shear K., Pini S., Maser J. (1999) The bipolar spectrum: a clinical reality in search of diagnostic criteria and an assessment methodology. *J. Affect. Disord.*, **54**: 319–328.

74. Cassano G.B., Akiskal H.S., Savino M., Musetti L., Perugi G., Soriani A. (1992) Proposed subtypes of bipolar II disorder: with hypomanic episodes and/or with hyperthymic temperament. *J. Affect. Disord.*, **26**: 127–140.

75. Akiskal H.S., Hantouche E.G., Allilaire J.F., Sechter D., Bourgeois M.L., Azorin J.M., Chatenêt-Duchêne L., Lancrenon S. (2001) Systematic comparison of major depression with spontaneous hypomania (bipolar II) versus those with antidepressant-associated hypomania in the French national EPIDEP study. *J. Affect. Disord.* (in press).

76. Bertelsen A., Harvald B., Hauge M. (1977) A Danish twin study of manic-depressive disorders. *Br. J. Psychiatry*, **130**: 330–351.

77. Fieve R.R., Go R., Dunner D.L., Elston R. (1984) Search for biological/genetic markers in a long-term epidemiological and morbid risk study of affective disorders. *J. Psychiatr. Res.*, **18**: 425–445.

78. Coryell W., Endicott J., Reich T., Andreasen N., Keller M (1984) A family study of bipolar II disorder. *Br. J. Psychiatry*, **145**: 49–54.

79. Heun R., Maier W. (1993) The distinction of bipolar II disorder from bipolar I and recurrent unipolar depression: results of a controlled family study. *Acta Psychiatr. Scand.*, **87**: 279–284.

80. Simpson S.G., Folstein S.E., Meyers D.A., McMahon F.J., Brusco D.M., DePaulo J.R. Jr. (1993) Bipolar II: The most common bipolar phenotype? *Am. J. Psychiatry*, **150**: 901–903.

81. Alda M., Grof P., Grof E., Zvolsky P., Walsh M. (1994) Mode of inheritance in families of patients with lithium-responsive affective disorders. *Acta Psychiatr. Scand.*, **90**: 304–310.

82. Akiskal H.S., Placidi G.F., Signoretta S., Liguori A., Gervasi R., Maremmani I., Mallya G., Puzantian V.R. (1998) TEMPS-I: Delineating the most discriminant traits of cyclothymic, depressive, irritable and hyperthymic temperaments in a nonpatient population. *J. Affect. Disord.*, **51**: 7–19.

83. Hirschfeld R.M., Williams J.B., Spitzer R.L., Calabrese J.R., Flynn L., Keck P.E. Jr., Lewis L., McElroy S.L., Post R.M., Rapport D.J. *et al* (2000) Development and validation of a screening instrument for bipolar spectrum disorder: the Mood Disorder Questionnaire. *Am. J. Psychiatry*, **157**: 1873–1875.

84. Petzel T.P., Rado E.D. (1990) Divergent validity evidence for Eckblad and Chapman's hypomanic personality scale. *J. Clin. Psychol.*, **46**: 43–46.

85. Williams J.B.W., Terman M., Link M.J., Amira L., Rosenthal N.E. (1999) Hypomania interview guide (including hyperthymia): retrospective assessment version (HIGH-R). *Depress. Anxiety*, **9**: 92–100.

86. Akiskal H.S., Bourgeois M.L., Angst J., Post R., Möller H.J., Hirschfeld R. (2000) Re-evaluating the prevalence of and diagnostic composition within the broad clinical spectrum of bipolar disorders. *J. Affect. Disord.*, **59**: S5–S30.
87. Taylor M.A., Abrams R. (1980) Reassessing the bipolar-unipolar dichotomy. *J. Affect. Disord.*, **2**: 195–217.
88. Akiskal H.S. (2000) Mood disorders: clinical features. In *Kaplan & Sadock's Comprehensive Textbook of Psychiatry* (Eds. B.J. Sadock, V.A. Sadock), pp. 1338–1377, Lippincott Williams & Wilkins, Philadelphia.
89. Bauer M.S., Crits-Christoph P., Ball W.A., Dewees E., McAllister T., Alahi P., Cacciola J., Whybrow P.C. (1991) Independent assessment of manic and depressive symptoms by self-rating: scale characteristics and implications for the study of mania. *Arch. Gen. Psychiatry*, **48**: 807–812.
90. Beigel A., Murphy D.L., Bunney W.E. (1971) The Manic-State Rating Scale: scale construction, reliability, and validity. *Arch. Gen. Psychiatry*, **25**: 256–262.
91. Bell L. (1849) On a form of disease resembling some advanced stages of mania and fever, but so contradistinguished from any ordinarily observed or described combination of symptoms as to render it probable that it may be an overlooked and hitherto unrecorded malady. *Am. J. Insanity*, **6**: 97–127.
92. Cowdry R.W., Goodwin F.K. (1981) Dementia of bipolar illness: diagnosis and response to lithium. *Am. J. Psychiatry*, **138**: 1118–1119.
93. Ghaemi S.N., Boiman E., Goodwin F.K. (2000) Insight and outcome in bipolar, unipolar, and anxiety disorders. *Compr. Psychiatry*, **41**: 167–171.
94. Peralta V., Cuesta M.J. (1998) Lack of insight in mood disorders. *J. Affect. Disord.*, **49**: 55–58.
95. Schneider K. (1959) *Clinical Psychopathology*. Grune and Stratton, New York.
96. Regier D.S., Farmer M.E., Rae D.S., Loskce B.Z., Keith S.D., Judd L.L., Goodwin F.K. (1990) Comorbidity of mental disorders with alcohol and other drug abuse. *JAMA*, **264**: 2511–2518.
97. Winokur G., Turvey C., Akiskal H.S., Coryell W., Solomon D., Leon A., Mueller T., Endicott J., Maser J., Keller M. (1998) Alcoholism and drug abuse in three groups—bipolar I, unipolars and their acquaintances. *J. Affect. Disord.*, **50**: 81–89.
98. Taylor M.A., Abrams R. (1973) The phenomenology of mania: a new look at some old patients. *Arch. Gen. Psychiatry*, **29**: 520–522.
99. Andreasen N.C., Akiskal H.S. (1983) The specificity of Bleulerian and Schneiderian symptoms: a critical re-evaluation. *Psychiatr. Clin. North Am.*, **6**: 41–54.
100. Welner A., Liss J.L., Robins E. (1973) Psychiatric symptoms in white and black inpatients. II. Follow-up study. *Compr. Psychiatry*, **14**: 483–488.
101. Bell C.C., Mehta H. (1981) Misdiagnosis of black patients with manic depressive illness: second in a series. *JAMA*, **73**: 101–107.
102. Strakowski S.M., McElroy S.L., Keck P.E., West S.A. (1996) Racial influence on diagnosis in psychotic mania. *J. Affect. Disord.*, **39**: 157–162.
103. Kirov G., Murray R.M. (1999) Ethnic differences in the presentation of bipolar affective disorder. *Eur. Psychiatry*, **14**: 199–204.
104. Perugi G., Akiskal H.S., Rossi L., Paiano A., Quilici C., Madaro D., Musetti L., Cassano G.B. (1997) Chronic mania. Family history, prior course, clinical picture and social consequences. *Br. J. Psychiatry*, **173**: 514–518.
105. Helzer J.E., Clayton P.J., Pambakian R., Reich T., Woodruff R.A. Jr., Reveley M.A. (1977) Reliability of psychiatric diagnosis. II. The test/retest reliability of diagnostic classification. *Arch. Gen. Psychiatry*, **34**: 136–141.
106. Young R., Biggs J., Meyer D. (1978) A rating scale for mania: reliability, validity, and sensitivity. *Br. J. Psychiatry*, **133**: 429–435.

107. Bech P., Bolwig T.G., Kramp P., Rafaelsen O.J. (1979) The Bech–Rafaelsen mania rating scale and the Hamilton depression scale. *Acta Psychiatr. Scand.*, **59**: 420–430.
108. Altman E. (1998) Rating scales for mania: is self-rating reliable? *J. Affect. Disord.*, **50**: 283–286.
109. Jamison K.R., Gerner R.H., Hammen C., Padesky C. (1980) Clouds and silver linings: positive experiences associated with primary affective disorders. *Am. J. Psychiatry*, **137**: 198–202.
110. Akiskal H.S., Djenderedjian A.H., Rosenthal R.H., Khani M.K. (1977) Cyclothymic disorder: validating criteria for inclusion in the bipolar affective group. *Am. J. Psychiatry*, **134**: 1227–1233.
111. Angst J. (1992) L'hypomanie: à propos d'une cohorte de jeunes. *Encéphale*, **18**: 23–29.
112. Hantouche E.G., Angst J., Akiskal H.S. (2001) A factor analysis of hypomania and cyclothymia. *J. Affect. Disord.* (in press).
113. Benazzi F. (2001) Is 4 days the minimum duration of hypomania in bipolar II disorder? *Eur. Arch. Psychiatry Clin. Neurosci.*, **251**: 32–34.
114. Manning J.S., Haykal R.F., Connor P.D., Akiskal H.S. (1997) On the nature of depressive and anxious states in a family practice setting: the high prevalence of bipolar II and related disorders in a cohort followed longitudinally. *Compr. Psychiatry*, **38**: 102–108.
115. Kretschmer E. (1936) *Physique and Character*. Kegan, Paul, Trench, Trubner, London.
116. Brieger P., Marneros A. (1997) Dysthymia and cyclothymia: historical origins and contemporary development. *J. Affect. Disord.*, **45**: 117–126.
117. Akiskal H.S. (2001) Dysthymia and cyclothymia in psychiatric practice a century after Kraepelin. *J. Affect. Disord.*, **62**: 17–31.
118. Akiskal H.S., Khani M.K., Scott-Strauss A. (1979) Cyclothymic temperamental disorders. *Psychiatr. Clin. North Am.*, **2**: 527–554.
119. Hantouche E.G., Akiskal H.S., Lancrenon S., Allilaire J.F., Sechter D., Azorin J.M., Bourgeois M., Fraud J.P., Châtenet-Duchêne L. (1998) Systematic clinical methodology for validating bipolar-II disorder: data in mid-stream from a French national multisite study (EPIDEP). *J. Affect. Disord.*, **50**: 163–173.
120. Placidi G.F., Signoretta S., Liguori A., Gervasi R., Maremmani I., Akiskal H.S. (1998) The Semi-Structured Affective Temperament Interview (TEMPS-I): reliability and psychometric properties in 1010 14–26 year students. *J. Affect. Disord.*, **47**: 1–10.
121. Akiskal H.S., Perugi G., Hantouche E., Haykal R., Manning S., Connor P. (2002) The affective temperament scales of Memphis, Pisa, Paris and San Diego: progress towards a self-rated auto-questionnaire version (TEMPS-A). *J. Affect. Disord.* (in press).
122. Depue R.A., Slater J.F., Wolfstetter-Kausch H., Klein D., Goplerud E., Farr D. (1981) A behavioral paradigm for identifying persons at risk for bipolar depressive disorder: a conceptual framework and five validation studies. *J. Abnorm. Psychol.*, **90**: 381–437.
123. Klein D.N., Depue R.A., Slater J.F. (1986) Inventory identification of cyclothymia. IX. Validation in offspring of bipolar-I patients. *Arch. Gen. Psychiatry*, **43**: 441–445.
124. Andreasen N.C. (1987) Creativity and mental illness: prevalence rates in writers and their first-degree relatives. *Am. J. Psychiatry*, **144**: 1288–1292.

125. Akiskal H.S., Akiskal K. (1988) Reassessing the prevalence of bipolar disorders: clinical significance and artistic creativity. *Psychiatr. Psychobiol.*, **3**: 29s–36s.
126. Richards R., Kinney D.K., Lunde I., Benet M., Merzel A.P. (1988) Creativity in manic-depressives, cyclothymes, their normal relatives, and control subjects. *J. Abnorm. Psychol.*, **97**: 281–288.
127. Akiskal H.S. (1992) Delineating irritable-choleric and hyperthymic temperaments as variants of cyclothymia. *J. Pers. Disord.*, **6**: 326–342.
128. Schneider K. (1958) *Psychopathic Personalities*. Thomas, Springfield.
129. Possl J., von Zerssen D. (1990) A case history analysis of the "manic type" and the "melancholic type" of premorbid personality in affectively ill patients. *Eur. Arch. Psychiatry Clin. Neurosci.*, **239**: 347–355.
130. Eckblad M., Chapman L.J. (1986) Development and validation of a scale for hypomanic personality. *J. Abnorm. Psychol.*, **95**: 214–222.
131. Klein D.N., Lewinsohn P.M., Seeley J.R. (1996) Hypomanic personality traits in a community sample of adolescents. *J. Affect. Disord.*, **38**: 135–143.
132. Kwapil T.R., Miller M.B., Zinser M.C., Chapman L.J., Chapman J., Eckblad M. (2000) A longitudinal study of high scorers on the hypomanic personality scale. *J. Abnorm. Psychol.*, **109**: 222–226.
133. Akiskal H.S., Hantouche E.G., Bourgeois M., Azorin J.M., Sechter D., Allilaire J.F., Lancrenon S., Fraud J.P., Châtenet-Duchêne L. (1998) Gender, temperament, and the clinical picture in dysphoric mixed mania: findings from a French national study (EPIMAN). *J. Affect. Disord.*, **50**: 175–186.
134. Perugi G., Maremmani I., Toni C., Madaro D., Mata B., Akiskal H.S. (2001) The contrasting influence of depressive and hyperthymic temperaments on psychometrically derived manic subtypes. *Psychiatry Res.*, **101**: 249–258.
135. Henry C., Lacoste J., Bellivier F., Verdoux H., Bourgeois M.L., Leboyer M. (1999) Temperament in bipolar illness: impact on prognosis. *J. Affect. Disord.*, **56**: 103–108.
136. Himmelhoch J.M. (1998) Social anxiety, hypomania and the bipolar spectrum: data, theory and clinical issues. *J. Affect. Disord.*, **50**: 203–213.
137. Bunney W.E., Jr, Goodwin F.K., Murphy D.L., House K.M., Gordon E.K. (1972) The "switch process" in manic-depressive illness, II: Relationship to catecholamines, REM sleep, and drugs. *Arch. Gen. Psychiatry*, **27**: 304–309.
138. Himmelhoch J.M. (2000) Biology of the switch process in bipolar disorders. In *Bipolar Disorders: Basic Mechanisms and Therapeutic Implications* (Eds J.C. Soares, S. Gershon), pp. 273–303, Dekker, New York.
139. Bunney W.E. (1978) Psychopharmacology of the switch process in affective illness. In *Psychopharmacology: A Generation of Progress* (Eds. M.A. Lipton, A. DiMascio, K.F. Killam), pp. 1249–1259, Raven Press, New York.
140. Stoll A.L., Mayer P.V., Kolbrener M., Goldstein E., Suplit B., Lucier J., Cohen B.M., Tohen M. (1994) Antidepressant-associated mania: a controlled comparison with spontaneous mania. *Am. J. Psychiatry*, **151**: 1642–1645.
141. Preda A., MacLean R.W., Mazure C.M., Bowers M.B., Jr (2001) Antidepressant-associated mania and psychosis resulting in psychiatric admissions. *J. Clin. Psychiatry*, **62**: 30–33.
142. Himmelhoch J.M., Mulla D., Neil J.F., Detre T.P., Kupfer D.J. (1976) Incidence and significance of mixed affective states in a bipolar population. *Arch. Gen. Psychiatry*, **33**: 1062–1066.
143. Himmelhoch J.M., Coble P., Kupfer K.J., Ingenito J. (1976) Agitated psychotic depression associated with severe hypomanic episodes: a rare syndrome. *Am. J. Psychiatry*, **133**: 765–771.

144. Perugi G., Akiskal H.S., Micheli C., Musetti L., Paiano A. Quilici C., Rossi L., Cassano B. (1997) Clinical subtypes of bipolar mixed states: validating a broader European definition in 143 cases. *J. Affect. Disord.*, **43**: 169–180.
145. Benazzi F. (2000) Depressive mixed states: unipolar and bipolar II. *Eur. Arch. Psychiatry Clin. Neurosci.*, **250**: 249–253.
146. Berner P., Gabriel E., Katschnig H., Kieffer W., Koehler K., Lenz G., Nutzinger D., Schanda H., Simhandl C. (1992) *Diagnostic Criteria for Functional Psychoses*, 2nd ed., Cambridge University Press, Cambridge.
147. Swann A.C., Secunda S.K., Katz M.M., Croughan J. Bowden C.L., Koslow S.H., Berman N., Stokes P.E. (1993) Specificity of mixed affective states: clinical comparison of dysphoric mania and agitated depression. *J. Affect. Disord.*, **28**: 81–89.
148. Mitchell P.B., Wilhelm K., Parker G., Austin M.P., Rutgers P., Malhi G.S. (2001) The clinical features of bipolar depression: a comparison with matched major depressive disorder patients. *J. Clin. Psychiatry*, **62**: 212–216.
149. Post R.M., Rubinow D.R., Uhde T.W., Roy-Byrne P.P., Linnoila M., Rosoff A., Cowdry R.W. (1989) Dysphoric mania: clinical and biological correlates. *Arch. Gen. Psychiatry*, **46**: 353–358.
150. Dell'Osso L., Placidi G.F., Nassi R., Freer P., Cassano G.B., Akiskal H.S. (1991) The manic-depressive mixed state: Familial, temperamental and psychopathologic characteristics in 108 female inpatients. *Eur. Arch. Psychiatry Clin. Neurosci.*, **240**: 234–239.
151. Dell'Osso L., Akiskal H.S., Freer P., Barberi M., Placidi G.F., Cassano G.B. (1993) Psychotic and nonpsychotic bipolar mixed states: comparisons with manic and schizoaffective disorders. *Eur. Arch. Psychiatry Clin. Neurosci.*, **243**: 75–81.
152. Dilsaver S.C., Swann A.C., Shoaib A.M., Bowers T.C., Halle M.T. (1993) Depressive mania associated with nonresponse to antimanic agents. *Am. J. Psychiatry*, **150**: 1548–1551.
153. Strakowski S.M., McElroy S.L., Keck P.E. Jr, West S.A. (1996) Suicidality among patients with mixed and manic bipolar disorder. *Am. J. Psychiatry*, **153**: 674–676.
154. Goldberg J.F., Garno J.L., Leon A.C., Kocsis J.H., Portera L. (1998) Association of recurrent suicidal ideation with nonremission from acute mixed mania. *Am. J. Psychiatry*, **155**: 1753–1755.
155. Bauer M.S., Whybrow P.C., Gyulai L., Gonnel J., Yeh H.S. (1994) Testing definitions of dysphoric mania and hypomania: prevalence, clinical characteristics and inter-episode stability. *J. Affect. Disord.*, **32**: 201–211.
156. McElroy S.L., Strakowski S.M., Keck P.E., Tugrul K.L., West S.A., Lonczak H.S. (1995) Differences and similarities in mixed and pure mania. *Compr. Psychiatry*, **36**: 184–194.
157. Hantouche E.G., Akiskal H.S. (1997) Outils d'évaluation cliniques des tempéraments affectifs. *Encéphale*, **23**: 27–34.
158. Akiskal H.S. (1992) The distinctive mixed states of bipolar I, II and III. *Clin. Neuropharmacol.*, **15**: 632–633.
159. Cassidy F., Murry E., Forest K., Carroll B.J. (1997) The performance of DSM-III-R major depression criteria in the diagnosis of bipolar mixed states. *J. Affect. Disord.*, **46**: 79–81.
160. Swann A.C., Bowden C.L., Morris D., Calabrese J.R., Petty F., Small J., Dilsaver S.C., Davis J.M. (1997) Depression during mania. Treatment response to lithium or divalproex. *Arch. Gen. Psychiatry*, **54**: 37–42.

161. Tohen M., Jacobs T.G., Grundy S.L., McElroy S.L., Banov M.C., Janicak P.G., Sanger T., Risser R., Zhang F., Toma V. *et al* (2000) Efficacy of olanzapine in acute bipolar mania: a double-blind placebo-controlled study. The Olanzapine HGGW Study Group. *Arch. Gen. Psychiatry*, **57**: 841–849.
162. Makanjuola R.O.A. (1985) Recurrent unipolar manic disorder in the Yoruba Nigerian: further evidence. *Br. J. Psychiatry*, **147**: 434–437.
163. Nurnberger J.I. Jr., Roose S.P., Dunner D.L., Fieve R.R. (1979) Unipolar mania: a distinct clinical entity? *Am. J. Psychiatry*, **136**: 1420–1423.
164. Keller M.B., Lavori P.W., Coryell W., Andreasen N.C., Endicott J., Clayton P.J., Klerman G.L., Hirschfeld R.M. (1986) Differential outcome of pure manic, mixed/cycling, and pure depressive episodes in patients with bipolar illness. *JAMA*, **255**: 3138–3142.
165. Krauthammer C., Klerman G.L. (1978) Secondary mania. *Arch. Gen. Psychiatry*, **35**: 1333–1339.
166. Carroll B.T., Goforth H.W., Kennedy J.C., Dueno O.R. (1996) Mania due to general medical conditions: frequency, treatment, and cost. *Int. J. Psychiatry Med.*, **26**: 5–13.
167. Brockington I. (1996) *Motherhood and Mental Health*. Oxford University Press, Oxford.
168. Dilsaver S.C., Chen R., Shoaib A.M., Swann A.C. (1999) Phenomenology of mania: evidence for distinct depressed, dysphoric, and euphoric presentations. *Am. J. Psychiatry*, **156**: 426–430.
169. Cassidy F., Forest K., Murry E., Carroll B.J. (1998) A factor analysis of the signs and symptoms of mania. *Arch. Gen. Psychiatry*, **55**: 27–32.
170. Rice J.P., McDonald-Scott P., Endicott J., Coryell W., Grove W.M., Keller M.B., Altis D. (1986) The stability of diagnosis with an application to bipolar II disorder. *Psychiatry Res.*, **19**: 285–296.
171. Dunner D.L., Tay L.K. (1993) Diagnostic reliability of the history of hypomania in bipolar II patients with major depression. *Compr. Psychiatry*, **34**: 303–307.
172. Perugi G., Akiskal H.S., Lattanzi L., Cecconi D., Mastrocinque C., Patronelli A., Vignoli S. (1998) The high prevalence of soft bipolar (II) features in atypical depression. *Compr. Psychiatry*, **39**: 73.
173. Benazzi F. (2000) Depression with DSM-IV atypical features: a marker for bipolar II disorder. *Eur. Arch. Psychiatry Clin. Neurosci.*, **250**: 53–55.
174. Ebert D., Barocka A., Kalb R., Ott G. (1993) Atypical depression as a bipolar spectrum disease. Evidence from a longitudinal study: the early course of atypical depression. *Psychiatria Danubina*, **5**: 133–136.
175. MacKinnon D., Xu J., McMahon F.J., Simpson S.G., Stine C., McInnis M.G., DePaulo J.R., (1998) Bipolar disorder and panic disorder in families: an analysis of chromosome 18 data. *Am. J. Psychiatry* **55**: 829–831.
176. Vieta E., Gasto C., Otero A., Nieto E., Vallejo J. (1997) Differential features between bipolar I and bipolar II disorder. *Compr. Psychiatry*, **38**: 98–101.
177. Rihmer Z., Pestality P. (1999) Bipolar II disorder and suicidal behavior. *Psychiatr. Clin. North Am.*, **22**: 667–673.
178. Egeland J.A. (1983) Bipolarity: the iceberg of affective disorders? *Compr. Psychiatry*, **24**: 337–344.
179. Koukopoulos A., Tundo A., Floris G.F., Reginaldi D., Minnai G.P., Tondo L. (1990) Changes in life habits that may influence the course of affective disorders. In *Psychiatry: A World Perspective*, Vol. 1 (Eds C.N. Stefanis, A.D. Rabavilas, C.R. Soldatos), pp. 478–483, Elsevier, Amsterdam.

180. Benazzi F. (1997) Prevalence of bipolar II disorder in outpatient depression: a 203-case study in private practice. *J. Affect. Disord.*, **43**: 163–166.
181. Lewis J.L., Winokur G. (1982) The induction of mania. A natural history study with controls. *Arch. Gen. Psychiatry*, **39**: 303–306.
182. Angst J. (1985) Switch from depression to mania—a record study over decades between 1920 and 1982. *Psychopathology*, **18**: 140–154.
183. Kupfer D.J., Carpenter L.L., Frank E. (1988) Is bipolar II a unique disorder? *Compr. Psychiatry*, **29**: 228–236.
184. Akiskal H.S., Rosenthal R.H., Rosenthal T.L., Kashgarian M., Khani M.K., Puzantian V.R. (1979) Differentiation of primary affective illness from situational, symptomatic, and secondary depressions. *Arch. Gen. Psychiatry*, **36**: 635–643.
185. Menchon J.M., Gasto C., Vallejo J., Catalan R. (1993) Rate and significance of hypomanic switches in unipolar melancholic depression. *Eur. Psychiatry*, **8**: 125–129.
186. Wehr T.A., Goodwin F.K. (1987) Can antidepressants cause mania and worsen the course of affective illness? *Am. J. Psychiatry*, **144**: 1403–1411.
187. Sultzer D.L., Cummings J.L. (1989) Drug-induced mania—causative agents, clinical characteristics and management. A retrospective analysis of the literature. *Med. Toxicol. Adv. Drug Exper.*, **4**: 127–143.
188. Altshuler L.L., Post R.M., Leverich G.S., Mikalauskas K., Rosoff A., Ackerman L. (1995) Antidepressant-induced mania and cycle acceleration: a controversy revisited. *Am. J. Psychiatry*, **152**: 1130–1138.
189. Howland R.H. (1996) Induction of mania with serotonin reuptake inhibitors. *J. Clin. Psychopharmacol.*, **16**: 425–427.
190. Boerlin H.L., Gitlin M.J., Zoellner L.A., Hammen C.L. (1998) Bipolar depression and antidepressant-induced mania: a naturalistic study. *J. Clin. Psychiatry*, **59**: 374–379.
191. Bottlender R., Rudolf D., Strauss A., Möller H.J. (1998) Antidepressant-associated maniform states in acute treatment of patients with bipolar I depression. *Eur. Arch. Psychiatry Clin. Neurosci.*, **248**: 296–300.
192. Jann M.W., Bitar A.H., Rao A. (1982) Lithium prophylaxis of tricyclic-antidepressant-induced mania in bipolar patients. *Am. J. Psychiatry*, **139**: 683–684.
193. Himmelhoch J.M., Thase M.E., Mallinger A.G., Houck P. (1991) Tranylcypromine versus imipramine in anergic bipolar depression. *Am. J. Psychiatry*, **48**: 910–916.
194. Rosenthal T.L., Akiskal H.S., Scott-Strauss A., Rosenthal R.H., David M. (1981) Familial and developmental factors in characterologic depressions. *J. Affect. Disord.*, **3**: 183–192.
195. Rihmer Z. (1990) Dysthymia: a clinician's perspective. In *Dysthymic Disorder* (Eds S.W. Burton, H.S. Akiskal), pp. 112–125, Gaskell, London.
196. Bauer M.S., Calabrese J.R., Dunner D.L., Post R.P., Whybrow P.C., Gyulai L., Tay L.K., Younkin S., Bynum D., Lavori P. *et al* (1994) Multi-site data re-analysis: validity of rapid cycling as a course modifier for bipolar disorder in DSM-IV. *Am. J. Psychiatry*, **151**: 506–515.
197. Maj M., Magliano L., Pirozzi R., Marasco C., Guarneri M. (1994) Validity of rapid cycling as a course specifier for bipolar disorder. *Am. J. Psychiatry*, **151**: 1015–1019.
198. Coryell W., Endicott J., Keller M. (1992) Rapidly cycling affective disorder: demographics, diagnosis, family history and course. *Arch. Gen. Psychiatry*, **49**: 126–131.

199. Wolpert E.A., Goldberg J.F., Harrow M. (1990) Rapid cycling in unipolar and bipolar affective disorders. *Am. J. Psychiatry*, **147**: 725–728.
200. Koukopoulos A., Reginaldi D., Laddomada P., Floris G., Serra G., Tondo L. (1980) Course of the manic-depressive cycle and changes caused by treatment. *Pharmakopsychiatr. Neuropsychopharmakol.*, **13**: 156–167.
201. Kilzieh N., Akiskal H.S. (1999) Rapid-cycling bipolar disorder: an overview of recent research and clinical experience. *Psychiatr. Clin. North Am.*, **22**: 585–607.
202. Tondo L., Baldessarini R.J. (1998) Rapid cycling in women and men with bipolar manic-depressive disorders. *Am. J. Psychiatry*, **155**: 1434–1436.
203. Perugi G., Micheli C., Akiskal H.S., Madaro D., Socci C., Quilici C., Musetti L. (2000) Polarity of the first episode, clinical characteristics, and course of manic depressive illness: a systematic retrospective investigation of 320 bipolar I patients. *Compr. Psychiatry*, **41**: 13–18.
204. McElroy S.L., Pope H.G., Jr., Keck P.E., Jr., Hudson J.I., Phillips K.A., Strakowski S.M. (1996) Are impulse-control disorders related to bipolar disorder? *Compr. Psychiatry*, **37**: 229–240.
205. Ten Have M., Vollebergh W., Bijl R., Nolen W.A. (2002) Bipolar disorder in the general population. *J. Affect. Disord.* (in press).
206. Ghaemi S.N., Sachs G.S., Chiou A.M., Pandurangi A.K., Goodwin K. (1999) Is bipolar disorder still underdiagnosed? Are antidepressants overutilized? *J. Affect. Disord.*, **52**: 135–144.
207. National Depressive and Manic-Depressive Association (2001) *Living with Bipolar Disorder: How Far Have We Really Come? A Constituency Survey*. DMDA, Chicago.
208. Ghaemi S.N., Boiman E.E., Goodwin F.K. (2000) Diagnosing bipolar disorder and the effect of antidepressants: a naturalistic study. *J. Clin. Psychiatry*, **61**: 804–808.
209. Lehmann H. (1970) The impact of the therapeutic revolution on nosology. In *The Schizophrenic Syndrome* (Ed. R. Cancro), pp. 136–153, Brunner/Mazel, New York.
210. Baldessarini R.J. (1970) Frequency of diagnoses of schizophrenia versus affective disorders from 1944–1968. *Am. J. Psychiatry*, **127**: 759–763.
211. Zisook S., Janowsky D.S., Overall J.E., Risch S.C. (1985) The dexamethasone suppression test and unipolar/bipolar distinctions. *J. Clin. Psychiatry*, **46**: 461–465.
212. Gurpegui M., Casanova J., Cervera S. (1985) Clinical and neuroendocrine features of endogenous unipolar and bipolar depression. *Acta Psychiatr. Scand.*, **320** (Suppl.): 30–37.
213. Rybakowski J.K., Twardowska K. (1999) The dexamethasone/corticotropin-releasing hormone test in depression in bipolar and unipolar affective illness. *J. Psychiatr. Res.*, **33**: 363–370.
214. Gershon E.S. (2000) Bipolar illness and schizophrenia as oligogenic diseases: implications for the future. *Biol. Psychiatry*, **47**: 240–244.
215. Taylor M.A., Amir N. (1994) Are schizophrenia and affective disorder related?: The problem of schizoaffective disorder and the discrimination of the psychoses by signs and symptoms. *Compr. Psychiatry*, **35**: 420–429.
216. Maj M., Pirotti R., Formicola A.M., Bartoli L., Bucci P. (2000) Reliability and validity of the DSM-IV diagnostic category of schizoaffective disorder: preliminary data. *J. Affect. Dis.*, **57**: 95–98.
217. Marneros A., Tsuang M.T. (Eds) (1990) *Affective and Schizoaffective Disorders: Similarities and Differences*. Springer, New York.

218. Sovner R.D., McHugh P.R. (1976)   Bipolar course in schizo-affective illness. *Biol. Psychiatry*, **11**: 195–204.
219. Van Eerdewegh M.M., Van Eerdewegh P., Coryell W., Clayton P.J., Endicott J., Koepke J., Rochberg N. (1987)   Schizo-affective disorders: bipolar-unipolar subtyping—natural history variables: a discriminant analysis approach. *J. Affect. Disord.*, **12**: 223–232.
220. Gunderson J.G., Phillips K.A. (1991)   A current view of the interface between borderline personality disorder and depression. *Am. J. Psychiatry*, **148**: 967–975.
221. Akiskal H.S., Chen S.E., Davis G.C., Puzantian V.R., Kashgarian M., Bolinger J.M. (1985)   Borderline: an adjective in search of a noun. *J. Clin. Psychiatry*, **46**: 41–48.
222. Hollander E., Allen A., Lopez R.P., Bienstock C.A., Grossman R., Siever L.J., Merkatz L., Stein D.J. (2001)   A preliminary, double-blind, placebo-controlled trial of divalproex sodium in borderline personality disorder. *J. Clin. Psychiatry*, **62**: 199–203.
223. Pinto O.C., Akiskal H.S. (1998)   Lamotrigine as a promising approach to borderline personality: an open case series without concurrent DSM-IV major mood disorder. *J. Affect. Disord.*, **51**: 333–343.
224. Kranzler H.R., Rounsaville B.J. (Eds) (1998)   *Dual Diagnosis and Treatment: Substance Abuse and Comorbid Medical and Psychiatric Disorders*. Dekker, New York.
225. Chengappa K.N., Levine J., Gershon S., Kupfer D.J. (2000)   Lifetime prevalence of substance or alcohol abuse and dependence among subjects with bipolar I and II disorders in a voluntary registry. *Bipolar Disord.*, **2**: 191–195.
226. Lemere F., Smith J.W. (1990)   Hypomanic personality trait in cocaine addiction. *Br. J. Addict.*, **85**: 575–576.
227. Rounsaville B.J., Anton S.F., Carroll K., Budde D., Prusoff B.A., Gawin F. (1991)   Psychiatric diagnoses of treatment-seeking cocaine abusers. *Arch. Gen. Psychiatry*, **48**: 43–51.
228. Mirin S.M., Weiss R.D. (1986)   Affective illness in substance abusers. *Psychiatr. Clin. North Am.*, **9**: 503–514.
229. Sonne S.C., Brady K.T. (1999)   Substance abuse and bipolar comorbidity. *Psychiatr. Clin. North Am.*, **22**: 609–627.

Commentaries

1.1

Terminology, History and Definition of Bipolar Spectrum

Jules Angst[1]

Hagop Akiskal has written a masterly review on bipolar disorder, which amply illustrates Heracleitus' view that all things are in a state of flux.

This volume of the World Psychiatric Association is devoted to bipolar disorders, making the history of the term and concept of central interest. The terms "unipolar" and "bipolar" disorder were coined by Karl Kleist [1] and were taken over by his pupils Neele [2] and Leonhard [3]. Apart from manic-depressive (circular) disorders, Kleist and Leonhard's bipolar concept included the three atypical (cycloid) psychoses. It is important to note that they classified both mania and melancholia as "homonomic" [4], "unipolar" [1, 2] or "monopolar" [3] disorders: in other words, the bipolar concept of the Kleist–Leonhard school excluded mania. Moreover, Kleist and Leonhard assumed the genetic load in monopolar disorders to be much lower than in bipolar disorders, as shown by the monographs of Neele [2] and Leonhard [3]. Kleist and Neele saw bipolar disorders as being a combination of the monopolar forms with a special affinity [5]. Leonhard himself did not follow Kleist completely; he accepted the existence of monopolar and bipolar (manic-depressive) disorders and positioned himself between Kleist and Kraepelin, who rejected the dichotomy of monopolar and bipolar disorders [5].

The term "unipolar depression" was redefined by Perris [6] as recurrent depression with a minimum of three depressive episodes; the purpose was as far as possible to exclude hidden bipolar disorders; the underlying assumption could not be confirmed, because highly recurrent depression is particularly at risk of a diagnostic change into bipolar illness [7]. The term "unipolar depression" was later used more broadly to mean non-bipolar depression.

The modern bipolar concept originates in the monographs of Angst [8], Perris [5], and Winokur *et al* [9]; it includes mania without depression, but it excludes the cycloid psychoses of Kleist and Leonhard. The three monographs differed very widely in their conclusions as to the overall morbidity risk among first-degree relatives. However, all three studies demonstrated

[1] *Psychiatrische Universitätsklinik, Lenggstrasse 31, Postfach 68, CH-8029 Zürich, Switzerland*

that there was a qualitative difference between bipolar disorder and depression, showing that a significant bipolar morbid risk was present only in the families of bipolar probands and not in the families of their depressive counterparts.

Whether mania really belongs to bipolar disorder is still a matter of debate; pure mania has a very low prevalence rate, although Kraepelin found it to be very frequent in Java. Every failure to obtain full information favours the diagnosis of a pure case; retrospective diagnoses are suspect.

Hagop Akiskal is an advocate of a broad spectrum concept of bipolar disorders, and in my view he is right. Psychiatric research into bipolar illness, including modern drug trials, continues to be dominated by studies on mania, which characterizes the most severe expression of the spectrum, but bipolar I disorder is no more prevalent than schizophrenia. There is relatively little research into bipolar II disorder and the wider spectrum, although in general practice and in the community bipolar II is probably five to 10 times more prevalent than bipolar I disorder.

The operational definition of the bipolar spectrum remains a knotty problem: What are the minimum requirements for a hypomanic syndrome, as determined from good data rather than the agreement of experts? What are the necessary symptoms and their minimum duration? Is the two days' minimum duration not too long? Is a case of ultrarapid cycling over months or years (24 hours depressed, 24 hours manic) only classified as bipolar after two years if it meets criteria of cyclothymia? How do we classify patients with major depression and brief hypomania of only one day's duration if it can be shown that subjects with one-day hypomania have the same positive family history for mania as DSM-IV hypomanics? Are there cases who manifest depression in the morning and hypomania in the evening, thereby failing even to meet a criterion of hypomania of one day's duration? Is the DSM-IV criterion of "clinically significant distress and impairment" applicable to hypomania? If there is "distress", is it not felt more by significant others than by the subjects manifesting hypomania themselves? Is hypomania always pathological? Can it not also be beneficial? Is hyperthymia chronic hypomania? Is cyclothymia—defined as a more chronic cycling state by analogy with dysthymia—a useful concept?

It is clear that the spectrum concept has raised more questions than it answers, which demonstrates its heuristic value. All things are indeed in a state of flux.

REFERENCES

1. Kleist K. (1953) Die Gliederung der neuropsychischen Erkrankungen. *Monatsschr. Psychiatr. Neurol.*, **125**: 526–554.

2. Neele E. (1949)   *Die phasischen Psychosen nach ihrem Erscheinungs- und Erbbild.* Barth, Leipzig.
3. Leonhard K. (1957)   *Aufteilung der Endogenen Psychosen.* Akademie, Berlin.
4. Kleist K. (1937)   Zustandsbilder und Krankheitsarten im Lichte der Gehirn- pathologie. *Psychiatr. Neurol. Wochenschr.,* **39**: 420–422.
5. Leonhard K. (1968)   Über monopolare und bipolare endogene Psychosen. *Nervenarzt,* **39**: 104–106.
6. Perris C. (1966)   A study of bipolar (manic-depressive) and unipolar recurrent depressive psychoses. *Acta Psychiatr. Scand.,* **194** (Suppl.).
7. Angst J., Felder W., Frey R., Stassen H.H. (1978)   The course of affective disorders. I. Change of diagnosis of monopolar, unipolar, and bipolar illness. *Arch. Psychiatr. Nervenkr.,* **226**: 57–64.
8. Angst J. (1966)   *Zur Aetiologie und Nosologie Endogener Depressiver Psychosen. Eine Genetische, Soziologische und Klinische Studie.* Springer, Berlin.
9. Winokur G., Clayton P.J., Reich T. (1969)   *Manic Depressive Illness.* Mosby, St. Louis.

1.2
Toward an Expansion of Bipolar Disorders in DSM-V

David L. Dunner[1]

The work group for mood disorders in DSM-IV and the group developing the ICD-10 classification for mood disorders expanded the concept of bipolar disorders to include bipolar II disorder and rapid cycling into the nomenclature. These two additions were based, at least from the DSM-IV perspective, on sufficient data to warrant their inclusion in the nomenclature. A multi-site data re-analysis was performed to provide validity for the inclusion of rapid cycling [1]. The validity was demonstrated by noting a change in gender frequency as episode frequency increased in bipolar patients. The inclusion of bipolar II disorder was based on a review of the literature involving clinical description, family studies, longitudinal course, biological factors and familial factors differentiating this condition from other forms of bipolar/unipolar disorders [2].

Hagop Akiskal comments that the criterion of four days or longer for hypomania seems too stringent. This criterion was actually determined by the ICD-10 committee and accepted by DSM-IV. There were no data provided to determine the proper duration of a hypomanic episode for its inclusion. ICD-10 planners indeed determined that a hypomanic episode would be four days or longer in duration.

[1] *Department of Psychiatry and Behavioral Sciences, University of Washington, 4225 Roosevelt Way NE, Suite 306C, Seattle, WA 98105, USA*

Akiskal notes quite correctly that there are still undefined affective conditions lying between the unipolar/bipolar distinction. These vary from individuals who are chronically hypomanic with brief depressive periods to unipolar patients found among relatives of bipolar probands. The Akiskal–Mallya proposal for a "soft bipolar spectrum" is presented in the review. Interestingly, support for broadening the concept of bipolar disorder comes from a series of international studies and enjoys a considerable database, particularly from the French National Collaborative Study and the Pisa–Memphis Collaborative Study.

Clearly, patients encountered in clinical and research settings have a greater degree of "spectrum" disorders than are permitted by the current classification systems. Are they all to be considered "bipolar, not otherwise specified" or can meaningful distinctions be made among patients in order to be more specific regarding their classification and perhaps treatment options?

The thrust of Akiskal's paper is descriptive. He describes the nuances of clinical features of the current bipolar disorders (bipolar I and bipolar II) as well as proposing expansion of the concept of bipolar disorder toward his proposed spectrum concept. This is an elegant and erudite argument. Whether it will carry the day with the planners for DSM-V and ICD-11 is unclear at this time.

It is my opinion that a few rather glaring problems persist in the DSM-IV regarding the classification of bipolar disorder. First of all, is the concept of mixed mania and its differentiation from rapid cycling and cyclothymic disorder. These terms are frequently used interchangeably and interestingly there are increasing numbers of patients in clinical settings who have dysphoric manic episodes. Whether this is the result of prior history of substance abuse, which was less likely to occur 30 years ago, or whether such patients are presenting more to academic medical centres because of treatment resistance is not entirely clear. However, clarification of the concept of mixed mania would seem to be a useful endeavour for the DSM-V/ICD-11 planners.

The second area has to do with treatment-induced hypomania. Currently patients who are depressed and become hypomanic in response to treatment are classified as major depression with (antidepressant) induced hypomania. This classification ignores the fact that many patients with bipolar disorder go through phasic cycles with mania or hypomania preceded by depressive states. Thus, the natural history of their disorder is to have a switch from depression to an elevated mood state. Why such patients were not considered bipolar in the DSM-IV/ICD-10 is unclear. However, data to clarify this point would seem to be an important contribution to the planners for the next nomenclature.

The third area which is highlighted by Akiskal's paper is the relationship of bipolar mood states to personality disorders and clarification of what is truly in the bipolar spectrum and what may not be. Data regarding this issue would be of considerable importance to our field.

REFERENCES

1. Dunner D.L. (1993) A review of the diagnostic status of "Bipolar II" for the DSM-IV work group on mood disorders. *Depression*, **1**: 2–10.
2. Bauer M.S., Calabrese J., Dunner D.L., Post R., Whybrow P.C., Gyulai L., Tay L.K., Younkin S.R., Bynum D., Lavori P. *et al* (1994) Multisite data reanalysis of the validity of rapid cycling as a course modifier for bipolar disorder in DSM-IV. *Am. J. Psychiatry*, **151**: 506–515.

1.3
Narrowing and Broadening Diagnostic Criteria for Bipolar Disorder: Competing Demands of Research and Clinical Practice

Stephen M. Strakowski[1]

Like most psychiatric, and many medical disorders, the diagnosis of a bipolar disorder remains fixed to clinical evaluation, symptom recognition and syndrome definition. Hagop Akiskal provides a comprehensive review of the evolution of this diagnosis during the previous two millennia, particularly the most recent 100 years. Additionally, he proposes a spectrum of bipolar disorders that incorporates broader coverage into primarily depressive states that have typically been included under the rubric of unipolar depression.

In the struggle to identify meaningful psychiatric diagnoses, two often competing demands infringe upon the effort. The first of these is the need to develop useful, pragmatic illness descriptions that permit clinicians to label the wide variety of patients that they face each day in their offices. Broad diagnostic guidelines serve the role of helping clinicians develop an initial treatment plan for the many different patients that they see. These diagnostic guidelines are most useful if they help clinicians identify a therapy that is more likely to be helpful than harmful in the treatment of a given patient. In this context, a broad spectrum approach to bipolar disorder is useful in order to maximize identification of patients who may benefit from mood stabilizers, yet be at risk if mis-labelled and assigned antidepressants (although the risk of antidepressants, particularly for "soft spectrum" bipolar

[1] *Department of Psychiatry, University of Cincinnati College of Medicine, Cincinnati, OH 45267–0559, USA*

conditions, remains incompletely defined) [1]. In such a plan it is preferable to expose unipolar depressed patients to mood stabilizers (which are not likely to be directly harmful and may even be beneficial) than bipolar patients to antidepressants. Within a purely clinical context, then, broadening diagnostic considerations in such a way that maximizes therapeutic options while minimizing risks is the most appropriate approach.

An often competing demand, however, is to narrow the diagnostic criteria of a patient sample in order to identify a more homogeneous patient group for biological study. Indeed, in order to develop external validators, neurobiological studies of patients with bipolar disorders are, of course, critical. As described by Feighner and colleagues in 1972 [2], in order to advance the study of many psychiatric conditions, narrowly defined patient groups are needed, and criteria that create these patient groups are critical. As an example, neuroimaging provides the most direct means to study human brain dysfunction *in vivo* and, in so doing, potentially define the neurophysiologic substrate of this condition. However, it has been difficult to replicate many neuroimaging studies in bipolar disorder [3]. We have recently examined this difficulty in our own data sets and found that failure to replicate appears strongly associated with the clinical and demographic constitution of the patient (and healthy comparison) groups [4]. Additionally, Drevets *et al* [5] recently demonstrated that by studying a narrowly defined group of familial depressives and bipolar patients, they were able to identify biological differences (using functional imaging) from healthy subjects that seem to have a histopathological basis [6] and have been replicated by others using a similar, narrow approach [7]. Of course, results from these narrowly defined patient groups will not generalize to all patients that clinicians treat, nor is this intended. The results will, however, help advance our understanding of the neurobiological substrates of these conditions which may then identify external validators of clinical types. Much of the quandary that criteria sets like DSM-IV and its predecessors have encountered has been the result of these sets evolving from research tools (in which narrowly defined criteria were the goal) into broad clinical application without accompanying external validation.

Akiskal's spectrum provides one solution to the competing needs between the clinical and research worlds. Specifically, by identifying subgroups within a broader definition, the researcher has a narrower patient population to permit more homogeneous samples, while the clinician has a broader umbrella to permit a starting point in treatment development. Ultimately, these symptom-based nosologies are only as valuable as they are useful for guiding patient treatment, diagnosis or prognosis. Over time, then, this spectrum can be validated, discarded, or moved under other major diagnostic headings by rigorously applying external validators, such as common neuroimaging abnormalities, shared genetic patterns, or predictable treatment response. In order for this to occur, however, these criteria will have to remain unmodified long enough to permit this research to actually occur, a recurring problem with the ever changing DSM system. Otherwise, the evolution of the diagnosis of bipolar disorder will persist indefinitely, to no useful end.

ACKNOWLEDGEMENT

Supported by a grant from the Theodore and Vada Stanley Foundation and an NIH award (MH 58170).

REFERENCES

1. Altshuler L.L., Post R.M., Leverich G.S., Mikalauskas K., Rosoff A., Ackerman L. (1995) Antidepressant-induced mania and cycle acceleration: a controversy revisited. *Am. J. Psychiatry*, **152**: 1130–1138.
2. Feighner J.P., Robins E., Guze S.B., Woodruff R.A., Jr., Winokur G., Munoz R. (1972) Diagnostic criteria for use in psychiatric research. *Arch. Gen. Psychiatry*, **26**: 57–63.
3. Strakowski S.M., DelBello M.P., Adler C.M., Cecil K.M., Sax K.W. (2000) Neuroimaging in bipolar disorder. *Bipolar Disord.*, **2**: 148–164.
4. Strakowski S.M., DelBello M.P., Zimmerman M.E., Getz G.E., Mills N.P., Jak A., Ret J., Shear P.K., Adler C.M. Subcortical and cerebellar MRI structural volumes in first-versus multiple-episode bipolar disorder. Submitted for publication.
5. Drevets W.C., Price J.L., Simpson J.R., Jr., Todd R.D., Reich T., Vannier M., Raichle M.E. (1997) Subgenual prefrontal cortex abnormalities in mood disorders. *Nature*, **386**: 824–827.
6. Rajkowska G., Halaris A., Selemon L.D. (2001) Reductions in neuronal and glial density characterize the dorsolateral prefrontal cortex in bipolar disorder. *Biol. Psychiatry*, **49**: 741–752.
7. Hirayasu Y., Shenton M.E., Salisbury D.F., Kwon J.S., Wible C.G., Fischer I.A., Yurgelun-Odd D., Zarate C., Kikinis R., Jolesz F.A. *et al* (1999) Subgenual cingulate cortex volume in first-episode psychosis. *Am. J. Psychiatry*, **156**: 1091–1093.

1.4

Is Phenomenological Dissection for Bipolar Disorders Spectrum Possible?

Samuel Gershon[1] and Joseph Levine[2]

Hagop Akiskal's review stresses the breadth and scope of the clinical picture involved in an inclusive spectrum view of bipolar disorders. Whichever perspective of this view one wishes to focus upon, the importance of the issues and questions described is undeniable. Such an inclusive view of bipolar spectrum poses an array of questions including: a) What is the scope of signs, symptoms and behaviours that ought to be taken into consideration (i.e., should it include behavioural patterns associated with certain personality traits or disorders?); b) How does one label certain constellations of behaviours as psychopathological and others as a normal variant in the population?; c) What is the nature of the criteria needed for a dissection of a given psychopathological phenomenological field (i.e., bipolar spectrum) into illness subgroups? In this regard, one asks whether course of illness, patterns of inheritance and treatment response are appropriate and sufficient tools for such dissection.

The answers to these questions are vital for such a phenomenological dissection.

As to the last question, it seems to us that solid pathophysiological and etiological data is necessary for the task of dissecting a suggested disorder/s spectrum into valid subgroups. However, with deficient knowledge as to the underlying pathophysiology and/or etiology of bipolar disorders at this time, one may use course of illness, patterns of inheritance and treatment response as dissecting tools. Once a spectrum is ordered into groups and/or subgroups, such subgroups may be researched for their shared and unshared pathophysiology.

Regrettably, there is a current lack of such research for several groups of the proposed bipolar spectrum (i.e., bipolar disorders II $\frac{1}{2}$; III; III $\frac{1}{2}$ and IV), and only few biological research studies comparing bipolar I and II. Therefore, it seems to us premature to conclude that a spectrum view with its proposed groups (subgroups) should be accepted, or refuted.

What about the scope of the psychopathological phenomenological field? It is clear that in the extreme, unipolar and bipolar disorders are discriminable clinically and familiarly; however, many observations have shown areas of overlap. There is data suggesting that there is overlap between anxiety and depressive disorders and recently Akiskal [1] stated

_____

[1] _Department of Psychiatry, Western Psychiatric Institute & Clinic, UPMC Health System, Pittsburgh, PA 15213, USA_
[2] _Beersheva Mental Health Center, P.O. Box 4600, Beersheva, Israel_

that "clinical observations have revealed complex associations between anxiety and bipolar disorders". These data suggest that the scope of the phenomenological field to be taken into consideration for a dissection into different disorders or subgroups may be even broader. And such suggestions do not consider the overlap between the schizophrenic spectrum and the affective spectrum manifested in the diagnosis of schizoaffective disorder.

Next, one may ask what is the potential importance of the spectrum view of bipolar illness to psychopharmacologic interventions and the shaping or modification of course of bipolar illness by pharmacological treatment.

As to the importance of the specific bipolar spectrum groups or subgroups presented by Akiskal in regard to biological treatment, much has still to be done. It is not clear enough whether bipolar II $\frac{1}{2}$, III, III $\frac{1}{2}$ and IV should be treated with mood stabilizers or whether they respond similarly to other pharmacological treatments as bipolar II and I disorders. Also, certain psychotropics, mainly antidepressant drugs, have been suggested to accelerate episode frequency in bipolar I and II patients and thus modify the course of the disorder, whereas this is not clear for bipolar II $\frac{1}{2}$, III, III $\frac{1}{2}$ and IV subgroups.

Finally, the task of defining a phenomenological field and the process involved in such dissection is considerable. A new theoretical framework for the spectrum of affective and anxiety disorders may need to be formulated. We suggest that such a theoretical framework will follow that of connective tissue immunological disorders (i.e., systemic lupus erythematosus, Sjogren's syndrome, etc.) showing a high co-occurrence on one hand, and having shared and unshared biological properties within the framework of the same system on the other.

REFERENCE

1. Akiskal H.S. (Ed.) (1999) *Bipolarity: Beyond Classic Mania.* Saunders, Philadelphia.

1.5
In Search for a Definition for Bipolar Disorder
Alan C. Swann[1]

We now lack any objective test that can determine whether an individual has, or does not have, bipolar disorder. Therefore, despite great recent advances in understanding the treatment and phenomenology of bipolar disorder, we are left with the vital and basic questions of a) what is bipolar disorder and b) what is not bipolar disorder. Hagop Akiskal, combining scholarship with an emphasis on clinical pragmatism, addresses these questions. There is no better person for this endeavour, since he has arguably done more than anyone else in the field to change the way in which we think about bipolar disorder.

One refreshing and useful feature of Akiskal's review is its emphasis on historical context. It is a common error to overemphasize the cross-sectional view of a patient. The same is true of bipolar disorder as an entity. Bipolar disorder is, we think, an old disease, but it is a relatively new and changing concept. There has been a trend toward viewing bipolar disorder as part of a spectrum, at the expense of viewing it as discrete diagnostic categories. Official nosology, both North American and European, has perhaps not kept pace with that trend.

There is a danger, however, of falling into the trap of generalizing bipolar disorder to the point of meaningless universality. This danger cannot be avoided, however, by clinging doggedly to outmoded and sometimes inaccurate diagnostic systems that sacrifice validity for reliability. Instead, we need a better idea of what is the *sine qua non* for bipolar disorder, and how it can be detected early.

Depression is responsible for much of the suffering associated with bipolar disorder [1]. Its role in the illness, however, is still not well understood, and many of the unresolved problems in diagnosis involve depression. Akiskal emphasizes these: the existence of mixed depressions as well as mixed manias, the prominent role of depression in bipolar II (and the higher bipolar numbers) [2], the identification of patients with bipolar disorder who have experienced depressive episodes but have not yet been manic or hypomanic. These questions have large practical treatment implications, since "antidepressant" treatments may have deleterious effects in at least some patients with bipolar disorder.

Our thinking about bipolar disorder has focused too much on episodes and not enough on the underlying illness. Yet, even so-called euthymic patients with bipolar disorder are worse off than stable patients with

[1] *Department of Psychiatry and Behavioral Sciences, University of Texas Medical School, Houston, 1300 Moursund St., Houston, Texas 77030, USA*

major depressive disorder or individuals without a psychiatric illness [3]. Akiskal has addressed this by emphasizing the role of temperament [4]. As pointed out earlier by Kraepelin, temperament shades gradually into normal variation. It may provide, however, the physiological substrate on which other aspects of bipolar disorder are potentially imposed. Akiskal and his coworkers have developed clinical instruments for measuring temperament, but the concept requires better validation with physiological or psychophysiological measures. The specificity of the relationship between temperament and other aspects of bipolar disorder is also not yet understood. For example, temperament may be something which interacts with bipolar disorder, but is inherited independently. Alternatively, temperament may represent a useful indicator of genetic predisposition [5].

Akiskal emphasizes a number of important features of bipolar disorder that are not adequately appreciated, including:

a) Most people with bipolar disorder were never manic.
b) Bipolar I and bipolar II disorders differ greatly in their course and are basically different types of illness: bipolar I has more severe manias and bipolar II has a more severe course. Not emphasized enough, however, is the fact that depressive episodes associated with bipolar II disorder can be quite severe, with psychotic features.
c) Depression, as well as mania, can have mixed features. The idea (in DSM-IV) that mixed states are possible only in bipolar I disorder is absurd.
d) Diagnosis of bipolar disorder is best made through multiple interviews rather than a single structured interview. Similarly, management and evaluation should emphasize longitudinal measurement. This will require changes in statistical design of studies and in the assumptions underlying treatment and evaluation [6].
e) Pharmacologic hypomania (or mania) is almost surely bipolar disorder, contrary to the DSM and ICD systems.

The numeric scheme now in use for classification of bipolar disorders is not yet satisfactory. Bipolar I through IV progresses, more or less, in the direction of less severe mania, but there is no orderly progression in terms of severity of depression or course of illness. Yet, Akiskal has argued convincingly that for most patients these aspects are more important than mania. Perhaps a more pragmatic and descriptive system could be devised using a multi-axial approach, possibly based on a) temperament, b) cyclicity/course, and c) intensity or type of episodes. We will ultimately need a system that can be validated by objective physiological measures. Until that (probably distant) goal is achieved, better understanding of bipolar disorder will depend on rigorous clinical description and logic.

REFERENCES

1. MacQueen G.M., Young L.T., Robb J.C., Marriott M., Cooke R.G., Joffe R.T. (2000) Effect of number of episodes on wellbeing and functioning of patients with bipolar disorder. *Acta Psychiatr. Scand.*, **101**: 374–381.
2. Perugi G., Akiskal H.S., Lattanzi L., Cecconi D., Mastrocinque C., Patronelli A., Vignoli S., Bemi E. (1998) The high prevalence of "soft" bipolar (II) features in atypical depression. *Compr. Psychiatry*, **39**: 63–71.
3. Robb J.C., Cooke R.G., Devins G.M., Young L.T., Joffe R.T. (1997) Quality of life and lifestyle disruption in euthymic bipolar disorder. *J. Psychiatr. Res.*, **31**: 509–517.
4. Akiskal H.S., Cassano G.B., Musetti L., Perugi G., Tundo A., Mignani V. (1989) Psychopathology, temperament, and past course in primary major depressions. 1. Review of evidence for a bipolar spectrum. *Psychopathology*, **22**: 268–277.
5. Niculescu A.B., III, Akiskal H.S. (2001) Proposed endophenotypes of psychiatry: evolutionary, clinical, and pharmacogenomic considerations. *Mol. Psychiatry*, **6**: 363–366.
6. Arndt S., Turvey C., Coryell W.H., Dawson J.D., Leon A.C., Akiskal H.S. (2000) Charting patients' course: a comparison of statistics used to summarize patient course in longitudinal and repeated measures studies. *J. Psychiatr. Res.*, **34**: 105–113.

1.6
What is Disordered in Bipolar Disorders?

Marc Louis Bourgeois[1]

Mania (euphoric or irritable), the clinical hallmark of bipolar disorder, is usually easy to recognize, whereas the limits of hypomania (the criterion for bipolar type II) with normality and mania proper are much more difficult to ascertain. But what is specific of bipolar disorder is still debated. It is not the symptoms: according to Kraepelin [1], all symptoms can be seen in all mental disorders; Pope and Lipinski [2] and Brockington *et al* [3] found schizophrenic symptoms as frequent in mania as in schizophrenia. It is not the prognosis: "terrible" for Falret [4], "good" for Kraepelin [1], and recently "bad" for Goldberg and Harrow [5, 6]. Finally, course (which was so important for Falret and Kraepelin) "should be dropped completely as a criterion for the classification of endogenous psychoses", according to Angst (quoted in [7]). The core of the disease is rather the instability and cyclicity of psychic processes, with swerves and switches, larger than normal oscillations of mood (and also) cognitions, psychomotor activity, instinctive and social life. Circularity and cyclicity are typical (for Delay [8]

[1] *Université Bordeaux II, Hôpital Charles Perrens, 121 rue de la Béchade, 33076 Bordeaux, France*

bipolar disorder was a *cyclophrenia*). The fragile and unstable balance is easily disturbed by life events and psychoactive drugs. This is well documented for antidepressants (the pharmacological moodswings defining bipolar disorder type III) [9–11] and for lithium abrupt interuption [12]. The course of the disease is altered by tricyclic antidepressants [13]. Recent data suggest that prescription of psychostimulants during childhood increases the risk of earlier onset of bipolar disorder [14].

Unlike Kraepelin, for whom stress and life events could play a role only in the very first episodes, whereas afterwards "manic depressive episodes can be surprisingly independent from external events", and in disagreement with Post's model of kindling [15], Hammen *et al* [16] and Swendsen *et al* [17] found that severe stress almost always triggers the episodes. These events are often induced by the patient's behaviour and personality and are unspecific [18].

Is mania always psychotic in essence, even in the absence of clear delusions and hallucinations? One can distinguish three (sometimes four) stages in the process of psychotization of mania (as for depression): 1) the patient is still aware of being (happily) boosted, driven, excited most of the time with a euphoric mood, with a relative control of behaviour; 2) insight and awareness disappear and the patient enters a psychotic phase, either abruptly or more slowly; 3) delusions, hallucinations and crazy behaviour submerge the patient who has lost all insight and control; 4) sometimes, there are even confusion, delirium and severe vegetative symptoms (which have been lethal in the past).

There is now evidence that bipolar temperaments, either depressive or manic, colour the acute episode [19–22]. One can also differentiate two subtypes of bipolar type I disorder: on the one hand, a subtype "with a predominance of manic psychopathology" [23] and on the other a "prevailing depressed" [23] or "depression prone" [24] type or a "poor prognosis subtype marked by a relative persistence of depressive symptoms" [25]. There are also differences between the DMD (or d) sequence of episodes and the MDM (or m) type [26]. There is a spectrum (even a continuum) of subcategories from pure manic disorder (unipolar mania) [27] to "pure depressive" [28] or "pseudo unipolar type" [29]. More research is required to determine what is the best choice of treatment for each of these subcategories, especially for the choice of mood stabilizers or antidepressants.

Finally, hypersensitivity, hypersyntony, extraversion, instability, suggestibility, loss of limits and proprieties, hyperesthesia, hyperreactivity, sensation seeking, disinhibition, intolerance to obstacles, excitation, acceleration, disorganization, disorder, chaos, whirling and swirling, twirling (*Wirbel*) characterize the mind and world of bipolar patients [30] and often confuse the differential diagnosis with hysteria, borderline personality and other cluster B axis II disorders.

REFERENCES

1. Kraepelin E. (1899/1921) *Manic Depressive Insanity and Paranoia*. Livingstone, Edinburgh.
2. Pope H.G., Lipinski J.S., Jr. (1978) Diagnosis in schizophrenia and manic-depressive illness: a reassessment of the specificity of "schizophrenic" symptoms in light of current research. *Arch. Gen. Psychiatry*, **35**: 811–828.
3. Brockington I.F., Wainwright S., Kendell R.E. (1980) Manic patients with schizophrenic or paranoid symptoms. *Psychol. Med.*, **10**: 73–83.
4. Falret J.P. (1854) Mémoire sur la folie circulaire, forme de la maladie mentale caracterisée par la reproduction successive et régulière de l'état maniaque, de l'état mélancolique, et d'un état lucide plus ou moins prolongé. *Bulletin de l'Académie de Médecine*, **19**: 382–415.
5. Goldberg J.F., Harrow M. (Eds) (1999) *Bipolar Disorders. Clinical Course and Outcome*. American Psychiatric Press, Washington.
6. Bourgeois M.L., Marneros A. (2000) The prognosis of bipolar disorders: course and outcome, In *Bipolar Disorders: 100 Years after Manic Depressive Insanity* (Eds A. Marneros, J. Angst), pp. 405–436, Kluwer, Dordrecht.
7. Goodwin F.K., Jamison K.R. (1990) *Manic-Depressive Illness*. Oxford University Press, New York.
8. Delay J. (1945) *Les Dérèglements de l'Humeur*, Vol. 1. Presses Universitaire de France, Paris.
9. Akiskal H.S. (1983) The bipolar spectrum. New concepts in classification and diagnosis. In *Psychiatry Update*, Vol. 2. (Ed. L. Grinspoon), pp. 271–292, American Psychiatric Press, Washington.
10. Wehr T.A., Goodwin F.K. (1987) Can antidepressants cause mania and worsen the course of affective illness? *Am. J. Psychiatry*, **144**: 1403–1411.
11. Angst J. (1985) Switch from depression to mania: a recorded study over decades between 1920 and 1982. *Psychopathology*, **18**: 140–154.
12. Maj M. (1999) Lithium discontinuation. *Am. J. Psychiatry*, **156**: 1130.
13. Koukopoulos A., Reginaldi D., Laddomada P., Floris G., Serra G., Tondo L. (1980) Course of the manic-depressive cycle and changes caused by treatments. *Pharmako-psychiatr. Neuropsychopharmakol.*, **13**: 156–167.
14. Reichart C. (2001) What are the risk factors for an early development of bipolar disorder in children? Presented at the 4th International Conference on Bipolar Disorder, Pittsburgh, June 14–16.
15. Post R.M., Kopanda R.T. (1976) Cocaine, kindling, and psychosis. *Am. J. Psychiatry*, **133**: 627–634.
16. Hammen C., Gitlin M. (1997) Stress reactivity in bipolar patients and its relation to prior history of disorder. *Am. J. Psychiatry*, **154**: 856–857.
17. Swendsen J., Hammen C., Heller T., Gitlin M. (1995) Correlates of stress reactivity in patients with bipolar disorder. *Am. J. Psychiatry*, **152**: 795–797.
18. Marneros A. (1999) *Handbuch der Unipolaren und Bipolaren Erkrandungen*. Thieme, Stuttgart.
19. Akiskal H.S., Akiskal K. (1992) Cyclothymic, hyperthymic and depressive temperaments as subaffective variants of mood disorders. In *Review of Psychiatry*, Vol. 11 (Eds A. Tasman, M.B. Ribas), pp. 43–62, American Psychiatric Press, Washington.
20. Akiskal H.S., Placidi G.F., Signoretta S., Liguori A., Gervasi R., Maremmani I., Mallya G., Puzantian V.R. (1998) TEMPS-I : Delineating the most discriminant

traits of cyclothymic, depressive, irritable and hyperthymic temperaments in a nonpatient population. *J. Affect. Disord.*, **51**: 7–19.

21. Henry C., Lacoste J., Bellivier F., Verdoux H., Bourgeois M.L., Leboyer M. (1999) Temperament in bipolar illness: impact on prognosis. *J. Affect. Disord.*, **56**: 103–108.

22. Perugi G., Maremmani I., Toni C., Madaro D., Mata B., Akiskal H.S. (2001) The contrasting influence of depressive and hyperthymic temperaments on psychometrically derived manic subtypes. *Psychiatry Res.*, **101**: 249–258.

23. Angst J. (1978) The course of affective disorders. II. Typology of bipolar manic depressive illness. *Arch. Psychiatr. Nervenkr.*, **226**: 65–73.

24. Quitkin F.M., Rabkin J.G., Prien R.F. (1986) Bipolar disorder: are there manic-prone and depressive-prone forms? *J. Clin. Psychopharmacol.*, **6**: 167–172.

25. Coryell W., Turvey C., Endicott J., Leon A.C., Mueller T., Solomon D., Keller M. (1998) Bipolar I affective disorder: predictors of outcome after 15 years. *J. Affect. Dis.*, **50**: 109–116.

26. Perugi G., Micheli C., Akiskal H.S., Madaro D., Socci C., Quilici C., Musetti L. (2000) Polarity of the first episode, clinical characteristics, and course of manic depressive illness: a systematic retrospective investigation of 320 bipolar I patients. *Compr. Psychiatry*, **41**: 13–18.

27. Abrams R., Taylor M.A. (1979) Unipolar mania revisted. *J. Affect. Disord.*, **1**: 59–68.

28. Winokur G., Clayton P. (1967) Family history studies : I. Two types of affective disorders separated according to genetic and clinical factors. In *Recent Advances in Biological Psychiatry*, Vol. 10 (Ed. J. Wortis), pp. 35–40, Plenum, New York.

29. Mendels J. (1976) Lithium in the treatment of depression. *Am. J. Psychiatry*, **133**: 373–378.

30. Ey H. (1950) Manie. In *Etudes Psychiatriques*, Vol. 3, pp. 47–116, Desclée de Brouwer, Paris.

1.7
How Prevalent is the Bipolar Spectrum?

Robert M.A. Hirschfeld[1]

Hagop Akiskal concisely provides us with a broad overview on what bipolar disorder is and what it is not. His paper dramatically describes the remarkable lack of consensus in the field on what constitutes bipolar disorder in light of very clear and cogent clinical descriptions of mania and depression dating back to the ancient Greeks. Curiously in light of this, the concept of bipolar disorder as a distinct nosologic entity is less than 50 years old.

[1] *Department of Psychiatry and Behavioral Sciences, University of Texas Medical Branch, 301 University Boulevard, Galveston, TX 77555–0188, USA*

Akiskal notes that the two major official classification systems in the world today, the DSM-IV and the ICD-10, denote a rather restrictive, narrow concept of bipolar disorder. The DSM includes bipolar I, bipolar II, cyclothymia, and bipolar not otherwise specified. ICD-10 includes bipolar I and cyclothymia.

Akiskal has been visionary in developing a view of the bipolar spectrum which includes a variety of clinical conditions. His most recent proposal includes four basic types, each with a subtype—a total of eight different diagnoses. In proposing this, Akiskal has given credit where credit is due to a variety of clinical theorists around the world in the last half century. Perhaps Akiskal is too modest in not emphasizing his leadership and vision in this process.

I find somewhat surprising that in defining that there is no clear statement of what is the core feature that defines bipolar spectrum. Stated differently, what is it that ultimately determines whether an individual's condition is within the circle of definition or outside. Is it "bipolarity"—that is, periods of highs and periods of lows? If so, then unipolar mania and hyperthymic temperament would be outside the circle. If it is the requirement of "highs" alone—that is mania or hypomania—then cyclothymia would not be included. For me the hallmark of bipolar disorder is dysregulation of mood, characterized by a periodic or continuous inability to regulate mood in an appropriate fashion.

Another issue, which has been the focus of some of my own work, is how often and why bipolar disorder is unrecognized and undiagnosed. As Akiskal points out in his review, a report of a survey of the national patient organization, the National Depressive and Manic-Depressive Association (DMDA), found that over one-third of the patients did not receive the correct diagnosis for over a decade [1]. Over half of these patients had consulted three or more professionals before receiving the correct diagnosis of bipolar disorder. Similar findings were reported by Suppes *et al* [2] for the Stanley Foundation: in a sample of 261 outpatients with bipolar disorder, the average time from the first symptoms of bipolar disorder to the first treatment averaged 10 years. Unfortunately, many of these patients received antidepressants without concurrent mood stabilizers. The situation, at least in the United States, does not appear to have improved. A repeat survey of DMDA members was conducted in 2000, and nearly the same results were found as in 1994.

One reason for this substantial delay in diagnosis and appropriate treatment is that the bipolar patient's initial diagnosis is often incorrect. In the 2000 National DMDA survey, 69% of the patients were misdiagnosed, most frequently as unipolar depression. Other frequent misdiagnoses included anxiety disorders, schizophrenia, personality disorders, and substance abuse.

An effective way to increase recognition of bipolar spectrum is to screen for it. Our group has developed a self-report screening instrument, the

Mood Disorder Questionnaire (MDQ). The MDQ is a 13-question survey which has been validated in a psychiatric outpatient clinic sample [3]. Sensitivity and specificity were found to be excellent. The MDQ has also been validated in a large general population sample in the United States [4]. Sensitivity and specificity in the general population were also very good. This instrument provides a way to help identify patients at risk for bipolar disorder, and to prevent the consequences of misdiagnosis, which include antidepressant-induced switch into mania and rapid cycling.

REFERENCES

1. Lish J.D., Dime-Meenan S., Whybrow P,C., Price R.A., Hirschfeld R.M.A. (1994) The National Depressive and Manic-depressive Association (DMDA) survey of bipolar members. *J. Affect. Disord.*, **31**: 281–294.
2. Suppes T., Leverich G.S., Keck P.E., Jr., Nolen W.A., Denicoff K.D., Altshuler L.L., McElroy S.L., Rush A.J., Kupka R., Frye M.A. *et al* The Stanley Foundation bipolar treatment outcome network: demographics and illness characteristics of the first 261 patients. Submitted for publication.
3. Hirschfeld R.M.A., Williams J.B.W., Spitzer R.L., Calabrese J.R., Flynn L., Keck P.E., Lewis L., McElroy S.L., Post R.M., Rapport D.J. *et al* (2000) Development and validation of a screening instrument for bipolar spectrum disorder: the Mood Disorder Questionnaire. *Am. J. Psychiatry*, **157**: 1873–1875.
4. Hirschfeld R.M.A., Calabrese J.R., Weissman M.M., Reed M., Davies M.A., Frye M.A., Keck P.E. Jr., Lewis L., McElroy S.L., McNulty J.P. *et al* Prevalence of bipolar spectrum disorder in the United States. Submitted for publication.

1.8
Broadening the Definition of Bipolar Disorder
Robert Boland and Martin B. Keller[1]

Hagop Akiskal has produced an important review, which elucidates well some of the major current issues concerning the diagnosis of bipolar disorder. As with most "current" debates, Akiskal demonstrates that the issues are hardly new. The tension between sensitivity and specificity—between defining the disorder such that it will capture all nuances, while yet maintaining confidence in the validity of the diagnosis—is clearly an old one. There remain a variety of disorders which may turn out to be subsyndromal forms of bipolar disorder. On the other hand, they may not.

[1] *Department of Psychiatry and Human Behavior, Brown University, Butler Hospital, 345 Blackstone Blvd, Providence, RI 02906, USA*

Akiskal makes several cases for broadening the definition of the disorder. In addition to the theoretical and historical arguments he advances, he also notes the practical value of widening the disorder's boundaries. Most obvious are the ramifications for treatment. To take one example that Akiskal gives, to broaden the criteria to include some patients currently diagnosed with personality disorders, could result in novel treatment approaches to this difficult population. If Akiskal's suggestions regarding relaxing the somewhat conservative symptom and time requirements were implemented, indeed many patients now diagnosed with other disorders would probably be considered bipolar.

In clinical practice, some of this broadening seems to have already occurred. Here in our corner of the northeastern United States, it seems difficult to find a patient with any sort of chronic psychiatric illness (be it a personality or even a chronic psychotic disorder) who is not already receiving some sort of mood stabilizer. As Akiskal wisely suggests, treatments drive diagnoses, and the availability of a number of new treatments for bipolar disorder has surely increased the enthusiasm for approaching any sort of mood instability from a bipolar perspective. One must also assume that medical economics, most notably third-party reimbursement, must drive diagnostic decisions as well. As managed care companies often will not cover treatment for Axis II or other complicated disorders, there may be a pressure to reconceptualize the patient from an Axis I perspective.

Is there any potential drawback to a broadening of these diagnoses? What is the purpose of devising the diagnoses, and subdiagnostic categories? Akiskal has highlighted one of the most important purposes: diagnoses guide treatment. There are other complementary purposes as well. For example, we need valid and reliable diagnoses in order to properly characterize the disorders, and better predict their likely outcome. In essence, for research on the disorders to advance (be it treatment or course related), we need a rigorous diagnostic system.

In contemplating this, one is reminded of the rationales that went into the major shift from the dimensional diagnoses of DSM-I and II to the categorical ones of DSM-III and beyond. Prior to DSM-III, the diagnoses were quite broad, and encompassing. However, these diagnoses tended to lack reliability and validity. Several factors contributed to the push for a better diagnostic system. First, the increasing importance of psychopharmacology treatments created a need for better specificity, to more accurately predict who would respond to pharmacotherapy. Other research, such as epidemiological data, was also stalemated by the lack of reliable diagnoses. Community studies of mental disorders using DSM-I criteria, such as the Baltimore Morbidity Study [1], yielded inconsistent findings. Attempts to assess the prevalence and incidence of psychiatric disorders suffered from this unreliability. The situation was such that, in the 1970s, the Carter Commission [2] concluded that goals for mental health treatment could not be formulated without a better understanding of the incidence of different psychopathologies. And that goal could not be met without better diagnostic instruments for the disorders. Thus, the changes that resulted in the current diagnostic system.

An example of how diagnosis aids clinical understanding can be seen in the research on the course of bipolar disorder. One important finding is that the course of the disorder is strongly related to the particular type of episode. This relationship was demonstrated in the National Institute of Mental Health (NIMH) Clinical Branch Collaborative Program on the Psychobiology of Depression–Clinical Studies, or the "Collaborative Depression Study" (CDS) [3]. The CDS was designed to study the natural course of unipolar and bipolar mood disorders. Almost 1000 patients from several sites were included; of these, about 175 subjects with bipolar disorders were followed for up to five years. This study found that the time to recovery from an index episode of the disorder was much longer for the group with mixed mania than other types of episodes [4, 5]. Specifically, the time to recovery was 14 weeks for the mixed group, compared with five weeks for the manic group and nine weeks for the depressed group. The overall probability of chronicity was different for both groups as well. After five years, all the patients with pure mania had recovered from their index episode, compared with 89% of patients with an index depressive episode and 83% of patients with a mixed episode. Time to relapse was longer for the manic group: by six months, the manic group had a 20% risk of relapse, compared with 33% in the depressed group and 36% in the mixed group.

Thus, proper definition of the particular type of bipolar episode has implications for the overall course of disease. Such an understanding can guide clinical judgement around treatment decisions. In the CDS study, conservative criteria (basically those from DSM-III as described by Akiskal) were used to define the different types of bipolar episodes. One must wonder whether such striking differences as those found above would have been apparent if more subsyndromal varieties of the disorders were included.

Clearly, it is possible to be both broad and rigorous. However, if the disorders were broadened, it would be important to ensure that we would continue to apply equal rigour. Field-testing of different criteria might be indicated, to ensure that we do not sacrifice specificity for the sake of sensitivity. Though we have also had the experience of seeing chronic disorders "melt away" when the underlying mood disorder was successfully treated, we have also observed patients undergo fruitless trials in the vain search for the "right pill", while missing out on more definitive psychotherapeutic treatments. In understanding bipolar disorder, we must continue to appreciate the importance of the varied manifestations of the disorder, both on treatment and on outcome, while investigating the limitations on that variance.

REFERENCES

1. Commission on Chronic Illness (1957) *Chronic Illness in the United States*, Vol. 4: *Chronic Illness in a Large City*. Harvard University Press, Cambridge.
2. President's Commission on Mental Health (1978) Report to the President. US Government Printing Office, Washington.
3. Katz M., Klerman G.L. (1979) Introduction: overview of the clinical studies program. *Am. J. Psychiatry*, **136**: 49–51.
4. Keller M.B., Lavori P.W., Coryell W., Andreasen N.C., Endicott J., Clayton P.J., Klerman G.L., Hirschfeld R.M.A. (1986) Differential outcome of pure manic, mixed/cycling, and pure depressive episodes in patients with bipolar illness. *JAMA*, **255**: 3138–3142.
5. Keller M.B., Lavori P.W., Coryell W., Endicott J., Mueller T.I. (1993) Bipolar I: a five-year prospective follow-up. *J. Nerv. Ment. Dis.*, **181**: 238–245.

1.9

Beyond Behavioural Boundaries: Redefining Mood and its Disorder Phenotype

Peter C. Whybrow[1]

In medicine the classification of disease is fundamental to therapeutic intervention—so fundamental, in fact, that classification has long had its own designation as "diagnosis". Accurate diagnosis helps predict the natural history of a patient's illness—based upon the cumulative experience of observing those individuals who have previously suffered similar affliction—while ordering in a useful fashion the empirical evidence gained from therapeutic trials, pharmacological and otherwise, that have advantageously modified the natural course of the disease. The opportunities for rational treatments are increased, although not uniformly so, when a knowledge of the basic morphology and pathophysiology of the disorder is available. And with growth in our understanding of the varied genetic templates that may underlie the phenotypic vulnerability to specific illness, there is the promise of further gains in treatment. Thus in precise diagnostic definition we weave the threads of new therapeutic cloth.

Nowhere in medicine today is this process more challenging than in defining the disorders of complex behaviour. In Hagop Akiskal's comprehensive review, the dimensions of that challenge are engaged and clearly delineated. First, as Akiskal emphasizes, because manic depressive illness disrupts the survival behaviours we call emotional regulation, the threads of

[1] *UCLA Neuropsychiatric Institute, 740 Westwood Plaza, Room C7-463, Los Angeles, CA 90024, USA*

the illness are woven inextricably through the weft of life. Emotional tone—individual temperament or habit of mind—like acuity of vision, hearing, athletic ability, or the functional output of any other *system* of complex brain function, varies among individuals.

Thus, while maniacal madness and the manifestations of melancholia may be readily agreed upon—and, as Akiskal notes, have been accepted for centuries—the boundary definitions of affective illness are annoyingly elusive. Such equivocation probably will, and perhaps should, remain so for it is social context and not medical science that defines pathology when a disability is mild or socially rewarding. In America, where restlessness and risk-taking are valued, an individual of hyperthymic temperament who experiences short sleep and high energy but who is also impulsive and aggressive is less likely to receive a diagnosis within the "bipolar spectrum" than is a dysthymic person who is of low energy and reticent in his inter-action with others. Beyond doubt, in American society today, Charles Darwin would simply not have made the grade and in Victoria's England many of our "dot-com" entrepreneurs would have been considered luna-tics. Thus the diagnoses at the "edges" of a behavioural spectrum or syn-drome are rarely "objective", but change with culture, time, and fashion.

None of this, however, should be seen as licence for physicians to pull back from scientific curiosity. Why is it, for example, that the architects of DSM-IV insist on distinguishing "substance-induced mood disorder" from a disturbance "better accounted for by a mood disorder that is not substance induced"? Why is it that hypomanic symptoms induced by antidepressants in some of those receiving such treatments for their depression should be dismissed when such a response may be the "smoking gun" that provides evidence for an underlying bipolar diathesis? Why is it so difficult to accept that a faltering thyroid economy can change the phenotypic expression of bipolar II disorder to the more malignant form of the illness called rapid cycling? And why does this phenomenon occur predominantly in women? [1] Why, in short, do we remain relatively disinterested in those aberrant threads which, although untidy, may lead to an elucidation of the genetic templates of mood and emotion?

In its complexity, emotional behaviour embraces at least three major subsystems of brain function, including social vigilance (the expression of emotion and the monitoring of the emotional communication of others), memory storage and retrieval, and the orderly circadian management of bodily function. It appears—as we learn more about the anatomical sub-strates of emotion—that these dynamic responsibilities are distributed among the limbic structures of the amygdala, the hippocampus together with the frontal lobe, and the hypothalamus, respectively [2]. Thus, in disorders of mood, we can reasonably expect to find a varied and oscillating pattern of disturbance of these behaviours among individuals, with the total number of activities compromised being greatest in those who suffer most severely. Furthermore, it is logical, given that our existing diagnostic categories are driven by the short-term observation of the phase and amplitude of behavioural disturbance, to expect that any one individual may have more than one "diagnosis" over time. It is also likely that those individuals will cluster disproportionately at the boundaries of our understanding.

Thus, in my own opinion, the exercise of sorting and resorting behavioural phenotypes will not weave the new therapeutic cloth we seek. I agree with Akiskal that we must now look beyond such sterile exercise to what we can learn at the diagnostic boundaries where disagreement is fierce. It is there that we will find new threads, as for example have Niculescu and Kelsoe and colleagues in employing a convergent functional genomics approach to potentially elucidate the permissive genetic substrate for maniacal behaviour [3]. Building on the observation that amphetamine will induce mania in those so predisposed and hypomania in many others—the increased activity of which can be modelled in mice—these investigators have refined their search for the candidate genes of mood and its disorder. In identifying one such contestant—the G protein-coupled receptor kinase 3 (GRK3)—they suggest that we must revise our concepts of pathogenesis seeking not only those genetic elements that permit but also those that protect. Such lateral thinking is important. Given the complexity of emotion it would make sense that no one gene codes for aberration. Rather, where one combination of genetic instruction may lead to the asylum, another constellation, differing only slightly, may open the door to an executive suite. A better understanding of such boundary conditions will not only elucidate pathophysiology, but also offer new insights both in prophylaxis and therapeutics. With the opportunities that lie ahead, one suspects a certain prescience in Akiskal's statement that "the weight of the reviewed evidence indicates that bipolar disorder is broader than what is included in DSM-IV and ICD-10".

REFERENCES

1. Bauer M.S., Whybrow P.C., Winokur A. (1990) Rapid cycling bipolar affective disorders, I: Association with grade I hypothyroidism. *Arch. Gen. Psychiatry*, **47**: 427–432.
2. Whybrow P.C. (1998) *A Mood Apart. The Thinkers Guide to Emotion and its Disorder*. Harper Perennial, New York.
3. Niculescu A.B., Segal D.S., Kuczenski R., Barrett T., Hauger R.L., Kelsoe J.R. (2000) Identifying a series of candidate genes for mania and psychosis: a convergent functional genomics approach. *Physiol. Genomics*, **4**: 83–91.

1.10

Towards a Unitary Framework for Mood Spectrum Beyond the Bipolar–Unipolar Dichotomy

Giovanni B. Cassano[1]

Based on epidemiological and family studies and clinical intuition, Akiskal estimated that 4–5% of the general population belongs to a broad bipolar spectrum with predominantly depressive phenomenology and muted bipolar features. These figures contrast the classical figure of 1–1.6% for bipolar disorder. This widening of bipolarity to the detriment of unipolar forms was corroborated by Angst [1], who demonstrated through epidemiological data that more than 5% of the general population might be affected by bipolar spectrum conditions. Akiskal proposes a number of syndromes as candidates for inclusion in a broadly conceived bipolar spectrum: mania, recurrent depressions with hypomania (irrespective of duration), pharmacologically induced hypomania, as well as depressions in association with cyclothymic and hyperthymic temperaments, and recurrent (pseudo-unipolar) depressions with bipolar family history or cyclic depressions responsive to lithium. He also argues that a substantial proportion of cases categorized as borderline personality disorder and many cases of alcohol abuse belong to the bipolar spectrum.

Akiskal's competent and comprehensive appraisal of contemporary classifications of mood disorders illustrates very elegantly the evolution of the nosology of bipolar disorder from the antiquity to current days, elucidating how, since before Kraepelin, the pendulum in mood disorders classification has moved back and forth between unitary (spectrum) and discontinuity (unipolar–bipolar) positions. He finally brings support to the spectrum position, even though he concludes that its ultimate range remains undefined.

With his distinguished mastery, Akiskal describes various categories of bipolar spectrum, namely mania, hypomania, cyclothymia and hyperthymia. Under the rubric of "atypical depression" Akiskal speculates on those conditions which are difficult to be accommodated in DSM or ICD diagnostic criteria, and are "liable to be consigned to some wastepaper basket category" or even ignored. He argues that the recognition of atypical mood signs/symptoms and atypical mood syndromes may represent a valuable adjunct to categorical methods of diagnosis and classification of bipolar spectrum.

Atypical presentations of depression may characterize "special populations" of patients [2], with less predictable clinical course and response to

_____

[1] Department of Psychiatry, Neurobiology, Pharmacology and Biotechnologies, University of Pisa, Via Roma 67, 56100 Pisa, Italy

treatment, or peculiar (often dangerous) behaviours and lifestyles. In these subjects, bipolar symptoms may remain undetected, masked or misdiagnosed by more "visible" manifestations. Stated differently, because many bipolar II patients have an underlying cyclothymic temperamental dysregulation, their clinical presentations are varied and inconsistent and often prove confusing in cross-section. That is, they could present with cross-sectional features of atypical depression, and lifelong history of anxiety states, bulimia, substance abuse, and cluster B personality disorders. Atypical depressive features are perhaps the most important clinical markers for bipolar II disorder. Akiskal points out that the ambiguities regarding the boundaries between unipolar and bipolar disorders, and the definition of relationships between polarity and cyclicity, still stand, raising practical problems for research and treatment choices. Using clinical data and case reports, Akiskal states that many major depressions in the DSM-IV schema are, in reality, part of the bipolar spectrum. This approach led to the formulation of a list of prototypes (BP-I, BP-I ½, BP-II, BP-II ½, BP-III, BP-III ½, BP-IV) along the continuum of mood dysregulations. The major implication of this theory is that the extension of the concept of bipolar spectrum would defend depressed patient unprotected by mood stabilizers from possible negative effects of antidepressants. Second, recognition of some attenuated forms of bipolarity pursuing sub-acute or chronic course may prevent from more prognostically unfavourable diagnoses, including borderline or antisocial personality disorder or schizophrenia. Furthermore, this model has shed light on the true prevalence of bipolar spectrum conditions.

This approach produced multiple subcategories of bipolar disorder, that are one phenomenologically different from another. This requires particular circumspection as far as treatment implications are concerned. In fact, the use of mood stabilizers for each prototype does not follow precise experimental data. A substantial proportion of depressed patients with mild bipolar features may show satisfactory and stable long-term outcome with antidepressants not necessarily associated with mood stabilizers. Treatment indications for "hyperthymic depression", the least severe bipolar spectrum form proposed, though reported to be at high risk of manic switches, still need to be tested.

Akiskal's proposals for distinguishing different bipolar–unipolar subtypes may lead to a diagnostic fragmentation which is in contrast with his fundamental unitary mood spectrum conceptualization. I wonder whether a parsimonious approach for assessing manic and depressive features within a unitary framework, encompassing the broad range of mood spectrum manifestations along a continuum, might be more appropriate.

In a recent paper, Baldessarini [3] recalls the extreme and inappropriate widening of the schizophrenia rubric in the middle of the past century.

Based on loose clinical criteria and on a psychodynamic stereotyped conceptualization, the expansion of the diagnosis of schizophrenia was detrimental to the diagnosis of various forms of psychoses belonging to the realm of mood and anxiety disorders and, in some cases, personality disorders. Analogously, clinicians and researchers should avoid any uncontrolled and widespread use of lithium and anticonvulsants in the absence of clear scientific evidence of their efficacy in soft bipolar conditions. At present, for instance, controlled studies and clinical experience do not exhaustively support a favourable cost-benefit ratio for the systematic use of mood stabilizers in individuals with subsyndromal bipolar features [4].

Nevertheless, the definition of the cut-off point between unipolar and bipolar forms—if it exists at all—still stems from a purely descriptive approach to the varying degrees of loading for depressive and manic dimensions. Clinicians often face complex arrays of co-occurring isolated or clustered mood symptoms that may be associated with one or more axis I or axis II conditions. Within this context, the spectrum model might be used to refer to a continuum of threshold and subthreshold mood phenomena related to a single mental disorder, including: a) core atypical symptoms of the primary axis I disorder, b) signs, isolated symptoms, symptom clusters and behavioural patterns related to the core symptoms that may be prodromal, may represent precursors of not yet fully expressed conditions, or may be sequelae of a previously experienced disorder, and c) temperamental or personality traits and lifestyles [5, 6]. The mood spectrum conditions should be better defined by fostering a unitary dimensional model to the detriment of a fragmentation in multiple subcategories. Actually, the combination of the categorical and the dimensional approach seems to be the most suitable solution to overcome such practical problems. The assessment of mood dysregulations in a life-long perspective, by focusing on distinct evolving steps of mood phenomenology, reduces the "entropy level" produced by the effort of splitting mood symptoms in "unipolar" versus "bipolar". If implemented and integrated with the categorical approach, the dimensional model permits the efforts to be directed to a different aim, and promotes a unitary view of mood disorders. In this perspective, in harmony with Akiskal's ideas, it would be worth wishing that a "mood spectrum" model substituted the "bipolar spectrum" model.

Akiskal argues that Baldessarini [3] and Cassano et al [7] converge in their requirement of methodological purity, which may be necessary for certain research operations versus practice considerations, that, Akiskal would contend, do not require pristine methodological designs, or unwieldy assessment instruments which are unrealistic in a clinical setting.

I believe that the detection of less classical mixtures of manic-depressive and unipolar depressive symptoms needs subtle diagnostic approaches, and can be improved by the introduction of refined assessment procedures also aimed at identifying vulnerability to recurrences or to the emergence of more severe forms of psychopathology. Moreover, the possibility to put into effect in clinical settings a systematic assessment of mood spectrum would add substantial educational impact by giving psychiatry professionals and residents an operational frame of reference for their clinical practice.

In conclusion, Akiskal authoritatively proposes a spectrum approach to mood disorders to override the unipolar–bipolar distinction. Indeed, the boundary between bipolar and unipolar disorders is still undefined. Akiskal's description of bipolar spectrum is firmly grounded on clinical observation and produced relevant nosographic advances. Certainly, this conceptual framework requires new research efforts which will result in advances in our understanding of the biological and genetic bases of manic-depressive illness, as well as in the treatment of these clinically challenging syndromes.

REFERENCES

1. Angst J. (1998) The emerging epidemiology of hypomania and bipolar II disorder. *J. Affect. Disord.*, **50**: 143–51.
2. Cassano G.B. , McElroy S.L. , Brady K., Nolen W.A. , Placidi G.F. (2000) Current issues in the identification and management of bipolar spectrum disorders in "special populations". *J. Affect. Disord.*, **59**: S69–S79.
3. Baldessarini R.J. (2000) A plea for integrity of the bipolar disorder concept. *Bipolar Disord.*, **2**: 3–7.
4. MacQueen G..M., Young L.T. (2001) Bipolar II disorder: symptoms, course, and response to treatment. *Psychiatr. Serv.*, **52**: 358–361.
5. Cassano G.B., Michelini S., Shear M.K., Coli E., Maser J.D., Frank E. (1997) The panic agoraphobic spectrum: a descriptive approach to the assessment and treatment of subtle symptoms. *Am. J. Psychiatry*, **154** (Suppl. 6): 27–38.
6. Frank E., Shear M.K., Rucci P., Cyranowski J.M., Endicott J., Fagiolini A., Grochocinski V.J., Houck P., Kupfer D.J., Maser J.D. *et al* (2000) Influence of panic-agoraphobic spectrum symptoms on treatment response in patients with recurrent major depression. *Am. J. Psychiatry*, **157**: 1101–1107.
7. Cassano G.B., Dell'Osso L., Frank E., Miniati M., Fagiolini A., Shear K., Pini S., Maser J.D. (1999) The bipolar spectrum: a clinical reality in search of diagnostic criteria and an assessment methodology. *J. Affect. Disord.*, **54**: 319–328.

1.11
The Diagnosis of Bipolar Disorder: Some Open Issues
Costas N. Stefanis[1]

The thorough and comprehensive review on the diagnosis of bipolar disorders by Hagop Akiskal, one of the leading clinical investigators in the field, leaves no room for new information. Nevertheless it warrants some comments on the main issues he has raised.

Since the diagnosis of bipolar disorders is still lacking a solid validation, derived from either an identifiable cause or from objectively measured neurobiological markers, the clinical insightful observation remains the only tool for their recognition and for assessing all those variables that could be utilized for their effective management. One issue that emerges from Akiskal's review is which of the two, the categorical or the dimensional approach, is better fitted for understanding and managing cases with mood disorders and bipolarity in particular. In reviewing diagnostic issues in depressive disorders [1], we have argued that both approaches have their merits and their limitations. Viewing bipolar disorders as a categorical entity, a line adopted in the formulation of operational criteria of DSM-IV and to a lesser degree of ICD-10, offers the advantage of being conceptually more acceptable and is more compatible to the medical thinking of the practising psychiatrists. On the other hand, the categorical approach may restrict the domain of bipolarity to only the typical bipolar I cases, ignoring the extent and the depth of bipolarity as depicted in Akiskal's review.

Regarding the core symptom construct of mania, Kraepelin identified two clinical dimensions: elation and accelerated psychomotor activity. Subsequently, a number of other symptoms, most of them deriving from the initial core symptom, were identified, and resulted in the expansion of bipolarity, which currently ranges from close to normal emotional variations of a temperamental nature to sustained emotional instability, to full-blown bipolar I disorder up to the opposite extreme that includes delusional and other psychotic features often clinically indistinguishable from paranoid schizophrenia.

Both the mood and the energy elements are interwoven in the process of developing a bipolar disorder. It is of clinical and research interest to access their interaction pattern and accommodate the treatment accordingly.

Thus far emphasis was given mainly to elevated mood and its behavioural manifestations. The abundance of energy expressed clinically in a variety of symptoms has largely been underrated, although it may very well be the primary driving force and as such may be more amenable to study, more specifically in the framework of the current system and chaos theories [2].

---

[1] *University Mental Health Research Institute, Eginition Hospital, 72 Vasilissis Sophias Avenue, Athens 11528, Greece*

The expansion of bipolarity to a spectrum that includes, in addition to bipolar I disorder, the temperamental disturbance, the "soft" or the sub-threshold bipolar states, the cycloid, the hyperthymic and the mixed states, is an attractive proposal advocated by many but substantiated clinically mainly by Akiskal's group in their many studies and publications [3].

The classical mania or bipolar I disorder in its current version seems to represent a quantitative exacerbation of normally distributed temperamental traits. This is a very plausible hypothesis which has significant clinical and theoretical implications, posing the age-long and still unresolved question of the relationship between personality and psychopathology, as well as of the boundaries between personality disorders and axis I psychopathology. Akiskal's view that a temperamental proneness lies in the roots of bipolarity has adequate empirical support from extensive clinical studies [4].

This view could be further strengthened if well-designed, large-scale, population-based, prospective studies assessing in frequent intervals personality traits, biological markers and psychopathological manifestations were available. Potentially they would further support the bipolar spectrum diagnostic scheme, by enriching it with empirically derived predictive validity. Such studies are also of great necessity due to the low reliability of retrospective assessments based on poor descriptive recollections, as well as to potential modifying effects on personality traits of internal and external impactors, among which prior episodes of affective disorder have to be included. The notion that psychopathology may induce personality changes is consistent with current knowledge on brain plasticity and more specifically with the experimentally proven hypothesis of synaptic restructuring by experience and learning. Such a possibility has been alluded to by Aretaeus already in the 5th century BC, by describing the post-manic personality changes. Furthermore, this type of study would better clarify the sequence and the possible interference of comorbid states in the evolutionary process of the primary "stem" disorder from which the many bipolar variants may eventually branch off.

Another issue that emerges from Akiskal's review and invites discussion is the distinction between non-bipolar and bipolar depressions. Despite the reported differences, mainly with regard to familial loading [5], to which I would add findings from our own genetic association studies [6, 7], the conclusive evidence that would validate their nosological separation is lacking. If we take into account the great number of false positive monopolars who have latter turned into bipolar and accept as legitimate bipolar signs drug induced mood changes, abrupt onset, impulsive eating disorders and extreme diurnal mood and psychomotor variations (retarded and desponded in the morning, euphoric and hyperactive in the evening), and we include in the bipolar spectrum all mixed states, then only a small minority of "tine" uncontaminated cases of non-bipolar depressions will retain their diagnostic purity. Should we therefore reconsider the currently available clinical, biological and epidemiological findings and proceed in comparative studies in which sampling is composed only by typical bipolars and "pure" monopolars? We may then obtain more reliable findings to substantiate or refuse the distinction and sort out the "true" from the "apparent" differences between the two types of depression.

REFERENCES

1. Stefanis C.N., Stefanis N.C. (1999) Diagnosis of depressive disorders: a review. In *Depressive Disorders* (Eds M. Maj, N. Sartorius), pp. 1–51, Wiley, Chichester.
2. Gottschalk A., Bauer M.S., Whybrow P.C. (1995) Evidence of chaotic mood variation in bipolar disorder. *Arch. Gen. Psychiatry*, 52: 947–959.
3. Akiskal H.S., Placidi G.F., Signoretta S., Liguori A., Gervasi R., Maremmani I., Mallya G., Puzantian V.R. (1998) TEMPS-I: delineating the most discriminant traits of cyclothymic, depressive, irritable and hyperthymic temperaments in a nonpatient population. *J. Affect. Disord.*, 51: 7–19.
4. Akiskal H.S., Maser J.D., Zeller P.J., Endicott J., Coryell W., Keller M., Warshaw M., Clayton P., Goodwin F.K. (1995) Switching from "unipolar" to bipolar II: an 11-year prospective study of clinical and temperamental predictors in 559 patients. *Arch. Gen. Psychiatry*, 52: 114–123.
5. Tsuang M.T., Faraone S.V., Fleming J.A. (1985) Familial transmission of major affective disorders. Is there evidence supporting the distinction between unipolar and bipolar disorders? *Br. J. Psychiatry*, 146: 268–271.
6. Papadimitriou G.N., Dikeos D.G., Karadima G., Avramopoulous D., Daskalopoulou E.G., Stefanis C.N. (2001) GABA-A receptor β3 and α5 subunit gene cluster on chromosome 15q11-q13 and bipolar disorder: a genetic association study. *Am. J. Med. Gen. (Neuropsychiatr. Genet.)*, 105: 317–320.
7. Dikeos D.G., Papadimitriou G.N., Avramopoulos D., Karadima G., Daskalopoulou E.G., Souery D., Mendlewicz J., Vassilopoulos D., Stefanis C.N. (1999) Association between the dopamine D3 receptor gene locus (DRD3) and unipolar affective disorder. *Psychiatr. Genet.*, 9: 189–195.
8. Hirschfeld R.M. (2001) Bipolar spectrum disorder: improving its recognition and diagnosis. *J. Clin. Psychiatry*, 62 (Suppl. 14): 5–9.
9. Angst J. (1999) Categorical and dimensional perspectives of depression. In *Depressive Disorders* (Eds M. Maj, N. Sartorius), pp. 54–56, Wiley, Chichester.

1.12
The Bipolar Spectrum: Focus on Core Personality Characteristics

David S. Janowsky[1]

Hagop Akiskal's review is both informative and provocative. He coherently supports the position that various manifestations of bipolar disorders exist on a spectrum ranging from temperament or personality to affectively loaded psychotic illness (i.e. "schizobipolar" or schizoaffective disorder). The glue holding this spectrum together appears to be the existence of and/ or the potential for manic, hypomanic or "sub-hypomanic" phenomena, the tendency for antidepressants to cause hypomanic episodes in these groups, and the observation that the entire spectrum is linked by increased loading for a family history of hyperthymia, hypomania, mania, and other manic-depressive phenomena of a variety of types.

In his review, Akiskal briefly mentions the differential ability of specific bipolar spectrum disorders to be helped by specific pharmacological agents. Thus, for example, patients with mixed mania appear to differentially improve on divalproex, as compared to lithium. Furthermore, some bipolar subgroups, such as patients with comorbid substance use disorder, generally do less well on psychotropic drugs than do more "pure" forms of bipolar disorder. All of the above speaks to a degree of pharmacological specificity, and implies that pharmacologically dissectable differences may exist among various bipolar diagnoses. Furthermore, Akiskal describes familial clustering of different bipolar subtypes, thus suggesting genetic heterogeneity. These observations, to some extent, challenge the "spectrum hypothesis" in its purest form, and beg for an explanation from future research.

This having been said, Akiskal presents a credible argument that clusters of entities found in the bipolar spectrum are at least loosely related genetically. What is not clear is how to explain those influences that determine the various subtypes that exist within the bipolar spectrum. Were the bipolar spectrum composed of a logical progression of psychopathology, ranging, for example, from hyperthymia to hypomanic symptoms to classic euphoric mania, an internally consistent spectrum would be obvious. However, differences between cyclothymic and hyperthymic individuals do exist at one end of the spectrum, and differences exist at the other end between "pure" mania, mixed mania, and schizoaffective disorder.

One perspective concerning the differences within bipolar spectrum comes from studies of underlying personality attributes [1–3]. Basic, core or underlying personality implies a set of well validated "normal" or "non-

[1] Department of Psychiatry, University of North Carolina at Chapel Hill, Chapel Hill, NC 27599, USA

pathological" personality characteristics, common to people in general. Thus, for example, all people range on a spectrum from introversion to extroversion. Such a perspective differs from the highly accepted categorical classifications of "personality disorders", based on symptom clusters, and is a cousin to the classification of personality and temperament used by Akiskal and others. Core personality characteristics are quite heritable, as shown in monozygotic/dizygotic twin studies, and are indeed as heritable as are bipolar disorders [4].

Several core personality variables studied to date have been shown to differentiate between bipolar and unipolar patients, both when these patients are symptomatic and when they are euthymic. Most studies have found that an overall group of bipolar patients of a variety of types are more extroverted than are unipolar patients, even when both groups are equally depressed [2, 5]. Furthermore, bipolar patients score higher on novelty seeking and its subcomponents, including impulsivity, than do unipolar patients and normative controls [2, 5]. Similarly, bipolar patients score as having greater intuitiveness on the Myers Briggs Type Indicator Sensing to Intuitive dimension, and on the related NEO-Personality Inventory (NEO-PI) personality characteristic of openness [5].

When one considers the nature of extroversion, intuitiveness/openness and novelty seeking, parallels are obvious between the phenomenology of hypomania and hyperthymia with respect to increased energy, increased interactions, gregariousness, risk taking, impulsiveness and creativity, all characteristics discussed in Akiskal's article. However, studies discriminating core personality differences in specific bipolar spectrum subtypes are lacking (i.e. bipolar mixed type, bipolar II patients, cyclothymic patients).

It is possible that differentiation of bipolar subtypes lies in understanding underlying personality traits. Therefore, bipolar spectrum disorder patients showing predominantly depressive symptoms and having characteristics more typical of the depressive personality disorder, such as might occur in mixed states, might be expected to have relatively high scores on neuroticism and/or introversion, as would their relatives. In contrast, individuals with pure mania would be expected to be more extroverted and novelty seeking.

Considering the above line of reasoning, it is conceivable that the bipolar spectrum may depend in part on the specific constellation of core personality variables. Possibly, the discrimination of "true unipolar" patients from "pseudo-unipolar" patients, and the identification of "phenotypically" unipolar and "genotypically" bipolar patients may be aided by defining the core personality profiles of these individuals and their families.

Thus, future studies of the bipolar spectrum might be enhanced by incorporating measurements of core personality as one set of easily measured variables, possibly having the potential for discriminating bipolar spectrum subtypes or bipolar versus unipolar patients, or the ultimate bipolar outcome of initially depressed patients.

REFERENCES

1. Costa P.T., Jr., McCrae R.R. (1992) Trait psychology comes of age. In *Nebraska Symposium on Motivation; Psychology and Aging* (Ed. T.B. Sonderegger), pp. 169–202, University of Nebraska Press, Lincoln.
2. Janowsky D.S., Morter S., Hong L., Howe L. (1999) Myers Briggs Type Indicator and Tridimensional Personality Questionnaire differences between bipolar patients and unipolar depressed patients. *Bipolar Disord.*, 2: 98–108.
3. Bagby R., Ryder A.G. (2000) Personality and the affective disorders: past efforts, current models, and future directions. *Curr. Psychiatr. Rep.*, 2: 465–472.
4. Bouchard T.J., Jr., Hur Y.M. (1998) Genetic and environmental influences on the continuous scales of the Myers-Briggs Type Indicator: an analysis based on twins reared apart. *J. Personality*, 66: 145–149.
5. Janowsky D., Hong L., Morter S., Howe L. (1998) Underlying personality characteristics related to affective disorders and suicidality. In *Neurobiology of Depression and Related Disorders* (Ed. J. Nomura), pp. 9–29, Mie Press, Tsu, Mie, Japan.

1.13

Rate of Detection and Care Utilization by People with Bipolar Disorder. Results from the Netherlands Mental Health Survey and Incidence Study (NEMESIS)

Willem A. Nolen[1], Margreet ten Have[2], Wilma Vollebergh[2]

In this comment we would like to add some information on what proportion of the people with bipolar disorder in the general population have been diagnosed, what proportion are receiving care and what factors motivate them to seek help. The data are derived from the Netherlands Mental Health Survey and Incidence Study (NEMESIS) [1]. NEMESIS is a prospective survey among 7076 respondents in the Dutch general population aged 18 to 64, with three assessment points in 1996, 1997 and 1999. The primary diagnostic instrument is the Composite International Diagnostic Interview 1.1 (CIDI), a fully structured interview for diagnosing psychiatric disorders. The CIDI generates the following DSM-III-R bipolar diagnoses: bipolar I disorder and bipolar disorder not otherwise specified (NOS). The results are from the first wave of NEMESIS in 1996 [2].

[1] *Altrecht Institute for Mental Health Care, Vrouwjuttenhof 18, 3512 PZ Utrecht, The Netherlands*
[2] *Netherlands Institute of Mental Health and Addiction, P.O. Box 725, 3500 AS Utrecht, The Netherlands*

The lifetime prevalence of bipolar disorder was 1.9% ($n = 136$, 1.6% for men, 2.2% for women, $\chi^2 = 3.20$, NS). The majority ($n = 93$; 68.6%) of the persons diagnosed with lifetime bipolar disorder had experienced bipolar I disorder, while a further 31.4% ($n = 43$) had experienced a bipolar disorder NOS. The average age at the first manic or hypomanic episode was 26.2 years, with 40.2% having their first episode between the ages of 18 and 24 and 29.4% between 25 and 34. Most people had been through at least five manic or hypomanic episodes and three depressive episodes in their lifetimes.

Of the people who had ever experienced bipolar disorder, 72.1% had sought help for mental health problems from a primary care provider, such as a general practitioner or a community social worker; 56.6% had called on a mental health care (MHC) provider, usually a community mental health institute or a psychiatrist in private practice. 25.5% had never sought any help at all for their mental health problems, either from the general health care or MHC sector or from the informal or alternative care circuit.

In the 12 months preceding the study, 27.2% had felt the need for professional help, but had not applied for it. The four most common reasons were: "I wanted to solve my problems by myself" (64.5%); "I thought the problem would go away by itself" (49.4%); "I had no confidence in the care providers I would have had to go to" (46.9%); and "I thought no one could help me anyway" (43.3%) (more than one answer was possible).

More than four out of 10 people with bipolar disorder ($n = 59$; 43.4%) had never sought any help at all in the MHC sector. They did not differ from the MHC-seekers in any of the sociodemographic characteristics, including gender, age, living conditions, employment status, education and income. The main apparent difference was that they were less severely ill. Non-MHC-seekers were significantly more likely to have a bipolar disorder NOS ($p < 0.01$) and experienced lower degrees of comorbidity, especially anxiety disorders ($p < 0.01$).

Contact with a MHC provider does not necessarily lead to a diagnosis or treatment of the bipolar disorder. If the (hypo)manic symptoms are reported to have been discussed, we consider that as a sign that the condition was recognized. Of the bipolar respondents who had ever sought help in the MHC sector ($n = 77$), 20% ($n = 14$) had never spoken to a professional there about one of their (hypo)manic episodes. Apparently they had sought help for other problems, and their bipolar disorder may have gone unnoticed.

Of those whose disorder did not remain undiscussed ($n = 63$), 39.7% had made no use of MHC services recently ($n = 25$). In view of the serious nature of bipolar disorder, we might justifiably argue that these respondents were lacking adequate treatment. Tallying these undertreated patients together with the respondents whose disorder went entirely unrecognized $(59 + 14 + 25 = 98)$, we conclude that nearly three out of four people with bipolar disorder at the time of the study were not receiving appropriate treatment. Even this estimate is conservative, because we still do not know whether the bipolar condition of those with recent MHC contact ($n = 38$) was truly being recognized as such and adequately treated. In view of their conspicuously low use of medication, it seems probable that they, too, were not optimally benefiting from the treatments available.

The finding that nearly three-quarters of those with bipolar disorder are failing to receive adequate treatment is in agreement with two US studies as well as with a Canadian general population study [3–5]. Some of the possible explanations for the degree of undertreatment we have encountered in our study could be sought in the mentally disturbed people themselves. They seem little inclined to seek help. That is partly because they have little confidence in the MHC services, and partly because they may have not yet suffered many serious consequences from their (hypo)manic episodes and therefore have seen no reason to consult a professional (at least not for their bipolar disorder). A further explanation is that bipolar disorder itself presumably stands in the way of a swift and adequate diagnosis. This is partly because it presents a complex psychiatric picture with many different manifestations, and partly because it is highly comorbid with other psychiatric syndromes. Finally, it is possible that the CIDI as a fully structured interview has led to some overestimation of the prevalence of bipolar disorder, when compared to diagnosis made by clinicians. Therefore, we are currently performing a follow-up study on NEMESIS, in which all persons with a lifetime diagnosed bipolar disorder as well as major depression are re-interviewed by clinicians with the Structured Clinical Interview for DSM-IV (SCID).

REFERENCES

1. Bijl R.V., Van Zessen G., Ravelli A. (1998) The Netherlands Mental Health Survey and Incidence Study (NEMESIS): objectives and design. *Soc. Psychiatry Psychiatr. Epidemiol.*, **33**: 581–586.
2. Ten Have M., Vollebergh W., Bijl R., Nolen W.A. (2002) Bipolar disorder in the general population. Prevalence, consequences and care utilisation. Results from the Netherlands Mental Health Survey and Incidence Study (NEMESIS). *J. Affect. Disord.* (in press).
3. Regier D.A., Narrow W.E., Rae D.S., Manderscheid R.W., Locke B.Z., Goodwin F.K. (1993) The de facto US mental and addictive disorders service system. Epidemiologic catchment area prospective 1-year prevalence rates of disorders and services. *Arch. Gen. Psychiatry*, **50**: 85–90.
4. Kessler R.C., Rubinow D.R., Holmes, C., Abelson J.M., Zhao S. (1997) The epidemiology of DSM-III-R bipolar I disorder in a general population survey. *Psychol. Med.*, **27**: 1079–1089.

5. Katz S.J., Kessler R.C., Frank R.G., Leaf P., Lin E., Edlund M. (1997) The use of outpatient mental health services in the United States and Ontario: the impact of mental morbidity and perceived need for care. *Am. J. Publ. Health*, **87**: 1136–1143.

1.14
Bipolar II is Bipolar, Too
Zoltan Rihmer[1]

The comprehensive review by Hagop Akiskal clearly shows that the prevalence and clinical significance of bipolar affective disorders is much greater than previously believed. This is particularly true for bipolar II disorder, which seems to be the most common phenotype of the full bipolar spectrum [1, 2]. Our previous findings in Hungary also showed that bipolar II illness was more common than bipolar I, either in clinical samples [3] or in the general population [4].

Akiskal also provides a lot of evidence supporting the separation of bipolar II from bipolar I disorder within the broad clinical spectrum of bipolar disorders. Reporting on a significant difference in the distribution of AB0 blood group types [5] and in the serum dopamine-β-hydroxylase level [6] between bipolar I and bipolar II patients, 20 years ago we concluded that these results indicated a possible genetic difference between these disorders. A few years later our conclusion was corroborated when it was published that levels of dopamine-β-hydroxylase activity were controlled by a gene linked to the AB0 blood group locus on chromosome 9 [7]. These results are also in good agreement with later family studies suggesting the possibility that bipolar I and bipolar II disorders are genetically distinct categories [8].

In psychiatry and, in particular, in the field of affective disorders, the cross-sectional clinical picture is hardly sufficient for making a precise clinical diagnosis. As demonstrated in Akiskal's review, not only depressed patients with past hypomania, but also those with premorbid cyclothymia or hyperthymia can correctly receive a diagnoses of bipolar II rather than unipolar depression.

The recognition of bipolar II disorder—besides its treatment implications—is quite important in the estimation of suicide risk. Reviewing the studies in which bipolar II, bipolar I and unipolar major depressive patients were analysed separately, it was found that the rate of lifetime history of suicide attempts was 24%, 17% and 12%, respectively, while, on the other

[1] *National Institute for Psychiatry and Neurology, Budapest 27 Pf. 1, 1281 Hungary*

hand, bipolar II patients were relatively overrepresented among consecutive suicide victims [9]. Our very recent (still unpublished) results also show that it is not only the personal history of suicide attempts, but also the family history of committed suicide (in first degree relatives) that was significantly higher in 28 bipolar II patients as compared to 85 unipolar major depressives (44% and 25% vs. 19% and 14%, respectively) [10].

The possible causes of the extremely high suicidality in bipolar II patients (common misdiagnosis resulting in a lack of adequate treatment, high rate of psychiatric and medical comorbidity, more frequent violent and serious suicide methods) have been discussed by us elsewhere [9]. Investigating the prevalence of marital instability in different subtypes of major affective disorders in a community sample of the Hungarian population aged between 25 and 64 years ($N = 3648$), we found recently the rate of persons with one or more divorce(s)/separation(s) to be 22.9% among those with no lifetime history of major affective disorders, while the corresponding figures for patients with history of bipolar II, bipolar I and unipolar depression were 40.4%, 27.3% and 33.0%, respectively [11]. These results suggest that interpersonal conflicts, marital instability and/or family breakdown are particularly frequent among bipolar II patients, which may also contribute to their high suicidality.

REFERENCES

1. Akiskal H.S., Mallya G. (1987) Criteria for the "soft" bipolar spectrum: treatment implications. *Psychopharmacol. Bull.*, **23**: 68–73.
2. Angst J. (1998) The emerging epidemiology of hypomania and bipolar II disorder. *J. Affect. Disord.*, **50**: 143–151.
3. Rihmer Z., Arató M. (1984) The DST as a clinical aid and research tool in patients with affective disorders. *Psychopharmacol. Bull.*, **20**: 174–177.
4. Szádóczky E., Papp Z., Vitrai J., Rihmer Z., Füredi J. (1998) The prevalence of major depressive and bipolar disorders in Hungary. Results from a national epidemiologic survey. *J. Affect. Disord.*, **50**: 153–162.
5. Rihmer Z., Arató M. (1981) AB0 blood groups in manic-depressive patients. *J. Affect. Disord.*, **3**: 1–7.
6. Rihmer Z., Bagdy G., Arató M. (1984) Serum dopamine-β-hydroxylase activity in female manic-depressive patients. *Biol. Psychiatry*, **19**: 423–427.
7. Wilson A.F., Alston R.C., Siervogel R.M. (1988) Linkage of gene-regulating dopamine-β-hydroxylase activity and the AB0 blood group locus. *Am. J. Hum. Genet.*, **42**: 160–166.
8. Coryell W. (1996) Bipolar II disorder: a progress report. *J. Affect. Disord.*, **41**: 159–162.
9. Rihmer Z., Pestality P. (1999) Bipolar II disorder and suicidal behavior. *Psychiatr. Clin. North Am.*, **22**: 667–673.

10. Rihmer Z., Schmidt V., Szádóczky E., Rózsa S. (2001) Suicide attempts and family history of suicide in patients with bipolar II and unipolar major depression (in preparation).
11. Rihmer Z., Szádócky E., Rózsa S., Füredi J. (2001) Marital instability in subtypes of major affective disorders: results from a population-based study in Hungary (in preparation).

1.15
The Clinical Spectrum of Mania
Per Bech[1]

In his authoritative review, Akiskal has used the spectrum of mania as the royal road to the field of bipolar disorders. When mapping the manic spectrum Akiskal, the trialblazer, has seen boundaries both in the current classification systems (DSM-IV and ICD-10) and in various rating scales and questionnaires [1]. Thus, the manic symptomatology goes from schizomania at the top to hyperthymia at the bottom. Between these extremes are the other categories from mania to hypomania.

The description of hypomania ranges from the hypomanic episode in bipolar II patients to states of hypomania induced by antidepressant treatment (bipolar III). The mood swings associated with substance and/or alcohol use are placed between hypomania and hyperthymia (bipolar III1/2). In accordance with ICD-10, cyclothymia is defined by episodes of hypomania, not by hyperthymia. In the description of hypomania Akiskal prefers ICD-10 to DSM-IV. However, if Akiskal had referred to the ICD-10 version with diagnostic criteria for research, the algorithm would be realized to be very close to DSM-IV.

A trailblazer like Akiskal has no need for DSM-IV algorithms. However, for the reliability of the marking of bipolar trails the proposed algorithms in his various tables are needed. The use of mania scales measuring severity of the manic spectrum such as the Mania Rating Scale (MAS) [2] might be superior to the many algorithms covering the various subcategories. Thus, the MAS has been standardized [3], showing that the extreme degrees range from 33 to 44 (schizomania), severe mania from 28 to 32, moderate mania from 15 to 27, hypomania from 10 to 14, hyperthymia from 6 to 9, and euthymia from 5 to 0. In a recent study by Henry et al. [4], an antidepressant-induced mania in bipolar patients typically scored 15, i.e. at the border between hypomania and moderate mania. Lithium seemed superior to

[1] Psychiatric Research Unit, Frederiksborg General Hospital, Dyrehavevej 48, DK-3400 Hillerod, Denmark

anticonvulsants in preventing this reaction [4]. It has also been shown that comorbid bipolar patients with alcohol dependence typically have MAS scores around 15 [5].

Self-rating scales are not applicable in severe mania, as the patients here will play the manic game. In states from euthymia over hyperthymia to hypomania it is relevant to use questionnaires completed by the patients themselves as is the case in states from anxiety over dysthymia to major depression.

It can be discussed to which extent there is a need for developing new scales to cover the milder forms of mania. Thus, the Hopkins Symptom Checklist (HSCL-90) includes a mania scale [6], and the Eysenck Personality Questionnaire includes the dimension of extraversion in which the choleric versus the sanguine temperaments are operating [7]. Both temperaments share the characteristic of being changeable, in contrast to the temperament of melancholia, which, as a photocopy, has minimal day-to-day variations.

In the clinical syndrome circle [8], depression and dysthymia are super-imposed on anxiety while mania and schizomania are superimposed on cyclothymia. When depression in bipolar II $\frac{1}{2}$ is superimposed on cyclothymia, states between "double depression" and hypomania fluctuate. Likewise, bipolar IV seems to be unipolar depression in patients with bipolar temperaments (extraversion). Such patients have a good outcome on long-term lithium therapy [9].

REFERENCES

1. Bech P. (1993) *Rating Scales for Psychopathology, Health Status and Quality of Life. A Compendium on Documentation in Accordance with the DSM-III-R and WHO Systems.* Springer, Berlin.
2. Bech P., Baastrup P.C., de Bleeker E., Ropert P. (2001) Dimensionality, responsiveness and standardization of the Bech–Rafaelsen Mania Scale in the ultra-short therapy with antipsychotics in patients with severe manic episodes. *Acta Psychiatr. Scand.*, **104**: 25–30.
3. Bech P. (1996) *The Bech, Hamilton and Zung Scales for Mood Disorders: Screening and Listening. A Twenty Years Update with Reference to DSM-IV and ICD-10*, 2nd ed., Springer, Berlin.
4. Henry C., Sorbara F., Lacoste J., Gindre C., Leboyer M. (2001) Antidepressant-induced mania in bipolar patients: identification of risk factors. *J. Clin. Psychiatry*, **62**: 249–255.
5. Salloum I.M., Cornelius J.R., Daley D.C., Kirisci L., Spotts C.R. (2000) The validity of the primary-secondary distinction among comorbid bipolar disorder and alcohol dependence. Presented at the 40th NCDEU Meeting, Boca Raton, May 30–June 2.
6. Hunter E.H., Powell B.J., Penick E.C., Nickel E.J., Othmer E., DeSouza C. (2000) Development and validation of a mania scale for the symptom checklist 90. *J. Nerv. Ment. Dis.*, **188**: 176–179.

7. Eysenck H.J. (1973) *Extraversion*. Crosby Lockwood Staples, London.
8. Bech P., Kastrup M., Rafaelsen O.J. (1986) Mini-compendium of rating scales for states of anxiety, depression, mania, schizophrenia with corresponding DSM-III syndromes. *Acta Psychiatr. Scand.*, **73** (Suppl. 326): 7–37.
9. Bech P., Shapiro R.W., Nielsen B.M., Sorensen B., Rafaelsen O.J. (1980) Personality in unipolar and bipolar manic-melancholic patients. *Acta Psychiatr. Scand*, **62**: 245–257.

1.16
The Relevance of a Clinical Approach Towards an Earlier Diagnosis of the Bipolar Spectrum

Maria Luisa Figueira[1]

In clinical settings, during the last decades, descriptive phenomenology has been progressively replaced by the pragmatic use of operational diagnostic criteria included in internationally accepted classification systems. Nevertheless, major problems might arise from the use of these criteria in clinical practice as the only diagnostic tool, with the reduction of complex psychopathological phenomena to the presence or absence of cross-sectionally assessed symptoms.

A critical example is that of a clinician observing a patient whose most evident symptoms are the manic and depressive ones. Presumably, he will not feel the need to go further in gathering the subtler clinical phenomenology, which would make his choice of therapeutic approach a wiser one. These considerations arise very clearly from recent research and clinical data supporting a broader bipolar concept. A major problem is the difficulty of recognizing subthreshold clinical expressions of this complex clinical entity. This is not a new issue. For long have several authors, like Weitbrecht [1], emphasized the need to search and evaluate hypomanic oscillations in the past history of the "endogenous depressive patients". Also Storring [2] described an "uncomplete manic syndrome", pointing out the difficulties in establishing a clear-cut separation from the depressive clinical picture. According to this author, some clinically relevant aspects of bipolarity "might already be present weeks, months or even years before the full blown clinically evident episode". Furthermore, he emphasizes that both "complexity" as well as "apparently contradictory aspects" during "emotional psychoses" might be due to "simultaneous bipolarity", i.e., to a complex mixture of both manic and depressive symptoms resulting "in an extended array of possible diagnostic errors".

[1] *Department of Psychiatry, Faculty of Medicine University of Lisbon, Av. Prof. Egas Moniz, P-1649-028 Lisbon, Portugal*

In the realm of bipolar disorders, bipolar II is the most under-recognized variant. The first episode has generally a depressive polarity, frequently with atypical features. To explore subthreshold expressions of mania or hypomania (*mania mitigata*) in the patient's past history, or to recognize partial manic elements intruded in the depressive symptoms, may be difficult or require a lot of clinical expertise. The prescription of an antidepressant in monotherapy is the common choice in this situation. If the patient has a bipolar II disorder, one may predict, on the basis of the available clinical evidence, an unstable and tumultuous course, or a tendency to non-response to antidepressants, or a switch to an excitable state with a mixture of both dysphoric and anxiety symptoms, or an increase of underlying affective dysregulation, or periods with brief hypomanic states or cyclothymic episodes, or eventually the full-blown picture of mixed states.

The introduction of the bipolar II diagnostic category, as well as the clinical studies of bipolar spectrum disorders, has generated marked changes in the diagnostic and treatment approaches to our bipolar patients. In a preliminary study by our group [3, 4], 60 bipolar patients (30 bipolar I and 30 bipolar II; DSM-IV criteria) were retrospectively evaluated. Patients included in the bipolar II subsample had a mean treatment duration of 18 years ($+/-$ 9 years), with a the mean time gap between the first clinical psychiatric evaluation and the diagnosis of bipolar II disorder of 11 years. During this period, depressive episodes dominated the clinical picture both in frequency and duration (more than four episodes in 70% of patients), but mixed depressive episodes were also present in 53.3% of cases. Dysphoric hypomania was recorded in 43.3% of patients. Compared with their bipolar I counterparts, bipolar II patients had a significantly higher frequency of polymorphic anxious symptoms (40% vs. 16.6%), generalized anxiety, panic attacks, episodic obsessive-compulsive disorder, phobias and dissociative symptoms. In the subsample of bipolar II patients, a significant positive correlation ($p < 0.001$) was observed between the frequency of mixed episodes, clinical instability, poor prognosis and the time to the diagnosis of bipolarity. A significant number of these patients, in whom instability and tumultuous course was the rule, became stabilized after the introduction of anticonvulsants.

The acceptance of the concept of spectrum in mood disorders should lead to a change of our clinical attitude from the anchorage to a rigid set of quantified rules to a more clinical comprehensive descriptive approach. This should include a more accurate process of diagnosis; an increased awareness that some of the clinical expressions can be caused by bipolar factors related to a basic affective temperament; the need to systematically re-evaluate changes in the clinical picture over time; and, last but not least, the necessity for a continuous training both in clinical phenomenology and in personality and temperament evaluation procedures.

Even if one is aware of the current controversies concerning the concept of bipolar disorder spectrum vs. a more categorical approach, clinical evidence imposes a more refined and cautious clinical judgement.

REFERENCES

1. Weitbrecht H.J. (1968) *Psychiatrie im Grundriss*, 2nd ed., Springer, Berlin.
2. Storring G. (1969) *Esquizofrenia e Ciclotimia*. Editiones Morata, Madrid.
3. Figueira M.L., Albuquerque R. (2000) Anxiety and bipolar disorders, diagnostic and treatment implications. Presented at the II Symposium Ibérico de Psiquiatria, Canary Islands, 14–16 June.
4. Severino L., Figueira M.L. (2000) The anxiety spectrum syndromes in bipolar disorder. Presented at the 6th Symposium on Bipolar Disorders, Lisbon, 17–18 November.

1.17
Syndromes, Symptoms and Spectra
Robert H. Belmaker[1]

My personal clinical experience of treating bipolar illness includes 27 years of continuous maintenance of an outpatient bipolar clinic with over 150 patients under treatment at any given time, along with innumerable consultations on inpatient stays mostly with mania. This experience agrees with that of Hagop Akiskal to the effect that many mixed syndromes occur, that hyperthymic and dysthymic intermorbid personalities have something to do with the course of illness, that relatives of patients often have bipolar II or cyclothymic syndromes, and that many unusual illnesses that come to me for consultation can be conceptualized as related to bipolar disorder. This much I know, but in the sense that I know how to ride a bicycle. I don't know how to make a bicycle nor do I know how to give detailed instructions to someone else as to how to ride a bicycle. I certainly do not know how my nerves and muscles work to ride a bicycle. A clinician armed with a wide, flexible spectrum concept of bipolar illness is probably a better clinician. Good clinical work involves interactive treatment trials in a given patient until something works, and Type I errors are less damaging than Type II errors. Scientific progress, however, is much more damaged by Type I errors and a sharp narrow definition of bipolar illness might be more useful for biochemical studies and imaging studies, for instance. The use of a large

[1] *Department of Psychiatry, Ben Gurion University of the Negev, P.O. Box 4600, Beersheva, Israel*

category of "undiagnosed" psychiatric disorder is often useful for the researcher although totally irrelevant to the clinician.

The role of culture in the milder forms of the bipolar spectrum cannot be overemphasized. Recently, we reported that Israeli bipolar patients had more manic episodes than depressive episodes, compared to European data which reported the opposite ratio [1]. Could this be related to the Mediterranean temperament?

Various aspects of the bipolar spectrum concept may or may not be useful for guiding genetic or therapeutic research. Does neuroleptic treatment clearly help schizotypal personality? Do stroke and cardiac infarction, with some common risk factors and genetic risk overlap, have similar treatments?

REFERENCE

1. Osher Y., El-Rom R., Belmaker R.H. (2000) Predominant polarity of bipolar patients in Israel. *World J. Biol. Psychiatry*, **1**: 187–189.

1.18
Atypical Psychosis: The Other Boundary of Bipolar Disorder
Tadafumi Kato[1]

The concept of bipolarity presented by Hagop Akiskal is a good clue for all psychiatrists to find an alternative and effective treatment strategy in patients who might have received a diagnosis of unipolar depression according to classical diagnostic systems. Since nothing should be added to his thorough and well-organized review, I would like to comment on one topic, the other boundary of bipolar disorder, which may be specific to Japan.

Although DSM-IV is generally used in research and education in Japan, many psychiatric experts are still influenced by traditional clinical diagnostic practice. In particular, the traditional diagnosis of "atypische Psychose" (atypical psychosis) still has some impact on clinical practice, especially in the Western part of Japan. The concept of atypical psychosis was proposed by Mitsuda [1] in Japan based on his hypothesis that there is a genetically different category between schizophrenia and manic-depressive illness. Its conceptual framework was subsequently established by Hatotani [2] in the 1960s. The Japanese concept of atypical psychoses focuses on the "alteration of consciousness" and the nosological relationship to epilepsy. This concept

[1] *Laboratory for Molecular Dynamics of Mental Disorders, Brain Science Institute, Riken, Hirosawa 2–1, Wako, Saitama, 351–0198, Japan*

is close to bouffèe dèlirante (French traditional diagnosis), Degenerationsp-sychose (according to Kleist), or zykloide Psychosen (according to Leonhard). These categories are characterized by acute onset, phasic course, complete remission between psychotic episodes, and confusion, just like that observed in mild delirium. Needless to say, these characteristics resemble those of bipolar disorder. Although it is true that some patients having these features should be diagnosed as "psychotic disorder not otherwise specified" accord-ing to DSM-IV, many other patients having such symptoms can receive a DSM-IV diagnosis of bipolar disorder. However, in the Western part of Japan, patients having psychotic features, catatonic features, or confusion during manic episodes may receive a diagnosis of "atypical psychosis" and no specific DSM-IV diagnosis. When they are diagnosed according to the ICD-10 system, they tend to receive a diagnosis of acute and transient psychotic disorder. In some Japanese psychiatric wards for acute psychotic patients, no patients with bipolar disorder are admitted. On the contrary, many patients with "atypical psychosis" are admitted. This may lead to an under-diagnosis of bipolar disorder, especially the one with catatonic features, in Japan [3].

The concept of atypical psychosis led to important clinical achievements in Japan, such as prophylactic treatment with thyroid hormone, and predic-tion of good prognosis of acute psychotic episodes based on their symptom-atology. However, the inter-rater reliability for this diagnosis was much lower than that for schizophrenia and bipolar disorder [4, 5]. If this diagno-sis is overused, it can cause confusion in clinical practice.

However, it is also true that some patients have recurrent psychotic epi-sodes that cannot be diagnosed as bipolar or as schizophreniform disorder, because they do not have any signs of mania or depression, or delusions and hallucinations. The diagnostic classification of these cases should be studied further.

REFERENCES

1. Mitsuda H. (1965) The concept of "atypical psychoses" from the aspect of clinical genetics. *Acta Psychiatr. Scand.*, **41**: 372–377.
2. Hatotani N. (1996) The concept of "atypical psychoses": special reference to its development in Japan. *Psychiatry Clin. Neurosci.*, **50**: 1–10.
3. Kato T., Takahashi S. (1997) Clinical characteristics of bipolar disorder with catatonic features in DSM-IV. *Seishin Igaku (Clinical Psychiatry)*, **39**: 593–600.
4. Takahashi S. (1985) [Classification of so-called endogenous psychoses and proposed diagnostic criteria]. *Seishin Shinkeigaku Zasshi*, **87**: 781–787.
5. Kitamura T., Fujinawa A., Okazaki H., Takahashi S, Kasawara Y. (1992) [Con-cept of diagnosis of atypical psychotic disorders in Japan and clinical symp-toms—results from multicenter studies]. *Seishin Shinkeigaku Zasshi*, **94**: 1194–1201.

2

Prognosis of Bipolar Disorder: A Review

Andreas Marneros and Peter Brieger

Department of Psychiatry and Psychotherapy, Martin-Luther-University, Halle-Wittenberg,
06097 Halle, Germany

INTRODUCTION

Bipolar disorders are severe and chronic diseases. Many researchers and clinicians tend to see only brief "snapshots" of the long-term course of these disorders: the weeks in which a patient is admitted to an acute hospital ward or takes part in a scientific study. Physicians and psychiatrists in primary care or community mental health professionals may get a longer perspective of the illness. But, most of all, the patients themselves and their families experience the burden of the disease. For them, the question of prognosis is essential.

There is a further, more theoretical, reason why course and outcome are essential aspects to understand bipolar disorders: in the mid- and late 19th century, Falret [1, 2], Kahlbaum [3], Kraepelin [4] and other authors expressed the view that long-term rather than cross-sectional observation is essential for a valid diagnosis. Quite often the diagnosis of bipolar disorder can be correctly made only *during* the long-term course of the illness, as in the majority of cases the first episode of the disorder is depressive [5]. Thus, the concept of bipolar disorder is fundamentally defined by its (further) course.

According to Kraepelin, essential to manic-depressive insanity is its more favourable prognosis, in contrast to dementia praecox, although he also observed, as modern research has confirmed, that persistent alterations in bipolar (and unipolar) disorders are not rare [6].

Is the "Kraepelinian binary system" indeed dead, as Tim Crow [7] stated some time ago? Kraepelin reported that episodes of manic-depressive insanity never lead to the same severe personality changes ("Verblödung") as

Bipolar Disorder. Edited by Mario Maj, Hagop S. Akiskal, Juan José López-Ibor and Norman Sartorius.
© 2002 John Wiley & Sons Ltd.

schizophrenic psychoses. Half a century earlier, Falret had described *folie circulaire* quite differently, as a "terrible ... incurable form of insanity" [1, 2]. According to Kraepelin, there is no regular pattern in the course, while Falret described a nearly perfect regularity. Both these authors regarded course, outcome and prognosis as essential for their definition, but they drew opposite conclusions. Modern research does not support fully either Kraepelin's or Falret's description. The truth lies somewhere in the middle. Several decades after the above contributions, the monographs of Jules Angst [8] and Carlo Perris [9] initiated a series of studies which have proved that bipolar disorder is neither an entirely benign nor a totally malign illness. The history of bipolar disorder constantly oscillates between these two poles, although all authors agree on one basic assumption: only the observation of course and outcome can adequately characterize bipolar illness.

DEFINITIONS AND METHODOLOGICAL ISSUES

There is some confusion in the literature concerning the terms *prognosis*, *course* and *outcome*. The term *prognosis* actually includes *course* and *outcome*. The term *course* has been used sometimes as an equivalent of *outcome*, but this is not appropriate, as outcome is only one aspect of course, the end-point of course in a defined period of time [6, 10]. The course of bipolar disorders (as of any other mental disorder) includes all phenomena which occur after the onset of the illness [11]. The most important features of the course are the following:

- onset of the disorder (i.e., type of onset, age of onset, precipitation)
- episodes (i.e., type of episode, number, frequency, length)
- cycles (i.e., number, length, frequency, intervals, persisting symptoms, stability of symptom constellation or syndrome shift)
- activity of the episodes (i.e., re-manifestation during a defined period of time)
- outcome (the end-point of course in a defined period of time).

In many studies course and outcome are grouped together under the heading "prognosis". Sometimes the expression "good prognosis" is used to mean few episodes; sometimes to mean full remission or recovery [5, 12–14]. Tohen *et al* [15] proposed criteria to differentiate between syndromic and functional recovery. Functional recovery was defined as the return to the premorbid level of psychosocial activity.

There are considerable differences concerning the definition of *episode*. The MacArthur Foundation Research Network [16] defines an episode as a period of a certain length "during which the patient is consistently within the full symptomatic range on a sufficient number of symptoms to meet syndromal criteria for the disorder". Nevertheless, in bipolar disorder there is the problem of the demarcation of two separate episodes. Concerning rapid cycling, the DSM-IV requires either a switch to a mood state of opposite polarity or a period of remission lasting two months to delineate a new episode. Quite differently, in the Research Diagnostic Criteria (RDC, [17]), one episode can consist of states of opposite polarity. Therefore, only if one disregards the DSM-IV definition, episodes can be viewed as mono-phasic, biphasic and polyphasic, as does for example the National Institute of Mental Health (NIMH) Collaborative Program on the Psychobiology of Depression. Then, a *monophasic* episode is exclusively manic or depressive. A *biphasic* episode consists of one (hypo)manic and one depressive episode, although not necessarily in that order. A *polyphasic* episode includes at least two switches in polarity.

Course and outcome can be assessed with different methodologies. A truly *prospective* design is obviously superior to a *retrospective* design, as prospective studies tend to lead to data with higher validity. But retrospec-tive studies or, preferably, studies with both a retrospective and a prospec-tive observation time are essential for the design and goals of purely prospective studies. Certain aspects of the prognosis of bipolar disorders, like the development of persisting alterations, syndrome shift etc., depend on the duration of the illness. At the same time, to perform a truly prospec-tive study is far more difficult (longer study duration, change of diagnostic systems over time, new therapies, etc.). A compromise may be the concept of a *catch-up study*. A "catch-up" design [18] means that index information, e.g. diagnosis or psychopathology, comes from case records and is therefore retrospectively assessed, while present data are assessed by "catching up" with the former patients and actively examining them. High *drop-out rates* limit the relevance of results significantly (low generalizability), as lost-to-follow-up subjects have been shown to be the most impaired ones in the context of psychiatric epidemiological studies [19].

The *observation time* (length of the follow-up) is crucial. Because of the long duration of the illness, some aspects can be observed only later during the course. Therefore, *long-term* studies (more than 10 years) have the highest validity regarding prognosis. For obvious reasons, they are difficult to carry out and consequently rather scarce. Therefore, *medium-term* (4–9 years) and *short-term* (1–3 years) studies complement our knowledge. With observation periods shorter than one year, it is very unlikely to come to relevant conclusions concerning the natural course of bipolar illness, as the natural duration of one episode lies in this interval. Therefore, such studies can only give information concerning the course of acute episodes [14, 20].

Finally, there is the distinction between *controlled* and *naturalistic* studies. The former "control" for certain variables, which may modify course and outcome, such as treatment. They aim to keep such modifying variables constant during the observation period. *Naturalistic* studies observe course and outcome without interfering with the natural course of the illness (including available treatment). Nevertheless, a strict distinction between *naturalistic* and *controlled* studies has its limits: on the one hand, it is impossible to control for all relevant variables that may influence course and outcome; on the other, the inclusion of a subject in a naturalistic study may already alter his behaviour. There is a great number of naturalistic studies, which stem from certain specialized outpatient clinics, mostly lithium clinics. Such studies are a good chance to collect data on course and outcome prospectively, especially as one confounding variable (treatment) is kept constant. At the same time, one has to be aware that subjects from such studies may be even more selected than in most other naturalistic studies, as motivation and compliance are bound to be better in the patients who attend such clinics, compared to those who fail to do so.

LONG-TERM NATURALISTIC STUDIES (Table 2.1)

"Classical" Studies Before 1966

Due to their great number of patients included, the long observation periods, and often an excellent clinical and psychopathological basis, some of the "older" long-term naturalistic studies on the prognosis of bipolar disorders are very valuable. Nevertheless, they have some obvious shortcomings, as for example the fact that the distinction between bipolar and unipolar illnesses was not always followed. Also, operational criteria or other explicit definitions were not available. Related to this is the fact that since the 1970s—especially in North America [21]—the concept of schizophrenia has become narrower [22], and the concept of bipolar disorder broader [23].

It is not always easy to draw a clear demarcation between "old" and "new" studies. We decided to use the year 1966 as a turning-point, as in that year the influential studies by Angst [8] and Perris [9] were published, which showed that the Kraepelinian unitary concept for affective disorders was not valid. These two studies supported the view of those who had regarded unipolar and bipolar disorders as separate entities before 1966, as for example Kleist [24] and Leonhard [25].

Some of the most well-known studies before 1966 were those by Wertham [26] (2000 patients!, 12 years of follow-up), Rennie [27] (66 patients, 26 years of follow-up), Lundquist [28] (103 patients, 30 years of follow-up), Kinkelin [29] (57 bipolar patients, 1–27 years), Hastings [30] (67 patients, 6–12 years) and Bratfos and Haug [31] (42 patients, 1–12 years). These studies showed that after a sufficiently long duration of the illness approximately 25% of

TABLE 2.1 Long-term naturalistic studies of the course and outcome of bipolar disorders

Study	Duration of observation (years)	No. subjects and diagnostic groups	Type of study	Results at follow-up
"Classical" Studies (26–31)	1–26	42–2000 Various diagnostic groups, mostly manic-depressive illness	Retrospective or catch-up	Among hospitalized manic-depressive patients, around 2/3 had a unipolar and 1/3 a bipolar course. Transient schizophrenic symptoms were not rare. 15–20% of bipolar patients had a markedly unfavourable course. Discrete impairments were frequent in bipolar patients (around 50%?)
Tsuang et al [47] (Iowa-500 Study)	35	100 Bipolar, first episode manic (RDC)	Catch-up, naturalistic Non-psychiatric control group	The course of bipolar illness was better than in schizophrenia but worse than in non-psychiatric controls. 64% good, 14% fair and 22% poor prognosis (clinical and social) in bipolar patients. Bipolar schizoaffective disorder had a more severe, but otherwise similar course to bipolar affective disorder.
McGlashan [50, 51] (Chestnut Lodge Follow-up Study)	16	19 Bipolar (DSM-III/RDC) Later report: comparison of 28 patients with adolescent-versus 26 with adult-onset mania	Catch-up, naturalistic	5 (26%) of bipolar patients lived in a "hospital or sheltered environment"; global functioning was poor ("continuously incapacitated") for 6 (32%), while 2 (11%) had fully recovered. Patients with adolescent-onset mania had more psychotic symptoms and greater chronicity than adult-onset manic patients.

(continues overleaf)

TABLE 2.1 (*continued*)

Study	Duration of observation (years)	No. subjects and diagnostic groups	Type of study	Results at follow-up
Marneros et al [52–58] (Cologne Study)	25	30 Bipolar affective (BP), 56 Bipolar schizoaffective (BISCH) (DSM-III)	Catch-up, naturalistic	Mild to moderate residual symptoms in 33% of the BP, 52% of the BISCH. Median of 5.0 (BP) and 5.7 (BISCH) episodes during 25 years. Median length of episode: 2 months. Median GAS score after 25 years: 85 (BP), 75 (BISCH). Disability was moderate to high in 20% (BP) and 36% (BISCH). 29% (BP) and 53% (BISCH) had a negative development concerning employment, 29% (BP) versus 26% (BISCH) concerning social situation. 12% (BP) and 28% (BISCH) did not live independently.
Angst [42–46] (Zurich Study)	28	220 Bipolar (DSM-III)	Prospective, naturalistic	The annual change rate from unipolar to bipolar was 1% per year. The only significant predictor was an earlier age of onset of depression. 21% of the bipolars developed mood-incongruent psychotic features. Bipolars (versus unipolars) had more and shorter episodes (0.2 versus 0.4 episodes per year, median length 4 versus 5–6 months). The median cycle length was 32 (''pure'' bipolar) and 35 (schizobipolar) versus 54 (pure unipolar) and 62 (schizodepressive) months. There was a decrease of cycle length with increasing cycle number. 16% of the bipolars showed chronicity. 5 year remission occurred in only 16% of all bipolar

Study	Years	Sample	Design	Findings
Coryell et al [39, 41] Akiskal et al [40] (NIMH Study)	10–11	559–605 with Unipolar depression; 186–231 with Bipolar I; 96 with Bipolar II (RDC)	Prospective, naturalistic	Switch rates from unipolar to bipolar I and to bipolar II were each 5% over 10 years. Switch rates from bipolar II to bipolar I were 14% over 10 years. Converters from unipolar to bipolar I had more severe index episodes. Initially, converters from unipolar to bipolar II exhibited more mood lability, more energy-activity and more daydreaming. They had a more unfavourable course with higher social withdrawal, more minor antisocial behaviours and more problems concerning employment. Only in the first 4 years progressively longer symptom-free periods were clearly associated with lower relapse risks. After 7 years the cumulative likelihood of recurrence was 4 in 5 for all bipolar patients. With sustained lithium prophylaxis, the likelihood of at least one recurrence exceeded 70% within 5 years of recovery.
Coryell et al [36] (NIMH Study)	15	114 Bipolar I (RDC)	Prospective, naturalistic	Clinically, 20% had poor prognosis. Functionally, 34% suffered from impairment in employment and 27% in friendship. Baseline variables were not predictive for poor prognosis. Poor outcome went along with high depression rates in the first 2 years.

(continues overleaf)

TABLE 2.1 (*continued*)

Study	Duration of observation (years)	No. subjects and diagnostic groups	Type of study	Results at follow-up
Turvey et al [33] (NIMH Study)	10	165 Bipolar I (RDC)	Prospective, naturalistic	16% had poor prognosis. Baseline variables were not predictive for poor prognosis. Poor prognosis went along with longer, but fewer episodes (RDC, not DSM-IV criterial), more delusions and more polyphasic episodes (RDC). Following DSM-IV criteria, poor-prognosis subjects had more and shorter cycles. No indication for shortening of cycle length during course.
Kessing et al [60–62]	23	2903 Bipolar (ICD-8/9)	Retrospective, case register	No indication for shortening of episodes during course, but indication for shortening of intervals between episodes. No effect of age or gender on length or frequency of cycles or episodes. A higher number of previous episodes was a predictor for further recurrence. During the 23 years, the mean length of hospitalisation increased.
Cusin et al [64]	14	244 Bipolar	Retrospective assessment of in-patients	Bipolar (versus unipolar) disorder and manic first episode were predictive for higher frequency of episodes. Other baseline variables were not predictive for course. During the course of the illness a shortening of cycle length was observed, which might be the result of an unrepresentative sample (inpatients!)

Harrow et al [63] (Chicago Follow-up Study)	10	26 with Psychotic bipolar mania (RDC) (overall 210 with Functional psychoses)	Prospective, naturalistic	Schizoaffective outcome was better than schizophrenic outcome and poorer than outcome for psychotic affective disorders. Mood-incongruent psychotic symptoms had negative prognostic implications. No separate analysis for the bipolar versus unipolar distinction was presented.
Tsai et al [65]	15	101 Bipolar (DSM-III-R)	15 years retrospective plus 2 years prospective observation of a cohort from a treatment centre	Mean age of 47 years, mean length of illness 25 years, a mean number of 9.2 episodes. 22% history of rapid cycling, 10% of substance abuse and 59% of psychotic symptoms. Overall outcome: poor 16%, fair 36% and good 48%. Predictors of good outcome were male gender, early age of onset and good compliance with pharmacotherapy. Compared to "Western studies" with much higher rates of comorbid substance abuse, the outcome was not much better in Taiwan.
MacQueen et al [66]	"Up to 15 years"	1450 Bipolar patients were pooled from 17 patient cohorts	Meta-analysis	30–60% of all patients had detectable levels of psychosocial impairment. Predictors of good psychosocial outcome found in several (but not all) studies were: high premorbid social and functional status, absence of psychosis during course, low number of prior admissions or past episodes, low number of past depressions, no history of alcohol/substance abuse.

RDC—Research Diagnostic Criteria
GAS—Global Assessment Scale

patients with a bipolar disorder developed persisting alterations concerning psychopathology and social functioning [14, 32].

"Modern" Studies

The NIMH Collaborative Program on the Psychobiology of Depression

The NIMH Collaborative Program on the Psychobiology of Depression observed bipolar patients prospectively up to 15 years in a large naturalistic study. One 10-year follow-up report of 165 patients with bipolar I disorder (drop-out rate 29%) focused on comparison of "poor-prognosis" and (non-poor-prognosis) "control" bipolar subjects [33]. Poor prognosis was defined as belonging to the highest quartile of a morbidity index for the last three consecutive years. 16% of the patients fulfilled this criterion. The poor-prognosis group had significantly lower levels of social functioning and satisfaction at the 10 year follow-up (for example, the mean Global Assessment Scale (GAS [34]) score was 40 versus 70). As in many other studies, baseline variables had little power to predict a poor outcome. On the other hand, some course variables were predictive: the poor-prognosis group had fewer (three versus five), but longer episodes (83 versus 28 weeks) and more polyphasic episodes (58% versus 24%) than controls. Here, one has to be aware that this study used RDC for an episode. Therefore, polyphasic episodes were counted as one episode (in DSM-IV they would make three or more episodes). Looking at cycles according to DSM-IV criteria, poor-prognosis subjects had more (7.6 versus 4.1) and shorter (66 versus 131 weeks) cycles. Furthermore, poor-prognosis subjects developed delusions during the course of the illness more often than controls (63% versus 31%). No differences concerning treatment were observed between the two groups. In contrast to the "kindling" or "sensitization" hypotheses [35], neither the poor-prognosis nor the control group showed a significant shortening of cycle length during the observation period.

Another report from the same cohort [36] included 15-year outcome results in 113 bipolar I patients (drop-out 37.2%). In this analysis, an unfavourable outcome was defined as suffering from symptoms of major depressive disorder (MDD), schizoaffective disorder or mania during the entire 15th year of follow-up. 20% of the patients had such a bad outcome. The study employed measures of social functioning in a subsample. Here, in some respects, the outcome was even worse: 34% of all patients suffered from moderate to marked impairment concerning employment and 27% concerning friendship. Again, all baseline variables failed to have any predictive power with respect to the 15-year outcome, while one course variable did so: a high rate of depression (but not mania) in the first two years of follow-up correlated with a less favourable outcome and higher rates of depression after 15 years. The authors therefore discussed—as others before [37, 38]—the existence of a depression-prone subtype of bipolar disorder with a less favourable course.

The NIMH study also presented data on the diagnostic stability of affective disorders [39]. In an analysis of the 10-year course, 5% of the initially non-bipolar probands developed mania (thus becoming bipolar I) and 5% developed hypomania (thus becoming bipolar II) during the observation period. The switch rates from bipolar II to bipolar I were higher: the Kaplan–Meyer survival analysis indicated a switch rate of over 14% in 10 years. In an analysis of the predictors of conversion from unipolar to bipolar [40], it was shown that conversion from unipolar to bipolar I correlated with more severe index episodes, while most other variables were non-predictive. In contrast, conversion from unipolar to bipolar II was predicted by a certain personality profile: such converters had exhibited more "mood lability", more "energy-activity" and more "daydreaming" at baseline. During the course of the illness, compared to unipolars, "bipolar II converters" were more socially withdrawn, they were more often engaging in minor antisocial acts and they showed evidence of poorer long-term occupational or educational adjustment (job changes, unemployment, etc.).

A further report [41] analysed 10-year recurrence rates in 186 bipolar patients. Although progressively longer symptom-free periods were clearly associated with lower relapse risks over the subsequent four years, thereafter this effect dissipated. Seven years after recovery, the cumulative likelihood of recurrence was four in five for all bipolar patients and two in three for those whose index episode had been followed by at least three years without symptoms. Even with sustained lithium prophylaxis, the likelihood of at least one recurrence exceeded 70% within five years of recovery.

The Zurich Study

In prospective observations [38, 42–46] of up to 220 bipolar patients over a period of—finally—28 years, Angst and coworkers' assessments were continued until finally the majority of the cohort had died (mostly for natural causes, though 8% committed suicide). The annual switch rate from unipolar to bipolar—186 unipolar patients were also followed-up—was 1% per year (24% during the whole observation period). The only significant predictor for a unipolar-to-bipolar switch was an earlier age of onset of depression. 21% of the bipolars developed mood-incongruent psychotic features during the follow-up and were reclassified as schizoaffective. Compared to unipolars, bipolars had more and shorter episodes (0.2 versus 0.4 episodes per year, median length 4 versus 5–6 months), which resulted in more frequent hospitalizations. The median cycle length was 32 ("pure" bipolar) and 35 (schizobipolar) versus 54 (pure unipolar) and 62 (schizodepressive) months. The fact that the schizoaffective forms resembled their affective counterparts so closely led the authors to the conclusion that "schizophrenic symptoms, present in schizodepressives or schizobipolars, do not change the length of a cycle". Interestingly, the overall medians of episode length were not different from those reported in the pre-pharmacological era, which supports the assumption that "modern pharmacotherapy does not really lead to shorter episodes, but only suppresses symptoms". Overall, there was a decrease of cycle length with increasing cycle number. 16% of the bipolars showed chronicity (defined as an episode lasting at least 24 months with GAS scores constantly under 61). A recovery (defined as 5-year remission) occurred in only 16% of all bipolar cases (versus 26% in unipolars). In an earlier report [44] on 95 bipolar patients (observation time 23.8 years), Angst found that 24% of all bipolar patients had residual symptoms, 82% had experienced another episode (mean number 9), with a median length of three months. All reports from this cohort compare affective and schizoaffective disorders and come to the conclusion that bipolar affective and schizoaffective disorders lie on a continuum, with schizoaffective bipolar disorder tending to be a quantitatively more severe form. For example, where 24% of bipolar patients developed residual symptoms, the percentage for bipolar schizoaffective patients was 57% [44]. To our knowledge this report was the first to distinguish between bipolar and unipolar schizoaffective disorder.

The Iowa-500 Study

Due to its methodological accuracy (for example, the use of a non-psychiatric control group) and its long observation period (35 years), the Iowa-500 Study [47] is one of the most important psychiatric follow-up studies carried out up to now. After 35 years, 100 patients originally admitted for mania showed a better course than well-matched schizophrenic patients; at the same time, their outcome was worse than that of surgical controls. Combining different measurements (both clinical and social), outcome was good in 64% of bipolar patients, fair in 14% and poor in 22%. Schizoaffective and bipolar affective disorders had in many respects a comparable course and outcome, but schizoaffective disorder was more severe [48, 49].

The Chestnut Lodge Follow-Up Study

Only a relatively small subsample ($n = 19$) of the Chestnut Lodge follow-up sample ($N = 226$) suffered from bipolar affective disorder [50]. After almost

16 years of follow-up, five (26%) of them lived in a "hospital or sheltered environment". Global functioning was poor ("continuously incapacitated") for six (32%), while two (11%) had fully recovered. In a later report [51], 28 patients with adolescent-onset mania were compared to 26 adult-onset manic patients. After a mean of 15 years, patients with adolescent-onset mania presented with more psychotic symptoms and greater chronicity than adult-onset ones. However, the long-term (15-year) outcome of the adolescent-onset patients was comparable to or better than that of the adult-onset patients. Nevertheless, this could have been an age effect, as at follow-up the age difference was significant.

The Cologne Study

The Cologne Study of Marneros et al [5, 52–58] is a long-term naturalistic study involving 402 patients, who were personally assessed by the authors. Additionally to the "catch-up" results, the course of the illness during a 25-year period was evaluated. Episodes were defined according to DSM-III-R criteria. The final diagnoses at catch-up were affective disorder ($n = 106$), schizoaffective disorder ($n = 101$) and schizophrenic disorder ($n = 148$). Affective disorders were dichotomized into bipolar ($n = 30$) and unipolar ($n = 76$) forms, as well as schizoaffective disorders (bipolar: $n = 56$; unipolar: $n = 45$). 33% of the bipolar affective patients (compared to 37% of the unipolar affectives) and 52% of the bipolar schizoaffectives (compared to 36% of the unipolar schizoaffectives) suffered from persisting alterations at catch-up. Bipolar affective patients had suffered from a median of 5.0 episodes, bipolar schizoaffectives from 5.7, both with a median length of two months. 17% of the bipolar affectives and 29% of the bipolar schizoaffectives had made suicide attempts during the observation period. The mean GAS score in the two groups was 85 (bipolar affective) versus 75 (bipolar schizoaffective) (median 95 versus 83) at catch-up. Social adjustment as assessed with the Disability Assessment Schedule (DAS, 59) was moderate to low for 20% of the bipolar affective and 36% of the bipolar schizoaffective patients. 29% of the bipolar affective and 53% of the bipolar schizoaffective subjects had a negative outcome concerning employment and 29% (bipolar affective) versus 26% (bipolar schizoaffective) concerning social situation. Overall, 12% of the bipolar affective and 28% of bipolar schizoaffective subjects did not live independently at catch-up.

A Danish Case Register Study

A Danish case register study [60–62] analysed retrospectively the data of more than 20 000 patients with affective disorders (ICD-8/ICD-9). Almost

9200 of these had recurrent episodes during an observation period of 23 years, with 2903 suffering from recurrent bipolar disorder. In the study, "admission to hospital" was equalled with "expression of episode". Such episodes did not become shorter during the course of the illness. The mean length of such an "episode"—or rather the mean duration of a hospital admission—was 5.3 weeks for patients with an initial manic episode. Interestingly, the only variable which predicted recurrence was a high number of previous episodes. Gender and age did not have predictive power in this respect. Finally, the authors came to the unexpected observation that, in spite of better treatment methods and a sharp reduction of available hospital beds during the 23 years of the observation period, the duration of hospital admission actually increased over time. Possible explanations might be the tendency to admit only severe cases, to admit them later in the episode (due to lower bed capacities) and thus prolong episodes or—and this might be a challenging hypothesis—a worsening of the natural history of bipolar disorders over time.

The Chicago Follow-Up Study

A 10-year outcome report from the Chicago Follow-Up Study [63], concerning 210 patients with schizophrenia, schizoaffective disorder, affective disorders and mood-incongruent psychotic disorder, found that the outcome of schizoaffectives was better than that of schizophrenics but poorer than that of patients with psychotic affective disorders. Mood-incongruent psychotic symptoms had negative prognostic implications. No separate analysis for unipolar versus bipolar patients was provided in this specific report.

A Retrospective Analysis from Milan

In a retrospective analysis of the prior course of 244 bipolar and 182 unipolar patients, who were admitted to inpatient treatment in Milan, Italy, the average duration of the illness was 14.4 years, with an average of 4.4 episodes [64]. A shortening of cycles during the course of the illness was noted. Furthermore, bipolar disorder (versus unipolar disorder) was predictive for a higher frequency of episodes, as was a manic first episode (although this effect "disappeared" after the third episode). Other baseline variables were unrelated to the cycle frequency. As in other studies, the risk of recurrence increased with the number of previous episodes. The authors acknowledge that their observations may be due to the fact that all subjects were recruited in a clinical setting and then retrospectively assessed. Therefore, unfavourable courses are likely to have been over-represented.

The Outcome Study of the Taipei City Psychiatric Centre

In an analysis from Taiwan [65], 101 bipolar patients were retrospectively (15 years) and prospectively (2 years) assessed. With a mean age of 47 years, the mean length of illness was almost 25 years. Patients had a mean number of 9.2 episodes. 22% had a history of rapid cycling, 10% of substance abuse and 59% of psychotic symptoms. The overall outcome was poor in 16% of cases, fair in 36% and good in 48%. Overall, the authors come to the conclusion that, in spite of the low prevalence of substance abuse in Taiwan, the overall outcome is not better than in Western cohorts with high rates of a history of comorbid substance abuse (30–50%).

A Meta-analysis

MacQueen and co-workers [66] have pooled data from 17 patient cohorts from already published studies. Their meta-analysis reports of 1450 bipolar patients observed for up to 15 years. Between 30 and 60% of these patients had detectable levels of psychosocial impairment at follow-up. Low premorbid social and functional status, presence of psychosis during course, a high number of prior admissions or past episodes, a high number of past depressions and a history of alcohol/substance abuse were found to be predictive for a negative psychosocial outcome in many but not all studies.

MEDIUM-TERM NATURALISTIC STUDIES (Table 2.2)

Further Analyses from the NIMH Collaborative Program on the Psychobiology of Depression

In a five-year outcome report for patients with "mixed/cycling" episodes [67], out of 172 subjects with bipolar I disorder, 76 had mixed or rapid cycling symptoms, with a clear preponderance of rapid cycling (more than 90% rapid cycling versus less than 10% mixed). A mixed/cycling index episode at study intake predicted a longer time to remission (median 17 weeks) than after a purely depressive (11 weeks) or a purely manic episode (5 weeks). As in nearly all studies reviewed so far, a greater number of previous affective episodes predicted further recurrence in all groups. Nevertheless, at the same time, the remission time from the index episode was shorter for patients with more previous episodes. Psychotic features during a mixed/cycling index episode were predictive for a later remission (37% probability of recovery after six months versus 65% for non-psychotic mixed/cycling patients). Chronicity (defined by non-remission) after five years occurred in none of the manic

TABLE 2.2 Medium-term naturalistic studies of the course and outcome of bipolar disorders

Study	Duration of observation (years)	No. subjects and diagnostic groups	Type of study	Results at follow-up
Coryell et al [68–70] (NIMH Study)	5	117–186 Bipolar (RDC) Different control groups (unipolar depressives, asymptomatic relatives)	Prospective, naturalistic	MDD, BPI and BPII exhibited similar times to recovery from index and subsequent depressive episodes. BPI and BPII had substantially higher relapse rates and developed more episodes than MDD. BPII were much less likely to be hospitalized than BPI. Work impairment was greater in BPII than in BPI (mild to severe work impairment: 42% versus 30%). Bipolars showed more declines in job status and income and fewer improvements. 55% of bipolars (vs. 27% of controls) experienced "decreased occupational status from lifetime best" at follow-up. 32% of bipolars (vs. 13% of controls) experienced a decrease of annual income. Married bipolars did *not* experience a poorer relationship with spouses (including sexual activities) (unipolars did). Subjects with remission sustained throughout the final 2 years of follow-up showed severe and widespread impairment in spite of this remission. Rapid cycling was associated with a significantly lower likelihood of recovery in the second year of follow-up (44% versus 68%) but not in the third, fourth, or fifth. The likelihood of a final follow-up year entirely free of affective symptoms was greater in the non-rapid cycling group (41% versus 26%).

Tohen et al [73–75]	4	75 with index episode of mania; 24 had first episode mania	Prospective, naturalistic	After 1 year 51% relapses, after 2 years 33%, after 4 years 28%. Psychosocial outcome was better after 4 years than after 6 months. After 4 years, 28% were unable to work or study. There was a marked correlation between interepisode symptoms and occupational and residential impairment. Predictors for an unfavourable outcome included poor occupational status prior to index episode; history of previous episodes; history of alcoholism, psychotic features and symptoms of depression during the index manic episode; male gender; and inter-episode affective symptoms at 6-month follow-up. Mood-incongruent psychotic manic episodes with Schneiderian first-rank symptoms were particularly predictive for an unfavourable outcome.
Gitlin et al [79] (UCLA Study)	4.3	82 Bipolar (DSM-III)	Prospective, naturalistic, all patients attended specialized clinic and received treatment	37% relapsed in the first year, 73% in 5 years. 66% had multiple relapses (mean "survival" time 2.9 years). Only 17% of all patients remained euthymic/minimally symptomatic throughout the follow-up. 15% were symptomatic for more than half of the follow-up time, another 15% were symptomatic for 25–50% of the follow-up time. Occupational outcome was good in 28% and poor in 35%. A greater number of previous episodes and a history of psychotic symptoms predicted an unfavourable course. There was a relation between low family and social outcome and more depressive (but not manic) episodes. Better job functioning avoided relapses.

(continues overleaf)

TABLE 2.2 (*continued*)

Study	Duration of observation (years)	No. subjects and diagnostic groups	Type of study	Results at follow-up
Goldberg et al [77, 78] (Chicago Follow-up Study)	4.5	51 Bipolar I (RDC)	Prospective, naturalistic	Only 41% had good outcome, more than half suffered from functional impairment, 45% were re-hospitalized. An affective episode in the year before assessment was a negative predictor. Unipolar patients (controls) did better than bipolars. Psychotic symptoms and more hospitalizations before index episodes were negative predictors. No other predictors could be identified.
Kröber et al [80]	5	71 Bipolar (DSM-III)	Prospective, naturalistic	48% were re-hospitalized, 37% repeatedly. 52% were able to work continuously in the last 2 years. 9% were off work for more than 9 months in last 2 years. The number of re-hospitalizations went along with a high number of previous episodes, a high mania versus depression ratio, and certain personality features, which may be seen as the expression of a residual syndrome.
Boland and Keller [67] (NIMH Study)	5	155 Bipolar I (RDC) 69 with mixed/cycling (more than 90% rapid cycling)	Prospective, naturalistic	Rapid-cycling patients remitted later than pure manic or pure depressive patients. Rapid-cycling patients showed more chronicity (non-remission, 17%) after 5 years than pure manic (0%) or pure depressive patients (11%). Rapid-cycling patients had a higher probability of relapse than purely manic patients.

| Winokur [72] (NIMH Study) | 5 | 231 Bipolar (RDC) 70 of these had alcoholism | Prospective, naturalistic | There were no significant differences with respect to course between bipolar patients with and without alcoholism. Primary alcoholism plus bipolar disorder occurred more often in men. It had a better 5-year course than primary bipolar disorder plus alcoholism, which occurred more often in women. During the course of bipolar disorder, remission of alcoholism was frequent. |

MDD—major depressive disorder
BPI—bipolar I disorder
BPII—bipolar II disorder

index patients, 11% of patients with depressive index episode and 17% of the mixed/cycling patients. Relapse during five years occurred in 81% of the manic index patients and 91% of patients with a mixed/cycling index episode.

Further analyses by Coryell and co-workers from the NIMH study focuses on different aspects of course and outcome of bipolar disorders. In one analysis [68], 64 bipolar II patients had a better course than 53 bipolar I patients. Compared to a large group with major depression ($n = 442$), all three groups exhibited similar times to recovery from index and subsequent major depressive episodes, but bipolar groups had substantially higher relapse rates and developed more episodes of major depression, hypomania and mania. The two bipolar groups differed by the severity of manic-like syndromes and thus remained widely diagnostically stable; the bipolar II patients were much less likely to develop full manic syndromes or to be hospitalized during follow-up. During five years, 64% of the bipolar I and 48% of the bipolar II patients were re-hospitalized. Nevertheless, like Akiskal *et al.*'s paper [40] proved later for unipolar to bipolar II converters, work impairment after five years was greater in the bipolar II than in the bipolar I group (mild to severe work impairment: 42% versus 30%). Concerning psychosocial outcome variables, no significant differences occurred between the two bipolar groups.

The psychosocial consequences of illness in 148 patients with bipolar and 240 with major affective disorder were assessed after a five-year follow-up and compared to matched relatives as a control group [69]. All affective disorder subjects were significantly more likely to report declines in job status and income at the end of follow-up and significantly less likely to report improvements. 55% of the bipolars and only 27% of the controls experienced a "decreased occupational status from lifetime best" at follow-up and 32% versus 13% had experienced a decrease of annual income since intake. Interestingly, while bipolar subjects were less likely to have ever been married (32% unmarried versus 15% in controls), the ones who were married did not report a poorer relationship with spouses (including sexual activities), while unipolars did experience such a worsening of "marital functioning". Subjects with remission sustained throughout the final two years of follow-up showed severe and widespread impairment in spite of this remission.

In an analysis of rapid cycling [70], it was shown that 45 bipolar patients, who developed a rapidly cycling bipolar course during the first year, were—in comparison with 198 patients who showed a non-rapidly cycling bipolar course— more likely to be female and to have exhibited depression, hypomania, or cycling between depression and hypomania within the index episode. Rapid cycling was associated with a significantly lower likelihood of recovery in the second year of follow-up (44% versus 68%) but not in the third, fourth, or fifth. Nevertheless, the likelihood of a final follow-up year entirely free of affective symptoms was greater in the non-rapid cycling group (41% versus 26%).

Two posthumously published analyses from the legacy of George Wino-kur [71, 72] looked at the NIMH data in the light of the hypothesis concerning the close link between substance abuse and bipolar disorder. A high comorbidity rate between alcoholism and bipolar disorder was found at study intake (more than one-third), with an impressive male preponderance. Nevertheless, during the five years of observation some unexpected results were found. The overall course of patients with alcohol plus bipolar disorder was no more unfavourable than the one of patients with bipolar disorder only concerning such outcome measures as number of episodes, number of weeks in hospital and frequency of psychotic features. If one distinguished between primary alcoholic patients (alcoholism before bipolar disorder) and primary bipolar patients (bipolar disorder before alcoholism), the latter were female in majority (63% versus 29%). Primary bipolar patients relapsed earlier than primary alcoholic patients (median 49 versus 73 weeks). Furthermore, primary bipolar patients tended to have a higher chronicity rate than primary alcoholic patients (17% versus 3%). Unexpectedly, the course of alcoholism during the observation time was rather favourable. After five years, 95% of the primary bipolar and 75% of the primary alcoholic patients had remitted concerning alcoholism. Data from the 10-year follow-up indicated that the rate of alcoholism had even decreased from 30% to 1%. Nevertheless, one has to be cautious concerning selection effects during the 10-year follow-up period, as it is well known that in drop-outs substance abuse tends to be over-represented. Nevertheless, Winokur's data do not support the conviction that comorbid alcoholism is a risk factor for an unfavourable course of bipolar disorder.

The McLean Outcome Study

Winokur's results may be seen as partly divergent from those of Tohen et al's [73] prospective study on manic patients. 75 patients with mania were prospectively assessed over four years. 51% had not relapsed after one year, 33% after two years and 28% after four years. The median time in remission was one year. The longer a patient was in remission, the better were the chances to remain in remission. Psychosocial outcome was better after four years than after six months. Nevertheless, after four years 28% were unable to work or study. There was a marked correlation between inter-episode symptoms and occupational and residential impairment. No baseline variable was found to be predictive for inter-episode changes. Predictors for an unfavourable outcome included poor occupational status prior to index episode, history of previous episodes, history of alcoholism, psychotic features and symptoms of depression during the index manic episode, male gender, and inter-episode affective symptoms at six-month follow-up. In a further analysis [74], it was clearly shown that a mood-incongruent psychotic manic episode with Schneiderian first-rank symptoms was particularly predictive for an un-favourable outcome. Overall, patients with a mood-incongruent index epi-sode relapsed earlier than patients with a mood-congruent index episode (median time 8 versus 33 months). In another subsample of 24 first-episode patients [75], again psychotic features during the index episode and a history of alcoholism were predictive for an earlier relapse. After four years, 58% of the patients had relapsed. Patients who had inter-episode symptoms after four years were psychosocially impaired in various areas.

The Chicago Follow-Up Study

One has to be aware that shorter follow-up periods "are associated with higher estimates of chronicity because they include patients while still in the episode who would eventually recover if followed long enough" [14]. The Chicago Follow-up Study [76–78] has supported this: in bipolar patients, the 4.5 year outcome was better than the 2-year outcome. The prospective and naturalistic observation of 51 bipolar patients showed that, after 4.5 years, 41% of the patients had good functioning, 37% moderate impairment and 22% poor functioning. Fewer than half of the bipolar patients were able to maintain adequate role performance (including work performance). A cohort of unipolar depressive patients ($n = 49$) as a comparison group did some-what better. 45% of the bipolars were re-hospitalized during the observation time. Patients who had a relapse in the year prior to the follow-up did worse at follow-up than the ones without a recurrence. Only two baseline variables had a (negative) effect on outcome measures: a higher number of hospitaliza-tions before the index episode and the presence of psychotic symptoms.

The UCLA Study

The UCLA Study [79] used a specialized outpatient clinic to observe a cohort of 82 bipolar patients prospectively for a mean of 4.3 years. Although they all received "aggressive pharmacological maintenance treatment", 37% relapsed in the first year, 73% in five years. 66% had multiple relapses. The mean "survival" time (until first relapse) was 2.9 years. Nevertheless, only 17% of all patients stayed euthymic or minimally symptomatic throughout the follow-up. 15% of all patients spent more than half of the follow-up time symptomatic and another 15% did so for 25–50% of the follow-up time. Occupational outcome was good in 28% and poor in 35%. Social, family interaction and functional outcome measures were somewhat better than occupational outcome. A greater number of previous episodes and a history of psychotic symptoms, but no other baseline variable, were predictive for an unfavourable course. A great number of previous depressive episodes correlated with low levels of family and social outcome. Furthermore, the authors tested the hypothesis that "poor social, work, and family functioning are also stressors that may contribute to further episodes". In a Cox regression, only one difference reached statistical significance: "those with better job functioning avoided relapses better over time than those with poor job functioning". In a hierarchical multiple regression analysis, psychosocial factors were significantly related to time of first relapse, although they did not explain more than 7% of the corresponding variance.

An Analysis from Heidelberg

In a study from the University of Heidelberg, Germany [80], 77 bipolar patients were assessed with standardized instruments after discharge from inpatient treatment for bipolar disorder. Five years later they were re-assessed with a drop-out rate of only 8%. 48% had been re-hospitalized during the observation period, 37% even repeatedly. 52% were able to work in the last two years before re-assessment, without having any days off, while 9% were off work for more than nine months in these two years. In their multivariate analysis, the authors found that the number of previous episodes was strongly correlated with the number of re-hospitalizations. There were additional factors, which were even more predictive for re-hospitalization: a high mania versus depression ratio, schizotypic features, low scores of initiative/ motivation, discrete negative symptoms and fewer signs of a syntonic personality, which the authors interpret altogether as persisting alterations.

The Duration of Mania: An Analysis from Pisa and San Diego

Perugi *et al* [81] analysed the duration of manic episodes in 155 subjects. Interestingly, despite state-of-the-art therapies, 13% had a chronic course (defined by an index episode longer than two years). For most baseline variables, there were no differences between chronic and non-chronic manic patients—except for the fact that chronic patients had more previous hospitalizations and more psychotic features than non-chronic patients.

SHORT-TERM NATURALISTIC STUDIES (Table 2.3)

Long-term changes in bipolar disorder are easily overlooked in short-term studies. The Cologne Study [5, 10, 57], for example, showed that persisting alterations were found in schizophrenic patients after a mean of one year, in

TABLE 2.3 Short-term studies of the course and outcome of bipolar disorders

Study	Duration of observation (years)	No. subjects and diagnostic groups	Type of study	Results at follow-up
Harrow et al [93]	2–4	47 Formerly manic patients	Prospective, naturalistic	Severe thought disorder persisted in 30% and were closely related to a more severe form of illness.
Harrow et al [94]	1.7	73 Formerly manic patients	Prospective, naturalistic	Many hospitalized manic patients had a severe, recurrent, and pernicious disorder.
Hunt et al [104]	2	62 Bipolars	Prospective, naturalistic	Relapses were more often preceded by a severe life event in the previous month, although this was only true for 19% of all relapses.
Maj et al [140]	2–5	37 Rapid cyclers (RC); 74 Nonrapid cyclers (NRC)	Prospective, naturalistic	RC had a longer illness, were more likely to be bipolar II, had more suicide attempts. RC had more episodes during the next 4 years than NRC, although the majority of RC no longer fulfilled criteria for RC at follow-up. RC with a pole-switching pattern before study intake were more likely to further fulfil criteria for RC.
Brown et al [91] (Chandigarh Acute Psychosis Study)	1	24 Bipolar (ICD-9) with considerable diagnostic instability	Prospective, naturalistic	75% had remitted and had no social impairment. Mean duration of index episode was 10 weeks.

| Strakowski et al [83, 84] (Cincinnati Studies) | 1 | 64 Bipolars after first hospitalization with mania (DSM-III-R) (35% mixed) (plus 19 lost-to-follow-up) | Prospective, naturalistic | 61% syndromatic, 39% symptomatic and 36% functional remission. Treatment compliance was full in 41%, partial in 26% and absent in 33% of the patients. Syndromatic remission was associated with higher treatment compliance. Symptomatic and functional remission went along with higher socioeconomic status and good premorbid function. Functional recovery was more often seen in mixed (52%) than in pure manic (28%) patients. The lost-to-follow-up group consisted of more patients with substance abuse and lower socioeconomic status. |
| Keck et al [85] Dunayevich et al [86] (Cincinnati Studies) | 1 | 106 Bipolars (DSM-III-R) after a hospitalization with mania (DSM-III-R) (43% mixed) (plus 28 lost-to-follow-up) | Prospective, naturalistic | 48% syndromatic, 26% symptomatic and 24% functional remission. Shorter duration of illness and treatment compliance predicted syndromatic remission. Medication treatment compliance was inversely associated with comorbid substance use disorders. Symptomatic and functional recovery occurred more rapidly and in a greater percentage of patients from higher social classes. Mixed mania patients showed no worse outcome than pure mania patients. Personality disorders led to a significantly less favourable outcome. |

(continues overleaf)

TABLE 2.3 (continued)

Study	Duration of observation (years)	No. subjects and diagnostic groups	Type of study	Results at follow-up
Tohen et al [82] (Harvard-McLean Study)	2	159 First-episode bipolar patients (DSM-IV) (26% mixed)	Prospective, naturalistic	99% achieved syndromal recovery, 40% functional recovery. "Mixed mania" did not have a less favourable outcome than "pure mania". Low depression severity at baseline, functional recovery by 6 months, a short length of hospital stay and an age of more than 30 years predicted earlier syndromal recovery. A short length of hospital stay and an age of more than 30 years predicted functional recovery.
Craig et al [89] (Suffolk County Psychosis Project)	2	119 First-admission bipolar patients with psychotic features (DSM-IV)	Prospective, naturalistic	16% partial remission, 4% continually ill. Compared to schizophrenic and psychotic depressive patients, first episode psychotic bipolar patients had a shorter period of untreated psychosis (84% hospitalization within 4 weeks, only 5% after 1 year). There was no effect of the duration of untreated psychosis on the 2-year outcome.

schizoaffective patients after a mean of five years and in affective patients after a mean of nine years. Therefore, most short- and medium-term studies would overlook such personality changes. As the number of medium- and long-term outcome studies has grown considerably during the last years, short-term studies are of interest when they focus on special aspects of bipolar disorders and thus complement our knowledge. Therefore, our following overview is not intended to be complete.

The Harvard–McLean First Psychosis Project

In a large and well-designed prospective study of 219 patients with a DSM-IV first-episode major affective disorder with psychotic features, 159 patients had a manic first episode (41 mixed manic) [82]. After two years, 99% of the bipolar patients had achieved syndromal recovery, but only 40% had reached functional recovery. The "mixed manic" versus "pure manic" episode distinction did not lead to significant differences concerning outcome. A shorter time to *syndromal recovery* was predicted by:

- low depression severity at baseline,
- functional recovery by six months,
- a short length of hospital stay,
- an age of more than 30 years at hospital stay,
- high GAS scores at six months,
- being employed,
- having bipolar (versus unipolar) disorder and
- being married.

Nevertheless, in multivariate analysis only the first four variables remained predictive. *Functional recovery* was predicted by:

- a short length of hospital stay,
- an age of more than 30 years at hospital stay,
- syndromal recovery by six months,
- no axis I comorbidity and
- high GAS scores at six months.

Here, in multivariate analysis only the first two variables remained predictive. All other baseline and course variables failed to reach significance.

The Cincinnati Studies

There are several studies from the University of Cincinnati, which investigate the short-term outcome of affective psychosis with a refined methodology. One analysis [83, 84] looked at the 12-month outcome after first hospitalization for bipolar disorder. The lost-to-follow-up group consisted of more patients with substance abuse and lower socioecononic status. Of the remaining 64 patients, 61% were in syndromatic, 39% in symptomatic and only 36% in functional remission after 12 months. Even one-third of these follow-up patients had exhibited poor treatment compliance (versus 41% with good compliance). Good treatment compliance was a predictor for syndromatic remission, but not for symptomatic or functional remission, which went along with higher socioeconomic status and good premorbid functioning. An unexpected finding was that functional recovery was better in mixed (52%) than in pure manic (28%) patients. Overall, the presence of a substance abuse disorder, although frequent, was not directly predictive for a poorer outcome in the follow-up group, although it was a risk factor to belong to the potentially more unfavourable lost-to-follow-up group. In a related report, Keck et al [85] observed the 12-month course of 106 bipolar patients, who were not necessarily first-episode patients. Although syndromatic recovery occurred in 48% of the overall group, symptomatic recovery occurred in only 26% and functional recovery in only 24%. Predictors of syndromatic recovery included shorter duration of illness and full treatment compliance. Treatment compliance was inversely associated with the presence of comorbid substance use disorders. Symptomatic and functional recovery occurred more rapidly and in a greater percentage of patients from higher social classes. Again, rather unexpectedly, mixed mania patients did by no means worse than pure mania patients. Rather, functional and syndromatic remission rates of mixed mania patients were numerically higher than those of pure mania patients, although this difference was non-significant. In another report from this cohort [86], in 59 bipolar patients the presence of a DSM-III-R personality disorder was a negative predictor for a 12-month syndromatic remission. In "ultra-short" follow-ups of eight months [87, 88] in two cohorts, it was shown that in first-episode manic patients different areas of psychosocial functioning (such as role performance, interpersonal relationships, sexual activity and recreational enjoyment) recovered rather independently from each other. Furthermore, in a cohort which consisted of first- and multiple-episode manic patients, mood-incongruent psychosis (versus no such a syndrome) resulted in a less favourable outcome.

The Suffolk County Psychosis Project

"Is there an association between duration of untreated psychosis and 24-month clinical outcome in a first-admission series?" asks a paper from the Suffolk County Psychosis Project [89] and comes to the answer "no", not only for 119 psychotic bipolar patients, but for all 349 patients with psychosis included in the study. In this epidemiological multicentre study, one-third of all schizophrenic patients were hospitalized only after one year or later of having been symptomatic, while two-thirds of all bipolar psychotic patients were hospitalized within the first month of being symptomatic. Nevertheless, the duration of the untreated symptomatic period was unrelated to the two-year outcome. In another analysis from this study, Schwartz *et al.* [90] looked at the diagnostic stability of DSM-IV diagnosis over two years. 83% of the index bipolar disorders ($N = 141$) retained their diagnosis after two years, 9% "shifted" to the schizophrenia spectrum and 8% to delusional disorder, substance abuse disorder and residual categories. Vice versa, 8% of the "other psychosis" cases and 3% of the schizophrenia spectrum subjects were reclassified as bipolar after two years.

The Chandigarh Acute Psychosis Study

Almost all studies reviewed here stem from Europe, North America or Australia/New Zealand. "Developing" countries are missing. One exception is a study from India [91]. 24 bipolar patients with an acute onset were observed for one year. At follow-up, 75% of all patients remitted and showed no social impairment. In some respect this positive result is difficult to interpret, as diagnoses were made according to ICD-9 and the definition of "social impairment" was not very clear. Furthermore, there was a considerable instability of diagnosis from index assessment to follow-up.

Further Analyses from the Chicago Study

Several studies of Grossman, Harrow and co-workers have looked at the development of thought disorder in manic patients [92, 93]. Two to four years after discharge, 30% of the manic patients showed severe thought disorder, which was most closely related to the presence of manic behaviour and psychosis. Thought disorder was more frequent in patients with poor post-hospital functioning and in those with multiple previous manic episodes or a more chronic course of illness. In this respect, compared to a schizophrenic control group, the manic patients did somewhat better, but the difference was not significant. The same research group reported [94] that many hospitalized manic patients may have a severe, recurrent, and pernicious disorder.

SPECIAL ASPECTS

Onset

Age at Onset

The exact definition of age at onset is difficult, because the age when symptoms first appear does not correspond to the age at first medical consultation or at first admission to hospital. Symptoms generally appear some time before medical consultation is first sought [5, 14, 95]. Bipolar affective patients usually become ill at a younger age than unipolar patients. There is good agreement in the literature that the peak onset occurs in the 20s (between 25 and 30) for bipolar disorders and in the late 30s for unipolar disorders [5, 8, 14, 32, 96–98].

Type of Onset

An acute onset of depressive symptomatology, in which the symptoms develop from a healthy state to a full-blown disorder within a few days, is rare. Usually the onset is subacute, with signs and symptoms beginning some weeks or even months before the full manifestation of the illness. More than 20% of patients have a gradual onset with prodromal signs between several months and some years before the full manifestation [5, 14, 99, 100]. A follow-up project of the Epidemiological Catchment Area Study [99] showed that average duration of prodromal signs was one year, but for dysphoria, as well as for anhedonia, psychomotor disturbances, feelings of guilt and insufficiency, it was five years.

Manic symptomatology is usually acute in onset, over a number of days, although in some cases long-lasting prodromal signs have been noted [101–103]. Quite differently than in schizophrenia, psychotic symptoms in bipolar disorder seem to lead to treatment within a few days [89].

The majority of first episodes in bipolar disorder are depressive: the Cologne Study found 85% depressive, 12% manic and 3% mixed first episodes in a sample of bipolar patients [5].

Precipitants

Kraepelin's observation [4] that the onset of affective episodes appears to be independent of external influences proved only partially correct. Research showed a partial relation of stressful life events and the manifestation of episodes [79, 104], although the influence of such factors was not all too great.

Some theories on the pathogenesis of affective disorders assign primary causal relevance to psychosocial environmental events [105, 106]. It is, however, now generally accepted that psychosocial or physical events contribute more to the timing of an episode than to causing it. Causality is likely to be largely biological and, especially, genetic. Precipitating events seemingly play an important role in the onset of the first episodes but not in the later ones. In the Cologne study, approximately 53% of the unipolar and 47% of the bipolar patients had stressful life events at the onset of an episode (the difference is statistically insignificant) [5, 54]. An analysis of all episodes of the long-term course (more than 25 years' duration) indicated that only in approximately 13% of all episodes stressful life events could be found in a period of six months before the onset of the episode. It is interesting that the difference between manic and melancholic episodes regarding the frequency of life events is not significant. The type of life event (bereavement, changing job, moving house, etc.) seems to be unspecific [107].

Cycle and Episode Length

Studies on the natural length of episodes which were published prior to introduction of effective treatments, like those of Mendel [108], Panse [109], Wertham [26], Rennie [27] and Kinkelin [29], described durations of episodes betweeen two months and more than one year [110]. Despite differences in the literature, it can be said that the duration of a full depressive episode is between two and five months [5, 99], although a longer duration is not exceptional [13, 14, 45]. The duration of manic episodes averages around two months [12, 32, 111, 112], although again much longer episodes are anything but rare [81]. Bipolar mixed episodes seem to be longer than all other episodes during the bipolar course—a mean length from over five months up to one year has been described [5, 113, 114].

The *number of episodes* during the long-term course of the illness depends on the duration of illness and the response to prophylactic treatment. Therefore, it does not make sense to compare the number of episodes reported by the various studies. Rather, for research purposes, it may be useful to assess the "Annual Frequency of Episodes" ("AFE"), defined as the number of episodes during the whole course divided by the duration of illness [115]. The Cologne Study found an AFE of 0.23, which was significantly higher than the AFE of unipolar affective disorder (0.12). The majority of bipolar patients have more than three episodes during an illness duration of 20 years. They have significantly more episodes than unipolar patients [8, 9, 14, 52, 54].

Much more reliable is the assessment of the length and frequency of *cycles*. A *cycle* is defined as the time from the onset of one episode to the onset of the next episode [11]. A variation of cycle length usually reflects variations in the length of intervals between episodes. The length of cycles in bipolar patients was found to be significantly shorter than in unipolar ones. Especially the length of the first cycle differs markedly between the two disorders. Subsequent cycles are usually shorter [5, 11, 45, 116]. The mean cycle length found in the various studies varied considerably between 68 weeks and many years [5, 33, 45, 117].

Some authors have postulated a shortening of cycle length during the course of the illness [6, 14, 110]. Nevertheless, there are some recent analyses [33, 62], which—with refined methodology— put these results in question. In some of the earlier studies, statistical artefacts may have led to the observation of the shortening of cycle length, as patients with more episodes tend to have shorter cycles. Other authors showed that a shortening of subsequent cycles occurred in some, but not all patients [5].

Predictors of Course and Outcome

Almost all studies from our above review, which have looked at predictors for outcome of bipolar disorders, agree on some basic observations, which we have summarized below. Nevertheless, one has to be aware that such predictors are not necessarily causal. Rather they reflect statistical correlations between two aspects of the illness.

- Outcome measures can only reliably be assessed after several years. Short-term studies tend to over-report negative outcome, possibly due to the fact that episode length varies so considerably that some episodes have not even remitted. Therefore—as an artefact—the study length is a positive predictor. Long-term studies report better outcomes [14].
- Most baseline variables—such as gender, age, age of onset and most socio-demographic variables—are surprisingly unpredictive for course and outcome. So many studies, which have set out to characterize such predictors, have failed to do so that this result is beyond doubt (for example [33, 36, 45, 46, 52, 54, 66, 118]).
- The seemingly tautological observation that a high number of previous episodes predicts a high number of future episodes emerges as one of the most robust predictors of a negative course and outcome. Maj et al [119] spoke of a biologically determined "driving force" of the illness, which seems highly variable between different individuals, but which is highly essential to understand bipolar illness. Therefore, it is not surprising that rapid cycling tends to predict a less favourable course and outcome.
- A high level of premorbid functioning [79, 82, 83, 85], which may overlap with the concept of a "syntonic" personality [80], has been shown to have some predictive power for a more favourable outcome. At the same

time, there is some indication that the presence of a personality disorder may worsen course and outcome [86].

- High levels of inter-episode impairments (for example [74, 75, 82]) and a chronic course make a further negative course more likely. On the other hand, good integration into work and a good social network during the course of the illness have a stabilizing effect.
- Good treatment compliance and a better course and outcome are correlated [120].
- Life events may enhance the risk of both a manic and a depressive episode. Nevertheless, this effect is small (although statistically robust) [79, 104].
- Comorbid substance abuse is correlated with a less favourable course and outcome. Again, the mechanism of this relation is unclear [66, 121, 122].
- Mood-incongruent features, which indicate a closer relation to the schizoaffective pole of the bipolar spectrum, are indicators for a less favourable course and outcome [5, 44, 48, 63, 66, 123].
- There may be a depression prone subtype with a less favourable course than other subtypes of bipolar disorder [36–38].

SPECIAL FORMS OF BIPOLAR DISORDER

Mixed States

Although the concept of mixed bipolar disorder is a very old one (for historical reviews see [124, 125]), it has only received greater attention in the last years. Nevertheless, there is evidence that in a clinical setting mixed bipolar disorders tend to be under-diagnosed [126]. Today there are different criteria for mixed bipolar disorders [124, 125, 127]. DSM-IV and ICD-10 use a rather narrow set, which make mixed episodes a relatively rare occurrence, with a frequency of 5–10% of all manic episodes. If one uses broader criteria, as for example working groups in Pisa and Cincinnati have done [113, 128], the frequency of mixed episodes may reach 50% of all manic episodes. The Cologne Study [5, 114] assessed—amongst other aspects—also the frequency of mixed episodes over 25 years. 101 of the patients with a bipolar affective or schizoaffective episode according to DSM-III-R criteria had 602 episodes. 8.3% of these episodes were affective mixed episodes and 9.2% schizoaffective mixed episodes. 43% of all bipolar patients had least one affective or schizoaffective mixed episode. A monomorphous mixed course (i.e. only mixed episodes during all 25 years) was observed in only 1% of the patients. Only 4–8% were found to have a long-term course with predominantly mixed episodes (narrowly defined in accordance with DSM-III-R criteria).

Until now there are no criteria that follow Kraepelin's suggestion to distinguish between "transitional forms" (mixed episodes representing a transitional point or interval during the switch from depression to mania or vice versa) and "autonomous forms" (mixed episodes as a separate disorder) of mixed episodes [4, 124]. While most contemporary authors regard mixed bipolar episodes as sub-forms of manic episodes, Koukopoulos and Koukoupoulos [129] have pointed out that this is not what Weygandt [130] and Kraepelin [4] had originally intended when describing mixed states ("Mischzustände"), and what today's clinical reality actually shows. Certainly, mixed states can also arise from depressive episodes. Indeed, Koukopoulos and Koukopoulos present evidence that agitated depression is a form of a mixed state.

Obviously, different definitions of mixed episodes influence results concerning course and outcome. Different studies have used such different criteria for mixed episodes and have looked at their course and outcome [5, 73, 82, 83, 85, 111, 113, 114, 131–134]. Virtually all of them agree on two basic facts: mixed episodes are more difficult to treat than pure manic episodes. Lithium is less effective in this group, while valproate and carbamazepine may be preferable. The duration of a mixed episode is longer than that of a pure manic episode. In the Cologne Study [5], the mean length of a mixed affective episode was twice as long (five months) than other affective, schizophrenic or schizoaffective episodes. In 15% of mixed episodes a suicidal symptomatology was present. Affective mixed episodes were also significantly longer than schizoaffective mixed episodes.

Although part of the available literature postulates a worse course and outcome of mixed episodes, this is not fully supported by the existing empirical studies. Some studies have indeed observed a worse outcome compared to pure manic episodes (for example [111, 131–134]), but others—especially the most recent ones—have failed to do so (for example [82, 113]). Two analyses from Cincinnati have even found a better outcome in some respects [83, 85]. To interpret such differences, one must not necessarily conclude that the most recent studies have used a better methodology; rather, it seems that some of the most recent studies have used broader concepts of "mixed episode" (which is also reflected by higher frequency rates), while most of the "older" literature used narrower DSM-III or DSM-III-R criteria. Narrowly defined mixed bipolar disorders may indeed have a less favourable outcome, while broadly defined ones may not differ significantly from pure bipolar disorders concerning short- and medium-term outcome. But this issue is still open to research.

Rapid Cycling

Although there are different definitions of "rapid cycling", the DSM-IV definition ("occurrence of at least four major depressive, manic, hypomanic, or mixed episodes during the previous year, demarcated either by a remission of at least two months' duration or by a switch to an episode of opposite polarity") has gained wide acceptance, especially as alternative definitions were not shown to be clearly superior [135]. The phenomenon has been known for several decades: Weitbrecht [136] described cases of ultra-rapid cycling (without using the term) with an extremely unfavourable course. In this respect, he referred to an earlier article of the Italian psychiatrist Bertozzi [137], who described unipolar rapid cycling. There are surprisingly few studies that have looked at the medium- or long-term outcome of rapid-cycling bipolar disorders (for reviews see [138, 139]). One reason might be that rapid cycling has a relatively low stability over time. For example, in the analysis of Coryell et al [70], only 3% of the patients retained the rapid-cycling pattern over four years. This general tendency was supported by other studies [140, 141], although an earlier study by Wehr et al [142] had reported—with an alternative definition of rapid cycling—a 41% stability during an average of five years. There is a more recent report from the NIMH Collaborative Program on the Psychobiology of Depression [67], which quite in contrast to its title presents data on the course of rapid cycling. The study showed that rapid-cycling episodes needed a longer time to remit (median five weeks for pure mania, nine weeks for depression, 14 weeks for "mixed/cycling") and that after five years such rapid-cycling patients had a higher rate of non-remission (0% for mania, 11% for depression, 13% for "mixed/cycling"). Overall, the existing literature indicates that to fulfil criteria for rapid cycling at one point is a risk factor to develop more future episodes than the "average bipolar patient". As a greater number of episodes is a risk factor for a less favourable outcome, rapid cycling is—at least indirectly—a risk factor for a less favourable outcome. Nevertheless, there is little evidence that rapid cycling is a separate entity; there are no "natural" boundaries and its diagnostic stability over time tends to be rather low: rapid cycling may not be a qualitatively distinct subtype of the illness but simply a severe variant [143]. Over time, most rapid-cycling patients tend to convert to non-rapid cyclers [139]. Finally, there is some indication that a pole-switching pattern during rapid cycling may be a predictor of a less favourable course [140].

Seasonal Affective Disorder

There is a long tradition linking recurrent affective disorders to the seasons of the year, which goes back to Ancient Greek medicine [144]. For the northern hemisphere, depression has been seen as related to winter, and mania as related to summer [14]. Although for (unipolar) seasonal affective disorder this relationship is well established [145, 146], for bipolar disorders the empirical evidence for the mania-in-summer-depression-in-winter-cycle is still weak. Most recent studies with a stringent methodology have failed to support such a pattern for manic episodes [147–153]. One study [149] looked with the same methodology at an English and a New Zealand cohort and found no support for seasonality either in southern or in northern hemisphere, except for an autumn preponderance of bipolar depressions in both centres. While there are some recent studies reporting an association between season and episode onset or hospitalization in bipolar disorder [154–157], their methodology may not always outweigh the above-mentioned studies, which found no correlation. Still there are some more "classical" observations that have found at least a trend towards seasonality in bipolar disorders [158–162]. As seasonality is obviously a dimensional construct, which affects virtually all human beings, it certainly occurs in bipolar patients with different intensity. Therefore, there might be sub-groups of more or less seasonal bipolar patients. Nevertheless, the seasonal effect on cyclicity is possibly not as strong as often thought. It is likely, as one study has pointed out, that bipolar patients, as far as seasonality is concerned, lie somewhere between patients with seasonal affective disorder and normal controls [163]. A general clear seasonal pattern for the majority of bipolar disorders is not supported by the literature.

Bipolar Schizoaffective Disorder

The nosological position of schizoaffective disorders is still unclear [49, 123, 164–166]. In the last 20 years, the question whether schizoaffective disorders can be dichotomized into unipolar and bipolar disorders in the same way as affective disorders has arisen and has been answered positively. It was found that the differences between unipolar and bipolar schizoaffective disorders parallel those between unipolar and bipolar affective disorders [11, 32, 44, 52–54, 167–170].

The international diagnostic systems (ICD-10 and DSM-IV) have now included the dichotomy unipolar versus bipolar in their criteria for schizo-affective disorder. Unipolar and bipolar schizoaffective disorders differ in regard to sociodemographic and premorbid features (gender distribution, premorbid personality), but also significant differences in longitudinal course have been shown [52–54, 170]. Unfortunately, research regarding the long- and medium-term course and outcome of schizoaffective dis-orders, taking into account the unipolar versus bipolar distinction, is very scarce. One exception is the Cologne Study [5, 52–54, 170], in which patients with bipolar schizoaffective disorders had significantly more episodes (median six episodes during 25 years), a higher annual frequency of epi-sodes, more cycles and a higher annual frequency of cycles than unipolar schizoaffective patients. The most frequent type of course of schizoaffective disorders is the "polyphasic" one with more than four episodes during the long-term course. The cycles in bipolar schizoaffective disorders are usually shorter than in unipolar schizoaffective disorder. Regarding long-term outcome—assessed by the GAS, the DAS and the Psychological Impairment Rating (PIRS)—no significant differences between unipolar and bipolar schizoaffective disorders have been reported. However, the long-term outcome is dependent on the number and frequency of episodes: more frequent episodes lead to a less favourable long-term outcome. Usually patients with bipolar schizoaffective disorders relapse more frequently than unipolars, have more episodes and then perhaps a more unfavourable outcome. However, this seems to be a consequence of the number of episodes rather than of "bipolarity".

Suicide and Mortality

Some comprehensive reviews [14, 171, 172] have agreed that between 15 and 19% of all bipolar patients die of suicide, while up to 25–50% have attempted to do so. As is generally the case in suicidology, there is a preponderance of female suicide attempters. Nevertheless, recent (re-)analyses of these suicide data have come to the conclusion that for methodological reasons these reviews might have overestimated suicide rates [173–175]. The new analyses of lifetime suicide rates for all affective disorders come to 5–7%. Standardized mortality ratio (SMR) for suicide in bipolar disorder was 15 (males) and 22 (females) in a large population study [176], indicating that the risk of dying from suicide is 20-fold greater for bipolar patients than the general population.
   Two results are confirmed by virtually all studies:

- A comorbidity of bipolar disorder and substance abuse increases the risk of suicide significantly [174, 177–179]. For example, in a sample of 251 subjects with bipolar disorder, the 99 subjects with comorbid alcoholism had a suicide attempt rate of 38% compared to 22% amongst those without alcoholism [177].
- While it is not clear whether psychotic symptoms increase the risk for suicide [180], mixed episodes (as compared to pure manic episodes) do so [181–186].

   Suicide attempters have more depressive episodes during their illness [187], while rapid cycling may not result in higher suicide attempt rates [188]. Furthermore, there is indication that the group of bipolar patients at highest risk of suicide are young men who are in an early phase of the illness, especially those who have made a previous suicide attempt, those abusing alcohol, and those recently discharged from the hospital [174].

Despite all discussions on the efficacy of lithium, there seems to be sufficient evidence for its anti-suicidal effect for "classical" bipolar cases (which might nevertheless exclude mixed bipolar cases and those with comorbid substance abuse, who are at special risk for suicide) [79, 189–192].

Furthermore, there is an excess mortality of bipolar disorders compared to the general population. Goodwin and Jamison [14] estimate a 2.3-fold increase, which was supported by more recent studies (for example [193, 194]). This excess mortality is not fully explained by suicides alone. Some studies have reported excess mortality from cardiovascular diseases [195, 196], but others have failed to do so or come to the conclusion that further evidence is needed [197, 198]. Nevertheless, all studies comparing lithium to non-lithium treated patients agree that lithium reduces the overall mortality—possibly beyond its anti-suicidal effect [192, 194, 197, 199, 200].

Comorbid Substance Abuse

Comorbid substance abuse disorders (SUD) are frequent in bipolar disorders [121, 122, 201, 202]. In epidemiological samples, the lifetime prevalence for SUD in bipolar disorder may be as high as 40–60% [177, 203, 204]. Compared to the general population, the odds ratio for a comorbid SUD has been found to be 2–3. The relation between SUD and bipolar disorders is not fully clear. Why is there such an "excess comorbidity"? Do bipolar disorders and SUD share common genetic causes? Is SUD an attempt of self-medication? Is bipolar disorder a risk factor for SUD?

Almost all studies on this topic agree that the co-occurrence of bipolar disorders and SUD has a negative impact on the further course and outcome of the former disorders (for example [84, 85, 133, 205–208]), leading to a higher number of episodes and hospitalizations and a poorer treatment compliance. Also, there may be a connection between SUD and a shortening of bipolar cycles and the development of the rapid-cycling pattern [202, 205]. At the same time, there is some indication that the course of substance abuse is more favourable if SUD is associated with bipolar disorder [72, 209]. Also, primary alcoholism (with secondary bipolar disorder) may have a better course than secondary alcoholism (with primary bipolar disorder) [71, 72, 206, 210]. One study [82, 121] showed that, amongst 219 first-episode manic patients, only 17% fulfilled criteria for SUD, which is far less than in manic patients as a whole (e.g., 42% reported by McElroy *et al* [202] in 288 patients). Nevertheless, also the first-episode bipolar patients with an antecedent SUD seem to have a less favourable course than the ones without SUD [211]. Mixed manic episodes have higher comorbidity rates with SUD than "pure" ones [121, 131, 133, 201, 205, 207], but again—as Tohen pointed out [121]—this observation depends on the definition of "mixed episode".

Overall, the question remains open whether the indisputable unfavourable effect of SUD on the outcome of bipolar disorder is an indirect consequence of the negative effects of SUD (such as poorer treatment compliance or unfavourable social and medical development), or it points in the direction of a genuine "bipolar plus SUD" syndrome, which has its own course. Some multivariate analyses (for example [85]) support the first assumption, showing that it is the variable "treatment non-compliance", rather than "SUD", which affects the outcome negatively.

SUMMARY

Consistent Evidence

- Bipolar disorders are long-lasting and usually lifelong diseases.
- In most cases bipolar disorders are recurrent with a polyphasic course, i.e., with more than three episodes.
- The duration of the individual episodes varies between several weeks to several months and is dependent on the type of episode (mixed episodes usually having the longest duration, manic episodes usually the shortest) and on treatment response.
- Although the majority of bipolar patients do not suffer from persisting alterations of personality or social interactions, or from persisting symptoms, there is a considerable proportion (between 15 to 30%) who do exhibit such forms of chronic impairment.
- Affective bipolar disorders have a better long-term prognosis than schizophrenic and schizoaffective disorders.
- Bipolar disorders have a frequent comorbidity especially with substance abuse disorder, which can influence the course of the illness unfavourably.
- The course of bipolar disorders can be unfavourably modified by stressful life events and failure to comply with prophylactic treatment.
- Bipolar patients have higher risks than healthy people of dying of suicide and of other causes.

Incomplete Evidence

- It is still uncertain whether modern treatments have changed substantially the length of episodes or the number of relapses with respect to the pre-pharmacological area.
- Although it is evident that the first cycle of the illness is longer than subsequent cycles, the findings regarding further shortening of cycles during the course of the recovery are not consistent.

- Recent studies and re-analyses have raised doubt on earlier assumptions that approximately 15–20% of bipolar patients commit suicide. Rather, significantly lower rates (in the range of 7–10%) are now being reported.
- Although there is evidence that mixed episodes and rapid cycling may influence course and outcome negatively, this has not been confirmed by all investigators.
- Although there is some evidence that mixed episodes can occur repeatedly during the course of bipolar disorder, the long-term stability of this pattern is doubtful. Long-term investigations with an observation time of more than two decades showed that a monomorphous course (i.e., only mixed episodes during the whole course) is extremely rare.
- It is evident that schizoaffective bipolar disorders occupy a position between schizophrenia and affective bipolar disorder regarding outcome. However, bipolar schizoaffective disorders are possibly heterogeneous.
- Although some factors have been outlined, there is an overall lack of knowledge concerning variables predicting the course and outcome of bipolar disorders.

Areas Still Open to Research

The most important questions regarding the course and outcome of bipolar disorders which are completely open to research are the following:

- What factors lead to a favourable versus an unfavourable outcome?
- What factors generate the various courses of bipolar disorders, i.e. the *extremely polyphasic* (i.e. more than 10 episodes), the *moderate polyphasic* (more than three episodes), the *oligophasic* (fewer than three episodes), and the rare *monophasic course* (only one episode during life)?
- Is there a relationship between biological parameters (e.g. structural or functional brain changes) and the type of course and outcome? Are there genetic influences on course and outcome such that genetical distinctions between patients with "good" and "poor" prognosis or patients having mixed episodes or rapid cycling versus patients with typical episodes and course can be made?
- Has the course of bipolar disorder changed over time? Some authors postulate a more unfavourable course and an earlier age of onset in recent years, but the overall evidence is anything but clear.

Bipolar disorders may result in individually different courses and outcomes—dark ones and bright ones. We feel that few persons have expressed that clearer than Kay R. Jamison, both in her personal report [212] and in her scientific work [14]. She told about a friend, whose "attacks of mania and depression became more frequent and severe. No breakthrough ever came; no happy ending ever materialized. (...) He had a terrible disease and it eventually cost him his life—as it does tens of thousands of people every year" [212]. But at the same time she personally admits that "the countless hypomanias, and mania itself, all have brought into my life a different level of sensing and feeling and thinking". Research on prognosis, course and outcome must never forget to listen to the ones who are affected by and who suffer from the illness.

REFERENCES

1. Falret J.-P. (1851) Marche de la folie (suite). *Gaz. Hop.*, **24**: 18–19.
2. Falret J.-P. (1854) Mémoire sur la folie circulaire, forme de maladie mentale characterisée par la reproduction successive et régulière de l'état maniaque, de l'état mélancholique, et d'un intervalle lucide plus ou moins prolongé. *Bull. Acad. Natl. Med. (Paris)*, **19**: 382–400.
3. Kahlbaum K.L. (1863) *Die Gruppirung der psychischen Krankheiten und die Eintheilung der Seelenstörungen.* Kafemann, Danzig.
4. Kraepelin E. (1899) *Psychiatrie. Ein Lehrbuch für Studirende und Aerzte. 6. Auflage.* Barth, Leipzig.
5. Marneros A., Deister A., Rohde A. (1991) *Affektive, schizoaffektive und schizophrene Psychosen. Eine vergleichende Langzeitstudie.* Springer, Berlin.
6. Bourgeois M.L., Marneros A. (2000) The prognosis of bipolar disorders: course and outcome. In *Bipolar Disorders: 100 Years after Manic-Depressive Insanity* (Eds A. Marneros, J. Angst), pp. 405–436, Kluwer, Dordrecht.
7. Crow T.J. (1998) From Kraepelin to Kretschmer leavened by Schneider: the transition from categories of psychosis to dimensions of variation intrinsic to homo sapiens. *Arch. Gen. Psychiatry*, **55**: 502–504.
8. Angst J. (1966) *Zur Ätiologie und Nosologie endogener depressiver Psychosen.* Springer, Berlin.
9. Perris C. (1966) A study of bipolar and unipolar recurrent depressive psychoses. *Acta Psychiatr. Scand.*, **42** (Suppl. 194): 172–188.
10. Marneros A., Rohde A., Deister A., Steinmeyer E.M. (1990) Behinderung und Residuum bei schizoaffektiven Psychosen—Daten, methodische Probleme und Hinweise für zukünftige Forschung. *Fortschr. Neurol. Psychiatr.*, **58**: 66–75.
11. Angst J. (1986) The course of schizoaffective disorders. In *Schizoaffective Psychoses* (Eds A. Marneros, M.T. Tsuang), pp. 63–93, Springer, Berlin.
12. Zarate C.A., Tohen M. (1996) Outcome of mania in adults. In *Mood Disorders Across the Life Span* (Eds K.I. Shulman, M. Tohen, S.P. Kutcher), pp. 281–298, Wiley, Chichester.
13. Boland R.J., Keller M.B. (1996) Outcome studies of depression in adulthood. In *Mood Disorders Across the Life Span* (Eds K.I. Shulman, M. Tohen, S.P. Kutcher), pp. 217–250, Wiley, Chichester.
14. Goodwin F.K., Jamison K.R. (1990) *Manic-Depressive Illness.* Oxford University Press, New York.

15. Tohen M., Stoll A.L., Strakowski S.M., Faedda G.L., Mayer P.V., Goodwin D.C., Kolbrener M.L., Madigan A.M. (1992) The McLean First-Episode Psychosis Project: six-month recovery and recurrence outcome. *Schizophr. Bull.*, **18**: 273–282.
16. Frank E., Prien R.F., Jarrett R.B., Keller M.B., Kupfer D.J., Lavori P.W., Rush A.J., Weissman M.M. (1991) Conceptualization and rationale for consensus definitions of terms in major depressive disorder. Remission, recovery, relapse, and recurrence. *Arch. Gen. Psychiatry*, **48**: 851–855.
17. Spitzer R.L., Endicott J., Robins E. (1978) Research Diagnostic Criteria. Rationale and reliability. *Arch. Gen. Psychiatry*, **35**: 773–782.
18. Weiss G. (1996) Research issues in longitudinal studies. In *Do They Grow Out of It? Long-Term Outcomes of Childhood Disorders* (Ed. L. Hechtman), pp. 1–16, American Psychiatric Press, Washington.
19. Cox A., Rutter M., Quinton D. (1977) Bias resulting from missing information: some epidemiological findings. *Br. J. Prev. Soc. Med.*, **31**: 131–136.
20. Coryell W., Winokur G., Solomon D., Shea T., Leon A., Keller M. (1997) Lithium and recurrence in a long-term follow-up of bipolar affective disorder. *Psychol. Med.*, **27**: 281–289.
21. Kendell R.E. (1975) *The Role of Diagnosis in Psychiatry*. Blackwell, Oxford.
22. Hegarty J.D., Baldessarini R.J., Tohen M., Waternaux C., Oepen G. (1994) One hundred years of schizophrenia: a meta-analysis of the outcome literature. *Am. J. Psychiatry*, **151**: 1409–1416.
23. Akiskal H.S., Bourgeois M.L., Angst J., Post R., Möller H., Hirschfeld R. (2000) Re-evaluating the prevalence of and diagnostic composition within the broad clinical spectrum of bipolar disorders. *J. Affect. Disord.*, **59** (Suppl. 1): S5–S30.
24. Kleist K. (1953) Die Gliederung der neuropsychischen Erkrankungen. *Monatsschr. Psychiatr. und Neurol.*, **125**: 526–554.
25. Leonhard K. (1957) *Aufteilung der endogenen Psychosen und ihre differenzierte Ätiologie*. Akademie-Verlag, Berlin.
26. Wertham F. (1929) A group of benign psychoses: prolonged manic excitements. With a statistical study of age, duration and frequency in 2000 manic attacks. *Am. J. Psychiatry*, **9**: 17–78.
27. Rennie T. (1942) Prognosis in manic-depressive psychoses. *Am. J. Psychiatry*, **98**: 801–814.
28. Lundquist G. (1945) Prognosis and course in manic-depressive psychoses: a follow-up study of 319 first admissions. *Acta Psychiatr. Scand.*, **35** (Suppl.): 1–96.
29. Kinkelin M. (1954) Verlauf und Prognose des manisch-depressiven Irreseins. *Schweiz Arch. Neurol. Psychiatrie*, **73**: 100–146.
30. Hastings D.W. (1958) Follow-up results in psychiatric illness. *Am. J. Psychiatry*, **114**: 1057–1066.
31. Bratfos O., Haug J.O. (1968) Course of manic-depressive psychosis. A follow-up investigation of 215 patients. *Acta Psychiatr. Scand.*, **44**: 89–112.
32. Marneros A. (Ed.) (1999) *Handbuch der unipolaren und bipolaren Erkrankungen* Thieme, Stuttgart.
33. Turvey C.L., Coryell W.H., Solomon D.A., Leon A.C., Endicott J., Keller M.B., Akiskal H. (1999) Long-term prognosis of bipolar I disorder. *Acta Psychiatr. Scand.*, **99**: 110–119.
34. Endicott J., Spitzer R.L., Fleiss J.L., Cohen J. (1976) The Global Assessment Scale. A procedure for measuring overall severity of psychiatric disturbances. *Arch. Gen. Psychiatry*, **33**: 766–771.

35. Post R.M. (1990) Sensitization and kindling perspectives for the course of affective illness: toward a new treatment with the anticonvulsant carbamazepine. *Pharmacopsychiatry*, **23**: 3–17.
36. Coryell W., Turvey C., Endicott J., Leon A.C., Mueller T., Solomon D., Keller M. (1998) Bipolar I affective disorder: predictors of outcome after 15 years. *J. Affect. Disord.*, **50**: 109–116.
37. Quitkin F.M., Rabkin J.G., Prien R.F. (1986) Bipolar disorder: are there manic-prone and depressive-prone forms? *J. Clin. Psychopharmacol.*, **6**: 167–172.
38. Angst J. (1978) The course of affective disorders. II. Typology of bipolar manic-depressive illness. *Arch. Psychiatr. Nervenkr.*, **226**: 65–73.
39. Coryell W., Endicott J., Maser J.D., Keller M.B., Leon A.C., Akiskal H.S. (1995) Long-term stability of polarity distinctions in the affective disorders. *Am. J. Psychiatry*, **152**: 385–390.
40. Akiskal H.S., Maser J.D., Zeller P.J., Endicott J., Coryell W., Keller M., Warshaw M., Clayton P., Goodwin F. (1995) Switching from "unipolar" to bipolar II. An 11-year prospective study of clinical and temperamental predictors in 559 patients. *Arch. Gen. Psychiatry*, **52**: 114–123.
41. Coryell W., Endicott J., Maser J.D., Mueller T., Lavori P., Keller M. (1995) The likelihood of recurrence in bipolar affective disorder: the importance of episode recency. *J. Affect. Disord.*, **33**: 201–206.
42. Angst J., Felder W., Frey R., Stassen H.H. (1978) The course of affective disorders. I. Change of diagnosis of monopolar, unipolar, and bipolar illness. *Arch. Psychiatr. Nervenkr.*, **226**: 57–64.
43. Angst J. (1980) Verlauf unipolar depressiver, bipolar manisch-depressiver und schizo-affektiver Erkrankungen und Psychosen. Ergebnisse einer prospektiven Studie. *Fortschr. Neurol. Psychiatr.*, **48**: 3–30.
44. Angst J., Felder W., Lohmeyer B. (1980) Course of schizoaffective psychoses: results of a followup study. *Schizophr. Bull.*, **6**: 579–585.
45. Angst J., Preisig M. (1995) Course of a clinical cohort of unipolar, bipolar and schizoaffective patients. Results of a prospective study from 1959 to 1985. *Schweiz Arch. Neurol. Psychiatrie*, **146**: 5–16.
46. Angst J., Preisig M. (1995) Outcome of a clinical cohort of unipolar, bipolar and schizoaffective patients. Results of a prospective study from 1959 to 1985. *Schweiz Arch. Neurol. Psychiatrie*, **146**: 17–23.
47. Tsuang M.T., Woolson R.F., Fleming J.A. (1979) Long-term outcome of major psychoses. I. Schizophrenia and affective disorders compared with psychiatrically symptom-free surgical conditions. *Arch. Gen. Psychiatry*, **36**: 1295–1301.
48. Tsuang M.T., Dempsey G.M. (1979) Long-term outcome of major psychoses. II. Schizoaffective disorder compared with schizophrenia, affective disorders, and a surgical control group. *Arch. Gen. Psychiatry*, **36**: 1302–1304.
49. Tsuang M.T., Simpson J.C., Fleming J.A. (2000) Schizoaffektive Erkrankungen. In *Psychiatrie der Gegenwart. 5. Schizophrene und affektive Störungen. 4. Auflage* (Eds H. Helmchen, F. Henn, H. Lauter, N. Sartorius), pp. 637–660, Springer, Berlin.
50. McGlashan T.H. (1984) The Chestnut Lodge follow-up study. II. Long-term outcome of schizophrenia and the affective disorders. *Arch. Gen. Psychiatry*, **41**: 586–601.
51. McGlashan T.H. (1988) Adolescent versus adult onset of mania. *Am. J. Psychiatry*, **145**: 221–223.
52. Marneros A., Deister A., Rohde A. (1990) The concept of distinct but voluminous groups of bipolar and unipolar diseases. I. Bipolar diseases. *Eur. Arch. Psychiatry Clin. Neurosci.*, **240**: 77–84.

53. Marneros A., Rohde A., Deister A. (1990) The concept of distinct but voluminous groups of bipolar and unipolar diseases. II. Unipolar diseases. *Eur. Arch. Psychiatry Clin. Neurosci.*, **240**: 85–89.

54. Marneros A., Deister A., Rohde A. (1990) The concept of distinct but voluminous groups of bipolar and unipolar diseases. III. Bipolar and unipolar comparison. *Eur. Arch. Psychiatry Clin. Neurosci.*, **240**: 90–95.

55. Marneros A., Deister A., Rohde A. (1990) Psychopathological and social status of patients with affective, schizophrenic and schizoaffective disorders after long-term course. *Acta Psychiatr. Scand.*, **82**: 352–358.

56. Marneros A., Deister A., Rohde A. (1991) Stability of diagnoses in affective, schizoaffective and schizophrenic disorders. Cross-sectional versus longitudinal diagnosis. *Eur. Arch. Psychiatry Clin. Neurosci.*, **241**: 187–192.

57. Marneros A., Rohde A. (1997) "Residual states" in affective, schizoaffective and schizophrenic disorders. In *Dysthymia and the Spectrum of Chronic Depression* (Eds H.S. Akiskal, G.B. Cassano), pp. 75–86, Guilford, New York.

58. Deister A., Marneros A. (1993) Predicting the long-term outcome of affective disorders. *Acta Psychiatr. Scand.*, **88**: 174–177.

59. World Health Organization (1988) *WHO Psychiatric Disability Assessment Schedule (WHO/DAS)*. World Health Organization, Geneva.

60. Kessing L.V., Andersen P.K., Mortensen P.B., Bolwig T.G. (1998) Recurrence in affective disorder. I. Case register study. *Br. J. Psychiatry*, **172**: 23–28.

61. Kessing L.V. (1998) Recurrence in affective disorder. II. Effect of age and gender. *Br. J. Psychiatry*, **172**: 29–34.

62. Kessing L.V., Mortensen P.B. (1999) Recovery from episodes during the course of affective disorder: a case-register study. *Acta Psychiatr. Scand.*, **100**: 279–287.

63. Harrow M., Grossman L.S., Herbener E.S., Davies E.W. (2000) Ten-year outcome: patients with schizoaffective disorders, schizophrenia, affective disorders and mood-incongruent psychotic symptoms. *Br. J. Psychiatry*, **177**: 421–426.

64. Cusin C., Serretti A., Lattuada E., Mandelli L., Smeraldi E. (2000) Impact of clinical variables on illness time course in mood disorders. *Psychiatry Res.*, **97**: 217–227.

65. Tsai S.M., Chen C., Kuo C., Lee J., Lee H., Strakowski S.M. (2001) 15-year outcome of treated bipolar disorder. *J. Affect. Disord.*, **63**: 215–220.

66. MacQueen G.M., Young L.T., Joffe R.T. (2001) A review of psychosocial outcome in patients with bipolar disorder. *Acta Psychiatr. Scand.*, **103**: 163–170.

67. Boland R.J., Keller M.B. (1999) Mixed-state bipolar disorders: outcome data from the NIMH Collaborative Program on the Psychobiology of Depression. In *Bipolar Disorders. Clinical Course and Outcome* (Eds J.F. Goldberg, M. Harrow), pp. 115–128, American Psychiatric Press, Washington.

68. Coryell W., Keller M., Endicott J., Andreasen N., Clayton P., Hirschfeld R. (1989) Bipolar II illness: course and outcome over a five-year period. *Psychol. Med.*, **19**: 129–141.

69. Coryell W., Scheftner W., Keller M., Endicott J., Maser J., Klerman G.L. (1993) The enduring psychosocial consequences of mania and depression. *Am. J. Psychiatry*, **150**: 720–727.

70. Coryell W., Endicott J., Keller M. (1992) Rapidly cycling affective disorder. Demographics, diagnosis, family history, and course. *Arch. Gen. Psychiatry*, **49**: 126–131.

71. Winokur G., Turvey C., Akiskal H., Coryell W., Solomon D., Leon A., Mueller T., Endicott J., Maser J., Keller M. (1998) Alcoholism and drug abuse in

three groups—bipolar I, unipolars and their acquaintances. *J. Affect. Disord.*, **50**: 81–89.

72. Winokur G. (1999)   Alcoholism in bipolar disorder. In *Bipolar Disorders. Clinical Course and Outcome* (Eds J.F. Goldberg, M. Harrow), pp. 185–197, American Psychiatric Press, Washington.

73. Tohen M., Waternaux C.M., Tsuang M.T. (1990)   Outcome in mania. A 4-year prospective follow-up of 75 patients utilizing survival analysis. *Arch. Gen. Psychiatry*, **47**: 1106–1111.

74. Tohen M., Tsuang M.T., Goodwin D.C. (1992)   Prediction of outcome in mania by mood-congruent or mood-incongruent psychotic features. *Am. J. Psychiatry*, **149**: 1580–1584.

75. Tohen M., Waternaux C.M., Tsuang M.T., Hunt A.T. (1990)   Four-year follow-up of twenty-four first-episode manic patients. *J. Affect. Disord.*, **19**: 79–86.

76. Goldberg J.F., Harrow M., Leon A.C. (1996)   Lithium treatment of bipolar affective disorders under naturalistic followup conditions. *Psychopharmacol. Bull.*, **32**: 47–54.

77. Goldberg J.F., Harrow M., Grossman L.S. (1995)   Recurrent affective syndromes in bipolar and unipolar mood disorders at follow-up. *Br. J. Psychiatry*, **166**: 382–385.

78. Goldberg J.F., Harrow M., Grossman L.S. (1995)   Course and outcome in bipolar affective disorder: a longitudinal follow-up study. *Am. J. Psychiatry*, **152**: 379–384.

79. Gitlin M.J., Swendsen J., Heller T.L., Hammen C. (1995)   Relapse and impairment in bipolar disorder. *Am. J. Psychiatry*, **152**: 1635–1640.

80. Kröber H.L., Adam R., Scheidt R. (1998)   Einflüsse auf die Rückfälligkeit bipolar Manisch-Depressiver. *Nervenarzt*, **69**: 46–52.

81. Perugi G., Akiskal H.S., Rossi L., Paiano A., Quilici C., Madaro D., Musetti L., Cassano G.B. (1998)   Chronic mania. Family history, prior course, clinical picture and social consequences. *Br. J. Psychiatry*, **173**: 514–518.

82. Tohen M., Hennen J., Zarate C.M., Jr., Baldessarini R.J., Strakowski S.M., Stoll A.L., Faedda G.L., Suppes T., Gebre-Medhin P., Cohen B.M. (2000)   Two-year syndromal and functional recovery in 219 cases of first-episode major affective disorder with psychotic features. *Am. J. Psychiatry*, **157**: 220–228.

83. Strakowski S.M., Keck P.E., Jr., McElroy S.L., West S.A., Sax K.W., Hawkins J.M., Kmetz G.F., Upadhyaya V.H., Tugrul K.C., Bourne M.L. (1998)   Twelve-month outcome after a first hospitalization for affective psychosis. *Arch. Gen. Psychiatry*, **55**: 49–55.

84. Strakowski S.M., Sax K.W., McElroy S.L., Keck P.E., Jr., Hawkins J.M., West S.A. (1998)   Course of psychiatric and substance abuse syndromes co-occurring with bipolar disorder after a first psychiatric hospitalization. *J. Clin. Psychiatry*, **59**: 465–471.

85. Keck P.E., Jr., McElroy S.L., Strakowski S.M., West S.A., Sax K.W., Hawkins J.M., Bourne M.L., Haggard P. (1998)   12-month outcome of patients with bipolar disorder following hospitalization for a manic or mixed episode. *Am. J. Psychiatry*, **155**: 646–652.

86. Dunayevich E., Sax K.W., Keck P.E., Jr., McElroy S.L., Sorter M.T., McConville B.J., Strakowski S.M. (2000)   Twelve-month outcome in bipolar patients with and without personality disorders. *J. Clin. Psychiatry*, **61**: 134–139.

87. Strakowski S.M., Williams J.R., Sax K.W., Fleck D.E., DelBello M.P., Bourne M.L. (2000)   Is impaired outcome following a first manic episode due to mood-incongruent psychosis? *J. Affect. Disord.*, **61**: 87–94.

88. Strakowski S.M., Williams J.R., Fleck D.E., DelBello M.P. (2000) Eight-month functional outcome from mania following a first psychiatric hospitalization. *J. Psychiatr. Res.*, **34**: 193–200.

89. Craig T.J., Bromet E.J., Fennig S., Tanenberg-Karant M., Lavelle J., Galambos N. (2000) Is there an association between duration of untreated psychosis and 24-month clinical outcome in a first-admission series? *Am. J. Psychiatry*, **157**: 60–66.

90. Schwartz J.E., Fennig S., Tanenberg-Karant M., Carlson G., Craig T., Galambos N., Lavelle J., Bromet E.J. (2000) Congruence of diagnoses 2 years after a first-admission diagnosis of psychosis. *Arch. Gen. Psychiatry*, **57**: 593–600.

91. Brown A.S., Varma V.K., Malhotra S., Jiloha R.C., Conover S.A., Susser E.S. (1998) Course of acute affective disorders in a developing country setting. *J. Nerv. Ment. Dis.*, **186**: 207–213.

92. Grossman L.S., Harrow M., Sands J.R. (1986) Features associated with thought disorder in manic patients at 2–4-year follow-up. *Am. J. Psychiatry*, **143**: 306–311.

93. Harrow M., Grossman L.S., Silverstein M.L., Meltzer H.Y., Kettering R.L. (1986) A longitudinal study of thought disorder in manic patients. *Arch. Gen. Psychiatry*, **43**: 781–785.

94. Harrow M., Goldberg J.F., Grossman L.S., Meltzer H.Y. (1990) Outcome in manic disorders. A naturalistic follow-up study. *Arch. Gen. Psychiatry*, **47**: 665–671.

95. Egeland J.A., Blumenthal R.L., Nee J., Sharpe L., Endicott J. (1987) Reliability and relationship of various ages of onset criteria for major affective disorder. *J. Affect. Disord.*, **12**: 159–165.

96. Angst J. (1987) Verlauf der affektiven Psychosen. In *Psychiatrie der Gegenwart. 5. Affektive Psychosen. 3. Auflage* (Eds K.P. Kisker, H. Lauter, J.-E. Meyer, C. Müller, E. Strömgren), pp. 115–133, Springer, Berlin.

97. Tohen M., Goodwin F.K. (1995) Epidemiology of bipolar disorder. In *Text-book in Psychiatric Epidemiology* (Eds. M.T. Tsuang, M. Tohen, G.E.P. Zahner), pp. 301–315, Wiley-Liss, New York.

98. Weissman M.M., Leaf P.J., Tischler G.L., Blazer D.G., Karno M., Bruce M.L., Florio L.P. (1988) Affective disorders in five United States communities. *Psychol. Med.*, **18**: 141–153.

99. Eaton W.W., Anthony J.C., Gallo J., Cai G., Tien A., Romanoski A., Lyketsos C., Chen L.S. (1997) Natural history of Diagnostic Interview Schedule/DSM-IV major depression. The Baltimore Epidemiologic Catchment Area follow-up. *Arch. Gen. Psychiatry*, **54**: 993–999.

100. Winokur G. (1976) Duration of illness prior to hospitalization (onset) in the affective disorders. *Neuropsychobiology*, **2**: 87–93.

101. Carlson G.A., Goodwin F.K. (1973) The stages of mania. A longitudinal analysis of the manic episode. *Arch. Gen. Psychiatry*, **28**: 221–228.

102. Jacobson J.E. (1965) The hypomanic alert: a program designed for greater therapeutic control. *Am. J. Psychiatry*, **1965**: 295–299.

103. Post R.M., Ballenger J.C., Rey A.C., Bunney W.E., Jr. (1981) Slow and rapid onset of manic episodes: implications for underlying biology. *Psychiatry Res.*, **4**: 229–237.

104. Hunt N., Bruce-Jones W., Silverstone T. (1992) Life events and relapse in bipolar affective disorder. *J. Affect. Disord.*, **25**: 13–20.

105. Brown G.W. (2000) Die Rolle von Lebensereignissen als Ursache affektiver Störungen. In *Psychiatrie der Gegenwart. 5. Schizophrene und affektive Störungen.*

4. Auflage (Eds H. Helmchen, F. Henn, H. Lauter, N. Sartorius), pp. 461–474, Springer, Berlin.

106. Paykel E.S., Cooper Z. (1992) Life events and social stress. In *Handbook of Affective Disorders* (Ed. E.S. Paykel), pp. 149–176, Churchill Livingstone, Edinburgh.

107. Aronson T.A., Shukla S. (1987) Life events and relapse in bipolar disorder: the impact of a catastrophic event. *Acta Psychiatr. Scand.*, **75**: 571–576.

108. Mendel E. (1881) *Die Manie. Eine Monographie*. Urban & Schwarzenberg, Wien.

109. Panse F. (1924) Untersuchung über Verlauf und Prognose beim manisch-depressiven Irresein. *Monatsschr. Psychiatr. Neurol.*, **56**: 15–82.

110. Angst J., Sellaro R. (2000) Historical perspectives and natural history of bipolar disorder. *Biol. Psychiatry*, **48**: 445–457.

111. Keller M.B. (1988) The course of manic-depressive illness. *J. Clin. Psychiatry*, **49** (Suppl.): 4–7.

112. Silverstone T., Hunt N. (1992) Symptoms and assessment of mania. In *Handbook of Affective Disorders* (Ed. E.S. Paykel), pp. 15–24, Churchill Livingstone, Edinburgh.

113. Perugi G., Akiskal H.S., Micheli C., Musetti L., Paiano A., Quilici C., Rossi L., Cassano G.B. (1997) Clinical subtypes of bipolar mixed states: validating a broader European definition in 143 cases. *J. Affect. Disord.*, **43**: 169–180.

114. Marneros A., Rohde A., Deister A. (1996) Bipolar mixed disorders. *Eur. Neuropsychopharmacol.*, **6**(Suppl. 3): 9.

115. Marneros A., Deister A., Rohde A., Sakamoto K. (1988) Nonpsychopathological features of K. Schneider's mania. *Jpn. J. Psychiatry Neurol.*, **42**: 17–21.

116. Marneros A., Rohde A., Deister A., Junemann H., Fimmers R. (1988) Long-term course of schizoaffective disorders. Part II: Length of cycles, episodes, and intervals. *Eur. Arch. Psychiatry Neurol. Sci.*, **237**: 276–282.

117. Winokur G., Coryell W., Akiskal H.S., Endicott J., Keller M., Mueller T. (1994) Manic-depressive (bipolar) disorder: the course in light of a prospective ten-year follow-up of 131 patients. *Acta Psychiatr. Scand.*, **89**: 102–110.

118. Marneros A., Andreasen N.C., Tsuang M.T. (Eds) (1991) *Negative versus Positive Schizophrenia*. Springer, Berlin.

119. Maj M., Pirozzi R., Magliano L. (1996) Late non-response to lithium prophylaxis in bipolar patients: prevalence and prediction. *J. Affect. Dis.*, **39**: 39–42.

120. Maj M., Pirozzi R., Magliano L., Bartoli L. (1998) Long-term outcome of lithium prophylaxis in bipolar disorder: a 5-year prospective study of 402 patients at a lithium clinic. *Am. J. Psychiatry*, **155**: 30–35.

121. Tohen M., Zarate C.A. (1999) Bipolar disorder and substance abuse. In *Bipolar Disorders. Clinical Course and Outcome* (Eds J.F. Goldberg, M. Harrow), pp. 171–184, American Psychiatric Press, Washington.

122. Brieger P. (2000) Comorbidity in bipolar disorder. In *Bipolar Disorders: 100 Years After Manic-Depressive Insanity* (Eds A. Marneros, J. Angst), pp. 215–229, Kluwer, Dordrecht.

123. Marneros A., Tsuang M.T. (Eds) (1990) *Affective and Schizoaffective Disorders*. Springer, Berlin.

124. Marneros A., Angst J. (2000) Bipolar disorders: roots and evolution. In *Bipolar Disorders: 100 Years After Manic-Depressive Insanity* (Eds A. Marneros, J. Angst), pp. 1–36, Kluwer, Dordrecht.

125. Marneros A. (2001) Origin and development of concepts of bipolar mixed states: focus on Wilhelm Weygandt. *J. Affect. Disord.* (in press).

126. Goldberg J.F., Garno J.L., Portera L., Leon A.C., Kocsis J.H. (2000) Qualitative differences in manic symptoms during mixed versus pure mania. *Compr. Psychiatry*, **41**: 237–241.

127. McElroy S.L., Freeman M.P., Akiskal H.S. (2000) The mixed bipolar disorders. In *Bipolar Disorders: 100 Years After Manic-Depressive Insanity* (Eds A. Marneros, J. Angst), pp. 63–88, Kluwer, Dordrecht.

128. McElroy S.L., Keck P.E., Jr., Pope H.G., Jr., Hudson J.I., Faedda G.L., Swann A.C. (1992) Clinical and research implications of the diagnosis of dysphoric or mixed mania or hypomania. *Am. J. Psychiatry*, **149**: 1633–1644.

129. Koukopoulos A., Koukopoulos A. (1999) Agitated depression as a mixed state and the problem of melancholia. *Psychiatr. Clin. North Am.*, **22**: 547–564.

130. Weygandt W. (1899) *Über die Mischzustände des manisch-depressiven Irreseins. Ein Beitrag zur klinischen Psychiatrie.* Lehmann, München.

131. Himmelhoch J.M., Mulla D., Neil J.F., Detre T.P., Kupfer D.J. (1976) Incidence and significance of mixed affective states in bipolar patients. *Arch. Gen. Psychiatry*, **33**: 1062–1066.

132. Cohen S., Khan A., Robison J. (1988) Significance of mixed features in acute mania. *Compr. Psychiatry*, **29**: 421–426.

133. Keller M.B., Lavori P.W., Coryell W., Andreasen N.C., Endicott J., Clayton P.J., Klerman G.L., Hirschfeld R.M. (1986) Differential outcome of pure manic, mixed/cycling, and pure depressive episodes in patients with bipolar illness. *JAMA*, **255**: 3138–3142.

134. Keller M.B., Lavori P.W., Coryell W., Endicott J., Mueller T.I. (1993) Bipolar I: a five-year prospective follow-up. *J. Nerv. Ment. Dis.*, **181**: 238–245.

135. Maj M., Pirozzi R., Formicola A.M., Tortorella A. (1999) Reliability and validity of four alternative definitions of rapid-cycling bipolar disorder. *Am. J. Psychiatry*, **156**: 1421–1424.

136. Weitbrecht H.J. (1972) Depressive und manische endogene Psychosen. In *Psychiatrie der Gegenwart. Forschung und Praxis. Klinische Psychiatrie I. Band II/ Teil 1* (Eds K.P. Kisker, J.-E. Meyer, M. Müller, E. Strömgren), pp. 83–140, Springer, Berlin.

137. Bertozzi S. (1941) Sulla melancolia periodica giornaliera. *Riv. Pat. Nerv. Ment.*, **57**: 411–422.

138. Calabrese J., Rapport D., Findling R., Shelton M., Kimmel S. (2000) Rapid-cycling bipolar disorder. In *Bipolar Disorders: 100 Years After Manic-Depressive Insanity* (Eds A. Marneros, J. Angst), pp. 89–109, Kluwer, Dordrecht.

139. Kilzieh N., Akiskal H. (1999) Rapid-cycling bipolar disorder. An overview of research and clinical experience. *Psychiatr. Clin. North Am.*, **22**: 585–607.

140. Maj M., Magliano L., Pirozzi R., Marasco C., Guarneri M. (1994) Validity of rapid cycling as a course specifier for bipolar disorder. *Am. J. Psychiatry*, **151**: 1015–1019.

141. Bauer M.S., Calabrese J., Dunner D.L., Post R., Whybrow P.C., Gyulai L., Tay L.K., Younkin S.R., Bynum D., Lavori P. et al (1994) Multisite data reanalysis of the validity of rapid cycling as a course modifier for bipolar disorder in DSM-IV. *Am. J. Psychiatry*, **151**: 506–515.

142. Wehr T.A., Sack D.A., Rosenthal N.E., Cowdry R.W. (1988) Rapid cycling affective disorder: contributing factors and treatment responses in 51 patients. *Am. J. Psychiatry*, **145**: 179–184.

143. Maj M. (1999) Lithium prophylaxis of bipolar disorder in ordinary clinical conditions: patterns of long-term outcome. In *Bipolar Disorders. Clinical Course*

and Outcome (Eds J.F. Goldberg, M. Harrow), pp. 21–38, American Psychiatric Press, Washington.

144. Koukopoulos A., Sani G., Koukopoulos A., Girardi P. (2000) Cyclicity and manic-depressive illness. In *Bipolar Disorders. 100 Years After Manic-Depressive Insanity* (Eds A. Marneros, J. Angst), pp. 315–334, Kluwer, Dordrecht.

145. Schwartz P.J., Brown C., Wehr T.A., Rosenthal N.E. (1996) Winter seasonal affective disorder: a follow-up study of the first 59 patients of the National Institute of Mental Health Seasonal Studies Program. *Am. J. Psychiatry*, **153**: 1028–1036.

146. Magnusson A. (2000) An overview of epidemiological studies on seasonal affective disorder. *Acta Psychiatr. Scand.*, **101**: 176–184.

147. Hunt N., Sayer H., Silverstone T. (1992) Season and manic relapse. *Acta Psychiatr. Scand.*, **85**: 123–126.

148. Hardin T.A., Wehr T.A., Brewerton T., Kasper S., Berrettini W., Rabkin J., Rosenthal N.E. (1991) Evaluation of seasonality in six clinical populations and two normal populations. *J. Psychiatr. Res.*, **25**: 75–87.

149. Silverstone T., Romans S., Hunt N., McPherson H. (1995) Is there a seasonal pattern of relapse in bipolar affective disorders? A dual northern and southern hemisphere cohort study. *Br. J. Psychiatry*, **167**: 58–60.

150. Partonen T., Lonnqvist J. (1996) Seasonal variation in bipolar disorder. *Br. J. Psychiatry*, **169**: 641–646.

151. Suhail K., Cochrane R. (1998) Seasonal variations in hospital admissions for affective disorders by gender and ethnicity. *Soc. Psychiatry Psychiatr. Epidemiol.*, **33**: 211–217.

152. Whitney D.K., Sharma V., Kueneman K. (1999) Seasonality of manic depressive illness in Canada. *J. Affect. Disord.*, **55**: 99–105.

153. Daniels B.A., Kirkby K.C., Mitchell P., Hay D., Mowry B. (2000) Seasonal variation in hospital admission for bipolar disorder, depression and schizophrenia in Tasmania. *Acta Psychiatr. Scand.*, **102**: 38–43.

154. Avasthi A., Sharma A., Gupta N., Kulhara P., Varma V.K., Malhotra S., Mattoo S.K. (2001) Seasonality and affective disorders: a report from North India. *J. Affect. Disord.*, **64**: 145–154.

155. Clarke M., Moran P., Keogh F., Morris M., Kinsella A., Larkin C., Walsh D., O'Callaghan E. (1999) Seasonal influences on admissions for affective disorder and schizophrenia in Ireland: a comparison of first and readmissions. *Eur. Psychiatry*, **14**: 251–255.

156. D'Mello D.A., McNeil J.A., Msibi B. (1995) Seasons and bipolar disorder. *Ann. Clin. Psychiatry*, **7**: 11–18.

157. Kerr-Correa F., Souza L.B., Calil H.M. (1998) Affective disorders, hospital admissions, and seasonal variation of mania in a subtropical area, southern hemisphere. *Psychopathology*, **31**: 265–269.

158. Faedda G.L., Tondo L., Teicher M.H., Baldessarini R.J., Gelbard H.A., Floris G.F. (1993) Seasonal mood disorders. Patterns of seasonal recurrence in mania and depression. *Arch. Gen. Psychiatry*, **50**: 17–23.

159. Myers D.H., Davies P. (1978) The seasonal incidence of mania and its relationship to climatic variables. *Psychol. Med.*, **8**: 433–440.

160. Symonds R.L., Williams P. (1976) Seasonal variation in the incidence of mania. *Br. J. Psychiatry*, **129**: 45–48.

161. Wehr T.A., Sack D.A., Rosenthal N.E. (1987) Seasonal affective disorder with summer depression and winter hypomania. *Am. J. Psychiatry*, **144**: 1602–1603.

162. Takei N., O'Callaghan E., Sham P., Glover G., Tamura A., Murray R. (1992) Seasonality of admissions in the psychoses: effect of diagnosis, sex, and age at onset. *Br. J. Psychiatry*, **161**: 506–511.
163. Thompson C., Stinson D., Fernandez M., Fine J., Isaacs G. (1988) A comparison of normal, bipolar and seasonal affective disorder subjects using the Seasonal Pattern Assessment Questionnaire. *J. Affect. Disord.*, **14**: 257–264.
164. Marneros A., Tsuang M.T. (Eds) (1986) *Schizoaffective Psychoses*. Springer, Berlin.
165. Marneros A., Andreasen N.C., Tsuang M.T. (Eds) (1995) *Psychotic Continuum*. Springer, Berlin.
166. Maj M., Pirozzi R., Formicola A.M., Bartoli L., Bucci P. (2000) Reliability and validity of the DSM-IV diagnostic category of schizoaffective disorder: preliminary data. *J. Affect. Disord.*, **57**: 95–98.
167. Marneros A., Deister A., Rohde A., Junemann H. (1989) Unipolar and bipolar schizoaffective disorders: a comparative study. III. Long-term outcome. *Eur. Arch. Psychiatry Neurol. Sci.*, **239**: 171–176.
168. Marneros A., Rohde A., Deister A. (1989) Unipolar and bipolar schizoaffective disorders: a comparative study. II. Long-term course. *Eur. Arch. Psychiatry Neurol. Sci.*, **239**: 164–170.
169. Marneros A., Deister A., Rohde A. (1989) Unipolar and bipolar schizoaffective disorders: a comparative study. I. Premorbid and sociodemographic features. *Eur. Arch. Psychiatry Neurol. Sci.*, **239**: 158–163.
170. Marneros A., Deister A., Rohde A. (2000) Bipolar schizoaffective disorders. In *Bipolar Disorders: 100 Years After Manic-Depressive Insanity* (Eds A. Marneros, J. Angst), pp. 111–126, Kluwer, Dordrecht.
171. Guze S.B., Robins E. (1970) Suicide and primary affective disorders. *Br. J. Psychiatry*, **117**: 437–438.
172. Jamison K.R. (1986) Suicide and bipolar disorders. *Ann. N.Y. Acad. Sci.*, **487**: 301–315.
173. Inskip H.M., Harris E.C., Barraclough B. (1998) Lifetime risk of suicide for affective disorder, alcoholism and schizophrenia. *Br. J. Psychiatry*, **172**: 35–37.
174. Simpson S.G., Jamison K.R. (1999) The risk of suicide in patients with bipolar disorders. *J. Clin. Psychiatry*, **60**: 53–56.
175. Bostwick J.M., Pankratz V.S. (2000) Affective disorders and suicide risk: a reexamination. *Am. J. Psychiatry*, **157**: 1925–1932.
176. Ösby U., Brandt L., Correia N., Ekbom A., Sparén P. (2001) Excess mortality in bipolar and unipolar disorder in Sweden. *Arch. Gen. Psychiatry*, **58**: 844–850.
177. Potash J.B., Kane H.S., Chiu Y.F., Simpson S.G., MacKinnon D.F., McInnis M.G., McMahon F.J., DePaulo J.R., Jr. (2000) Attempted suicide and alcoholism in bipolar disorder: clinical and familial relationships. *Am. J. Psychiatry*, **157**: 2048–2050.
178. Tondo L., Baldessarini R.J., Hennen J., Minnai G.P., Salis P., Scamonatti L., Masia M., Ghiani C., Mannu P. (1999) Suicide attempts in major affective disorder patients with comorbid substance use disorders. *J. Clin. Psychiatry*, **60**: 63–69.
179. Waller S.J., Lyons J.S., Costantini-Ferrando M.F. (1999) Impact of comorbid affective and alcohol use disorders on suicidal ideation and attempts. *J. Clin. Psychol.*, **55**: 585–595.
180. Black D.W., Winokur G., Nasrallah A. (1988) Effect of psychosis on suicide risk in 1,593 patients with unipolar and bipolar affective disorders. *Am. J. Psychiatry*, **145**: 849–852.

181. Cassidy F., Murry E., Forest K., Carroll B.J. (1998) Signs and symptoms of mania in pure and mixed episodes. *J. Affect. Disord.*, **50**: 187–201.
182. Dilsaver S.C., Chen Y.W., Swann A.C., Shoaib A.M., Krajewski K.J. (1994) Suicidality in patients with pure and depressive mania. *Am. J. Psychiatry*, **151**: 1312–1315.
183. Dilsaver S.C., Chen Y.W., Swann A.C., Shoaib A.M., Tsai-Dilsaver Y., Krajewski K.J. (1997) Suicidality, panic disorder and psychosis in bipolar depression, depressive-mania and pure-mania. *Psychiatry Res.*, **73**: 47–56.
184. Goldberg J.F., Garno J.L., Leon A.C., Kocsis J.H., Portera L. (1998) Association of recurrent suicidal ideation with nonremission from acute mixed mania. *Am. J. Psychiatry*, **155**: 1753–1755.
185. Goldberg J.F., Garno J.L., Portera L., Leon A.C., Kocsis J.H., Whiteside J.E. (1999) Correlates of suicidal ideation in dysphoric mania. *J. Affect. Disord.*, **56**: 75–81.
186. Strakowski S.M., McElroy S.L., Keck P.E., Jr., West S.A. (1996) Suicidality among patients with mixed and manic bipolar disorder. *Am. J. Psychiatry*, **153**: 674–676.
187. Oquendo M.A., Waternaux C., Brodsky B., Parsons B., Haas G.L., Malone K.M., Mann J.J. (2000) Suicidal behavior in bipolar mood disorder: clinical characteristics of attempters and nonattempters. *J. Affect. Disord.*, **59**: 107–117.
188. Wu L.H., Dunner D.L. (1993) Suicide attempts in rapid cycling bipolar disorder patients. *J. Affect. Disord.*, **29**: 57–61.
189. Schou M. (1999) Perspectives on lithium treatment of bipolar disorder: action, efficacy, effect on suicidal behavior. *Bipolar Disord.*, **1**: 5–9.
190. Greil W., Ludwig-Mayerhofer W., Erazo N., Schochlin C., Schmidt S., Engel R.R., Czernik A., Giedke H., Müller-Oerlinghausen B., Osterheider M. *et al* (1997) Lithium versus carbamazepine in the maintenance treatment of bipolar disorders—A randomised study. *J. Affect. Disord.*, **43**: 151–161.
191. Coppen A., Farmer R. (1998) Suicide mortality in patients on lithium maintenance therapy. *J. Affect. Disord.*, **50**: 261–267.
192. Kallner G., Lindelius R., Petterson U., Stockman O., Tham A. (2000) Mortality in 497 patients with affective disorders attending a lithium clinic or after having left it. *Pharmacopsychiatry*, **33**: 8–13.
193. Nilsson A. (1995) Mortality in recurrent mood disorders during periods on and off lithium. A complete population study in 362 patients. *Pharmacopsychiatry*, **28**: 8–13.
194. Müller-Oerlinghausen B., Wolf T., Ahrens B., Glaenz T., Schou M., Grof E., Grof P., Lenz G., Simhandl C., Thau K. *et al* (1996) Mortality of patients who dropped out from regular lithium prophylaxis: a collaborative study by the International Group for the Study of Lithium-treated patients (IGSLI). *Acta Psychiatr. Scand.*, **94**: 344–347.
195. Sharma R., Markar H.R. (1994) Mortality in affective disorder. *J. Affect. Disord.*, **31**: 91–96.
196. Pratt L.A., Ford D.E., Crum R.M., Armenian H.K., Gallo J.J., Eaton W.W. (1996) Depression, psychotropic medication, and risk of myocardial infarction. Prospective data from the Baltimore ECA follow-up. *Circulation*, **94**: 3123–3129.
197. Ahrens B., Müller-Oerlinghausen B., Schou M., Wolf T., Alda M., Grof E., Grof P., Lenz G., Simhandl C., Thau K. *et al* (1995) Excess cardiovascular and suicide mortality of affective disorders may be reduced by lithium prophylaxis. *J. Affect. Disord.*, **33**: 67–75.

198. Barrick C.B. (1999) Sad, glad, or mad hearts? Epidemiological evidence for a causal relationship between mood disorders and coronary artery disease. *J. Affect. Disord.*, **53**: 193–201.

199. Müller-Oerlinghausen B., Wolf T., Ahrens B., Schou M., Grof E., Grof P., Lenz G., Simhandl C., Thau K., Wolf R. (1994) Mortality during initial and during later lithium treatment. A collaborative study by the International Group for the Study of Lithium-treated Patients. *Acta Psychiatr. Scand.*, **90**: 295–297.

200. Ahrens B., Grof P., Moller H.J., Müller-Oerlinghausen B., Wolf T. (1995) Extended survival of patients on long-term lithium treatment. *Can. J. Psychiatry*, **40**: 241–246.

201. Sonne S.C., Brady K.T. (1999) Substance abuse and bipolar disorder. *Psychiatr. Clin. North Am.*, **22**: 609–627.

202. McElroy S.L., Altshuler L.L., Suppes T., Keck P.E., Jr., Frye M.A., Denicoff K.D., Nolen W.A., Kupka R.W., Leverich G.S., Rochussen J.R. *et al* (2001) Axis I psychiatric comorbidity and its relationship to historical illness variables in 288 patients with bipolar disorder. *Am. J. Psychiatry*, **158**: 420–426.

203. Regier D.A., Farmer M.E., Rae D.S., Locke B.Z., Keith S.J., Judd L.L., Goodwin F.K. (1990) Comorbidity of mental disorders with alcohol and other drug abuse. Results from the Epidemiologic Catchment Area (ECA) Study. *JAMA*, **264**: 2511–2518.

204. Kessler R.C., Nelson C.B., McGonagle K.A., Edlund M.J., Frank R.G., Leaf P.J. (1996) The epidemiology of co-occurring addictive and mental disorders: implications for prevention and service utilization. *Am. J. Orthopsychiatry*, **66**: 17–31.

205. Sonne S.C., Brady K.T., Morton W.A. (1994) Substance abuse and bipolar affective disorder. *J. Nerv. Ment. Dis.*, **182**: 349–352.

206. Feinman J.A., Dunner D.L. (1996) The effect of alcohol and substance abuse on the course of bipolar affective disorder. *J. Affect. Disord.*, **37**: 43–49.

207. Goldberg J.F., Garno J.L., Leon A.C., Kocsis J.H., Portera L. (1999) A history of substance abuse complicates remission from acute mania in bipolar disorder. *J. Clin. Psychiatry*, **60**: 733–740.

208. Kessing L.V. (1999) The effect of comorbid alcoholism on recurrence in affective disorder: a case register study. *J. Affect. Disord.*, **53**: 49–55.

209. O'Sullivan K., Rynne C., Miller J., O'Sullivan S., Fitzpatrick V., Hux M., Cooney J., Clare A. (1988) A follow-up study on alcoholics with and without co-existing affective disorder. *Br. J. Psychiatry*, **152**: 813–819.

210. Winokur G., Coryell W., Akiskal H.S., Maser J.D., Keller M.B., Endicott J., Mueller T. (1995) Alcoholism in manic-depressive (bipolar) illness: familial illness, course of illness, and the primary-secondary distinction. *Am. J. Psychiatry*, **152**: 365–372.

211. Strakowski S.M., McElroy S.L., Keck P.E., Jr., West S.A. (1996) The effects of antecedent substance abuse on the development of first-episode psychotic mania. *J. Psychiatr. Res.*, **30**: 59–68.

212. Jamison K.R. (1995) *An Unquiet Mind. A Memoir of Mood and Madness.* Vintage Books, New York.

Commentaries

2.1
Studies of Course and Outcome in Bipolar Disorder: What is the Real-World Clinical Significance?

Peter P. Roy-Byrne and John Neumaier[1]

Over the past decade, there has been an increasing focus on specifying the applicability of research findings for routine clinical practice [1]. Most of these efforts have focused on treatment studies, where narrowly circumscribed patient populations and intensive clinical trial assessment and monitoring usually do not resemble the wider groups of patients and modes of service delivery typically seen in most clinical settings. However, this perspective likely has broader significance, and might also apply to findings generated in studies of phenomenology, experimental psychopathology, neurobiology and genetics.

In this vein, we ask the question: what is the real-world significance of the extensive body of knowledge on prognosis in bipolar illness, masterfully reviewed by Marneros and Brieger? To be sure, this is one of the most relevant research areas for both patients and clinicians. The major concern all bipolar patients have, almost from the first consultation, is what course their illness will take over time and what their chances are for recovery. For clinicians, knowledge of course of illness is indispensable for making a proper diagnosis, as well as for evaluating the effects of any treatments.

These studies, in their naturalistic form, are probably much more reflective of routine clinical practice than more tightly controlled and internally valid treatment studies. As the feasibility of entering bipolar patients in randomized clinical trials decreases [2], at least in the United States, such studies will take on more importance as a major tool to promote evidence-based medical treatment for this complex patient population. At the same time, the focus on treatment-seeking patients, the increasingly shorter term perspective and mirror-image design of more modern studies, the use of research centres which do not reflect real-world clinical practice, and a study intensity which creates subject burden that eliminates patients with more malignant illness, all compromise the generalizability of such studies.

[1] Department of Psychiatry and Behavioral Sciences, University of Washington at Harborview Medical Center, Box 359911, 325 9th Avenue, Seattle, Washington 98104, USA

What do these studies tell us? Marneros and Brieger provide a laundry list of summary statements out of which several relevant issues can be distilled. Regardless of the type of study, the era it came from, or the presence or absence of lithium treatment, there seems to be a subgroup of 15–30% of patients with chronic illness and poor outcome. This certainly makes sense and is consistent with the proportion of poor prognosis patients in other areas of medicine. However, the specific clinical characteristics of this group remain unclear. Suggestions that patients with depression-predominant bipolar disorder disproportionately fall into this group may be an artefact of the relatively poor antidepressant efficacy of commonly used mood stabilizers and could change with the introduction of newer agents with more antidepressant potency (e.g. lamotrigine). In fact, the inconsistent evidence implicating mixed states as a poor prognostic sign may reflect not just variations in definition, as the authors suggest, but also newer treatments (US centres failing to find that mixed states had a poorer outcome were among those with high utilization of sodium valproate, suggested by some studies as having particular efficacy in mixed and rapid-cycling subtypes). Similarly, determining whether comorbid substance abuse worsens prognosis will likely depend on patients' access to, and the availability of, state-of-the-art dual diagnosis treatment programmes [3]. Clearly we are at a point where carefully documenting the presence and adequacy of treatment will be a part of future naturalistic studies. However, the tendency for sicker patients to increasingly receive more intensive treatment, at least in the managed care markets in the US, will continue to confound study interpretations.

The authors nicely summarize the somewhat overblown controversy about whether lithium is effective in day-to-day practice. Clearly it is, although true relapse rates appear to be more consistent with the naturalistic Italian studies than earlier more tightly controlled and selective studies. The Chicago studies also highlight the fact that, when adherence is poor, comorbidity is extensive, and available resources are limited (as seen in this largely public-sector financed setting), outcome may be quite poor, even in the presence of recommendation and initiation of lithium treatment. Nonetheless, the number of studies supporting an effect of lithium on the most important of all outcomes, suicide, is impressive.

A few important areas were not touched on, in large part because available studies have not included them. Comorbid anxiety is more prevalent in bipolar patients than previously appreciated, and may be particularly associated with mixed states or other atypical forms of illness and longer time to recovery. Recent data suggests that over 40% of patients may have a comorbid anxiety disorder [4] and the more prominent anxiety presentation may obscure the true diagnosis and confuse clinicians, especially non-specialists, such as primary care medical providers, who likely see a large number of bipolar II patients who have not been hospitalized and do not present with frank manic symptoms. While it is clear that many patients have worsened cycling when exposed to antidepressants [5], these drugs remain an important component of current treatment of bipolar patients. It is not at all clear whether all bipolar patients have the same risk of antidepressant-induced cycling. The effect of antipsychotic medications on course of illness is a subject of controversy: while these medications are good anti-manic agents, they may promote or intensify depressive swings over the long haul, although recent evidence suggests that the atypical antipsychotic agents may be less likely to have this effect. Finally, the presence of cognitive impairment in bipolar patients, even when euthymic, is an understudied area that may have particular association with course and duration of illness, and be more likely to occur in later stages of the illness. Indeed, cognitive impairment may be either a symptom of bipolar disorder [6] or a consequence of treatment with mood stabilizer medications.

What is needed to move this area along and provide a firm scientific foundation for future investigations? Longer term studies, which might be less information intensive so that they can include a wider spectrum of patients, would be highly desirable. It is likely that the absence of any relationship between socio-economic status (SES) and prognosis is due to the absence of many low SES patients with malignant course of illness in many studies. It is highly unlikely that bipolar illness would stand alone, in contrast to depression and schizophrenia, as a condition that is not more prevalent or malignant in course in low SES patients [7]. More careful documentation and consideration of treatment effects on course of illness in naturalistic studies will be crucial to maximize generalizability and interpretability of results. While studies in specialty treatment clinics can describe patients receiving uniform treatment and therefore be more able to discern relationships between other predictors and course of illness, such studies may be less applicable to the broad range of patients who present to routine clinical settings and adhere to treatment to varying degrees. At least in the US, many bipolar patients will continue to have deficient access to appropriate treatment (i.e. sufficient specialist skill and intensity of monitoring), being followed in either case management intensive community mental health clinics with marginal psychiatric coverage or primary care settings with limited specialist access. Even patients being treated directly by private psychiatrists, depending on their level of illness acuity, may receive less optimal treatment as clinicians develop a siege mentality, trying to somehow survive successive crisis without time to appreciate the overall course of illness and the effects of treatment on it. We have not yet defined type and proper balance of expert psychopharmacology, psychosocial and case management services, and substance abuse treatment to meet the needs of a broad spectrum of individuals. While we now presume that careful observation of clinical phenomenology will lead to reliable predictors of prognosis, it is possible that, when we have a better grasp of the biological determinants of bipolar symptoms, we will discover that these are a family of disorders that can be better organized based on factors closer to cellular pathology underlying the illness, than behavioural symptoms [8].

REFERENCES

1. Wells K.B. (1999) Treatment research at the crossroads: the scientific interface of clinical trials and effectiveness research. *Am. J. Psychiatry*, **156**: 5–10.
2. Calabrese J.R., Rapport D.J., Shelton M.D., Kimmel S.E. (2001) Evolving methodologies in bipolar disorder maintenance research. *Br. J. Psychiatry*, **178**: 157–163.
3. Sonne S.C., Brady K.T. (1999) Substance abuse and bipolar comorbidity. *Psychiatr. Clin. North Am.*, **22**: 609–627.
4. McElroy S.L., Altshuler L., Suppes T., Keck P.E., Jr., Frye M.A., Denicoff K.D., Nolen W.A., Kupka R.W., Leverich G.S., Rochussen J.R. *et al* (2001) Axis I psychiatric comorbidity and its relationship with historical illness variables in 288 patients with bipolar disorder. *Am. J. Psychiatry*, **158**: 420–426.
5. Altshuler L.L., Post R.M., Leverich G.S., Mikalauskas K., Rosoff A., Ackerman L. (1995) Antidepressant-induced mania and cycle acceleration: a controversy revisited. *Am. J. Psychiatry*, **152**: 1130–1138.
6. Van Gorp W.G., Altshuler L., Theberge D.C., Wilkins J., Dixon W. (1998) Cognitive impairment in euthymic bipolar patients with and without prior alcohol dependence. *Arch. Gen. Psychiatry*, **55**: 41–46.
7. Kessler R.C., Rubinow D.R., Holmes C., Abelson J.M., Zhao S. (1997) The epidemiology of DSM-III-R bipolar disorder in a general population survey. *Psychol. Med.*, **27**: 1079–1089.
8. Manji H.K., Lenox R.H. (2000) Signaling: cellular insights into the pathophysiology of bipolar disorder. *Biol. Psychiatry*, **48**: 518–530.

2.2
Understanding Outcome Differences in Bipolar Disorder

Ming T. Tsuang and William S. Stone[1]

Marneros and Brieger provide an interesting and informative state-of-the-art perspective on the prognosis of bipolar disorder. At this juncture, converging evidence from multiple studies supports an interim consensus on several points. Among the more fundamental of these are that bipolar

[1] *Harvard Department of Psychiatry at Massachusetts Mental Health Center, 74 Fenwood Road, Boston, MA 02115, USA*

disorder is a recurring, lifelong disorder that shows striking individual differences in the severity and duration of its symptoms, and in its course, response to treatment, and prognosis. Another fundamental feature is that our concept of the disorder is defined largely by its course. For example, higher numbers of previous episodes predict higher numbers of future episodes, and more negative outcomes. Rapid cycling, low premorbid levels of function, comorbid substance abuse, and schizoaffective symptoms also predict more negative courses of illness, as might be expected. Interestingly, however, many social and demographic variables, like age, age of onset, and gender, have little predictive power.

Our current reliance on clinical symptoms for the diagnosis of bipolar disorder has been extremely useful. The major classification systems, including DSM and ICD, have greatly increased both the reliability and the validity of psychiatric diagnosis, generally. Moreover, unlike the situation for schizophrenia, which relies more heavily on the presence of psychotic symptoms for diagnosis [1], bipolar disorder may also be diagnosed in the presence or absence of psychosis. This reduces the risk for florid, relatively non-specific psychotic symptoms to obscure more subtle etiological differences between individuals. Nevertheless, many features of bipolar disorder remain unclear, such as the identification of factors that lead to positive or negative outcomes, and even more generally, the sources of broad differences in individual outcomes. This is particularly salient for an eventual understanding of the biological etiology and development of the disorder, and ultimately, for the development of strategies aimed at early intervention and prevention. Thus, while our current conception of bipolar disorder reflects considerable progress, especially in its diagnostic reliability, perhaps its validity can be improved upon.

A brief perspective on the biological etiology of bipolar disorder illustrates these points further. Data from family, twin and adoption studies provide clear evidence for a significant genetic component to the disorder; concordance rates in monogygotic twins, for example, are approximately three times higher than they are in dizygotic twins [2]. Yet, while molecular genetic studies (e.g., linkage studies) have identified chromosomal regions of interest, individual genes that underlie the inheritance of bipolar disorder have yet to be identified. While there are many reasons for this state of affairs [2, 3], one of them involves the use of relatively non-specific clinical symptoms in genetic studies to determine whether subjects are or are not "affected". Tsuang et al [4] have argued for the use of heritable phenotypes in genetic studies, particularly in light of the variable phenotypic expression inherent in many clinical syndromes. Future genetic investigations of bipolar disorder may thus benefit from a focus on subclinical conditions or symptoms that share underlying genetic etiological factors. The goal of this strategy is to facilitate the detection of heritable features that are more proximal to their genetic underpinnings. The strategy could be implemented in several ways. Among these, milder disorders such as dysthymia and cyclothmia, or other conditions in the affective spectrum, may be considered. Another approach would be to study more biologically based measures such as neuropsychological, psychophysiological or neurochemical functions, or brain structures and function through neuroimaging.

These subclinical syndromes and potential neurobiological markers may have a genetic etiology that is simpler than DSM or ICD bipolar disorder. If so, their use could facilitate the detection of genes for the disorder, and eventually of the proteins they code for. This will likely advance our understanding of the biological basis of individual differences in bipolar disorder. Hopefully, it will also lead to new treatments, in at least two ways. First, the identification of previously unidentified proteins in the disorder will provide new treatment targets. Second, the use of neurobiological markers and subclinical syndromes may help identify individuals who are more or less vulnerable to different types of symptoms. More broadly, it will also aid in the identification of premorbid syndromes that reflect the liability for bipolar disorder. This is a research direction that is receiving considerable attention in schizophrenia [1], but less so in affective disorders. Eventually, the identification of more homogeneous treatment groups will facilitate efforts to develop strategies aimed at the early intervention, and even prevention, of bipolar disorder. Clearly, we are not yet at that point. Nevertheless, as Marneros and Brieger's review reminds us, we now have very good clinical descriptions of the disorder to guide our next steps.

REFERENCES

1. Tsuang M.T., Stone W.S., Faraone S.V. (2000) Towards reformulating the diagnosis of schizophrenia. *Am. J. Psychiatry*, **157**: 1041–1050.
2. Tsuang M.T., Faraone S.V. (2000) The genetic epidemiology of bipolar disorder. In *Bipolar Disorders: 100 Years After Manic-Depressive Insanity* (Eds A. Marneros, J. Angst), pp. 231–242, Kluwer, Dordrecht.
3. Tsuang M.T., Stone W.S., Faraone S.V. (1999) Schizophrenia: a review of genetic studies. *Harvard Rev. Psychiatry*, **7**: 185–207.
4. Tsuang M.T., Faraone S.V., Lyons M.J. (1993) Identification of the phenotype in psychiatric genetics. *Eur. Arch. Psychiatry Clin. Neurosci.*, **243**: 131–142.

2.3
The Effect of Affective Episodes in Bipolar Disorder

Lars Vedel Kessing[1]

Marneros and Brieger present a broad review of the course and outcome of bipolar disorder and its predictors. The present commentary focuses on the effect of episodes on the risk of recurrence and on predictors of outcome. Longer term studies of patients with bipolar disorder are hampered by numerous methodological problems: selection bias in inclusion of the most ill patients, bias in recall of prior affective episodes, information bias due to selective drop out from studies of the most ill patients, confounding by comorbidity, diagnostic change over time, the effect of treatment, etc., which may affect the results in unpredictable ways [1]. The most serious drawback is, however, that most studies do not pay attention to the number of affective episodes in the analyses of predictors of course and outcome. The importance of considering the effect of prior episodes in analyses of the predictive effect of a variable has been emphasized by Hahighat [2] and Kessing [1, 3] and illustrated by Kessler and Magee [4], who presented examples of how the inclusion of the episode number in statistical analyses in various studies changed the results. Not paying attention to the number of episodes in the analyses is an error (the so-called "Slaters fallacy" [2]), due to two factors: a) within a given observation period, the time under risk for experiencing new events (episodes or outcome) will be reduced for every new episode; b) patients with many episodes will dominate the analyses. Regarding analyses of time to recurrence, each factor will have the implication that the average time between episodes will decrease with each new episode and thus analyses will result in artificially findings of a progressive course with decreasing intervals between affective episodes. The first factor may be compensated for by using survival statistics in the analyses, as time under risk hereby is considered, and the second factor by using analyses which take the individual heterogeneity into account.

Marneros and Brieger claim, as Angst et al [5] and Winokur et al [6], that it is more reliable to assess length of cycles than length of intervals between episodes, as they find it more reliable to assess the onset of an episode than the end. However, cycle lengths cannot be used in proper analyses of time to recurrence in which survival statistics have to be used, as a patient cannot be under risk for experiencing recurrence as long as he has an episode. Furthermore, it is not possible to discriminate between time to relapse and time to recurrence with cycle lengths, since cycle lengths provide a combined

[1] Department of Psychiatry, Rigshsopitalet University of Copenhagen, Blegdamsvej 9, 2100 Copenhagen Ø, Denmark

measure of relapse (into previous episodes) and recurrence (into new episodes). Finally, with the extensive modern outpatient treatment, the onset will often be less abrupt and symptoms will be suppressed both at the beginning and at the end of an episode, which is why the interval length is likely to be as reliable a measure as the cycle length [7].

Two studies of bipolar disorder have paid attention to the number of episodes in the analyses, however, not using survival analyses. In the international co-operative study reported by Angst et al [5] and in re-analyses of the Zurich study [8], it was found that the length of cycles decreased with increasing number of episodes when data were analysed within strata of patients with a similar number of episodes. So far only one long-term study has been published paying attention to the number of episodes and using survival statistics in the analyses of the risk of recurrence in patients with bipolar disorder [7]. This study identified all patients in Denmark who were first ever hospitalized with a bipolar disorder during 23 years and analysed time to recurrence (readmission after having been discharged eight weeks) following each new episode. The risk of recurrence was consistently found to increase with every new episode. Analyses with the use of frailty models, which take the individual tendency (the frailty) toward recurrence into account, confirmed the findings, although the effect of episodes was found to be moderately reduced [3].

Data from the Zurich and from the National Institute of Mental Health (NIMH) studies are currently being re-analysed with similar methods taking the individual liability into account. Such analyses from the NIMH study have recently been published regarding patients with recurrent depression and revealed an effect of episodes even after adjustment for the individual heterogeneity [9] and for both genders [10].

Several studies have consistently found that the risk of recurrence is greater for bipolar patients than for unipolar patients, although several findings suggest that the difference vanishes during the course of illness, so that the risk of recurrence is similarly high for the two disorders following the fourth or fifth episode [7]. It should be noted that the effect of episodes seems to be greater for unipolar patients than for bipolar patients. In the Danish case register study, the risk of recurrence increased 15% for unipolar and 9% for bipolar patients with each episode [11]. Angst [12] found the same relationship in his 16-year prospective study of 159 unipolar and 95 bipolar patients: the length of each cycle shortened 10% in unipolar disorder and 5% in bipolar disorder with each episode. Time to death or time to dropout caused by loss of follow-up were not included in Angst's calculations, while these were included in the survival analyses in the Danish study.

The question of whether there is an effect of episodes on the course and outcome is crucial for the understanding of affective disorder and for guidance of the patients. As Marneros and Brieger conclude, there is still a need for more studies regarding the effect of episodes (however, using the interval between episodes as a measure rather than cycle lengths). The studies should include analyses with advanced survival statistics taking the individual heterogeneity of the course of the disorder into account.

Another central aspect of the disorder is the demarcation in relation to unipolar disorder (single and recurrent depressive episodes). The intriguing problem of having an illness defined according to time is nearly unbearable (a patient is diagnosed as unipolar as long as he has not developed a manic or mixed episode and from that time he is diagnosed as bipolar). Apparently there are some patients with unipolar disorder who behave like patients with bipolar disorder, even before they develop their first manic episode—with an early age of onset at first episode and with a tendency to fast recurrence from onset of the illness [13, 14]. Are these patients "false" bipolars as long as they have not presented with mania? The central question whether unipolar and bipolar disorder constitute two different illnesses remains unanswered.

REFERENCES

1. Kessing L.V. (2001)   Course and cognitive outcome in major affective disorder. Doctoral dissertation. Lægeforeningens forlag, Copenhagen.
2. Haghighat R. (1996)   Lifelong development of risk of recurrence in depressive disorders. *J. Affect. Disord.*, **41**: 141–147.
3. Kessing L.V., Olsen E.W., Andersen P.K. (1999)   Recurrence in affective disorder—analyses with frailty models. *Am. J. Epidemiol.*, **149**: 404–411.
4. Kessler R.C., Magee W.J. (1994)   The disaggregation of vulnerability to depression as a function of the determinants of onset and recurrence. In *Stress and Mental Health. Contemporary Issues and Prospects for the Future* (Eds W.R. Avison, I.A. Gotlieb), pp. 239–258, Plenum Press, New York.
5. Angst J., Baastrup P., Grof P., Hippius H., Pöldinger W., Weiss P. (1973)   The course of monopolar depression and bipolar psychoses. *Psychiatry Neurol. Neurochir.*, **76**: 489–500.
6. Winokur G., Coryell W., Akiskal H.S., Keller M., Mueller T. (1994)   Manic-depressive (bipolar) disorder: the course in the light of a prospective ten-year follow-up of 131 patients. *Acta Psychiatr. Scand.*, **89**: 102–110.
7. Kessing L.V., Andersen P.K., Mortensen P.B., Bolwig T.G. (1998)   Recurrence in affective disorder. I—A case register study. *Br. J. Psychiatry*, **172**: 23–28.
8. Angst J., Preisig M. (1995)   Course of a clinical cohort of unipolar, bipolar and schizoaffective patients. Results from a prospective study from 1959 to 1985. *Schweiz Arch. Neurol. Psychiatrie*, **146**: 5–16.
9. Solomon D.A., Keller M.B., Leon A.C., Mueller T.I., Lavori P.W., Shea M.T., Coryell W., Warshaw M., Turvey C., Maser J.D. *et al* (2000)   Multiple recurrences of major depressive disorder. *Am. J. Psychiatry*, **157**: 229–233.
10. Solomon D.A., Leon A.C., Mueller T.I., Shea M.T., Keller M.B. (2001)   Dr. Solomon and colleagues reply. *Am. J. Psychiatry*, **158**: 5.

11. Kessing L.V., Andersen P.K. (1999) The effect of episodes in affective disorder—a case register study. *J. Affect. Disord.*, **53**: 225–231.
12. Angst J. (1981) Course of affective disorders. In *Handbook of Biological Psychiatry. Part 5. Brain mechanisms and abnormal behaviour* (Ed. E.J. Sachar), pp. 225–242, Dekker, New York.
13. Kessing L.V. (1999) The effect of the first manic episode in affective disorder—a case register study. *J. Affect. Disord.*, **53**: 233–239.
14. Winokur G. Tsuang M.T. (1996) *The Natural History of Mania, Depression, and Schizophrenia*. American Psychiatric Press, Washington.

2.4
Bipolar Disorder: A Longitudinal Perspective

Gabriele S. Leverich[1]

As Marneros and Brieger's comprehensive review of the differentiation and classification of affective disorders demonstrates, no single definition can accurately describe or quantify the pleomorphic and frequently progressive course of bipolar disorder. As the authors point out, differing approaches to episode delineation (e.g. monophasic, biphasic, polyphasic), the definition of remission (e.g. syndromatic, symptomatic, and functional recovery), and the categorization of cycling frequency represent only some examples of the divergent concepts applied to the study of bipolar illness. Many assessment tools are available that arrive at a comprehensive Axis I diagnosis, such as the Structured Clinical Interview for DSM-III-R (SCID), the Schedule for Affective Disorders and Schizophrenia (SADS), the Research Diagnostic Criteria (RDC) and others, as well as scales that intermittently measure depressive or manic symptoms for predetermined time periods, such as the Hamilton Rating Scale for Depression (HRSD) or the Young Mania Rating Scale (YMRS). The continuous assessment of the long-term course of bipolar disorder, however, has been hindered by lack of a methodology to record and codify systematically and comprehensively the retrospective and prospective course of illness to facilitate evaluation of the longitudinal unfolding of the affective disorders, the relationship of psychosocial stressors to illness onset and episode recurrence, and, most importantly, the degree of response to treatment. This, in turn, has led to significant controversies in the design of clinical trials appropriate to the variegated course of bipolar disorder and thus to a paucity of clinical trials in this potentially lethal medical illness.

[1] *National Institute of Mental Health, Biological Psychiatry Branch, Bethesda, Maryland 20892–1272, USA*

Based on the Kraepelinian concept of life charting [1], we developed the retrospective and prospective National Institute of Mental Health (NIMH)-Life Chart Method (NIMH-LCM℠) or LCM, which implements a schema of manic and depressive severity based on the degree of mood-related functional incapacity [2, 3]. Life charts make no *a priori* assumptions about course of illness, but allow for a continuous precise delineation, which helps confirm diagnosis, identify subtypes of the disorder, and promote elucidation of illness patterns that do not meet traditional criteria, such as brief recurrent depressions or hypomanias, including ultrarapid and ultradian cycling.

Briefly, course of illness is charted at three severity levels retrospectively and four levels prospectively, with manic episodes above and depressive episodes below a date line, which also signifies baseline or euthymic mood. Treatments are coded above the episodes, while comorbidities and psychosocial stressors are intercalated below. The time domain for retrospective assessment is a month, while prospective ratings are daily and are based on the patient's self-rated daily LCM when available or reconstructed with the clinician in an integrative interview. Manuals and a software program have been created for the LCM. Its utility has been demonstrated in clinical trials [4], together with its ability to allow for attribution of dysfunction separately to manic and depressive illness phases by providing a comprehensive topography of the illness based on daily ratings in prospective follow-up. A detailed portrayal of the degree of morbidity is provided by the LCM ratings, and it is interesting to note that in the study of Denicoff *et al* (1997) even a monthly administered HRSD missed six of eight moderately severe depressions in a moderately cycling patient over a one-year period [5]. In another study, using careful retrospective life charting, we found that bipolar patients with a more severe prior course of illness and a greater number of affective episodes performed more poorly (although in a relatively euthymic state at the time of testing) on performance tests of abstraction, attention, and memory [6].

The LCM has been validated against cross-sectional scales such as the HDRS, the Inventory of Depressive Symptomatology, Clinician Version (IDS-C), the YMRS, and the Global Assessment of Functioning (GAF) (5, 7) as part of our Stanley Foundation Bipolar Network (SFBN), a large, multisite network under the direction of Robert M. Post, which is dedicated to the assessment and treatment of bipolar disorders [8, 9]. The SFBN is now following 400 to 500 patients with bipolar disorder (approximately 78% are bipolar I) in naturalistic follow-up with open and blinded randomized clinical trials available for illness re-emergence.

Daily life charting is the core longitudinal instrument in the network and has enabled us to make detailed continuous observations of the pattern and severity in the first 258 outpatients during naturalistic treatment (according to prevailing standards in the community) followed for a year [10]. Marneros and Brieger elucidate and highlight the significant degree of morbidity in bipolar illness in many studies they reviewed. Our findings confirm the tremendous illness burden experienced by many bipolar patients; 26.8% of our outpatients were ill for more than three-quarters of the year, and 40.3% were intermittently ill. The remaining one-third of patients were relatively well for most of the year; however, only 11.2% were virtually illness free.

As part of the network's naturalistic follow-up we have also been able to examine the relationship of high severity early life stresses involving physical or sexual abuse in childhood and adolescence to the subsequent course of bipolar illness [11]. Of the 631 network patients who were evaluated, 24% endorsed a history of childhood/adolescent physical abuse and 25% a history of early sexual abuse. These individuals had experienced a more severe retrospective course of illness with a progressive increase in severity of mania and depression, an earlier illness onset, greater cycling frequencies, a higher incidence of suicide attempts, and increased Axis I and II comorbidities. The self-reports of a difficult prior course of illness were prospectively validated in a subgroup of 373 patients who had been followed prospectively for a mean of 2.8 years (range 1–5.7 years) with the daily LCM as well as cross-sectional ratings. In comparison to the non-abused group they experienced a greater percentage of time ill on the daily LCM and also on the IDS-C and YMRS. They also had more days of ultradian cycling as delineated on the LCM.

Studies in the network continue to look at prognosticators of course of illness, comorbidities, and novel treatment interventions. The hope is that the longitudinal description of the illness provided by the LCM can help resolve many of the ongoing controversies in the design of studies in bipolar illness and the assessment of treatments, so that this illness with its high degree of morbidity and mortality can be addressed in the most effective way to help ameliorate the suffering of our patients.

REFERENCES

1. Kraepelin E. (1921) *Manic-Depressive Insanity and Paranoia*. Livingstone, Edinburgh.
2. Leverich G.S., Post R.M. (1996) Life charting the course of bipolar disorder. *Current Review of Mood Disorders*, 1: 48–61.
3. Leverich G.S., Post R.M. (1998) Charting of affective illness. *CNS Spectrums*, 3: 21–37.
4. Denicoff K.D., Ali O.S., Sollinger A.B., Smith-Jackson E.E., Leverich G.S., Post R.M. (2001) Utility of the daily prospective National Institute of Mental Health Life Chart Method (NIMH-LCM) ratings in clinical trials of bipolar disorder. *Depress. Anxiety* (in press).

5. Denicoff K.D., Smith-Jackson E.E, Disney E.R., Suddath R.L., Leverich G.S., Post R.M. (1997) Preliminary evidence of the reliability and validity of the prospective life-chart methodology (LCMp). *J. Psychiatr. Res.*, **31**: 593–603.
6. Denicoff K.D., Ali S.O., Mirsky A.F., Smith-Jackson E.E., Leverich G.S, Duncan C.C., Connell E.G., Post R.M. (1999) Relationship between prior course of illness and neuropsychological functioning in patients with bipolar disorder. *J. Affect. Dis.*, **56**: 67–73.
7. Denicoff K.D., Leverich G.S., Nolen W.A., Rush A.J., McElroy S.L., Keck P.E., Jr., Suppes T., Altshuler L.L., Kupka R., Frye M.A. et al (2000) Validation of the prospective NIMH-Life Chart Method (NIMH-LCM^{TM}p) for longitudinal assessment of bipolar illness. *Psychol. Med.*, **30**: 1391–1397.
8. Leverich G.S., Nolen W.A., Rush A.J., McElroy S.L., Keck P.E., Jr., Denicoff K.D., Suppes.T., Altshuler L.L., Kupka R., Kramlinger K.G. et al (2001) The Stanley Foundation Bipolar Treatment Outcome Network: I. Longitudinal methodology. *J. Affect. Disord.* (in press).
9. Suppes T., Leverich G..S., Keck P.E., Jr., Nolen W.A., Denicoff K.D., Altshuler L.L., McElroy S.L., Rush A.J., Kupka R., Frye M.A. et al (2001) The Stanley Foundation Bipolar Treatment Outcome Network: II. Demographics and illness characteristics in the first 261 patients. *J. Affect. Disord.* (in press).
10. Post R.M., Denicoff K.D., Leverich G.S., Altshuler L.L., Frye M.A., Suppes T.M., Rush A.J., Keck P.E., Jr., McElroy S.L., Pollio C. et al (2001) Morbidity in 258 bipolar outpatients followed for one year with daily prospective ratings on the NIMH-LCM. Submitted for publication.
11. Leverich G.S., McElroy S.L., Suppes T., Keck P.E., Jr., Denicoff K.D., Nolen W.A., Altshuler L.L., Rush A.J., Kupka R., Frye, M.A. et al (2001) Early physical or sexual abuse and the course of bipolar illness. *Biol. Psychiatry* (in press).

2.5
Issues in the Assessment of Course of Illness in Bipolar Disorder

Leonardo Tondo[1]

Bipolar disorder is a recurrent, often severe, and sometimes disabling psychiatric illness marked by characteristic mood instability accompanied by changes in thinking and behaviour. Characterization of the course of the illness and the effects of maintenance treatment on long-term morbidity require prolonged longitudinal observations, as emphasized by Marneros and Brieger. The course can vary widely, from a single episode of mania to many recurrences of mania, depression, or mixed states, with or without psychotic features. Although even a single episode may have disruptive and lethal consequences, prognosis is best indicated by the number and severity of recurrences.

[1] *Department of Psychiatry, Harvard University—McLean Hospital, MRC 306, 115 Mill Street, Belmont, MA 02478, USA*

Marneros and Brieger review methods for clinical assessment and research on course and outcome in bipolar disorder, considering both the limitations and advantages of controlled vs. naturalistic study designs, and appropriately emphasizing the need to define and differentiate episodes and cycles, as well as to distinguish clinical and functional outcomes. They evaluate representative naturalistic studies of the course of bipolar disorder, including older and more recent studies of varying duration. The evaluation of course and outcome can be influenced not only by methodological and clinical factors, as well as setting of the study, but in the current psychopharmacological era it is also invariably confounded by treatments, especially long-term therapies, that surely affect the natural course of the illness [1].

The design of outcome and experimental therapeutic studies, to an extent, predetermines the results obtained [2]. For example, in controlled trials, patient-subjects must be competent to evaluate and accept some risk of new illness, and clinicians and review boards must weigh the greater risks in patient-subjects with a more severe past history. These requirements tend to exclude currently or previously severely manic or depressed and suicidal patients, or may bias toward less severely ill samples. Naturalistic studies may include a broader spectrum of illness severity and type than in controlled trials, but both study types are subject to uncontrolled, *differential* losses and retention of subjects over time as effects of emerging illness or intolerability of the specific treatment provided. Both study types also risk potential erosion of the quality and quantity of data, as well as rising logistical and cost considerations, with longer follow-up, as is required to fairly assess long-term course in an inherently unstable illness. Moreover, treatment-crossover designs and other protocols commonly involve rapid withdrawal from an ongoing active treatment. Consequences of such abrupt interruptions include increased probability of earlier recurrences or mania, depression, and suicidal acts than those occurring naturally in untreated illness, and far greater risks than when treatment remains uninterrupted [3].

Outcome measures in treatment-effectiveness studies in bipolar disorder usually rate occurrence of an episode of illness, time to a first recurrence of illness, or meeting a fixed criterion of response, commonly 50% reduction of episode frequency or of time ill during observation. Though such measures are attractive for their relatively simple quantifiability, they may be excessively narrow for an illness of variable course, with typically incomplete protection from future morbidity or disability regardless of the treatment provided. They can also miss clinically important, and common, partial responses, particularly as reflected in reduced frequency, duration, and severity of recurrences, and improved functional status [4].

The setting of a study will also affect the results obtained. Some settings involving opportunistic observations in moderately ill patients self-selected to remain in a closely supervised treatment programme may over-represent subjects with better prognoses, treatment adherence, and treatment responses. In some ordinary clinical settings or public institutions that manage a high proportion of very ill, highly comorbid, treatment-resistant, uncooperative, or infrequently followed patients, outcomes are often highly unfavourable [4]. However, either setting can yield highly misleading conclusions, particularly when compliance with treatment is a major uncontrolled variable [5].

In conclusion, studies of course and prognosis in bipolar disorder need to consider methodological, clinical, and treatment-related aspects of their designs very closely. Important considerations include sample characteristics, comorbidities, and methods of assessing and recording morbidity over time, as well as the type and duration of both specific and nonspecific therapeutic interventions, and finally treatment adherence. All these factors may ultimately influence the selection of the sample populations; therefore the published findings may not be generalized to all patients. Readers of reports of such studies should be able to estimate their quality in order to compare the results to their own experience and apply the findings to their practice.

REFERENCES

1. Koukopoulos A., Reginaldi D., Laddomada P., Floris G., Serra G., Tondo L. (1980) Course of the manic-depressive cycle and changes caused by treatments. *Pharmakopsychiat. Neuropharmakol.*, **13**: 156–167.
2. Guscott R., Taylor L. (1994) Lithium prophylaxis in recurrent affective illness. Efficacy, effectiveness and efficiency. *Br. J. Psychiatry*, **164**: 741–746.
3. Baldessarini R.J., Tondo L., Viguera A.C. (1999) Discontinuing lithium maintenance treatment in bipolar disorders: risks and implications. *Bipolar Disord.*, **1**: 17–24.
4. Baldessarini R.J., Tohen M., Tondo L. (2000) Maintenance treatment in bipolar disorder. *Arch. Gen. Psychiatry*, **57**: 490–492.
5. Brodersen A., Licht R.W., Vestergaard P., Olesen A.V., Mortensen P.B. (2000) Sixteen-year mortality in patients with affective disorder commenced on lithium. *Br. J. Psychiatry*, **176**: 429–433.

2.6
The Sustained Prospective Study: Is it Worth the Effort?

William Coryell[1]

Marneros and Brieger's comprehensive review reveals, among many other things, the scarcity of prospective follow-up studies with multiple assessments and a sustained observation beyond 10 years. Of nine studies listed as modern and long-term, only two meet these criteria—the National Institute of Mental Health (NIMH) Collaborative Depression Study (CDS) [1, 2] and the Zurich Study [3, 4]. The lengthy commitment required to conduct such studies accounts for their rarity. Why is it important that there be, nevertheless, more of them?

The advantages of a naturalistic design lie in feasibility and generalizability. The selection biases resulting from efforts to control treatment through protocols of even one or two months' duration are widely appreciated. Because clinicians deal almost exclusively with treatment-seeking patients, they easily forget that many individuals with major affective disorder seek treatment for some episodes but not others. Though all patients in the CDS study were recruited at treatment facilities during their index episodes, nearly one-third (31.8%) of those with major depressive disorders received no somatic treatment in their next prospectively observed episode [1]. The decision to seek treatment is, of course, not a random one and is driven largely by episode severity and persistence [2]. This gives rise to the "clinician's illusion" in which clinicians perceive illnesses as more chronic than, in fact, they are [5].

Moreover, certain patient characteristics, such as substance abuse and impulsivity, will influence both the course of illness, under any treatment circumstance, and the likelihood of compliance with, for instance, lithium. The increase in mortality described for patients who leave lithium clinics may therefore reflect factors other than the absence of lithium.

The term "prospective" generally implies that a uniform assessment of patient characteristics took place at the beginning of follow-up. Retrospective follow-ups must ascertain the variables necessary for diagnosis and outcome prediction from medical records. The irregular omission of specific variables makes the generation of replicable results much less likely.

Most of the lengthier, prospective, studies have employed repeated assessments during follow-up. The presence of memory artefacts makes this an extremely important feature if the course of a remitting illness is to be mapped accurately. Evidence for this is of several sorts.

In the CDS, a large group of relatives and spouses of probands, as well as a group of unrelated controls, were interviewed as the probands entered the

[1] University of Iowa College of Medicine, Psychiatry Research/2–205 MEB, Iowa City, IA 52242–1000, USA

study, and again six years later, this time by a rater blind to the results of the first interview. Of those who described a lifetime history of major depressive disorder, mania or hypomania at the first interview, 3 in 4, 1 in 2, and 1 in 3, respectively, described such a history again six years later [6]. In an earlier, test-retest, reliability study, Andreasen et al [7] showed that the kappa for a lifetime diagnosis of mania fell from 1.0 for a same-day re-interview, to 0.88 and 0.48 when the interval between interviews was increased to six months and five years, respectively.

Prevalence data provide a particularly striking illustration of this problem. In the two largest American efforts to establish the prevalence of mental disorders, Weissman et al [8] reported the 12-month and lifetime prevalence rates of bipolar disorder were 1.0 and 1.2%, respectively. Using a very different study design, Kessler et al [9] likewise found that 12-month and lifetime rates for mania were nearly identical (1.3 and 1.6%, respectively).

The above findings underscore the intuitively obvious fact that the remoteness of an event will correlate with its memorability. Thus, in addition to the general inaccuracy introduced by asking patients about time distant episodes, a foreshortening effect on cycle length or interval between episodes is very provable. Because episodes from the distant past will be preferentially forgotten, the intervals between more recent episodes will appear to shorten. The widely discussed kindling effect [10] is based on assessments which were largely retrospective. It is not surprising, then, that Angst [11], whose follow-up was "predominantly prospective", found only shortening between the first and second cycles and none between cycles 2–5. Turvey et al [12], using data which was purely prospective, found no evidence for increasing episode frequency over time.

An extended observation period offers other unique opportunities when combined with a suitable assessment interval. As Marneros and Brieger note, short-term follow-ups underestimate the likelihood of remission and produce an inaccurately grim view of prognosis. All experienced clinicians have faced chronically depressed patients who desperately want to know if there is hope for recovery. Only an extended follow-up could show, as Mueller et al [13] did, that 38% of patients with five years of a perspectively documented and unrelenting major depressive disorder recovered at some point in the next five years of follow-up.

Only extended follow-ups can show whether a recurrent illness "burns out" over the years, whether and how certain subgroups gradually worsen, and whether life stages, i.e. early adulthood, middle age, and old age, have predictable effects on the persistence and quality of affective symptoms. Marneros and Brieger listed a number of well-designed, prospective follow-ups under "medium-term naturalistic studies". Hopefully, most of these investigators will find the funding and the resolve to extend their efforts beyond 10 years.

REFERENCES

1. Coryell W., Akiskal H.S., Leon A.C., Winokur G., Maser J.D., Mueller T.I., Keller M.B. (1994) The time course of nonchronic major depressive disorder. *Arch. Gen. Psychiatry*, **51**: 405–410.
2. Coryell W., Endicott J., Winokur G., Akiskal H., Solomon D., Leon A., Mueller T., Shea T. (1995) Characteristics and significance of untreated major depressive disorder. *Am. J. Psychiatry*, **152**: 1124–1129.
3. Angst J., Preisig M. (1995) Course of a clinical cohort of unipolar, bipolar and schizoaffective patients. Results of a prospective study from 1959 to 1985. *Schweiz Arch. Neurol. Psychiatrie*, **146**: 5–16.
4. Angst J., Preisig M. (1995) Outcome of the clinical cohort of unipolar, bipolar and schizoaffective patients. Results of a prospective study from 1959 to 1985. *Schweiz Arch. Neurol. Psychiatrie*, **146**: 17–23.
5. Cohen P., Cohen J. (1984) The clinician's illusion. *Arch. Gen. Psychiatry*, **41**: 1178–1182.
6. Rice J.P., Rochberg N., Endicott J., Lavori P.W., Miller C. (1992) Stability of psychiatric diagnoses. *Arch. Gen. Psychiatry*, **49**: 824–830.
7. Andreasen N.C., Grove W.M., Shapiro R.W., Keller M.B., Hirschfeld R.M., McDonald-Scott P. (1981) Reliability of lifetime diagnosis. A multicenter collaborative perspective. *Arch. Gen. Psychiatry*, **38**: 400–405.
8. Weissman M., Leaf P., Tischler G., Blazer D., Karno M., Bruce M., Forio L. (1988) Affective disorders in five United States communities. *Psychol. Med.*, **18**: 141–153.
9. Kessler R.C., McGonagle K.A., Zhao S., Nelson C.B., Hughes M., Eshleman S., Wittchen H.U., Kendler K.S. (1994) Lifetime and 12–month prevalence of DSM-III-R psychiatric disorders in the United States. *Arch. Gen. Psychiatry*, **51**: 8–19.
10. Goodwin F.K., Jamison K.R. (1990) *Manic-Depressive Illness*. Oxford University Press, New York.
11. Angst J., Sellaro R. (2000) Historical perspectives and natural history of bipolar disorder. *Biol. Psychiatry*, **48**: 445–457.
12. Turvey C.L., Coryell W.H., Solomon D.A., Leon A.C., Endicott J., Keller M.B., Akiskal H. (1999) Long-term prognosis of bipolar I disorder. *Acta Psychiatr. Scand.*, **99**: 110–119.
13. Mueller T.I., Keller M.B., Leon A.C., Solomon D.A., Shea M.T., Coryell W., Ednicott J. (1996) Recovery after 5 years of unremitting major depressive disorder. *Arch. Gen. Psychiatry*, **53**: 794–799.

2.7

Prognosis—When and for Whom?

Thomas A. Wehr[1]

Before the era of modern treatments, one of the most valuable services that medical science could provide was the formulation of a prognosis, based on

[1] *Section on Biological Rhythms, Mood and Anxiety Disorders Program, National Institute of Mental Health, 10 Center Drive, MSC 1390, Bethesda, MD 20892–1390, USA*

a diagnosis. Sometimes this information was reassuring. When it was not, it would have confirmed one's fears, but it might also have given a feeling of control by reducing uncertainty. To be sure, the comfort afforded by such knowledge must have been meagre in many instances.

Given the severity of untreated mania or psychotic depression, and given the duration of untreated episodes, it must have seemed remarkable to our 19th-century colleagues that such episodes could remit spontaneously and patients could be discharged from their asylums, ostensibly well. To speak of the possibility of such a favourable outcome at the outset of an episode must have provided comfort to patients' loved ones and a feeling of power and usefulness to psychiatrists who had little else to offer besides custodial care. It is not surprising then that prognosis became one of the foundations of the diagnostic system bequeathed to us by Kraepelin and other psychiatrists of that era.

For contemporary psychiatrists, what is the relevance of the literature on prognosis to clinical practice? The answer to this question will depend on when a psychiatrist is asked to make a prognosis for bipolar illness. Frequently, patients and their families wish to know the prognosis when the illness is first diagnosed. As Marneros and Brieger point out, it is clear that good prognosis and bad prognosis do not invariably distinguish affective disorders and schizophrenia. For bipolar illness, the spectrum of outcomes is broad, from sustained, total remission to sustained, total disability, with significant numbers at either extreme. But the psychiatrist is asked to provide a prognosis for an individual, not a population. In light of this fact, the literature might not be particularly helpful, except to alert all interested parties to the diversity of possible outcomes.

The issue of prognosis can arise again later in the course of illness, when, for example, the patient has had unsatisfactory responses to treatment, or when marriage, children, or new professional responsibilities are contemplated. Sometimes, psychiatrists are asked to make prognoses for insurance applications or forensic purposes. In most of these situations, prognoses will surely differ, depending on prior course, response to treatment, and assessments of the patient's compliance with, and access to treatment. What is the prognosis of the treatment-resistant patient? What is the prognosis of the compliant patient? What is the prognosis of the stable patient? What is the prognosis of the patient with inadequate health care? In many of these instances, one suspects the prevailing opinion—for which the literature provides some support—is that the past is often the best predictor of the future.

In the modern era, formulation of a prognosis will usually reflect the clinician's expectation that the course of illness will be moderated by treatment. The extent to which this expectation proves to be true depends on several patient factors, such as compliance, comorbid substance abuse, and others, as enumerated by Marneros and Brieger. To this list, we undoubtedly will add genetic factors that predict response to treatment, as was recently reported for antidepressant-induced mania [1]. Factors external to the patient have received relatively less attention in research on course of illness and outcome of treatment. For example, access to and quality of care must profoundly affect these variables. Pharmacological treatment of bipolar illness is an art that requires persistence, vigilance and empiricism—persistence in trying new approaches to treatment, vigilance in detecting and treating the earliest symptoms of an episode, and empiricism in finding combinations of treatments that are effective for a given patient and in avoiding those that prove to be deleterious [2–5]. To be sure, the patient plays an important role as collaborator in this enterprise, but the patient's capacity to play this role depends in turn on the clinician's willingness to provide the information and the type of relationship that are conducive to collaboration. In these respects, prognosis is not only an inherent property of bipolar illness; it is also a function of the quality of care that will be provided.

REFERENCES

1. Mundo E., Walker M., Cate T., Macciardi F., Kennedy F.L. (2001) The role of serotonin transporter protein gene in antidepressant-induced mania in bipolar disorder. *Arch. Gen. Psychiatry*, **58**: 539–544.
2. Peselow E.D., Fieve R.R., Difiglia C., Sanfilipo M.P. (1994) Lithium prophylaxis of bipolar illness. The value of combination treatment. *Br. J. Psychiatry*, **164**: 208–214.
3. Frye M.A., Ketter T.A., Leverich G.S., Huggins T., Lantz C., Denicoff K.D., Post R.M. (2000) The increasing use of polypharmacotherapy for refractory mood disorders: 22 years of study. *J. Clin. Psychiatry*, **61**: 9–15.
4. Wehr T.A., Goodwin F.K. (1987) Can antidepressants cause mania and worsen the course of affective illness? *Am. J. Psychiatry*, **144**: 1403–1411.
5. Ghaemi S.N., Boiman E.E., Goodwin F.K. (2000) Diagnosing bipolar disorder and the effect of antidepressants: a naturalistic study. *J. Clin. Psychiatry*, **61**: 804–808.

2.8

Prognosis and Manic-Depressive Cycle

Athanasios Koukopoulos[1]

Manic-depressive illness is essentially a cyclic phenomenon. Its cyclicity is not simply a type of course such as can be observed, for instance, in malarial fevers or epileptic attacks, but is probably its fundamental component,

[1] *Centro Lucio Bini, Via Crescenzio 42, 00193 Roma, Italy*

because the disorder in its core manifestations appears closely related to cyclic biological rhythms like sleep, and to environmental, circadian and seasonal variations. From a clinical point of view, it is the single most distinguishing feature of the disorder and is more significant than any symptom or cluster of symptoms.

The unit of this cyclic course is the manic-depressive cycle, composed of an episode of mania, one of depression, and an interval in varying sequences. The word "cycle" was used for the first time in psychiatry in 1845, by W. Griesinger: "Not rarely the whole disease consists of a cycle of both forms (mania and melancholia), which often regularly alternate with each other" [1]. Many authors since antiquity have intuited the intrinsic link between mania and melancholia. Aretaeus said: "Once the attack of mania is over the sick person becomes slowed down, taciturn and sad and when they recall the illness they have been through they feel anguish at their wretchedness" [2]. Alexander of Tralles maintained that "nothing else is mania than the mounting of melancholia towards aggressive excitation" [3]. Thomas Willis writes: "These two, melancholy and mania, mutually exclude and replace each other like smoke and flame" [4]. Since then, however, the alternation between the two phases and their inner relation was never seen as a regular occurrence, intrinsic to the disease. It was viewed as accidental or random.

The credit for first describing a single disease entity must go to Falret, who described in 1851 a form he named *folie circulaire*, characterized by an alternation between mania and melancholia followed by a "lucid" interval [5]. He conceived these three stages as a "circle", hence the name *folie circulaire*. In 1854 Baillarger described his *folie à double forme* [6]. Unlike Falret's *folie circulaire*, the *folie à double forme* does not include a free interval after each cycle (*accès*) but only intermissions between the two episodes (*periodes*). For Falret, this new entity was a distinct disease, while for Baillarger it was a syndromal alternation of melancholia and mania.

In the 20th century the concept of cyclicity of mood disorders and of its relation to the seasons declined for various reasons: psychoanalysis, the change of perception of time from cyclical to linear, but also because of Kraepelin who, probably in his efforts to deny the precise regularities of the French authors, neglected the study of the manic-depressive cycle in his treatises.

In an investigation of the course of manic-depressive cycles, published in 1980 [7], and involving 434 bipolar patients, we found the following patterns. In 119 patients (28%), the cycle started with a manic episode which was followed by a depressive episode and then by a free interval (MDI pattern); 101 patients (85%) were bipolar I (BPI), and of all the 207 BPI patients, 50% had the MDI pattern. In 106 patients (25%), the cycle started with depression, followed by mania or more often by hypomania and then by a free interval (DMI pattern). 78% were bipolar II (BPII) patients. Eighty-seven patients

(20%) were rapid cyclers (RC), 83 (19%) had a continuous circular course (CC) with long cycles and 39 patients had irregular patterns.

The intrinsic link between the two phases of the cycle becomes evident in the different response to treatment. The MDI cycles respond far better to prophylactic treatments than the DMI cycles [7–11]. Our explanation is that in the first case lithium acts upon a mania that emerges gradually and without the interference of antidepressants. The prevention of mania prevents the onset of the depression. In the case of DMI cycles, the mania or hypomania is more resistant to lithium, because it is activated by the antidepressants given for the depression and often this results in a switch. The continuation of antidepressants may result eventually in rapid cyclicity [12].

These different types of manic-depressive cycle have also a different prognosis as far as frequency of relapse is concerned. We found that the BPI type, made up mainly of MDI cycles, had a frequency of 0.63 episodes per year, while the BPII type, made up mainly of depression-hypomania-free interval (DMI) cycles, had a frequency of 1.80 episodes per year [13]. To underline is the finding of Maj [14]: the patients who had a switch in their course (Dm or DM cycles) are more likely to become rapid cyclers.

These findings suggest a primacy of the mania in the structure and evolution of the manic-depressive cycle. In fact all the prophylactic treatments (neuroleptics, lithium, anticonvulsants, atypical antipsychotics) are antimanic treatments.

REFERENCES

1. Griesinger W. (1845) *Pathologie und Therapie der psychischen Krankheiten*. Krabbe, Stuttgart.
2. Aretaeus of Cappadocia (II C. AD, 1735) *De causis et signis acutorum et diuturnorum morborum*. Vander, Lugduni Batavorum.
3. Alexander of Tralles (VI C.AD, 1878) *Della Melancholia*. Wilhelm Braumueller, Wien.
4. Willis T. (1676) *De Anima Brutorum*. Lyon.
5. Falret J.P. (1851) *Marche de la folie*. Gaz. Hop., **24**: 18–19.
6. Baillarger J.G.F. (1854) Note sur un genre de folie dont l'accès sont caractérisés par deux périodes régulières, l'une de dépression et l'autre d'excitation. *Bull. Acad. Impériale Méd. Séance*, January 31.
7. Koukopoulos A., Reginaldi D., Laddomada P., Floris G., Serra G., Tondo L. (1980) Course of the manic-depressive cycle and changes caused by treatments. *Pharmakopsychiatr. Neuropsychopharmakol.*, **13**: 156–167.
8. Grof E., Haag M., Grof P., Haag H. (1987) Lithium response and the sequence of episode polarities: preliminary report on a Hamilton sample. *Progr. Neuropsychopharmacol. Biol. Psychiatry*, **11**: 199–203.
9. Haag H., Heidorn A., Haag M., Greil W. (1987) Sequence of affective polarity and lithium response: preliminary report on the Munich sample. *Progr. Neuropsychopharmacol. Biol. Psychiatry*, **11**: 205–208.

10. Maj M., Pirozzi R., Starace F. (1989)   Previous pattern of course of the illness as a predictor of response to lithium prophylaxis in bipolar patients. *J. Affect. Disord.*, **17**: 237–241.
11. Faedda G.L., Baldessarini R.J., Tohen M., Strakowski S.M., Waternaux C., (1991)   Episode sequence in bipolar disorder and response to lithium treatment. *Am. J. Psychiatry*, **148**: 1237–1239.
12. Koukopoulos A., Caliari B., Tundo A., Minnai G., Floris G., Reginaldi D., Tondo L. (1983)   Rapid cyclers, temperament and antidepressants. *Compr. Psychiatry*, **24**: 249–258.
13. Koukopoulos A. (1997)   The role of antidepressant treatment in rapid cycling. Presented at the 2nd International Conference on Bipolar Disorder, Pittsburgh, June 19–21.
14. Maj M., Magliano L., Pirozzi R., Marasco C., Guarneri M. (1994)   Validity of rapid cycling as a course specifier for bipolar disorder. *Am. J. Psychiatry*, **151**: 1015–1019.

2.9
The Importance of Natural Course and Depression in Bipolar I Disorder

Carolyn L. Turvey[1]

Marneros and Brieger's comprehensive review of the prognosis of bipolar I disorder offers considerable evidence that the most consistent and powerful predictor of long-term course is prior morbidity. Marneros and Brieger summarize several studies that fail to find baseline variables that predict long-term course. Candidate subtypes such as rapid cycling and mixed episodes show poor stability over time and support for their prognostic value is equivocal. Furthermore, evidence comparing pre-treatment and treatment-era studies suggest that the prophylactic efficacy of lithium may be less powerful than once thought. In contrast, studies with as widely disparate samples and methods as the National Institute of Mental Health (NIMH) Collaborative Study of Depression, and the Zurich, Danish, Naples and University of California at Los Angeles (UCLA) studies all draw the somewhat bland conclusion that morbidity predicts morbidity. These findings converge in support of the claim that the natural course of the illness specific to each individual patient is the most important determinant of long-term prognosis.

Marneros and Brieger carefully explain the potential bias towards an overrepresentation of more severe bipolar disorder in both clinical and research experience with this illness. However, the underrepresentation of the less severe forms of bipolar disorder should be emphasized more. Although Kraepelin is often cited in his discussion of the acceleration of

[1] *Department of Psychiatry, University of Iowa, Psychiatry Research-MEB, Iowa City, IA 52242–1000, USA*

relapse over the course of the illness, he also describes at length the enormous individual variability in course for manic-depressive illness [1]. Even in the pre-treatment era, patients could experience periods of remission for five years or more. In the context of my clinical research and practice, particularly in genetic family studies where untreated family members of bipolar I probands are evaluated, it has become clear that some bipolar I individuals can have a history of a single manic episode, but no follow-up treatment and no documented recurrence. The patient and family later attribute the manic episode to situational factors such as excessive travel or drug use, even though the treating physicians ruled out these explanations, made a diagnosis of bipolar I disorder and hospitalized the patient.

An understanding of this less severe end of severity spectrum for bipolar disorder enriches our understanding of the importance of the wide variability of individual differences in determining course for this illness as well as the prophylactic efficacy of our treatments. The heated controversy around the prophylactic efficacy of lithium is perhaps unnecessarily polemic. The repercussions of an untreated relapse and the demonstrated efficacy of lithium in clinical trials offers sufficient rationale for a conservative and preventive treatment approach for patients functioning at the severity level most commonly found in our clinics. Presumably, those who could function without prophylactic treatment are more likely to self-select out of treatment.

Although several studies have attempted to delineate meaningful subtypes of bipolar disorders, the prognostic importance of these subtypes is not clear. Mixed states, rapid cycling and seasonal affective disorder have failed to garner solid support as stable and prognostically relevant subtypes in spite of clinical accounts of their importance. To date, research in this area has been hampered by the variation in criteria used to define subtypes and site differences in how broadly the criteria are applied. More elaborate and methodologically rigorous diagnostic methods are needed before this research can progress. This cannot occur until the field decides which symptoms of irritability and agitation occurring during a depressive phase of an episode are "true" indications of mania. Otherwise, depending on the investigator's clinical bent, different investigators will label the same clinical presentation as a mixed episode, rapid cycling, agitated depression or one of the impulsive personality disorders.

Of the many demographic, baseline and phenomenological variables tested for their prognostic value, two have emerged as consistently significant: depression and psychosis. Admittedly, much of the support for the prognostic value of depression comes from the NIMH Collaborative Study of Depression and is a specific focus of our group. Coryell *et al* [2] found that persistence of depressive symptoms in the first two years of follow-up predicted poor long-term prognosis, yet persistence of mania did not. This finding is extraordinary and needs further independent replication because it suggests that not all types of morbidity are created equal. How is it that depression is relevant to later course but mania is not?

Some posit that mood stabilizers are more effective in treating mania than depression [3, 4]. However, it is difficult to tease this apart from the possibility that depression has a more chronic natural course than mania. Patients may be more inclined to report chronic subsyndromal depression than subsyndromal mania because the former causes more subjective distress. On a more speculative note, a chronic depressive course may indicate an end-stage or more severe form of the illness where the capacity to upregulate mood to achieve euthymia or even mania is no longer intact. Future research can examine whether patients' course becomes more depressive over time or with age. In addition, it would be important to test whether the prognostic significance of mixed or rapid cycling episodes is due primarily to the presence of chronic depressive symptoms. For example, Strakowski et al. [5] found that mixed episodes were predictive of later suicidality, but when the relative contribution of depressive versus manic symptoms was examined, only the depressive symptoms remained significant. Comparable studies should be conducted using poor long-term prognosis as the outcome.

Marneros and Brieger end their thorough review with a reminder of the potential benefits of this illness as well as the importance of including the personal reports of those suffering the illness in our general understanding of bipolar disorder. The potential benefits are most often attributed to hypomanic or manic symptoms with the paralysis associated with chronic depression left unmentioned. Although bipolar depression is less immediately exciting than the concept of rapid cycling, or kindling theory, we must turn our attention to the clinical and theoretical importance of the less beneficent pole of manic-depressive illness.

REFERENCES

1. Kraepelin E. (1921) *Manic-Depressive Insanity and Paranoia*. Livingstone, Edinburgh.
2. Coryell W., Turvey C., Endicott J., Leon A.C., Mueller T., Solomon D., Keller M. (1998) Bipolar I affective disorder: predictors of outcome after 15 years. *J. Affect. Disord.*, **50**: 109–116.
3. Koukopoulos A., Reginaldi D. (1980) Recurrences of manic-depressive episodes during lithium treatment. In *Handbook of Lithium Therapy* (Ed. F.N. Johnson), pp. 109–117. University Park Press, Baltimore.
4. Koukopoulos A., Tondo L. (1980) Lithium non-responders and their treatment In *Handbook of Lithium Therapy* (Ed. F.N. Johnson), pp. 109–117, University Park Press, Baltimore.
5. Strakowski S.M., McElroy S.L., Keck P.E., Jr., West S.A. (1996) Suicidality among patients with mixed and manic bipolar disorder. *Am. J. Psychiatry*, **153**: 674–676.

2.10
Analysing Course of Illness in Bipolar Disorder
David A. Solomon[1] and Andrew C. Leon[2]

Bipolar disorder is usually a lifelong illness, marked by multiple recurrences of mood episodes, persisting prodromal or residual subsyndromal symptoms, comorbid psychiatric disorders, and psychosocial impairment. In reviewing these and other aspects of the illness, Marneros and Brieger have organized their work around the length of follow-up for the many studies they have examined, rightfully giving more weight to findings from studies with a longer observation time. However, it is important to note that, although longitudinal follow-up is necessary for studying the course of illness in recurrent diseases such as mood disorders, what the follow-up data reveal is in large measure a function of the statistical models that are used to analyse the data. Different statistical models vary in their capacity to make full use of follow-up data.

Typically, for bipolar disorder, the outcome of interest includes recurrence of mania and major depression, and recovery from these mood episodes. Older studies treated recurrence and recovery as a dichotomous variable: the study patient had a recurrence or did not, and likewise, recovered from a mood episode or did not. Problems arise with this approach when subjects drop out of the study or ultimately when the study ends. Taking recurrence as an example, if subjects withdraw prior to recurrence, the rate of recurrence may be underestimated. Similarly, termination of the study may lead to underestimating the rate of recurrence simply because the length of follow-up was inadequate.

To avoid these problems, one can use the statistical method known as survival analysis to examine the outcomes of recurrence and recovery [1]. Survival analysis examines the *time that elapses until the event of interest occurs*. Since at least 1974 [2], it has been used to analyse longitudinal data in psychiatry. For several reasons, survival analysis is well suited to examine course of illness data. One reason is that survival analysis uses all available data from all subjects, including those who withdraw before completing the study. Second, survival analysis accounts for varying lengths of follow-up, and third, it estimates the changing probability of the event, for example recurrence, at different times over the course of follow-up [3]. The time to recurrence may be incomplete for many or even most subjects because not all of them are followed long enough to directly

[1] *Mood Disorders Program, Rhode Island Hospital, Brown University School of Medicine, 593 Eddy Street, Providence, RI 02067, USA*
[2] *Weill Medical College of Cornell University, Department of Psychiatry, 525 East 68th Street, New York, NY, USA*

measure the length of time to recurrence. For these subjects, time to recurrence is classified as "censored".

The Kaplan–Meier product-limit estimate [4] is a fundamental aspect of survival analysis which estimates the proportion of subjects who remain well, that is, survive without a recurrence up to a given time point or assessment. This quantity incorporates all available data, including data from subjects who drop out. Drop-outs are classified as censored cases at the point at which they withdraw from the study, and survival analysis assumes that drop-out is due to reasons unrelated to the event of interest. The validity of that assumption is not always clear; for example, subjects may drop out of a study or refuse further follow-up as they begin to suffer prodromal symptoms leading to recurrence. Survival analysis can be used to analyse course of illness data for many phenomena, such as time to recovery from a mood episode, time to return to work, or time to suicide attempt. The Cox proportional hazards model [5] is a regression approach to survival analysis that is used to examine the strength of the association between prognostic factors and the event of interest. A limitation of such survival analyses is that it restricts the analysis to one survival interval (for example, time to recurrence or well interval) per subject.

In contrast, a mixed-effects survival strategy can incorporate multiple survival intervals per subject. For instance, one subject may have five recurrences, another subject may have three. Regardless, one mixed-effects model can examine prognostic factors incorporating all of these survival intervals. To take full advantage of longitudinal data, one cannot arbitrarily restrict the analyses to one event (for example, the first recurrence or recovery) per subject. Rather, one ideally would examine the event in the context of prior events.

As Marneros and Brieger amply show, bipolar disorder is marked by the same event occurring repeatedly, such as multiple recurrences and recoveries. Unfortunately, up until recently, the statistical models available to examine multiple mood episodes have been restricted to analysing one mood episode per subject. Taking multiple recurrence as an example, these models do not allow one to analyse the effect of successive mood episodes on the risk of recurrence. Rather, these fixed-effects models can include only one well interval per subject. Thus, the researcher must arbitrarily select one of many possible well intervals. The result is that the findings are vulnerable to selection bias. This is because the median episode duration for a group of study patients may be dominated by patients with brief recurrences. To avoid this selection bias, one can now make use of a mixed-effects survival strategy such as mixed-effects, grouped-time survival analysis [6]. This analytic strategy allows one to construct an analytic model that accounts for within-subject variation in risk of recurrence of mood episodes, and does so by including multiple well intervals per subject. By accounting for individual heterogeneity or propensity toward recurrence, one can better gauge the effect of prior mood episodes, and better understand the overall course of illness and outcome. This strategy can be extended beyond multiple recurrences to other aspects of bipolar disorder, such as multiple recoveries, the course of prodromal and residual symptoms, and the return to productive functioning.

REFERENCES

1. Leon A.C., Friedman R.A., Sweeney J.A., Brown R.P., Mann J.J. (1990) Statistical issues in the identification of risk factors for suicidal behavior: the application of survival analysis. *Psychiatry Res.*, **31**: 99–108.
2. Klerman G.L., Dimascio A., Weissman M., Prusoff B., Paykel E.S. (1974) Treatment of depression by drugs and psychotherapy. *Am. J. Psychiatry*, **131**: 186–191.
3. Kalbfleisch J.D., Prentice R.L. (1980) *The Statistical Analysis of Failure Time Data.* Wiley, New York.
4. Kaplan E.L., Meier P. (1958) Nonparametric estimation from incomplete observations. *J. Am. Stat. Assoc.*, **53**: 457–481.
5. Cox D.R. (1972) Regression models and life tables. *J. Roy. Stat. Soc., Series B*, **34**: 187–220.
6. Hedeker D., Siddiqui O., Hu F.B. (2000) Random-effects regression analysis of correlated grouped-time survival data. *Stat. Methods Med. Res.*, **9**: 161–179.

2.11
Outcome in Bipolar Disorder: How Much Have We Learned?

Mauricio Tohen[1]

Bipolar disorder has been known for many centuries, However, our understanding of its course and outcome still remains incomplete. As Marneros and Brieger point out, the main problem has been the "snapshot" approach taken by both clinicians and researchers when approaching the disorder. The cross-sectional approach is no doubt flawed not only in the prediction of outcome, but also in the selection of treatment. Kraepelin emphasized a longitudinal approach more than a century ago.

Perhaps an aspect that has not been emphasized enough is the value of observing patients starting at the onset of their illness, which could be labelled a *complete longitudinal* approach. In recent years, there has been an emphasis in the non-affective psychosis, primarily schizophrenia, to conduct first-episode or prodromal studies. Research groups in the US, Europe and Australia have been conducting first-episode or prodromal studies for more than a decade. However, there are few first-episode studies of bipolar

[1] *Lilly Research Laboratories, Indianapolis, IN 46285, USA*

disorder. Although studies describing the outcome of a first-episode cohort are not new, most contemporary bipolar outcome studies have included multiple episode populations, which are prone to have a poor outcome. Two studies in the United States, however, have focused on first-episode cohorts: the McLean/Harvard First Episode Mania Study [1, 2] and the University of Cincinnati Study [3]. By assessing a first episode population, confounding factors such as chronicity itself may be controlled, providing more generalizable findings. It is possible that the current rather pessimistic portrayal of outcome in bipolar disorder stems from multiple episode cohorts recruited from academic institutions that may not be representative of most clinical samples.

The study of prodromal cases in bipolar disorder deserves more attention and may even provide the key to prevention. To test the concept of neuro-protection of pharmacological agents, the ideal population is no doubt first-episode and prodromal patients. Another contemporary approach that needs to be implemented to further understand the course of bipolar disorder is the use of neuroimaging and neuropsychological assessments.

A major contribution of Marneros and Brieger's review is the comprehensive description of the terminology utilized in outcome research in bipolar disorder. Terms such as recovery and relapse are frequently loosely utilized. To enable the comparison of different studies and even to be able to pool data from different cohorts when appropriate, it is of paramount importance for investigators to utilize common terminology. The classification of observation time into long-term, medium-term and short-term is a valuable contribution considering that length of the follow-up often affects many of the findings. Researchers and clinicians reviewing outcome research in bipolar disorder are encouraged to make these helpful distinctions.

One of the limitations of many studies in bipolar disorder is the lack of clarity on how outcome is defined. It is not appropriate to define outcome as a unidimensional parameter. Rather, multidimensional outcome studies are needed to describe the course of an illness. The inherent risk of multidimensional outcomes would be an overly complex definition of outcome. The challenge that outcome researchers have is to present the most parsimonious assessment of outcome—precise but not multiple to the risk of losing clarity.

An issue that remains unclear is the value of clinical trials with a reasonable duration (at least one year) in outcome research. The main advantage of clinical trials is that one of the most important confounding factors of outcome, treatment, is standardized. It is no doubt helpful to clinicians to know the expected outcome in patients who have been maintained in a commonly used treatment such as lithium. Another perhaps undervalued opportunity is the outcome of patients randomized to placebo—if washout of previous treatment was done appropriately, this represent a unique "naturalistic" observation. Of course, the main limitation of outcome findings in clinical trials is the potential lack of representativeness of clinical trial populations. However, no doubt outcome research on clinical trial populations can be generalized to other clinical trial populations. For clinical investigators or ethical board members, outcome research in clinical trial populations is of immense value, especially when outcomes such as suicide are considered.

An ongoing debate about outcome research in general is the value of one site versus multiple site studies. The main advantage of one site studies is the presence of a homogeneous sample and the uniformity of assessment methods, which are key to ensure internal validity. The main challenge is the smaller number of study subjects and the possible limitations in the generalizability of the results. No doubt to study rare events, large samples are needed. A recent major attempt has been taken by the National Institute of Mental Health, which will recruit 5000 patients in order to study the course and effectiveness of different pharmacological treatments. Finally, the determination of predictors of outcome in bipolar disorder is essential for clinicians, investigators, patients and their families. New technologies such as neuroimaging and genetics will no doubt enrich our knowledge of outcome in bipolar disorder.

REFERENCES

1. Tohen M., Waternaux C.M., Tsuang M.T., Hunt A.T. (1990) Four year follow-up of twenty-four first-episode manic patients. *J. Affect. Disord.*, **19**: 79–86.
2. Tohen M., Hennen J., Zarate C., Baldessarini R., Strakowski S., Stoll A., Faedda G., Suppes T., Gebre-Medhin P., Cohen B. (2000) The McLean/Harvard First Episode Project: two-year syndromal and functional recovery in 219 cases of major affective disorders with psychotic features. *Am. J. Psychiatry*, **157**: 220–228.
3. Strakowski S.M., Keck P.E., Jr., McElroy S.L., West S.A., Sax K.W., Hawkins J.M., Kmetz G.F., Upadhyaha V.H., Tugrul K.C., Bourne M.H. (1998) Twelve-month outcome following a first hospitalization for affective psychosis. *Arch. Gen. Psychiatry*, **55**: 49–55.

2.12

Heterogeneity of Course and Outcome in Bipolar Disorder: Can Genetics Help?

Bernard Lerer and Avraham Yakir[1]

One of the aspects of bipolar disorder that is most striking to clinicians is the remarkable clinical heterogeneity of the illness. The spectrum of patients

[1] *Biological Psychiatry Laboratory, Department of Psychiatry, Hadassah–Hebrew University Medical Center, Ein Karem, Jerusalem 91120, Israel*

runs the full range from highly functional, well-adjusted individuals who are almost completely symptom free for decades, to socially dysfunctional, chronically ill people who have repeated relapses from which they never recover fully. During the acute phase of the illness, patients may be severely psychotic, with mood elements that are barely sufficient to meet diagnostic criteria, or may manifest mood symptoms that are the epicentre of the episode and range in polarity from deep depression to expansive manias. According to currently accepted criteria, this entire clinical spectrum falls within the realm of bipolar disorder and also within the province of the comprehensive, systematic review by Marneros and Brieger.

Presenting the evidence with methodological precision, Marneros and Brieger inexorably lead us to a number of disturbing conclusions. Bipolar disorder is a recurrent illness characterized by a mean of three acute episodes during the lifetime course. Close to a third of patients have significant personality and social impairment; comorbidity with substance abuse is high and so is the risk of suicide, even if previously over-estimated. Most disturbing of all to the dedicated psychopharmacologist is that it is uncertain whether modern treatments have changed the length of episodes or the number of relapses essentially in comparison to the pre-pharmacological era.

The data summarized by Marneros and Brieger make it clear that demographic and clinical features, which have emerged from decades of research, have little power to predict course and outcome. Is there a different perspective that can help us to resolve the clinical heterogeneity of bipolar disorder? Since the 1970s an intriguing series of studies has suggested that there may be a subtype of bipolar disorder that is characterized by excellent response to lithium [1–3]. This may be a more heritable form, since patients who respond well to lithium have an excess of family members affected by bipolar disorder. Segregation analyses of lithium responsive families suggest that a major gene effect may be operative, possibly as an autosomal recessive trait [4]. Molecular genetic studies of such families, including a recently completed whole genome scan, point to a number of possible susceptibility loci [5]. If correct, this approach could help to resolve some of the heterogeneity and identify a genetically valid subtype of the illness with a better prognosis.

Other molecular genetic studies of major psychotic disorders, while potentially consistent with this proposal, mandate that it be considered at a greater level of complexity. There are now a number of linkage studies that point to loci which may be implicated *both* in schizophrenia and bipolar disorder. These loci are located in the chromosomal regions 18p11, 13q22, 10p14 and 22q13. Although a detailed consideration of these findings is beyond the scope of this commentary (for a review and references, see [6]), two caveats should be noted. The first is that none of the linkage findings are at a level that can be regarded as definitive or sufficiently replicated; the second is that there are also negative linkage findings for schizophrenia and bipolar disorder in all the regions noted. Nevertheless, the findings are of considerable interest and permit novel genetic hypotheses to be considered.

One such hypothesis is outlined in Figure 2.12.1. It is well recognized that the genetic basis of both schizophrenia and bipolar disorder is most likely polygenic, involving the additive and epistatic contribution of a number of different loci of small effect as well as an environmental contribution [7, 8]. The view put forward in Figure 2.12.1 suggests that some of these loci predispose to psychotic symptoms that are characteristic of schizophrenia while others predispose to mood disorder manifestations such as are seen in bipolar disorder. The combination of susceptibility loci carried by an individual would (in concert with environmental effects) determine the predominant phenotype that he manifests. Depending on the combination of genes carried by the individual, this could run the full range from lithium-responsive, pure bipolar disorder that has an excellent prognosis to pure schizophrenia, with schizoaffective disorder falling between. Family studies that show an increased risk of schizoaffective disorder in the relatives of schizophrenic as well as bipolar probands are consistent with this view (e.g. [9, 10]). Further support comes from the data reviewed by Marneros and Brieger, which show that mood incongruent features predict a worse prognosis and that patients with schizoaffective disorder occupy a position mid-way between schizophrenia and bipolar disorder in terms of course and outcome.

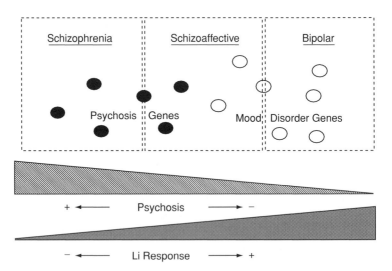

Figure 2.12.1 Hypothesized polygenic contribution of "psychosis" and "mood disorder" genes to schizophrenia, schizoaffective disorder and bipolar disorder, with severity of psychosis and responsiveness to lithium treatment dependent upon the additive and epistatic effects of the combination of genes carried by the individual

Unitary, or in their more modern version, continuum hypotheses of psychosis are not new. They existed before Kraepelin and have been advanced by numerous authors since Kraepelin dichotomized psychotic illness. A particularly influential view was proposed by Crow [11]. The ideas expressed in this commentary build on these approaches but are not identical with them. The suggestions outlined are decidedly speculative and require empirical testing. Nevertheless, they provide a route that may allow us to resolve the substantial heterogeneity of course, outcome and response to treatment that is presently one of the most vexing features of bipolar disorder and to better conceptualize the ill-understood construct of schizoaffective disorder.

REFERENCES

1. Mendlewicz J., Fieve R.R., Stallone F. (1973) Relationship between the effectiveness of lithium therapy and family history. *Am. J. Psychiatry*, **130**: 1011–1013.
2. Maj M., Del Vecchio M., Starace F., Pirozzi R., Kemali D. (1984) Prediction of affective psychoses response to lithium prophylaxis: the role of socio-demographic, clinical, psychological and biological variables. *Acta Psychiatr. Scand.*, **69**: 37–44.
3. Alda M. (2001) Genetic factors and response to prophylactic treatment in bipolar disorder. In *Pharmacogenetics of Psychotropic Drugs* (Ed. B. Lerer), Cambridge University Press, Cambridge (in press).
4. Alda M., Grof E., Cavazzoni P., Duffy A., Martin R., Ravindran L., Grof P. (1997) Autosomal recessive inheritance of affective disorders in families of responders to lithium prophylaxis? *J. Affect. Disord.*, **44**: 153–157.
5. Turecki G., Grof P., Cavazzoni P., Duffy A., Grof E., Ahrens B., Berghofer A., Müller-Oerlinghausen B., Dvorakova M., Libigerova E. *et al* (1998) Evidence for a role of phospholipase C-gamma1 in the pathogenesis of bipolar disorder. *Mol. Psychiatry*, **3**: 534–538.
6. Berrettini W.H. (2000) Are schizophrenic and bipolar disorders related? A review of family and molecular genetic studies. *Biol. Psychiatry*, **48**: 531–538.
7. McGue M., Gottesman I.I., Rao D.C. (1985) Resolving genetic models for the transmission of schizophrenia. *Genet. Epidemiol.*, **2**: 99–110.
8. Cox N., Reich T., Rice J., Elston R., Schober J., Keats B. (1989) Segregation and linkage analyses of bipolar and major depressive illnesses in multigenerational pedigrees. *J. Psychiatr. Res.*, **23**: 109–123.
9. Gershon E.S., Hamovit J., Guroff J.J., Dibble E., Leckman J.F., Sceery W., Targum S.D., Nurnberger J.I., Jr., Goldin L.R., Bunney W.E., Jr. (1982) A family study of schizoaffective, bipolar I, bipolar II, unipolar, and normal control probands. *Arch. Gen. Psychiatry*, **39**: 1157–1167.
10. Maier W., Lichtermann D., Minges J., Hallmayer J., Heun R., Benkert O., Levinson D.F. (1993) Continuity and discontinuity of affective disorders and schizophrenia. Results of a controlled family study. *Arch. Gen. Psychiatry*, **50**: 871–883.
11. Crow T.J. (1986) The continuum of psychosis and its implication for the structure of the gene. *Br. J. Psychiatry*, **149**: 419–429.

2.13
Chronicity, Milder Forms and Cognitive Impairment in Bipolar Disorder

Eduard Vieta, Francesc Colom and Anabel Martínez-Arán[1]

Bipolar disorders are severe illnesses, chronic and lifelong. This could be, in their own words, the summary of the excellent review by Marneros and Brieger on the course and prognosis of manic-depressive illness. However, if we look at the way we treat our patients (or the way they accept to be treated), it does not look like we really assume that. In Europe, many psychiatrists would wait until the second or even the third episode before they prescribe prophylactic treatment. Interruption of prophylactic pharmacotherapy is more the rule than the exception [1], and even in the context of sophisticated psychoeducational programmes the rate of non-compliance is close to 40% [2].

In this commentary we would like to deal with three important issues: a) as Marneros and Brieger emphasize, bipolar disorders are associated with high rates of recurrences and impairment: treatment, therefore, has to be early and lifelong; b) impairment and suicide risk are not exclusive of the most severe forms of the disorder: bipolar II and other apparently milder clinical presentations may indeed carry on high relapse rates and disability; c) one important source of impairment is cognitive dysfunction: contrary to Kraepelin's belief, many bipolar patients show neuropsychological disturbances, which may be associated to poor occupational and social functioning.

- Chronic illness means chronic treatment. Since in this book there is a complete chapter on therapies for bipolar disorder, we will just put emphasis on how important is to share this information with our patients. The younger ones are generally very reluctant to admit the chronicity of their illness and to be compliant with pharmacotherapy for long periods [3]. Denial is a common problem among bipolar patients, but the attitude of the treating physician is crucial to help the patient deal with it. The role of the family is essential as well. The family should be involved in the therapeutic process to help the patient understand and work actively towards achieving complete remission and effective prevention of new episodes [4]. Overall, the treatment should be vigorous and sustained, in order to achieve not only syndromal recovery, but functional recovery and prevention of recurrences [5].
- Milder forms are severe as well. Impairment is not only a consequence of psychosis, mania or hospitalizations. Many patients with bipolar II subtype suffer the consequences of an extremely high recurrence rate.

[1] *Bipolar Disorders Program, Clinical Institute of Psychiatry and Psychology, Hospital Clinic, University of Barcelona, Villarroel 170, 08036 Barcelona, Spain*

Several studies have reported that bipolar II disorder is less severe than bipolar I with regard to symptom intensity, but is more severe with respect to episode frequency [6, 7]. The incidence of rapid cycling is, consistently, higher in bipolar II disorder [8]. Comorbidity rates, often a supplementary source of impairment, are also higher [9], and so is suicide risk [10]. Since underdiagnosis and misdiagnosis are more the rule than the exception in bipolar II disorder [8], it is unclear whether these high relapse, suicide, and comorbidity rates are related to inadequate treatment. The regular use of mood stabilizers and psychoeducation may reverse the higher cyclicity and suicidality of bipolar II compared to bipolar I [11, 12].

• Cognitive impairment is an issue in bipolar disorder. Cognitive impairment has been believed to make a big difference in the outcome of schizophrenia versus bipolar disorder. However, there is a growing body of evidence that about one-third of bipolar patients show persistent and clinically significant neuropsychological disturbances [13]. These dysfunctions may involve changes in the fluency of thought and speech, learning, memory, sustained and selective attention and executive function [14]. Cognitive disturbances may have a great impact on occupational and social functioning, and on quality of life as well. There is some evidence that the presence of subthreshold symptoms is closely related to cognitive disability [15]. This leads again to the need of lifelong effective treatment and achievement of full remission as the main goal of therapy.

REFERENCES

1. Maj M. (1999) Lithium prophylaxis of bipolar disorder in ordinary clinical conditions: patterns of long-term outcome. In *Bipolar Disorders: Clinical Course and Outcome* (Eds J.F. Goldberg, M. Harrow), pp. 21–37, American Psychiatric Press, Washington.
2. Colom F., Vieta E., Corbella B., Martínez-Arán A., Reinares M., Benabarre A., Gastó C. (2000) Clinical factors associated to treatment non-compliance in euthymic bipolar patients. *J. Clin. Psychiatry*, **61**: 549–555.
3. Colom F., Vieta E., Martínez A., Jorquera A., Gastó C. (1998) What is the role of psychotherapy in the treatment of bipolar disorder? *Psychother. Psychosom.*, **67**: 3–9.
4. Reinares M., Colom F., Martínez-Arán A., Benabarre A., Vieta E. (2001) Therapeutic interventions focused on the family of bipolar patients. *Psychother. Psychosom.* (in press).
5. Tohen M., Hennen J., Zarate C.M., Baldessarini R.J., Strakowski S.M., Stoll A.L., Faedda G.L., Suppes T., Gebre-Medhin P., Cohen B.M. (2000) Two-year syndromal and functional recovery in 219 cases of first-episode major affective disorder with psychotic features. *Am. J. Psychiatry*, **157**: 220–228.

6. Ayuso-Gutiérrez J.L., Ramos-Brieva J.A. (1982) The course of manic depressive illness. A comparative study of bipolar I and bipolar II patients. *J. Affect. Disord.*, **4**: 9–14.

7. Vieta E., Gastó C., Otero A., Nieto E., Vallejo J. (1997) Differential features between bipolar I and bipolar II disorder. *Compr. Psychiatry*, **38**: 98–101.

8. Akiskal H.S. (1996) The prevalent clinical spectrum of bipolar disorders: beyond DSM-IV. *J. Clin. Psychopharmacol.*, **16** (Suppl. 1): 4–14.

9. Vieta E., Colom F., Martínez-Arán A., Benabarre A., Reinares M., Gastó C. (2000) Bipolar II disorder and comorbidity. *Compr. Psychiatry*, **41**: 339–343.

10. Rihmer Z., Barsi J., Arato M., Demeter E. (1990) Suicide in subtypes of primary major depression. *J. Affect. Disord.*, **18**: 221–225.

11. Vieta E. (1999) Diagnosis and classification of psychiatric disorders. In *Anticonvulsants in Psychiatry* (Ed. N. Sussman), pp. 3–8, Royal Society of Medicine Press, London.

12. Vieta E., Benabarre A., Colom F., Gastó C., Nieto E., Otero A., Vallejo J. (1997) Suicidal behavior in bipolar I and bipolar II disorder. *J. Nerv. Ment. Dis.*, **185**: 407–409.

13. Altshuler L. (1993) Bipolar disorder: are repeated episodes associated with neuroanatomic and cognitive changes? *Biol. Psychiatry*, **33**: 563–565.

14. Martínez-Arán A., Vieta E., Colom F., Benabarre A., Reinares M., Gastó C., Salamero M. (2000) Cognitive dysfunctions in bipolar disorder: evidence of neuropsychological disturbances. *Psychother. Psychosom.*, **69**: 2–18.

15. Martínez-Arán A., Penadés R., Vieta E., Colom F., Reinares M., Benabarre A., Salamero M., Gastó C. (2001) Executive function in remitted bipolar and schizophrenic patients and its relationship with functional outcome. *Psychother. Psychosom.* (in press).

2.14
Poor Clinical Course and Suicide Risk for Bipolar Disorders

Martin Harrow, Kalman Kaplan and Joseph F. Goldberg[1]

Marneros and Brieger's scholarly and comprehensive review of bipolar course and prognosis points to a variety of potential difficulties in bipolar outcome and adjustment over the years. Despite the newer advances in treatment, there is still a question of how much improvement there is in the current clinical course as compared to that prior to the modern treatment era. Thus, a large number of studies have provided data indicating that despite the use of lithium for many years and the more recent use of depakote, the great majority of bipolar patients experience at least some recurrences of full affective syndromes.

[1] *Department of Psychiatry, University of Illinois College of Medicine, 1601 W. Taylor St., Chicago, Illinois 60612, USA*

Among the many potential outcome difficulties associated with affective disorders, completed suicide has long been a danger and one often linked to both unipolar and bipolar disorders [1]. Marneros and Brieger cite evidence providing empirical support concerning this danger.

The issue of what factors predict risk for suicide in bipolar disorders has not been solved completely, since suicide is a complex behavioural event which can be influenced by many variables, with depression-related factors being among the most prominent ones. There are multiple factors each of which can increase, incrementally, the risk for suicide.

Affective disorders are not the only ones with increased risk for suicide. Both patients with affective disorders and schizophrenia show a high rate of suicide. Data from the Chicago Follow-up Study [2, 3] and from other major research groups indicate a 10% risk for completed suicide in schizophrenics, a high suicide risk among substance abusers, and possibly some other disorders as well [1]. Clearly, even in patients who suicide who do not have full depressive syndromes, depressive types of symptoms (e.g., despair, hopelessness and disappointment over failed-life expectations) can be an influence.

In regard to depression, low mood influences cognition and influences which aspects of memory are accessed into consciousness. Thus, depressed mood and associated feelings of despair often influence the *accessing* of memories about the course of one's life. Depressed mood, by making patients "aware" of their negative memories, and leading patients to focus on depressed memories, can bias patients to believe their lives have been one long series of miserable experiences, leading to further despair and hopelessness and increasing suicide risk.

The high risk for suicide in patients with schizophrenia and in substance abusers raises questions about what other factors are involved and why they increase risk for completed suicide. As one example of factors which may be involved, data indicating a high risk for suicide in early, young schizophrenics has led to the hypothesis that one factor is the contrast between previous higher expectations and current feelings of disappointment and frustration about their reduced level of functioning and the potential chronic nature of their disorder [2].

There are general predictors of suicide risk which apply to other major disorders and to people of all types. Most of these risk factors also apply to bipolar disorders. Cultural trends and styles within a country can increase risk for suicide. Both hopelessness and hostility have been studied as potential risk factors for suicide. A decline in functioning is also a risk factor for suicide. Additional risk factors include being a male, being elderly, especially being an elderly male living alone, and being Caucasian (rather than African-American). Other factors include higher education and higher socio-economic class. Research from the Chicago Follow-up Study tends to confirm these risk factors across major diagnostic groups [2, 3].

Fawcett et al [4] have suggested that different risk factors also may emerge for different diagnostic groups. Thus, in addition to the general factors described above, there may also be diagnosis-specific risk factors. Bipolar and unipolar affective disorders, in addition to the general factors, may have one suicidal risk profile, schizophrenia may have another such profile, and substance abusers a third profile.

Research from the Chicago Follow-up Study has suggested some suicide risk factors cut across major psychiatric diagnostic groups (e.g., declines in general functioning, being male, having a better educational level, and being Caucasian). Risk factors such as chronicity of psychosis may be more specific to early stages of schizophrenia, while some types of declines in cognitive functioning [4], and mixed states [5], may be risk factors for affective disorders. Overall, while our data suggest that most risk factors are general ones, there appear to be select diagnosis-specific ones (for some, involving the early presence in patients of symptoms most syntonic to their disorder). This research on diagnosis-specific factors needs to be confirmed with further empirical work.

REFERENCES

1. Miles C.P. (1997) Conditions predisposing to suicide: a review. *J. Nerv. Ment. Dis.*, **164**: 231–246.
2. Westermeyer J.F., Harrow M., Marengo J.T. (1991) Risk for suicide in schizophrenia and other psychotic and nonpsychotic disorders. *J. Nerv. Ment. Dis.*, **179**: 259–266.
3. Kaplan K.J., Harrow M. (1996) Positive and negative symptoms as risk factors for later suicidal activity in schizophrenics versus depressives. *Suicide Life Threat. Behav.*, **26**: 105–121.
4. Fawcett J., Scheftner W., Clark D., Hedeker D., Gibbons R., Coryell W. (1987) Clinical predictors of suicide in patients with major affective disorders: a controlled prospective study. *Am. J. Psychiatry*, **144**: 35–40.
5. Goldberg J.F., Garno J.L., Leon A.C., Kocsis J.H., Portera L. (1998) Association of recurrent suicidal ideation with nonremission from acute mixed mania. *Am. J. Psychiatry*, **155**: 1753–1755.

2.15
The Role of Seasonal Changes in the Course of Bipolar Disorder

Trevor Silverstone[1]

Bipolar disorder was, as Marneros and Brieger remind us in their comprehensive and scholarly review, originally described by Hippocrates some two and a half thousand years ago. It is a sobering thought that, despite all the scientific, clinical and therapeutic advances made since that time, we understand so very little about what determines its course and outcome. All we can say with any confidence is that the more episodes a patient has experienced, the more likely he or she is to have another [1].

A number of initially promising potential prognostic features have been examined in an impressive number of follow-up studies of varying duration. They have included the pattern of illness (rapid cycling vs. non-rapid cycling) [2], comorbidity (particularly with regard to substance abuse) [3] and seasonal factors [4]. None have been found to show *consistent* predictive reliability. Furthermore, despite our best efforts, it is only in a minority of patients that treatment with lithium and other mood stabilizing drugs stave off further episodes [5].

Our inability to define reliable and clinically useful prognostic indicators is, I believe, largely due to the lack of objective biological markers to confirm or refute a diagnosis of bipolar disorder. All we have to go on are clinical and demographic features. Another confounding influence has been the recent tendency to subdivide the illness into more and more subcategories, each with its own prognosis. For example, according to DSM-IV, bipolar I disorder can take one of six possible forms, with, in addition, the separate category of bipolar II disorder. Such nosological fragmentation is reminiscent of the catalogue of dramatic forms presented to Hamlet by Polonius: "...tragedy, comedy, history, pastoral, pastorical-comical, historical-pastoral, tragical-historical, tragical-comical-historical-pastoral...".

Contemporaneously with this practice of chopping the disease into ever smaller diagnostic subcategories ("splitting"), a counter-movement has taken place in the opposite direction. The term *bipolar spectrum disorders* [6] has been coined to cover a wide range of episodic mood changes of variable severity: from full-blown mania at one extreme, to the mild positive and negative fluctuations in mood experienced by many normal people at the other ("lumping"). Thus, when we discuss prognosis we must be clear about what it is we are talking; the prognosis may vary considerably from one subcategory to another.

[1] *Department of Psychological Medicine, Dunedin School of Medicine, University of Otago, New Zealand*

In addition to the various diagnostic subtypes described, there are a number of "longitudinal course specifiers" listed in DSM-IV which can influence prognosis. Of particular interest to me is the *seasonal pattern specifier* which can be applied to bipolar I, bipolar II or major depressive disorder. This relates to the onset of depressive episodes occurring at characteristic times of the year, typically in autumn or winter, with remission in spring/summer. Although not given the status of a diagnostic category in DSM-IV, this pattern of illness has been widely regarded as if it were a discrete condition, usually referred to as *seasonal affective disorder* (SAD). Here too, a number of variants have been described: "winter SAD", which is the most common and the one first described [7]; "summer SAD", a worsening of mood occurring mainly in summer rather than winter; sub-syndromal SAD, applying to less severe depressive mood swings which do not reach diagnostic criteria for depressive disorder. It is worth noting, in the context of a discussion on the prognosis of bipolar disorder, that the original description of SAD arose from clinical observations made in the context of "a clinic of patients with bipolar disorders"—we appear to have come full circle [7].

Reflecting the ambiguity of its diagnostic status, Marneros and Brieger place their discussion of seasonal factors under the heading "seasonal affective disorder". While they believe that the relationship between season and relapse is "well-established" for (unipolar) seasonal affective disorder, they caution that, for bipolar disorders, "the empirical evidence for the mania-in-summer-depression-in-winter cycle is still weak....A general clear seasonal pattern for the majority of bipolar disorders is not supported by the literature." This is an important matter, because if it can be shown, even in a subgroup of patients with bipolar disorder, that mood is consistently entrained with the seasons, close study of the neurobiological changes accompanying the passage of the seasons would offer a potential key to help us in our search for the biological basis of mood fluctuations.

Unfortunately, the relationship between mood and the seasons is not as clear cut as is often supposed, and the prevalence of SAD appears to be lower than previously reported [8]. Furthermore, epidemiological studies in both the northern and southern hemispheres have shown that the predicted geographical variation in the prevalence of SAD (i.e., that it should be commoner at greater degrees of latitude which have a correspondingly shorter photoperiod in the winter months) is small [9]. In fact, what has emerged is that personality variables, particularly neuroticism, are more closely related to SAD than latitude [10]. Such findings are in keeping with the notion that, for most people living in temperate and sub-arctic zones, winter, with its accompanying cold temperatures and unsettled climate, is a moderate stressor. Those who show a greater dysphoric reaction to stressful events (i.e., high neuroticism) are consequently more likely to become depressed in the winter. In keeping with this analysis are the reports of greater seasonal dysphoria in summer among people living nearer the equator, where summer is more uncomfortable (i.e., a more severe stressor) than winter.

We can only conclude that the relationship between mood and season is not as clear as Hippocrates originally supposed, but nor is that between mood and the colour of bile.

REFERENCES

1. MacQueen G.M., Young L.T., Robb J.C., Marriott M., Cooke R.G., Joffe R.T. (2000) Effect of number of episodes on wellbeing and functioning of patients with bipolar disorder. *Acta Psychiatr. Scand.*, **101**: 374–381.
2. Coryell W.E., Endicott J., Keller M. (1992) Rapid cycling affective disorder. *Arch. Gen. Psychiatry*, **49**: 126–131.
3. Strakowski S.M., DelBello M.P., Fleck D.E., Arndt S. (2000) The impact of substance abuse on the course of bipolar disorder. *Biol. Psychiatry*, **48**: 477–485.
4. Silverstone T., Romans S., Hunt N., McPherson H. (1995) Is there a seasonal pattern of relapse in bipolar affective disorder? A dual northern and southern hemisphere cohort study. *Br. J. Psychiatry*, **167**: 58–60.
5. Silverstone T., McPherson H., Hunt N., Romans S. (1998) How effective is lithium in the prevention of relapse in bipolar disorder? A prospective naturalistic follow-up study. *Aust. N.Z. J. Psychiatry*, **32**: 61–66.
6. Akiskal H.S., Bourgeois M.L., Angst J., Post R., Moller H., Hirschfeld R. (2000) Re-evaluating the prevalence of and diagnostic composition within the broad clinical spectrum of bipolar disorders. *J. Affect. Disord.*, **59** (Suppl. 1): S5–S30.
7. Rosenthal N.E., Sack D.A., Gillin J.C., Lewy A.J., Goodwin F.K., Davenport Y., Mueller P.S., Newsome D.A., Wehr T.A. (1984) Seasonal affective disorder. A description of the syndrome and preliminary findings with light therapy. *Arch. Gen. Psychiatry*, **41**: 72–80.
8. Partonen T., Lonnqvist J. (1998) Seasonal affective disorder. *Lancet*, **352**: 1369–1374.
9. Magnusson A. (2000) An overview of epidemiological studies on seasonal affective disorder. *Acta Psychiatr. Scand.*, **101**: 176–184.
10. Murray G.W., Hay D.A. (1997) Seasonal affective disorder in Australia: is photoperiod critical? *Aust. N.Z. J. Psychiatry*, **31**: 279–284.

3

Pharmacological Treatment of Bipolar Disorder: A Review

Charles L. Bowden

Department of Psychiatry, University of Texas Health Science Center at San Antonio, 7703 Floyd Curl Drive, San Antonio, TX 78229–3900, USA

INTRODUCTION

Definition of mood stabilizers

As the array of pharmacological treatments for bipolar disorder has expanded, implementation of treatment has become more complex, as have notions of the concept of mood stabilization. The first efforts at definition of mood stabilizers referred to drugs that benefited at least one primary aspect of bipolar illness (mania, depression, cycling frequency, number of episodes, subthreshold symptoms) without worsening any other aspect of the illness [1]. This definition focused on the developing evidence that an "ideal" mood stabilizer, one that would aid all aspects of the illness, was not likely to become available [2]. The definition has had some heuristic value since. Principally, it conforms to the increasing evidence that bipolar disorder is composed of a small number, perhaps four to six, of primary behavioural domains [3–7]. Some of these dimensions, or symptom groups, do not occur in every bipolar patient. Impulsivity appears to be the closest to a universal symptom complex in bipolar disorder [3, 8].

With increasing evidence that no drug eliminates all symptoms, and that a substantial portion of bipolar patients are more effectively treated with two or more medications, the rationale for holding to an ideal definition of a mood stabilizer is even weaker than in 1997. However, my sense is that the implied definition used by psychiatrists in practice differs somewhat from that initially proffered. Psychiatrists generally expect a mood stabilizer to be a fundamental component of the acute and maintenance treatment of the

Bipolar Disorder. Edited by Mario Maj, Hagop S. Akiskal, Juan José López-Ibor and Norman Sartorius.
© 2002 John Wiley & Sons Ltd.

patient with bipolar disorder. Surprisingly, only one study has tested the question of whether the treatment effective for an acute episode was effective for the maintenance phase of treatment [9]. However, the expanded definition would require that the drug have evidence of maintenance benefit. An updated definition then would be a drug that benefited at least one primary aspect of bipolar illness (mania, depression, cycling frequency, number of episodes, subthreshold symptoms), has been shown effective in acute and maintenance phase treatment, and does not worsen any aspect of the illness.

As of this writing, this definition would encompass lithium, valproate, lamotrigine, and, probably, carbamazepine.

Primary and Adjunctive Drugs

An additional useful distinction is between medications that have primary roles in treatment of, bipolar disorder, vs. those with roles that are *per se* adjunctive. Primary medications include mood stabilizers, but also include medications that are effective in the manic or depressive phase of the illness. Antipsychotic medications are effectively antimanic. Antidepressant drugs that are approved for major depression are probably effective in alleviating acute bipolar depression, although few have been systematically studied in even one adequate clinical trial. These drugs would qualify as primary treatments.

Drugs that are beneficial for component symptoms that are common in, but not diagnostic of, bipolar disorder, plus ones that may augment response to a primary or mood-stabilizing drug are better viewed as secondary, or adjunctive drugs. Examples include supplementation of antidepressant regimens with thyroid medications or other adjuncts such as pindolol or pramipexole. Others are medications that control anxious symptoms, and/ or improve sleep. These are principally benzodiazepines, or similar agents with GABAergic mechanisms. These are quite important, given the high comorbidity of anxious disorders with bipolar disorder, the high prevalence of anxious symptoms in manic states, and the frequency of sleep disturbance, especially in manic states. This last has probably contributed to early positive reports of antimanic effects of clonazepam and gabapentin [10, 11]. More systematic tests of these drugs has failed to provide evidence of monotherapy effectiveness in mania [12, 13]. It is likely that the improvement in sleep secondarily contributed to some improvement in manic symptoms with these drugs, but that the investigators interpreted the improvement as a primary antimanic or mood-stabilizing benefit. Failure to make this distinction will lead to the fallacy of treating the part of the disorder as the whole.

Tolerability Drives Drug Selection and Patient Adherence

Although no psychiatrist would employ ineffective medications to treat bipolar disorder, tolerability occupies a more important role in decisions to initiate, or continue, a drug than occurs with most mental disorders. Part of this stems from the excellent efficacy of many treatments for a substantial portion of the bipolar spectrum. Additionally, it is related to the inherent characteristics of bipolar disorder. Evidence of expanded creativity in the arts, sciences, politics and probably most work venues is substantial [14, 15]. Bipolar patients have evidence of enhanced educational achievement in first-degree relatives [16]. The bipolar patient expects to be able to operate at a high level of function. I have suggested that a little hyperthymia is not a bad thing, and that psychiatrists sometimes err in overmedicating with mood stabilizers to the point that cognitive dulling occurs. In effect, with this illness, we deal with patients who will often be exquisitely sensitive to subjective functionally impairing side effects. Compare this with the circumstance of numerous patients with epilepsy, who often are treated with the same group of drugs widely employed as mood stabilizers for bipolar disorder. Many such patients are unable to drive and are out of the work force because of their epilepsy. Cognitive side effects therefore are of somewhat lesser concern in the aggregate for such patients, compared with the circumstances in bipolar disorder.

Methodological Issues

In so far as possible this review takes an evidence-based approach in recommending treatments for bipolar disorder. The levels of evidence are divided into four categories. Category I, also referred to in the final summary as "consistent evidence", includes treatments whose efficacy and safety are supported by at least one randomized, double-blind, parallel-group, placebo-controlled study, conducted with a sufficient number of patients that at least one of the major planned analyses provided over a 50% likelihood of identifying a significant difference between groups. Category II has the same criteria as level I, except that no placebo control is required. Category III includes prospective, open trials that employ systematic inclusion and exclusion criteria, utilize behavioural ratings for which raters are trained, and involve a sufficient number of subjects that planned comparisons between two or more groups are possible. These allow comparison, for example, of patients with and without psychosis, or patients who achieved a good response with those who did not [17, 18]. Categories II and III are grouped as providing "incomplete evidence" in the final summary. Category IV, referred to as "areas still open to research" in the final summary, includes smaller open studies, retrospective studies and case reports.

Although the quality of many studies is high, several factors have contributed to past as well as present limitations of clinical trials in bipolar disorder. Early studies with lithium were nearly all discontinuation designs, wherein patients taking stable doses of lithium were randomized to continue lithium or placebo. Lithium was terminated abruptly among patients randomized to placebo in all of the studies before the mid-1980s. Investigators at the time did not know that rebound worsening of illness course, with short-term increases in rates of both manic or hypomanic symptoms, could occur. Following publication of studies characterizing this phenomenon [19–21], current studies provide some form of taper that appears to reduce or eliminate rebound increases in episodes with placebo assignment [9].

The diagnostic criteria for bipolar disorder have evolved rapidly over the past 50 years. The concepts of bipolar disorder, mixed episodes, rapid cycling, and ultra-rapid cycling have all originated during this period, although earlier descriptions citing such phenomena have been identified [22]. Early studies usually included a mix of bipolar and schizoaffective patients for manic presentations, and a mix of bipolar and unipolar patients for studies of depression [23–25].

The dramatic benefits of lithium observed following its introduction tended to lull psychiatrists and research pharmaceutical companies into an unfortunate sense of satisfaction that all that was needed for fundamental management of bipolar disorder was provided by lithium. Only from the mid-1980s did controlled [26] and open studies begin to indicate that outcomes, while positive compared to historical experience without treatment, were limited in many patients [25, 27–30].

The case with antidepressants was complicated by the fact that the DSM essentially utilized the criteria for major depression to define bipolar depression, despite evidence, dating back prior to introduction of the DSM system, that symptom pattern and other illness course features, while overlapping, allowed substantial differentiation [22, 31, 32]. Pivotal trials for currently approved antidepressants have included few bipolar depressed patients, and no drug is specifically approved for bipolar depression [24].

An additional factor has been the difficulty in conducting large sample size, placebo-controlled trials, even in recent years. Sample size is influenced by the impaired insight and judgement of some patients with bipolar disorder, especially attendant to manic states. Often the patient is unwilling to participate when assessed, or terminates prematurely, due to the continued impairment of judgement [33, 34]. The difficulties with placebo-controlled studies have several origins. The consequences of the illness when untreated are sufficiently serious that investigators, patients, and ethics boards are, ethically and practically, cautious about enrolling patients into long-term studies. Maintenance studies therefore have tended to enrol patients with less severe expression of bipolar disorder, as an understandable consequence of concerns about risks associated with placebo-based treatment [35]. This detriment is much less a factor in acute trials of 3–7 weeks [36–38]. European authorities have, until recently, been particularly reluctant to authorize placebo-controlled studies [38].

Placebo-controlled data from randomized trials are essential to establishment of efficacy. Furthermore, they also provide the only meaningful indication of the benefit that the medication tested adds to that of usual care without medication, or with a simpler medication regimen. Open trials generally attribute all of the benefit to the medication, or other regimen under study. However, placebo-controlled data indicate that a substantial proportion of patients improve with the benefits of the non-medication components of care. This fact has received insufficient recognition. Ethically, this provides a basis for proposing studies in which no active medication is provided initially. Scientifically, it allows a way of comparing non-specific treatment effects across studies, and serves as an indicator of the severity of patients enrolled. There is evidence that non-specific benefits of an effective therapeutic relationship are essentially the same across the spectrum of severity of a disorder [39, 40]. Therefore, a greater drug–placebo difference can generally be expected if patients with moderate to severe illness features are enrolled.

The use of placebo in recent mania trials indicates that from 18 to 44% of patients meet relatively stringent criteria for improvement (50% or greater improvement in baseline mania rating scale) [36, 37, 41]. It is likely that an 18 to 25% range of response on placebo can be expected with enrolment of a cohort of patients with generally quite severe mania. The 44% rate may be what can be expected with enrolment of somewhat less severely ill patients. It is also possible that other factors have influenced these improvement rates. For example, threshold severity criteria for inclusion could cause a rating psychiatrist to score a patient higher than was objectively warranted. Once enrolled, subsequent, uninflated ratings on the same scale would yield lower scores independent of actual treatment. The initial inflation of score would tend to magnify the apparent improvement over the course of treatment, particularly the first rating on blinded treatment.

DRUGS PRIMARILY ALLEVIATING MANIA

Lithium

Lithium was superior to placebo in four early crossover studies in manic patients (level II) [42–45]. The crossover designs contributed to artefactually low response rates on placebo, due to lithium withdrawal induced relapse, which was not recognized until after completion of the first series of trials [20]. Additionally, criteria for patient selection were unclear, and patients were largely assigned in a non-random manner. The 1994 study of Bowden *et al.* provides the only randomized, parallel-group, double-blind test of lithium in mania (level I) [36]. The study also utilized structured diagnostic assessments and ratings for mania, and was not confounded by concurrent medications, except for small doses of lorazepam during the first week of the three-week study. Lithium was significantly superior to placebo, and, overall, equivalent to divalproex. The study confirmed earlier impressions that serum levels of 0.8 mEq/1 or greater are associated with significantly better response in bipolar I manic patients.

Lithium has been compared with standard antipsychotic agents in mania in six controlled trials, none of which included a placebo group. In the aggregate, lithium was superior to antipsychotics in reducing manic symptomatology (level II) [46–51]. Antipsychotics had a more rapid onset of action, and were notably effective in alleviating agitation [52].

Lithium was superior to placebo in several early studies of prophylaxis (level II) [53–57]. These studies lacked clear diagnostic criteria, and in most of them stable doses of lithium were abruptly discontinued in patients randomized to placebo, thereby artefactually increasing relapse rate in that group [20, 21]. Large, well-conducted naturalistic studies of the 1990s consistently showed low rates of patients achieving good outcomes with lithium therapy (level III) [30, 58–64].

Two recent large, placebo-controlled, randomized, parallel-group, double-blind studies provide good evidence for effectiveness of lithium in prophylaxis, albeit on a limited aspect of the illness. A one-year study comparing divalproex, lithium and placebo reported that lithium extended time to a 25% rate of relapse to mania by 55% over placebo (Table 3.1).

TABLE 3.1 Time to relapse in bipolar I patients treated with divalproex, lithium or placebo (from Bowden *et al* [9])

	Treatment group		
	Divalproex ($n = 187$)	Lithium ($n = 91$)	Placebo ($n = 94$)
Time to 50% relapse to any mood episode, days (95% CL)	275 (167–NC)	189 (88–NC)	173 (101–NC)
Time to 25% relapse to mania, days (95% CL)	>365 (NC)	293 (71–NC)	189 (84–NC)
Time to 25% relapse to depression, days (95% CL)	126 (100–204)	81 (33–234)	101 (55–190)

However, on other indices of prophylaxis, especially time to relapse to depression, lithium was either ineffective or only modestly effective [9]. An 18-month study of bipolar patients who had experienced a recent manic episode reported that lithium extended time to relapse for any affective episode or to use of additional pharmacotherapy, and was generally equivalent to lamotrigine. Lithium significantly extended time to a manic episode, but not time to a depressive episode (level I) [65, 66]. These data are consistent with the randomized, crossover, one-year study by Denicoff *et al.* [67], showing that lithium reduced time spent in mania from 26% of the year to 9%. However, lithium did not change time spent in depression [67]. Similarly, a randomized, parallel-group maintenance study found that lithium reduced the number of manic episodes in both non-rapid cycling and rapid-cycling bipolar patients. In contrast, the number of depressive episodes was greater with lithium treatment than placebo among both non-rapid cycling and rapid-cycling patients [68].

Lithium was compared to carbamazepine in a 30-month randomized, open trial of bipolar I patients. On most measures, lithium was significantly superior to carbamazepine [69]. Lithium was also associated with fewer suicidal acts than was carbamazepine, consistent with open, naturalistic reports [21, 70]. As with most recent maintenance studies, the planned primary analysis did not indicate significant difference between the two groups, in part as a function of inadequate power. Taken in the aggregate, these data indicate definite prophylactic benefits of lithium, but in a relatively small percentage of bipolar patients who commence treatment, and largely limited to manic symptomatology.

Background factors associated with increased likelihood of response to lithium in mania include classical or pure manic symptoms, a previous positive response to lithium when manic, and fewer previous mood episodes (level I) [71]. Even as few as three depressive episodes predicted non-response to lithium among manic patients (level I) [72]. Mixed or depressive mania, concurrent substance abuse, mania secondary to general medical conditions, and rapid cycling have also been associated with poor response to lithium [23, 36, 73–75].

The characteristic side effects of lithium are, in the aggregate, less problematic during acute treatment. Gastrointestinal irritability and tremor occur early. Lithium reduces manic-associated hyperactivity to levels well below those seen in healthy controls [76]. However, cognitive dulling and sedation may be useful, or at least adequately tolerated during a manic episode. Most organ system toxicity develops gradually and becomes problematic only during maintenance phase treatment. Attention to weight gain, renal complications, thyroid function, cognitive function and degree of lethargy/inactivity are especially important in long-term use.

Valproate

Valproate as divalproex was superior to placebo in two randomized, double-blind studies in hospitalized manic patients (level I). The first study enrolled only patients intolerant to lithium, and found over a 5-fold greater response among divalproex- than placebo-treated patients [37]. The second study included lithium as an active comparator. Divalproex was superior to placebo, equivalent overall to lithium, and resulted in significant improvement somewhat sooner than lithium (level I). Improvement in sleep, psychosis, elevated mood, and elation/grandiosity was greater among divalproex- than lithium-treated patients [7]. Divalproex was better tolerated than lithium, a result that has been confirmed in all studies of substantial numbers of subjects [9, 25, 77].

Valproate was superior to carbamazepine in a randomized, double-blind study, with earlier improvement, less use of rescue medications, and fewer adverse effects (17% vs. 67%). Valproate produced greater improvement than carbamazepine on elevated mood, irritability, rapid speech, and thinking disturbance [78]. In a randomized, open study of acute psychotic manic patients, divalproex and haloperidol were comparable in reduction of both manic and psychotic symptoms (level II) [79]. Valproate plus haloperidol or other standard antipsychotic was superior in reduction of manic symptoms to the antipsychotic alone in a randomized, double-blind study of hospitalized manic patients. Additionally, patients receiving the combined regimen were treated with lower doses of antipsychotic by the end of the three-week study than were patients treated with antipsychotic alone (level I) [80].

Valproate has been studied in two randomized maintenance phase trials. The first, open 18-month study indicated somewhat fewer episodes among valpromide-treated patients than lithium-treated patients, as well as fewer discontinuations for ineffectiveness or intolerance among valpromide-treated patients [25]. The study is flawed by inclusion of some recurrent unipolar patients. The second study was a one-year comparison of divalproex, lithium and placebo. On most secondary measures of efficacy, divalproex was superior to placebo. However, the preponderance of benefit was in extending time to manic recurrence, rather than depressive recurrence. The time to 25% rate of relapse into mania was extended in excess of 93% compared with placebo, whereas the time to 25% relapse to depression was extended 25% (Table 3.1). The magnitude of effectiveness of divalproex during the maintenance phase was greater among the subset of patients whose manic episode at study entry had been brought under control with open, psychiatrist's choice divalproex. Among patients whose manic episode had been brought under control with lithium, lithium was no more or less effective during the blinded maintenance phase than it was among patients who had been treated with divalproex when manic (Table 3.2).

TABLE 3.2   Outcome measures among patients receiving divalproex or lithium in the open phase of one-year maintenance study (from Bowden *et al* [9])

	Randomized treatment group		
	Divalproex	Lithium	Placebo
Divalproex in open period (*n* = 149)	(*n* = 70)	(*n* = 41)	(*n* = 38)
Days in maintenance phase of study	209 ± 155*	162 ± 146	143 ± 123
Early termination for mania or depression	20 (29%)†	15 (37%)	19 (50%)
Early termination for intolerance to study drug or noncompliance	12 (17%)	14 (34%)	7 (19%)
Early termination for any reason	41 (59%)‡	31 (76%)	33 (87%)
Lithium in open period (*n* = 142)	(*n* = 79)	(*n* = 31)	(*n* = 32)
Days in maintenance phase of study	188 ± 150	130 ± 146	183 ± 151
Early termination for mania or depression	12 (15%)	10 (32%)	12 (38%)
Early termination for intolerance to study drug or noncompliance	16 (20%)§	10 (32%)‖	1 (3%)
Early termination for any reason	51 (65%)	25 (81%)	21 (66%)

*F (1,145) = 5.01, P = 0.027, divalproex vs. placebo
†P = 0.036, Fisher's exact test, divalproex vs. placebo
‡P = 0.002, Fisher's exact test, divalproex vs. placebo
§P = 0.022, Fisher's exact test, divalproex vs. placebo
‖P = 0.003, Fisher's exact test, lithium vs. placebo

This is the only published study that provides data about open, acute phase treatment and blinded, maintenance treatment with the same regimens, thereby addressing the important question of continued benefits of a treatment that was effective during an acute episode. The planned primary analysis in this study, time to recurrence of any mood episode, did not differ significantly between the treatments. The power to identify a significant difference with this analysis was an inadequate 30%, vs. the anticipated power of 80%. The discrepancy resulted largely from failing to take into account that the high relapse rate into mania in early placebo-controlled studies of lithium for prophylaxis had much higher rates of manic relapse, as a function of abrupt discontinuation of lithium.

Most factors associated with reduced likelihood of response to lithium among manics are not associated with differential response to valproate. Number of episodes is unrelated to response; mixed and pure manic patients have similar rates of response; and, though less secure, evidence suggests that patients with mania secondary to general medical conditions, mania associated with substance abuse, and rapid-cycling manics appear to respond relatively similarly to manics overall [17, 36, 75, 81]. Divalproex is more effective than lithium for mixed mania [36, 82]. In the aggregate, these studies indicate a broader spectrum for valproate than lithium in mania.

Serum levels of 45–50 μg/ml or higher are associated with efficacy in the treatment of mania [83]. Serum levels are not well established for management of hypomania, bipolar spectrum conditions, or even maintenance treatment. Patients in the largest and best designed maintenance study of valproate had mean serum levels of 85 μg/ml; higher levels (especially over 125 μg/ml) were associated with greater frequency of reported weight gain, reduction in platelet and white blood counts, and with less effective control of manic symptoms. The study therefore supports a somewhat lower serum level range for maintenance than for treatment of mania. Two reports suggest that patients with cyclothymia respond at lower serum levels than those needed for mania [84, 85]. The recently introduced extended release form of divalproex yields 10–15% lower serum levels than the initial divalproex formulation. Most patients therefore will need some dosage increase if changed to this better tolerated form of divalproex [86]. Valproate is highly protein bound. Women and elderly patients will tend to have higher relative free valproate levels, which is the active moiety. In these groups, slower dosage escalation, and reduction of dosage to yield a lower and better- tolerated serum level is often indicated.

Manic patients have tolerated well initial doses of 20–30 mg/kg body weight [87, 88], yielding an onset of response within 2–3 days. In one randomized study, this regimen was equivalent in efficacy to haloperidol, and better tolerated [79]. Intravenous valproate was well tolerated and usually effective within 24 hours in a small number of manic patients [89].

As with lithium, overall side-effect burden is less for treatment of mania than for maintenance treatment, with gastrointestinal irritability, tremor and reduced platelet and leucocyte counts being among the most common side effects in early treatment [36]. Gastrointestinal tolerability and overall side-effect burden is better with divalproex, and probably other sustained release forms of valproate, than with immediate release valproic acid [86]. Platelet counts below $150\,000/mm^3$ warrant closer follow-up, but bleeding complications are rare at levels above $75\,000/mm^3$. Hair loss may be managed by supplemental zinc and selenium, and by separating valproate dosage from meals or vitamin ingestion. During maintenance use, weight gain, cognitive dulling and lethargy bear special attention.

Lithium and valproate have additive effects on some signal transduction processes that are indirectly implicated as involved in the pathophysiology of bipolar disorder [90, 91]. Several open series and one blinded, randomized study indicate that the combination of lithium and divalproex may often improve response over that seen with either agent as monotherapy [17, 92].

Antipsychotic Drugs

Three atypical antipsychotic drugs have been shown superior to placebo in randomized, placebo-controlled studies in mania. Olanzapine was superior to placebo in hospitalized manic patients in two studies (level I) [41]. Response was similar among patients with and without psychotic symptoms at the point of study entry. The modal dose of olanzapine was 15 mg/day in the first study and 16 mg/day in the second [41, 93]. Olanzapine was equivalent in efficacy to divalproex in two randomized, double-blind studies [94]. Tolerability of divalproex was somewhat better. Ziprasidone has similarly been shown superior to placebo in short-term trials (level I) [95]. None of these monotherapy trials included an active comparator drug.

Two studies have demonstrated that an antipsychotic drug added to an ongoing regimen of either lithium or valproate that had not prevented a breakthrough manic episode provides greater improvement than continuing the mood stabilizer as monotherapy (level I). The olanzapine study showed equivalent additive benefits among patients with and without psychotic features [41, 96]. Risperidone was studied in a similar design, but haloperidol was included as an active comparator. Both risperidone and haloperidol plus mood stabilizer yielded greater improvement than continuation of the mood stabilizer alone. Risperidone was somewhat better tolerated than haloperidol, particularly on extrapyramidal adverse effects [97]. The risperidone study allowed patients to enter whose manic episode had developed while unmedicated. Among the patients for whom the mood stabilizer was started concurrently with the antipsychotic, no significant difference was noted for the combination treatment over the mood stabilizer plus placebo. This result suggests that combination therapy utilizing an atypical antipsychotic added to a mood stabilizer should be limited to those patients who develop mania while taking the mood stabilizer.

Antipsychotic drugs have been minimally studied systematically for maintenance treatment. The one placebo-controlled study of a standard antipsychotic added to lithium vs. lithium alone did not find a difference in efficacy between the two treatments. The fluphenthixol plus lithium group had an increase in depressive symptoms, consistent with open reports [98, 99]. A substantial percentage of patients who have psychotic features during a manic episode continue to have psychotic symptoms when followed prospectively for several years [100]. There is therefore interest in the efficacy and tolerability of atypical antipsychotics in maintenance phase treatment. Clozapine was superior to treatment as usual in rate of change in psychotic and manic scores in a randomized, open, one-year study of 38 bipolar and schizoaffective patients (level III) [101]. No randomized maintenance study of these drugs has been published.

Dosing regimens of antipsychotic drugs beyond treatment for mania are not established, but lower doses are generally used. Olanzapine and clozapine, and probably other antipsychotics with a basic dibenzodiazepine structure, have been demonstrated to increase serum glucose and low density lipids. There is inferential evidence that these increases may increase patient morbidity. The prevalence of these complications, and strategies to recognize risks and reduce them have not been established.

Carbamazepine

Carbamazepine has been studied in several trials in mania, but design weaknesses limit conclusions. Other antimanic agents were employed in most studies. One small, placebo-controlled crossover study reported that the majority of patients improved significantly in manic symptoms, and a switch to, or initial treatment with placebo was associated with poor response (level II). Of two randomized comparisons with lithium, one reported lithium superior, the other reported comparable, but low efficacy for the two drugs [102, 103]. As reviewed earlier, valproate was superior to carbamazepine in acute mania in a recent randomized, double-blind study [78]. Two studies compared carbamazepine with chlorpromazine and reported no differences between the drugs in efficacy [104, 105].

The few studies of carbamazepine in prophylaxis suggest that it is less effective than lithium, and associated with high rates of premature discontinuation [106]. Lithium was more effective than carbamazepine in a randomized, open, 2.5-year study [69]. Trends for carbamazepine to be more effective than lithium were present for mood incongruent delusions, comorbidity with other diseases, bipolar II features, and mixed states [70]. Carbamazepine may be more effective in combination treatment than alone [67, 107].

There are few guidelines as to features that might be associated with greater or lesser likelihood of response to carbamazepine other than those regarding atypical features of mania mentioned above.

Carbamazepine has been dosed at 600 to 2600 mg/day in trials in mania, with a mean dose around 1000 mg/day. There is no evidence of a threshold serum level significantly associated with response. Because of cognitive and neuromuscular side effects, carbamazepine requires a slow increase in dosage. Once a steady-state dosage is achieved and pharmacokinetic interactions avoided or effectively managed, carbamazepine is often better tolerated during maintenance use than acutely. This is in part because several of the side-effect complexes associated with it occur principally during dosing incrementation. Carbamazepine induces the 3A4 oxidative enzyme system in liver. As carbamazepine is also metabolized via 3A4, a dosing increase is required after several weeks of treatment to adjust for increased clearance rates. The 3A4 system metabolizes the largest range of drugs of all the oxidative enzyme isoforms. Unless drugs can be assayed by serum level measurement, it is inadvisable to combine drugs metabolized via 3A4 with carbamazepine. Software that can be loaded into palm-held computing devices now allow convenient checking of potential interactions between drugs, thereby allowing treatment decisions that can avoid regimens that are ineffective with concurrent carbamazepine use. One of two recent risperidone plus mood stabilizer trials in mania allowed entry of patients whose mania developed while taking carbamazepine [108]. Carbamazepine lowered risperidone serum levels dramatically, essentially precluding any effective dosage in the carbamazepine plus risperidone subjects. Carbamazepine causes a range of relatively severe rashes, requiring discontinuation in approximately 10% of patients from acute trials [67]. The limited evidence of efficacy of carbamazepine, coupled with pharmacokinetic and tolerability problems acutely, has resulted in some lowering of recommended priority of usage in recent expert guidelines [109].

A congener of carbamazepine, oxcarbazepine, is also marketed for treatment of epilepsy. Although minimally studied in mania, it appears to have a similar efficacy and tolerability. Magnitude of induction of 3A4 enzymes appears somewhat less, but it remains inadvisable to use the drug with any medication metabolized by this enzyme isoform.

DRUGS PRINCIPALLY AFFECTING DEPRESSION

Lamotrigine

Lamotrigine was significantly superior to placebo in a double-blind, randomized, placebo-controlled, seven-week study of bipolar I depressed patients (level I). Significant improvement was noted from the point at which lamotrigine-treated patients received 50 mg/day for one week [38]. The study is the only high quality designed monotherapy study conducted for bipolar depression. The planned primary test of efficacy yielded only trends for superiority of lamotrigine over placebo. The primary reason is that the instrument selected, the Hamilton Rating Scale for Depression, provides less sensitivity to assess the principally affective and cognitive symptoms of depression than did the secondary measure, the Montgomery Asberg Rating Scale [110]. Lamotrigine was studied at both 50 and 200 mg/day. Both doses were effective, but in the aggregate response was greater with the 200 mg/day dose. One double-blind, placebo-controlled crossover study also found lamotrigine superior to placebo as well as to gabapentin in bipolar depressed patients (level I) [13]. Systematic open study supports efficacy of lamotrigine as monotherapy and in combination with other mood stabilizers in bipolar I and II depressed patients [38]. One negative study of lamotrigine in bipolar depression enrolled both bipolar I and II patients. Lamotrigine was superior to placebo among bipolar I, but not bipolar II patients. Lamotrigine did not differ from placebo in treatment of bipolar I manic patients.

Lamotrigine was superior to placebo in a randomized, double-blind, 18-month study in bipolar patients who had experienced a recent manic episode (level I) [65, 66]. The study included a lithium comparator group. Although the drugs did not differ significantly from one another on efficacy measures, lamotrigine significantly extended time to a depressive episode, but not a manic episode, whereas lithium extended time to mania, but not depression. Additionally, lamotrigine was superior to placebo on most measures in a six-month maintenance study of rapid-cycling bipolar patients. The greatest advantage of lamotrigine over placebo was noted in bipolar II patients, not bipolar I patients. In the aggregate, these studies suggest that lamotrigine has marked efficacy in bipolar depression and no or low efficacy in mania, which is the converse of the profile of efficacy of lithium and valproate.

Lamotrigine requires slow dosage titration, due to the risk of serious rash. As monotherapy, an initial dose of 25 mg/day can generally be increased in 25 mg increments weekly until a dose of 100 mg/day is reached, after which dosage may be increased by up to 100 mg increments to a maximum of 600 mg/day. Lamotrigine is metabolized by glucuronidation, as principally is valproate. Lamotrigine used in the presence of valproate requires essentially half the starting dose, and a somewhat slower rate of titration [111].

Headache is the only side effect consistently more common with lamotrigine than placebo. In acute and maintenance studies to date, rates of development of mania or hypomania have been equivalent in lamotrigine- and placebo-treated groups.

Selective Serotonin Reuptake Inhibitors

Selective serotonin reuptake inhibitors (SSRIs) are safer in overdose than tricyclic antidepressants and have a better side-effect profile. However, as with all of the drugs other than lamotrigine in this section, there has been limited systematic study in bipolar depression. Cohn et al reported a higher response with fluoxetine treatment than with imipramine or placebo [112]. Nemeroff et al found paroxetine or imipramine plus standard lithium no different overall from lithium plus placebo (level I) [113]. Paroxetine plus lithium and imipramine plus lithium were superior to lithium alone in the subset of patients with serum levels of lithium below 0.8 mEq/l. Retrospective studies of fluoxetine, venlafaxine, and paroxetine suggest response rates above 50% (level III) [114–116]. Rates of mania/hypomania during treatment appear lower with SSRIs than with TCAs [112, 117].

Bupropion

Small open studies and one small, placebo-controlled study indicate that bupropion is effective in bipolar depression (level III) [118, 119]. Additionally, a small study found equal efficacy for bupropion and desipramine, but lower rates of manic switching with bupropion [120]. Another study did not report low rates of switching with bupropion [121].

Tricyclic Antidepressants and Other Principally Norepinephrine Uptake Inhibiting Drugs

The largest study of tricyclic antidepressants (TCAs) in unipolar and bipolar depressed patients found equal rates of efficacy in the two forms of depression (level II) [122]. In the aggregate, response rates to TCAs have been about 50 to 70% [123]. The one prospective, randomized study of TCAs in bipolar disorder indicated higher switch rates than have been reported with other antidepressant drugs [124].

Monoamine Oxidase Inhibitors

The reversible, type A selective monoamine oxidase inhibitor (MAOI) moclobemide was effective in 60% of bipolar depressed patients, compared with a 49% response rate for various comparator drugs (level III) [125]. In two studies of bipolar patients with anergic depression, tranylcypromine was more effective than imipramine in both a randomized and a crossover trial [126, 127]. Switch rates to hypomania have been 11% or greater in short-term studies [126, 127].

Antidepressant Induced Mood Instability

The paucity of studies allows at best tentative statements on the subject of induction of mania/hypomania, increase in cycling frequency, or symptomatically milder mood instability. The one randomized, prospective, on-off design of antidepressants in bipolar disorder indicated a marked increase in cycling frequency while taking the antidepressant (level II) [124]. The thoughtful study of Altshuler et al indicates a direct link between switching and increased frequency of cycling [128]. The only published studies that have not identified some increased rate of switching have imposed selection criteria on the subjects that tended to exclude at the outset all patients with evidence of mood instability, and, in fact, to require evidence of mood stability as a requirement for study eligibility [129, 130]. Additionally, a never-ending number of case reports of mania developing shortly following addition of an antidepressant, in some cases with confirmatory re-exposure, are available for practically all marketed antidepressants [131]. Only lamotrigine of the drugs reviewed appears, at this point, not to be associated with rates of mania/hypomania greater than those seen with placebo. The case is clearer with lamotrigine, as it is the only one of the drugs reviewed above for which good quality, placebo-controlled, randomized, parallel-group data are available. My assessment of the evidence is that bipolar patients have an inherent tendency to mood instability, from a wide range of internal and external factors, and that currently approved antidepressants do contribute to mood instability. Further, this mood instability is only in part ameliorated by concurrent use of a mood stabilizer [132]. Therefore, most bipolar patients who are prescribed antidepressants for depressive episodes should be tapered off the antidepressant within a period of several weeks following alleviation of depression (level III).

Mood Stabilizers in Bipolar Depression

Although eight of nine placebo-controlled, crossover-designed studies of lithium were reported as supporting superiority to placebo in treatment of bipolar depression, the study designs were consistently flawed, with abrupt discontinuation contributing in part to apparent lithium advantage. A systematic review of these studies, utilizing more realistic criteria of response, reported the response rate to be 36% (level II) [24]. This evidence of, at best, modest antidepressant effects in bipolar depression is in contrast to the consistent evidence that lithium can augment antidepressant effects in both unipolar and bipolar depressed patients [133, 134].

Divalproex yielded an aggregate 30% response rate in four open studies in depressed patients (level III) [135]. In the absence of adequate studies, the efficacy of divalproex in acute bipolar depression appears modest (level III). The 2000 study of divalproex, placebo and lithium in maintenance treatment of bipolar I patients allowed for treatment of patients who became clinically depressed with either paroxetine or sertraline [9]. Rates of patients developing depression did not differ across the three treatment groups. However, the combination of divalproex plus SSRI was associated with significantly greater likelihood of completion of the study than was placebo plus SSRI, with an intermediate result for lithium plus SSRI (divalproex = 90%, placebo = 55%, $P = .003$; lithium = 71%) [136]. This provides the most direct evidence that an antidepressant alone is an ineffective treatment strategy for depression occurring in bipolar disorder (level II). Further, it indicates that the combination of divalproex plus an SSRI is an effective strategy for management of breakthrough depression during maintenance treatment of bipolar I disorder.

Carbamazepine has been studied in 78 patients in controlled trials. The studies have design flaws such as enrolment of both unipolar and bipolar depressed patients. Approximately one-third of patients responded. The limited data suggest mild to moderate antidepressant effects for carbamazepine in bipolar depression (level III) [137, 138].

PUTATIVE TREATMENTS FOR BIPOLAR DISORDER

Many drugs are proposed conceptually, or presented in print as effective, in some aspect of treatment of bipolar disorder. Rarely is it possible to assess adequately a drug for bipolar disorder in other than a placebo-controlled, randomized, parallel-group study, enrolling patients who have common illness characteristics at the start of the study. The inherently changing symptomatology of bipolar disorder probably contributes to a greater likelihood of positive open reports in bipolar disorder than most other mental disorders, but ones wherein the improvement reflects inherent changes in symptomatology, rather than an effect of drug. The following drugs have case reports that suggest efficacy in some patients, but have not been tested in the above paradigms, or have had largely negative studies conducted that may have methodological constraints that reduced capacity to identify drug efficacy. Topiramate is a fructopyranose that has been reported as beneficial principally as add-on to mood stabilizers, and principally for manic symptomatology. Omega-3 fatty acids, naturally occurring branched chain fatty acids that may aid in stabilization of key components of intracellular membranes in brain, extended time in study when added to lithium, but no consistent baseline characteristics were present in the sample. Atypical antipsychotics that have not undergone adequate testing in bipolar disorder have been used because of their availability for treatment of schizophrenia. Antidepressants that have not undergone specific testing in bipolar disorder have also been used in that disorder because of their marketed status.

TREATMENT STRATEGY

Mania

Drug selection needs to take into account whether the patient has classical (euphoric, elated) or mixed (depressive, dysphoric) mania. The definition of mixed mania is in need of further study. Recent studies indicate that mixed mania may be a composite of patients with depressive, anxious, and irritable features [3, 6]. It is unclear whether this represents one coherent subgroup, or two or more subgroups that may have differing treatment response to antimanic drugs. Also, evidence of psychotic symptoms needs to be established, as does current rapid cycling. Severity of symptoms, especially in terms of irritability, agitation and psychosis needs to be determined. Concurrent medical or psychiatric disorders need to be identified. Past treatment, and response thereto must be clarified. Current medications need to be reviewed. With this set of information, a rational treatment plan can be implemented. In general, lithium may be a reasonable choice in patients with classical symptomatology and relatively mild manic severity. Divalproex, or other forms of valproate, may be considered over lithium in patients with mixed mania, psychotic mania or more severe forms of mania. Divalproex may also be suitable for classical forms of mania. Divalproex may be preferable where rapid control of symptoms is needed, due to ease of commencing treatment with a quickly therapeutic dose. Olanzapine or ziprasidone, or other atypical antipsychotics, may be suitable as monotherapy for some patients. Their effectiveness is equivalent for psychotic and non-psychotic manic patients. They have not been adequately assessed in regard to other illness course factors. They may be particularly suitable for patients with marked agitation, in whom rapid control of symptoms is critical.

Recent evidence provides assurance that combinations of any two, or possibly more, of these agents may be more effective than a single agent. There are no clear guidelines as to when in the scheme of treatment combination therapy should be considered. Most expert treatment guidelines recommend combination treatments at the third decision point, after two agents have been inadequate as monotherapy.

If the patient is taking a medication that may have destabilized mood, and is therefore contributing to the manic symptomatology, discontinuation is warranted. This approach should extend to stopping antidepressants used in low doses as sleep aids.

Depression

In addition to establishing that the patient has depression, evidence of any current manic symptomatology needs to be carefully assessed. Even though official nomenclature does not recognize depressive mixed states, it is possible that the patient will have sufficient manic symptomatology to warrant treatment as a mixed manic case. Clarifying whether the patient has bipolar I or II disorder is important. There is increasing evidence that bipolar II disorder is predominantly depressive in symptomatology, is more frequent in women, and is associated with rapid-cycling symptomatology

[139]. Based on the evidence for marked efficacy as maintenance monotherapy in a small cohort of bipolar II rapid-cycling patients, lamotrigine warrants consideration as a first treatment for such patients, although further studies are needed on the point.

Most practice guidelines recommend as a first step increasing current mood stabilizers if the doses are submaximal. The evidence for this strategy is minimal. In concept, equal attention might be paid to any possible obtundation or lethargy that the mood stabilizer might be producing. If this is the case, some reduction of the mood stabilizer dose should be considered.

The dearth of adequate studies of antidepressant treatments for bipolar depression places the psychiatrist in a quandary. At present, SSRIs and, where it is marketed, bupropion are often the agents of first choice. This is largely based on modest data suggesting better tolerability and possibly somewhat lower risk of mood destabilization. The positive, well-designed studies with lamotrigine make it an increasingly justifiable drug for consideration as initial, or second-stage treatment. History of mood destabilization while taking an antidepressant would generally discourage re-challenge with that drug.

Maintenance

Most patients are continued on medications that were effective during an acute episode. As discussed throughout this review, there is very little evidence to support this practice, essentially limited to one study [9]. If the acute episode was principally manic, some consideration of lowering the dose of the mood stabilizer is justified. For lithium and divalproex, there are some data supporting dose and serum levels as much as 25% below those required for control of mania [9, 30, 64].

Continued characterization of the relative proportion of time spent in depression vs. the time spent in mania is important. More attention to revising mood stabilizer use is indicated if symptomatology or time ill is principally manic. Alternatively, if symptomatology is principally depressive, consideration of antidepressants, including, especially, lamotrigine, is warranted.

Patients need to be apprised of characteristic side effects, and assured that the treating psychiatrist will work to reduce side effects to a fully tolerable range. Many patients will wish to discontinue drug treatments, not only for reasons of side effects but for various reasons associated with a belief that the illness is, at the least, in remission and does not require continued treatment. Often this will be evidence *per se* of inadequate control of symptomatology of the illness, rather than a rational consideration. Dealing with this in a proactive way, especially including use of educational approaches and involvement of significant other persons to the patient, can be helpful.

Many patients will be best treated with combination regimens. Attention to the target symptoms that are the focus of the combination is essential. Unless the patient obtains definite benefit with the combination, the added drug should be tapered, rather than risk some extra adverse effect burden unnecessarily. Combination treatments may include some adjunctive agents that are not discussed in detail in this chapter. These include supplemental T4, especially for lithium-treated patients; low dose antipsychotics; benzodiazepines, antidepressant augmenting agents, and, increasingly, a variety of herbal remedies, which at the least need to be assessed regarding generally understood spectrum of effects.

SPECIAL SITUATIONS

Sleep

Disturbed sleep is a common, and pathophysiologically important component of bipolar disorder. Persons with bipolar disorder often escalate their interest, elation and energy levels in the evening hours, into the early hours of the next day. It is important to counsel patients regarding this diurnal phase disturbance, but medications are often needed. No systematic studies have been conducted regarding comparative benefits of various strategies. Benzodiazepines are most commonly employed. Benzodiazepines vary along dimensions of speed of onset and half-life. It is best to tailor the drug in a trial-and-error fashion to the patient's unique sleep problems. Some patients may have side effects from benzodiazepines, principally carryover sedation, or less frequently disinhibition of affect and action. In such instances, alternative medications can be used. Despite lack of direct testing for insomnia, gabapentin, at doses of 100 to 400 mg, is often helpful for sleep induction. Although sedative antidepressants are often employed for insomnia, they are to be discouraged due to risks of mood destabilization.

Mood stabilizers can often be prescribed fully or largely at bedtime, and thereby have their sedative properties facilitate sleep. This can be a useful strategy for lithium, divalproex, atypical antipsychotics, and topiramate, but rarely for carbamazepine.

Children

Few and inadequate studies of treatments for bipolar disorder have been conducted in children. A small study comparing lithium with placebo in adolescents with manic symptoms who also had substance abuse reported lithium superior to placebo [140]. Other studies of lithium have yielded mixed results, with tolerability generally problematic. Divalproex has been reported effective in manic children and adolescents in two open studies, with most patients receiving either concomitant antipsychotics or stimulants for psychotic or attention deficit symptoms concurrent with manic symptoms [141, 142]. Although side effects of bipolar drugs are generally similar in children, the consequences may be different as a function of age-specific tasks. Tremor may be particularly interfering with sports and musical instruments. Obesity or acne may be acutely discomfiting in relationship to peers. Effective use of medications generally requires active cooperation from parents. However, parents often have elements of bipolar disorder, which may in turn impede their effective collaboration in the treatment process. Depressive episodes are much more common than manic episodes; psychotic and mixed manic episodes are common [143].

Elderly

Bipolar disorder occasionally has its onset in late life. More often, bipolar disorder that presented earlier becomes more difficult to treat in association with ageing processes. These factors include slower elimination of drugs, greater organ system sensitivity to untoward effects of the mood stabilizer, and concurrent general medical diseases. Bipolar disorder is often more difficult to diagnose in the elderly, since patient reporting is less accurate and symptoms of concurrent disorders blur diagnostic criteria. It is often therefore necessary to settle for treating symptomatic features of bipolar disorder, rather than having unequivocal bipolar episodes to treat. Divalproex appears to be somewhat better tolerated than lithium in elderly bipolar or bipolar spectrum patients [144, 145]. Although some studies have reported dosage ranges and serum levels consistent with those used in younger adult manic patients [146], other studies report that somewhat lower doses are effective, and are better tolerated [147].

Comorbid General Medical Disorders

Comorbid general medical disorders can predispose to bipolar disorder, generally presenting with mixed manic, especially irritable features. Such patients generally do not tolerate lithium well. Evidence suggests that divalproex and carbamazepine tend to be more effective in the spectrum of syndromes seen in such patients.

Pregnancy

Lithium, valproate and carbamazepine each poses some increased risk of teratogenic effects. Fortunately, with the approval of atypical antipsychotics, and the evidence of efficacy of lamotrigine, there are non-teratogenic alternatives to consider during the critical first trimester.

Breast Feeding

Lithium is excreted in breast milk. It is inadvisable for a woman taking lithium to breast feed. Concentrations of carbamazepine and especially valproate are low in breast milk [148]. Therefore, each of these drugs can be considered for use in women who desire to breast feed.

SUMMARY

Consistent Evidence

The following treatments reviewed here have consistent evidence of efficacy. For treatment of mania: divalproex, lithium, olanzapine, ziprasidone, risperidone combined with lithium or valproate, olanzapine combined with lithium or valproate, valproate combined with antipsychotics. For treatment of bipolar depression: lamotrigine. For maintenance treatment of bipolar disorder—principal effects on extending time to mania: lithium, divalproex; principal effects on extending time to depression: lamotrigine.

Incomplete Evidence

The following treatments have inconclusive evidence of efficacy. For treatment of mania: carbamazepine, standard antipsychotic drugs. For treatment of bipolar depression: SSRIs, bupropion, TCAs, MAOIs, carbamazepine. For maintenance treatment of bipolar disorder: carbamazepine, combination of lithium and carbamazepine, combination of lithium and valproate.

Areas Still Open to Research

The following treatments have limited evidence of efficacy, and thus should be considered as areas still open for research. For treatment of mania: topiramate, omega-3 fatty acids, levetiracetam, atypical antipsychotic drugs other than those listed above, oxcarbamazepine. For treatment of bipolar depression: reboxetine, duloxetine, fluvoxamine, citalopram. For maintenance treatment of bipolar disorder: topiramate, omega-3 fatty acids, levetiracetam. The level of evidence and the numbers of drugs within a category are likely to increase over the next decade, consequent to active drug development and testing currently in progress.

REFERENCES

1. Sachs G.S. (1996)   Treatment-resistant bipolar depression. *Psychiatr. Clin. North Am.*, **19**: 215–236.
2. Bowden C.L. (1997)   Treatment of bipolar disorder. *Current Review of Mood & Anxiety Disorders*, 1: 167–176.
3. Swann A.C., Janicak P.L., Calabrese J.R., Bowden C.L., Dilsaver S.C., Morris D.D., Petty F., Davis J.M. (2001)   Structure of mania: depressive, irritable, and psychotic clusters with distinct course of illness in randomized clinical trial participants. *J. Affect. Disord.* (in press).
4. Dilsaver S.C., Swann A.C., Shoaib A.M. (1993)   The manic syndrome: factors which may predict a patient's response to lithium, carbamazepine and valproate. *J. Psychiatry Neurosci.*, **18**: 61–66.
5. Chen Y.W., Dilsaver S.C. (1995)   Comorbidity of panic disorder in bipolar illness: evidence from the Epidemiologic Catchment Area survey. *Am. J. Psychiatry*, **152**: 280–282.
6. Cassidy F., Carroll B.J. (2001)   The clinical epidemiology of pure and mixed manic episodes. *Bipolar Disord.*, **3**: 35–40.
7. Bowden C.L., Davis J., Morris D., Swann A., Calabrese J., Lambert M., Goodnick P. (1997)   Effect size of efficacy measures comparing divalproex, lithium and placebo in acute mania. *Depress. Anxiety*, **6**: 26–30.
8. Janowsky D.S., Morter S., Hong L., Howe L. (1999)   Myers Briggs Type Indicator and Tridimensional Personality Questionnaire differences between bipolar patients and unipolar depressed patients. *Bipolar Disord.*, **1**: 98–108.
9. Bowden C.L., Calabrese J.R., McElroy S.L., Gyulai L., Wassef A., Petty F., Pope H.G., Jr., Chou J.C.-Y., Keck P.E., Jr., Rhodes L.J. *et al* (2000)   A randomized, placebo-controlled 12-month trial of divalproex and lithium in treatment of outpatients with bipolar I disorder. *Arch. Gen. Psychiatry*, **57**: 481–489.
10. Chouinard G. (1987)   Clonazepam in the acute and maintenance treatment of bipolar affective disorder. *J. Clin. Psychiatry*, **48** (Suppl. 10): 29–36.
11. McElroy S.L., Soutullo C.A., Keck P.E., Jr., Kmetz G.F. (1997)   A pilot trial of adjunctive gabapentin in the treatment of bipolar disorder. *Ann. Clin. Psychiatry*, **9**: 99–103.
12. Pande A.C., Crockatt J.G., Janney C.A., Werth J.L., Tsaroucha G. and Gabapentin Bipolar Disorder Study Group (2000)   Gabapentin in bipolar disorder: a placebo-controlled trial of adjunctive therapy. *Bipolar Disord.*, **2**: 249–255.
13. Frye M.A., Ketter T.A., Kimbrell T.A., Dunn R.T., Speer A.M., Osuch E.A., Luckenbaugh D.A., Cora-Locatelli G., Leverich G.S., Post R.M. (2000)   A placebo-controlled study of lamotrigine and gabapentin monotherapy in refractory mood disorders. *J. Clin. Psychopharmacol.*, **20**: 607–614.

14. Jamison K.R. (1993) *Touched with Fire.* Free Press, New York.
15. Bowden C.L. (1994) Bipolar disorder and creativity. In *Creativity and Affect* (Eds M.P. Shaw, M.A. Runco), pp. 73–86, Ablex Publishing Corporation, New Jersey.
16. Andreasen N.C. (1987) Creativity and mental illness: prevalence rates in writers and their first-degree relatives. *Am. J. Psychiatry,* **144**: 1288–1292.
17. Calabrese J.R., Delucchi G.A. (1990) Spectrum of efficacy of valproate in 55 patients with rapid-cycling bipolar disorder. *Am. J. Psychiatry,* **147**: 431–434.
18. Bowden C.L., Calabrese J.R., McElroy S.L., Rhodes L.J., Keck P.E., Jr., Cookson J., Anderson J., Bolden-Watson C., Ascher J., Monaghan E. *et al* (1999) The efficacy of lamotrigine in rapid cycling and non-rapid cycling patients with bipolar disorder. *Biol. Psychiatry,* **45**: 953–958.
19. Faedda G.L., Baldessarini R.J., Tohen M., Strakowski S.M., Waternaux C. (1991) Episode sequence in bipolar disorder and response to lithium treatment. *Am. J. Psychiatry,* **148**: 1237–1239.
20. Suppes T., Baldessarini R.J., Faedda G.L., Tohen M. (1991) Risk of recurrence following discontinuation of lithium treatment in bipolar disorder. *Arch. Gen. Psychiatry,* **48**: 1082–1088.
21. Baldessarini R.J., Tondo L., Faedda G.L., Suppes T.R., Floris G., Rudas N. (1996) Effects of the rate of discontinuing lithium maintenance treatment in bipolar disorders. *J. Clin. Psychiatry,* **57**: 441–448.
22. Swann A.C., Bowden C.L., Morris D., Calabrese J.R., Petty F., Small J., Dilsaver S.C., Davis J.M. (1997) Depression during mania: treatment response to lithium or divalproex. *Arch. Gen. Psychiatry,* **54**: 37–42.
23. Goodwin F.K., Jamison K.R. (1990) *Manic-Depressive Illness.* Oxford University Press, New York.
24. Zornberg G.L., Pope H.G. (1993) Treatment of depression in bipolar disorder: new directions for research. *J. Clin. Psychopharmacol.,* **13**: 397–408.
25. Lambert P.A., Venaud G. (1992) Comparative study of valpromide versus lithium as prophylactic treatment in affective disorders. *Nervure,* **5**: 57–65.
26. Prien R.F., Kupfer D.J., Mansky P.A., Small J.G., Tuason V.B., Voss C.B., Johnson W.E. (1984) Drug therapy in the prevention of recurrences in unipolar and bipolar affective disorders. Report of the NIMH Collaborative Study Group comparing lithium carbonate, imipramine, and a lithium carbonate–imipramine combination. *Arch. Gen. Psychiatry,* **41**: 1096–1104.
27. Markar H.R., Mander A.J. (1989) Efficacy of lithium prophylaxis in clinical practice. *Br. J. Psychiatry,* **155**: 496–500.
28. Moncrieff J. (1995) Lithium revisited. A re-examination of the placebo-controlled trials of lithium prophylaxis in manic-depressive disorder. *Br. J. Psychiatry,* **167**: 569–573.
29. Blackwell B. (1971) Lithium prophylaxis in recurrent affective disorders. *Br. J. Psychiatry,* **118**: 131–132.
30. Maj M., Pirozzi R., Magliano L., Bartoli L. (1998) Long-term outcome of lithium prophylaxis in bipolar disorder: a 5-year prospective study of 402 patients at a lithium clinic. *Am. J. Psychiatry,* **155**: 30–35.
31. Bowden C.L. (2001) Strategies to reduce misdiagnosis of bipolar depression. *Psychiatr. Serv.,* **52**: 51–55.
32. Bowden C.L. (1999) A two-illness model of bipolar disorder. *Bipolar Disord.,* **1**: 31–35.
33. Bowden C.L., Swann A.C., Calabrese J.R., McElroy S.L., Morris D., Petty F.L., Hirschfeld R.M.A., Gyulai L. (1997) Maintenance clinical trials in bipolar

disorder: design implications of the divalproex–lithium–placebo study. *Psychopharmacol. Bull.*, **33**: 693–699.

34. Gelenberg A.J., Kane J.M., Keller M.B., Lavori P., Rosenbaum J.F., Cole K., Lavelle J. (1989) Comparison of standard and low serum levels of lithium for maintenance treatment of bipolar disorder. *N. Engl. J. Med.*, **321**: 1489–1493.

35. Baldessarini R.J., Tohen M., Tondo L. (2000) Maintenance treatment in bipolar disorder. *Arch. Gen. Psychiatry*, **57**: 490–492.

36. Bowden C.L., Brugger A.M., Swann A.C., Calabrese J.R., Janicak P.G., Petty F., Dilsaver S.C., Davis J.M., Rush A.J., Small J.G. *et al* (1994) Efficacy of divalproex vs lithium and placebo in the treatment of mania. *JAMA*, **271**: 918–924.

37. Pope H.G., Jr., McElroy S.L., Keck P.E., Jr., Hudson J.I. (1991) Valproate in the treatment of acute mania: a placebo-controlled study. *Arch. Gen. Psychiatry*, **48**: 62–68.

38. Calabrese J.R., Bowden C.L., Sachs G.S., Ascher J.A., Monaghan E., Rudd D.G. (1999) A double-blind placebo-controlled study of lamotrigine monotherapy in outpatients with bipolar I depression. *J. Clin. Psychiatry*, **60**: 79–88.

39. Fisher S., Lipman R.S., Uhlenhuth E.H., Rickels K., Park L.C. (1965) Drug effects and initial severity of symptomatology. *Psychopharmacologia*, **7**: 57–60.

40. Uhlenhuth E.H., Matuzas W., Warner T.D., Thompson P.M. (1997) Methodological issues in psychopharmacological research. Growing placebo response rate: the problem in recent therapeutic trials? *Psychopharmacol. Bull.*, **33**: 31–39.

41. Tohen M., Jacobs T.G., Grundy S.L., McElroy S.L., Banov M.C., Janicak P.G., Sanger T., Risser R., Zhang F., Toma V. *et al* (2000) Efficacy of olanzapine in acute bipolar mania: A double-blind, placebo-controlled study. *Arch. Gen. Psychiatry*, **57**: 841–849.

42. Schou M., Juel-Nielsen N., Stromgren E., Voldby H. (1954) The treatment of manic psychoses by the administration of lithium salts. *J. Neurol. Neurosurg. Psychiatry*, **17**: 250–260.

43. Maggs R. (1963) Treatment of manic illness with lithium carbonate. *Br. J. Psychiatry*, **109**: 56–65.

44. Goodwin F.K., Murphy D.L., Bunney W.E., Jr. (1969) Lithium carbonate treatment in depression and mania: a longitudinal double-blind study. *Arch. Gen. Psychiatry*, **21**: 486–496.

45. Stokes P.E., Shamoian C.A., Stoll P.M., Patton M.J. (1971) Efficacy of lithium as acute treatment of manic-depressive illness. *Lancet*, **i**: 1319–1325.

46. Platman S.R. (1970) A comparison of lithium carbonate and chlorpromazine in mania. *Am. J. Psychiatry*, **127**: 351–353.

47. Spring G., Frankel M. (1981) New data on lithium and haloperidol incompatibility. *Am. J. Psychiatry*, **138**: 818–821.

48. Johnson G., Gershon S., Burdock E.I., Floyd A., Hekimian L. (1971) Comparative effects of lithium and chlorpromazine in the treatment of acute manic states. *Br. J. Psychiatry*, **119**: 267–276.

49. Prien R.F., Caffey E.M., Klett C. (1972) Comparison of lithium carbonate and chlorpromazine in the treatment of mania. *Arch. Gen. Psychiatry*, **26**: 146–153.

50. Shopsin B., Gershon S., Thompson H., Collins P. (1975) Psychoactive drugs in mania: a controlled comparison of lithium carbonate, chlorpromazine, and haloperidol. *Arch. Gen. Psychiatry*, **32**: 34–42.

51. Takahashi R., Sakuma A., Itoh K., Itoh H., Kurihara M., Saito M., Watanabe M. (1975) Comparison of efficacy of lithium carbonate and chlorpromazine in mania. *Arch. Gen. Psychiatry*, **32**: 1310–1318.

52. Keck P.E. Jr., McElroy S.L., Strakowski S.M. (1998) Anticonvulsants and anti-psychotics in the treatment of bipolar disorder. *J. Clin. Psychiatry*, **59** (Suppl. 6): 74–81.

53. Baastrup P.C., Poulsen J.C., Schou M., Thomsen K., Amdisen A. (1970) Prophy-lactic lithium: Double-blind discontinuation in manic-depressive and recurrent-depressive disorders. *Lancet*, **ii**: 326–330.

54. Melia P.I. (1970) Prophylactic lithium: A double-blind trial in recurrent affect-ive disorders. *Br. J. Psychiatry*, **116**: 621–624.

55. Coppen A., Peet M., Bailey J., Noguera R., Burns B., Swani M., Maggs R., Gardner R. (1973) Double-blind and open prospective studies of lithium prophylaxis in affective disorders. *Psychiatria, Neurologia, Neurochirurgia*, **76**: 500–510.

56. Cundall R.L., Brooks P.W., Murray L.G. (1972) A controlled evaluation of lithium prophylaxis in affective disorders. *Psychol. Med.*, **2**: 308–311.

57. Prien R.F., Caffey E.M., Klett C.J. (1973) Prophylactic efficacy of lithium car-bonate in manic-depressive illness. *Arch. Gen. Psychiatry*, **28**: 337–341.

58. Dickson W.E., Kendell R.E. (1986) Does maintenance lithium therapy prevent recurrences of mania under ordinary clinical conditions? *Psychol. Med.*, **16**: 521–530.

59. Harrow M., Goldberg J.F., Grossman L.S., Meltzer H.Y. (1990) Outcome in manic disorders: a naturalistic follow-up study. *Arch. Gen. Psychiatry*, **47**: 665–671.

60. O'Connell R.A., Mayo J.A., Flatow L., Cuthbertson B., O'Brien B.E. (1991) Out-come of bipolar disorder on long-term treatment with lithium. *Br. J. Psychiatry*, **159**: 123–129.

61. Keck P.E., Jr., McElroy S.L. (1996) Outcome in the pharmacologic treatment of bipolar disorder. *J. Clin. Psychopharmacol.*, **16** (Suppl.): 155–235.

62. Coryell W., Endicott J., Maser J.D., Mueller T., Lavori P., Keller M. (1995) The likelihood of recurrence in bipolar affective disorder: the importance of episode recency. *J. Affect. Disord.*, **33**: 201–206.

63. Coryell W., Winokur G., Solomon D., Shea T., Leon A., Keller M. (1997) Lith-ium and recurrence in a long-term follow-up of bipolar affective disorder. *Psychol. Med.*, **27**: 281–289.

64. Vestergaard P., Licht R.W., Brodersen A., Rasmussen N.A., Christensen H., Arngrim T., Gronvall B., Kristensen E., Poulstrup I. (1998) Outcome of lithium prophylaxis: a prospective follow-up of affective disorder patients assigned to high and low serum lithium levels. *Acta Psychiatr. Scand.*, **98**: 310–315.

65. Calabrese J., Bowden C., DeVeaugh-Geiss J., Earl N., Gyulai L., Sachs G., Montgomery P. (2001) Lamotrigine demonstrates long term mood stabiliza-tion in recently manic patients. Presented at the American Psychiatric Associ-ation Annual Meeting, New Orleans, 5–10 May.

66. Bowden C.L., Calabrese J.R., Rapaport M., Akthar S., Fieve R., DeVeaugh-Geiss J., Montgomery P. (2001) Lamotrigine demonstrates long-term mood stabil-ization in manic patients. Presented at the New Clinical Drug Evaluation Unit (NCDEU) Meeting, Phoenix, 29–31 May.

67. Denicoff K.D., Smith-Jackson E.E., Disney E.R., Ali S.O., Leverich G.S., Post R.M. (1997) Comparative prophylactic efficacy of lithium, carbamazepine, and the combination in bipolar disorder. *J. Clin. Psychiatry*, **58**: 470–478.

68. Dunner D.L., Stallone F., Fieve R.R. (1976) Lithium carbonate and affective disorders. *Arch. Gen. Psychiatry*, **33**: 117–120.

69. Greil W., Ludwig-Mayerhofer W., Erazo N., Schöchlin C., Schmidt S., Engel R.R., Czernik A., Giedke H., Müller-Oerlinghausen B., Osterheider M. *et al*

(1997)   Lithium versus carbamazepine in the maintenance treatment of bipolar disorders—a randomised study. *J. Affect. Disord.*, **43**: 151–161.
70.   Greil W., Kleindienst N., Erazo N., Müller-Oerlinghausen B. (1998)   Differential response to lithium and carbamazepine in the prophylaxis of bipolar disorder. *J. Clin. Psychopharmacol.*, **18**: 455–460.
71.   Swann A.C., Bowden C.L., Calabrese J.R., Dilsaver S.C., Morris D.D. (1999)   Differential effect of number of previous episodes of affective disorder on response to lithium or divalproex in acute mania. *Am. J. Psychiatry*, **156**: 1264–1266.
72.   Swann A.C., Bowden C.L., Calabrese J.R., Dilsaver S.C., Morris D.D. (2000)   Mania: differential effects of previous depressive and manic episodes on response to treatment. *Acta Psychiatr. Scand.*, **101**: 444–451.
73.   Secunda S., Katz M.M., Swann A., Koslow S.H., Maas J.W., Chuang S., Croughan J. (1985)   Mania: diagnosis, state measurement and prediction of treatment response. *J. Affect. Disord.*, **8**: 113–121.
74.   Prien R.F., Caffey E.M., Klett C.J. (1972)   Relationship between serum lithium level and clinical response in acute mania treated with lithium. *Br. J. Psychiatry*, **120**: 109–414.
75.   Brady K.T., Sonne S.C. (1995)   The relationship between substance abuse and bipolar disorder. *J. Clin. Psychiatry*, **56**: 19–24.
76.   Bowden C., Katz M., Swann A. (2000)   Impulsivity and aggression in unipolar and bipolar depression, mania and controls. Presented at the American College of Neuropsychopharmacology Annual Meeting, Puerto Rico, 10–14 December.
77.   Emilien G., Maloteaux J.M., Seghers A., Charles G. (1996)   Lithium compared to valproic acid and carbamazepine in the treatment of mania: a statistical meta-analysis of controlled trials. *Neuropsychopharmacology*, **6**: 245–252.
78.   Vasudev K., Goswami U., Kohli K. (2000)   Carbamazepine and valproate monotherapy: feasibility, relative safety and efficacy, and therapeutic drug monitoring in manic disorder. *Psychopharmacology*, **150**: 15–23.
79.   McElroy S.L., Keck P.E., Stanton S.P., Tugrul K.C., Bennett J.A., Strakowski S.M. (1996)   A randomized comparison of divalproex oral loading versus haloperidol in the initial treatment of acute psychotic mania. *J. Clin. Psychiatry*, **57**: 142–146.
80.   Müller-Oerlinghausen B., Retzow A., Henn F.A., Giedke H., Walden J. (2000)   Valproate as an adjunct to neuroleptic medication for the treatment of acute episodes of mania: a prospective, randomized, double-blind, placebo-controlled, multicenter study. *J. Clin. Psychopharmacol.*, **20**: 195–203.
81.   Sovner R. (1989)   The use of valproate in the treatment of mentally retarded persons with typical and atypical bipolar disorders. *J. Clin. Psychiatry*, **50**: 40–43.
82.   Freeman T.W., Clothier J.L., Pazzaglia P., Lesem M.D., Swann A.C. (1992)   A double-blind comparison of valproate and lithium in the treatment of acute mania. *Am. J. Psychiatry*, **149**: 108–111.
83.   Bowden C.L., Janicak P.G., Orsulak P., Swann A.C., Davis J.M., Calabrese J.R., Goodnick P., Small J.G., Rush A.J., Kimmel S.E. *et al* (1996)   Relation of serum valproate concentration to response in mania. *Am. J. Psychiatry*, **153**: 765–770.
84.   Lambert P.A. (1984)   Acute and prophylactic therapies of patients with affective disorders using valpromide (dipropylacetamide). In *Anticonvulsants in Affective Disorders* (Eds H.M. Emrich, T. Okuma, A.A. Muller), pp. 33–44, Excerpta Medica, Amsterdam.
85.   Jacobsen F.M. (1993)   Low dose valproate: a new treatment for cyclothymia, mild rapid cycling disorders, and premenstrual syndrome. *J. Clin. Psychiatry*, **54**: 229–234.

86. Zarate C.A., Jr., Tohen M., Narendran R., Tomassini E.C., McDonald J., Sederer M., Madrid A.R. (2000) The adverse effect profile and efficacy of divalproex sodium compared with valproic acid: a pharmacoepidemiology study. *J. Clin. Psychiatry*, **60**: 232–236.

87. McElroy S.L., Keck P.E., Tugrul K.C., Bennet J.A. (1993) Valproate as a loading treatment in acute mania. *Neuropsychobiology*, **27**: 146–149.

88. Hirschfeld R.M., Allen M.H., McEvoy J.P., Keck P.E. Jr., Russell J.M. (1999) Safety and tolerability of oral loading divalproex sodium in acutely manic bipolar patients. *J. Clin. Psychiatry*, **60**: 815–818.

89. Grunze H., Erfurth A., Amann B., Giupponi G., Kammerer C., Walden J. (1999) Intravenous valproate loading in acutely manic and depressed bipolar I patients. *Clin. Psychopharmacol.*, **19**: 303–309.

90. Manji H.K., Chen G., Hsiao J.K., Masana M.I., Potter W.Z. (1996) Regulation of signal transduction pathways by mood stabilizing agents: implications for the delayed onset of therapeutic efficacy. *J. Clin. Psychiatry*, **57** (Suppl. 13): 34–46.

91. Lenox R.H., Manji H.K. (1995) Lithium. In *The American Psychiatric Press Textbook of Psychopharmacology* (Eds A.F. Schatzberg, C.B. Nemeroff), pp. 303–349, American Psychiatric Press, Washington.

92. Solomon D.A., Ryan C.E., Keitner G.I., Miller I.W., Shea M.T., Kazim A., Keller M.B. (1997) A pilot study of lithium carbonate plus divalproex sodium for the continuation and maintenance treatment of patients with bipolar I disorder. *J. Clin. Psychiatry*, **58**: 95–99.

93. Tohen M., Sanger T.M., McElroy S.L., Tollefson G.D., Chengappa K.N.R., Daniel D.G., Petty F., Centorrino F., Wang R., Grundy S.L. *et al* (1999) Olanzapine versus placebo in the treatment of acute mania. *Am. J. Psychiatry*, **156**: 702–709.

94. Zajecka J., Weisler R., Sommerville K.W. (2000) Divalproex sodium vs. olanzapine for the treatment of mania in bipolar disorder. Presented at the 39th Annual Meeting of the American College of Neuropsychopharmacology, San Juan, 10–14 December.

95. Keck P.E., Jr., Ice K. (2000) A 3–week, double-blind, randomized trial of ziprasidone in the acute treatment of mania. *Eur. Neuropsychopharmacol.*, **10** (Suppl. 3): S297.

96. Tohen M., Chengappa K.N.R., Suppes T.R., Baker R.W., Zarate C.A., Jr., Calabrese J.R., Sachs G.S., Bowden C.L., Jacobs T.G., Timpe T.M. *et al* (2002) Efficacy of olanzapine in combination with valproate or lithium in the treatment of mania (in preparation).

97. Grossman F., Okamoto A., Bowden C. (2000) Risperidone plus mood stabilizer versus placebo plus mood stabilizer for manic episodes in bipolar disorder: a combined efficacy analysis. Presented at the 39th Annual Meeting of the American College of Neuropsychopharmacology, San Juan, 10–14 December.

98. Esparon J., Kolloori J., Naylor G.J., McHarg A.M., Smith A.H., Hopwood S.E. (1986) Comparison of the prophylactic action of flupenthixol with placebo in lithium treated manic-depressive patients. *Br. J. Psychiatry*, **148**: 723–725.

99. Koukopoulos A., Reginaldi D., Laddomada P., Floris G., Serra G., Tondo L. (1980) Course of the manic-depressive cycle and changes caused by treatment. *Pharmakopsychiatr. Neuropsychopharmakol.*, **13**: 156–167.

100. Harrow M., Grossman L.S., Silverstein M.L., Meltzer H.Y., Kettering R.L. (1986) A longitudinal study of thought disorder in manic patients. *Arch. Gen. Psychiatry*, **43**: 781–785.

101. Suppes T., Webb A., Paul B., Carmody T., Kraemer H., Rush A.J. (1999)   Clinical outcome in a randomized 1-year trial of clozapine versus treatment as usual for patients with treatment-resistant illness and a history of mania. *Am. J. Psychiatry*, **156**: 1164–1169.
102. Lerer B., Moore N., Meyendorff E., Cho S.R., Gershon S. (1987)   Carbamazepine versus lithium in mania: a double-blind study. *J. Clin. Psychiatry*, **48**: 89–93.
103. Small J.G., Klapper M.H., Milstein V., Kellams J.J., Miller M.J., Marhenke J.D., Small I.F. (1991)   Carbamazepine compared with lithium in the treatment of mania. *Arch. Gen. Psychiatry*, **48**: 915–921.
104. Okuma T., Inanaga K., Otsuki S., Sarai K., Takahashi R., Hazama H., Mori A., Watanabe M. (1979)   Comparison of the antimanic efficacy of carbamazepine and chlorpromazine: a double-blind controlled study. *Psychopharmacology*, **66**: 211–217.
105. Lenzi A., Lazzerini F., Grossi E., Massimetti G., Placidi G.F. (1986)   Use of carbamazepine in acute psychosis: a controlled study. *J. Int. Med. Res.*, **14**: 78–84.
106. Post R.M., Denicoff K.D., Frye M.A., Leverich G.S. (1997)   Re-evaluating carbamazepine prophylaxis in bipolar disorder. *Br. J. Psychiatry*, **170**: 202–204.
107. Stromgren L.S. (1990)   The combination of lithium and carbamazepine in treatment and prevention of manic-depressive disorder: a review and a case report. *Compr. Psychiatry*, **31**: 261–265.
108. Yatham L. (2000)   Safety and efficacy of risperidone as combination therapy for the manic phase of bipolar disorder: preliminary findings of a randomized, double-blind study. Presented at the 13th European College of Neuropsychopharmacology Congress, Munich, 9–13 September.
109. Sachs G.S., Printz D.J., Kahn D.A., Carpenter D., Docherty J.P. (2000)   The Expert Consensus Guideline Series: Medication Treatment of Bipolar Disorder 2000. *Postgrad. Med.*, special issue.
110. Bowden C.L., Mitchell P., Suppes T. (1999)   Lamotrigine in the treatment of bipolar depression. *Eur. Neuropsychopharmacol.*, **9** (Suppl. 4): S113–S117.
111. Messenheimer J., Mullens E.L., Giorgi L., Young F. (1998)   Safety of adult clinical trial experience with lamotrigine. *Drug Safety*, **18**: 281–296.
112. Cohn J.B., Collins G., Ashbrook E., Wernicke J.F. (1989)   A comparison of fluoxetine imipramine and placebo in patients with bipolar depressive disorder. *Int. Clin. Psychopharmacol.*, **4**: 313–322.
113. Nemeroff C.B., Evans D.L., Gyulai L., Sachs G.S., Bowden C.L., Gergel I.P., Oakes R., Pitts C.D. (2001)   A double-blind, placebo-controlled comparison of imipramine and paroxetine in the treatment of bipolar depression. *Am. J. Psychiatry* (in press).
114. Amsterdam J. (1998)   Efficacy and safety of venlafaxine in the treatment of bipolar II major depressive episode. *J. Clin. Psychopharmacol.*, **18**: 414–417.
115. Amsterdam J.D., Garcia-Espana F., Fawcett J., Quitkin F.M., Reimherr F.W., Rosenbaum J.F., Schweizer E., Beasley C. (1998)   Efficacy and safety of fluoxetine in treating bipolar II major depressive episodes. *J. Clin. Psychopharmacol.*, **18**: 435–440.
116. Baldassano C.F., Sachs G.S., Stoll A.L. (1995)   Paroxetine for bipolar depression: outcome in patients failing prior antidepressant trials. *Depression*, **3**: 182–186.
117. Peet M. (1994)   Induction of mania with selective serotonin re-uptake inhibitors and tricyclic antidepressants. *Br. J. Psychiatry*, **164**: 549–550.
118. Haykal R.F., Akiskal H.S. (1990)   Bupropion as a promising approach to rapid cycling bipolar II patients. *J. Clin. Psychiatry*, **51**: 450–455.

119. Merideth C.H., Feighner J.P. (1983)   The use of bupropion in hospitalized depressed patients. *J. Clin. Psychiatry*, **44**: 85–87.
120. Sachs G.S., Lafer B., Stoll A.L., Banov M., Thibault A.B., Tohen M., Rosenbaum J.F. (1994)   A double-blind trial of bupropion versus desipramine for bipolar depression. *J. Clin. Psychiatry*, **55**: 391–393.
121. Fogelson D.L., Bystritsky A., Pasnau R. (1992)   Bupropion in the treatment of bipolar disorders: the same old story? *J. Clin. Psychiatry*, **53**: 443–446.
122. Croughan J.L., Secunda S.K., Katz M.M., Robins E., Mendels J., Swann A., Harris-Larkin B. (1988)   Sociodemographic and prior clinical course characteristics associated with treatment response in depressed patients. *J. Psychiatr. Res.*, **22**: 227–237.
123. Montgomery S.A., Schatzberg A.F., Guelfi J.D., Kasper S., Nemeroff C., Swann A., Zajecka J. (2000)   Pharmacotherapy of depression and mixed states in bipolar disorder. *J. Affect. Disord.*, **59** (Suppl. 1): S39–S56.
124. Wehr T.A., Goodwin F.K. (1987)   Can antidepressants cause mania and worsen the course of affective illness? *Am. J. Psychiatry*, **144**: 1403–1411.
125. Angst J., Stabl M. (1992)   Efficacy of moclobemide in different patient groups: a meta-analysis of studies. *Psychopharmacology*, **106**: S109–S113.
126. Himmelhoch J.M., Thase M.F., Mallinger A.G., Houck P. (1991)   Tranylcypromine versus imipramine in anergic bipolar depression. *Am. J. Psychiatry*, **148**: 910–916.
127. Pickar D., Cowdry R.W., Zis A.P. (1984)   Mania and hypomania during antidepressant pharmacotherapy: clinical research implications. In *Neurobiology of Mood Disorders* (Eds R.M. Post, J.C. Ballenger), pp. 836–845, Williams and Wilkins, Baltimore.
128. Altshuler L.L., Post R.M., Leverich G.S., Mikalauskas K., Rosoff A., Ackerman L. (1995)   Antidepressant-induced mania and cycle acceleration: a controversy revisited. *Am. J. Psychiatry*, **152**: 1130–1138.
129. Lewis J.L., Winokur G. (1982)   The induction of mania: a natural history study with controls. *Arch. Gen. Psychiatry*, **39**: 303–306.
130. Kupfer D.J., Carpenter L.L., Frank E. (1988)   Possible role of antidepressants in precipitating mania and hypomania in recurrent depression. *Am. J. Psychiatry*, **145**: 804–808.
131. Shulman R.B., Scheftner W.A., Nayudu S. (2001)   Venlafaxine-associated mania. *J. Clin. Psychopharmacol.*, **21**: 239–241.
132. Quitkin F.M., Kane J., Rifkin A., Ramos-Lorenzi J.R., Nayak D.V. (1981)   Prophylactic lithium carbonate with and without imipramine for bipolar I patients: a double-blind study. *Arch. Gen. Psychiatry*, **38**: 902–907.
133. Austin M.P., Souza F.G., Goodwin G.M. (1991)   Lithium augmentation in antidepressant-resistant patients. A quantitative analysis. *Br. J. Psychiatry*, **159**: 510–514.
134. Ebert D., Jaspert A., Murata H., Kaschka W.P. (1995)   Initial lithium augmentation improves the antidepressant effects of standard TCA treatment in non-resistant depressed patients. *Psychopharmacology*, **118**: 223–225.
135. McElroy S., Keck P.E. Jr. (1993)   Treatment guidelines for valproate in bipolar, schizoaffective disorders. *Can. J. Psychiatry*, **38**: S62–S66.
136. Gyulai L., Bowden C.L., McElroy S.L., Calabrese J.R., Petty F., Swann A.C., Chou J.C.Y., Wassef A., Risch C.S., Hirschfeld R.M.A. *et al* (2002)   Maintenance efficacy of divalproex in the prevention of bipolar depression (in preparation).
137. Post R.M., Uhde T.W., Roy-Byrne P.P., Joffe R.T. (1986)   Antidepressant effects of carbamazepine. *Am. J. Psychiatry*, **143**: 29–34.

138. Kramlinger K.G., Post R.M. (1989) The addition of lithium carbonate to carbamazepine: antidepressant efficacy in treatment-resistant depression. *Arch. Gen. Psychiatry*, **46**: 794–800.
139. Coryell W., Endicott J., Keller M. (1992) Rapidly cycling affective disorder: demographics, diagnosis, family, and course. *Arch. Gen. Psychiatry*, **49**: 126–131.
140. Geller B. (1999) Lithium in bipolar adolescents with secondary substance dependency. *J. Am. Acad. Child Adolesc. Psychiatry*, **38**: 513–516.
141. Papatheodorou G., Kutcher S.P., Katic M., Szalai J.P. (1995) The efficacy and safety of divalproex sodium in the treatment of acute mania in adolescents and young adults. *J. Clin. Psychopharmacol.*, **15**: 110–116.
142. Wagner K.D., Weller E., Sachs G., Carlson G., Bowden C. (2000) Safety and efficacy of divalproex in childhood bipolar disorder. Presented at the Annual Meeting of the American Academy of Child and Adolescent Psychiatry, New York, 24–29 October.
143. Lewinsohn P.M., Klein D.N., Seeley J.R. (1995) Bipolar disorders in a community sample of older adolescents: prevalence, phenomenology, comorbidity, and course. *J. Am. Acad. Child Adolesc. Psychiatry*, **34**: 454–463.
144. McFarland B.H., Miller M.R., Straumfjord A.A. (1990) Valproate use in the older manic patient. *J. Clin. Psychiatry*, **51**: 479–481.
145. Kahn D., Stevenson E., Douglas C.J. (1988) Effect of sodium valproate in three patients with organic brain syndromes. *Am. J. Psychiatry*, **145**: 1010–1011.
146. Narayan M., Noaghiul S., Nelson J. C. (1997) Divalproex treatment of mania in elderly patients. Presented at the American Society of Clinical Psychopharmacology Annual Meeting, Barbados, 14–16 February.
147. Kando J.C., Tohen M., Castillo J., Zarate C.A. (1996) The use of valproate in an elderly population with affective symptoms. *J. Clin. Psychiatry*, **57**: 238–240.
148. Wisner K.L., Perel J.M. (1998) Serum levels of valproate and carbamazepine in breastfeeding mother–infant pairs. *J. Clin. Psychopharmacol.*, **18**: 167–169.

Commentaries

3.1
Pursuit of the Ideal Mood Stabilizer:
Time to Give Up and Move to Combination Trials

Joseph R. Calabrese, Daniel J. Rapport and Melvin D. Shelton[1]

Charles Bowden's authoritative and comprehensive description of the various pharmacotherapies currently being utilized in the medical management of bipolar disorder suggests that we have failed to develop an agent which possesses the capacity to simultaneously "stabilize mood from both above and below baseline" (terms proposed by Terry Ketter, personal communication). In addition, we do not have agents that exert their therapeutic effects quickly and without significant side-effect burden. Our patients find these conclusions demoralizing. We must do better. We must meet this unmet need, and Bowden's review would suggest that we are not going to achieve this goal without informed combination therapy.

The available data suggest that lithium remains the "gold standard" in the long-term management of bipolar disorder. However, despite being viewed as our best prophylactic treatment for bipolar disorder, lithium has never been shown with contemporary methodology to prevent both manic and depressive episodes. Indeed, a recent trial that compared lamotrigine to both placebo and lithium reported that lithium accomplished its long-term effects by preventing episodes of mania, not depression [1]. Past trials of lithium usually employed "enriched" discontinuation designs that compared the proportion of patients relapsing on lithium to that of placebo after random assignment to parallel arms. With the exception of the most recently completed trial [1], there exists no placebo-controlled maintenance study in patients with classic bipolar disorder that has successfully employed survival analyses in a comparison of any putative mood stabilizer to lithium and placebo. In Bowden's maintenance study [2], significant secondary differences were shown between divalproex and placebo, but the lack of superiority of lithium over placebo questioned the validity of these findings [2]. Survival analyses in bipolar disorder maintenance studies are now required by regulatory agencies around the world for approval of

[1] *Case Western Reserve University School of Medicine, 11400 Euclid Ave., #200, Cleveland, Ohio 44106, USA*

maintenance claims. Surprisingly, up until the recently completed lamotrigine study [1], lithium had never been shown to possess prophylactic efficacy through survival analyses. I believe these data suggest that lithium stabilizes mood through its antimanic properties primarily. These observations also call into question the scientific validity of requiring the use of survival analyses as primary outcome measures in bipolar disorder maintenance studies [3]. Since bipolar disorder is a disorder of impulse, these studies are inherently complicated by premature discontinuations. Since these drop outs are due to poor compliance, regulatory agencies argue these drop outs are frequently "unusable" study endpoints, and as a result, compromise data analysis plans that rely heavily on survival methodology.

There have been three large placebo-controlled maintenance studies conducted in bipolar disorder over the last 30 years ([2], divalproex vs. lithium vs. placebo), ([4], lamotrigine vs. placebo), ([1], lamotrigine vs. lithium vs. placebo). These studies have all employed survival analyses as the primary outcome measure to explore the mood-stabilizing properties of lithium, divalproex, and lamotrigine. Unfortunately, none of the medications evaluated in these studies have been shown to meet the definition of an "ideal" mood stabilizer—the possession of prophylactic efficacy in both phases of the disorder. I believe Bowden's review suggests that we should discard our primary pursuit of mood stabilizers for use in monotherapy and begin placebo-controlled combination therapy trials that achieve the desired objective of bimodal prophylactic efficacy with a more rapid rate of onset through use of combinations of medications that possess a spectrum of combined activity that is complementary. Since it is unlikely that these trials will be primarily funded by the pharmaceutical industry, the burden of these scientific studies will have to be assumed by government agencies.

We propose a nomenclature for mood stabilizers. Class A: Mood stabilizers that exert their primary acute and prophylactic effect by stabilizing mood from "above baseline". These agents appear to possess marked acute and prophylactic efficacy, but modest antidepressant properties. Class B: Mood stabilizers that exert their primary acute and prophylactic effect by stabilizing mood from "below baseline". These agents appear to possess marked acute and prophylactic efficacy, but modest antimanic properties. This nomenclature would facilitate the development of agents that possess complementary efficacy [5].

In conclusion, Bowden's review suggests that building upon the achievements of scientific forefathers our discipline has made tremendous progress over the last 25 years. In addition to having lithium and the typical antipsychotic agents, we now have antiepileptic drugs (carbamazepine, valproate, lamotrigine, and gabapentin) and the atypical antipsychotics (olanzapine and risperidone). These agents have been evaluated in large-scale, placebo-controlled studies and appear to have complementary spectra of efficacy. We believe the time has come to give up our hope of developing a single agent that possesses bimodal efficacy in both the acute and prophylactic setting and to move clinical research towards controlled combination therapy studies involving two or three mood-stabilizing agents.

REFERENCES

1. Calabrese J.R., Bowden C.L., DeVeaugh-Geiss J., Earl N., Gyulai L., Sachs G., Montgomery P. (2001) Lamotrigine demonstrates long term mood stabilization in recently manic patients. Presented at the American Psychiatric Association 154th Annual Meeting, New Orleans, 5–10 May.
2. Bowden C.L., Calabrese J.R., McElroy S.L., Hirschfeld R.M.A., Petty F., Gyulai L., Pope H.G., Chou J.C.Y., Keck P.E., Rhodes L.J. *et al* (2000) A randomized, placebo-controlled 12-month trial of divalproex and lithium in treatment of outpatients with bipolar I disorder. *Arch. Gen. Psychiatry*, **57**: 481–489.
3. Montgomery S., van Zwieten-Boot B., Angst J., Bowden C.L., Calabrese J.R., Chengappa R., Goodwin G., Lecrubier Y., Licht R., Nolen W.A. *et al* (2001) ECNP Nice consensus guidelines for investigating efficacy in bipolar disorder. *Eur. Neuropsychopharmacol.*, **11**: 79–88.
4. Calabrese J.R., Suppes T., Bowden C.L., Kusumakar V., Sachs G.S., Swann A.C., McElroy S.L., Ascher J.A., Earl N.L., Greene P.L. *et al* (2000) A double-blind, placebo-controlled, prophylaxis study of lamotrigine in rapid cycling bipolar disorder. *J. Clin. Psychiatry*, **61**: 841–850.
5. Calabrese J.R., Ketter T.A., Shelton M.D., Rapport D.J., Kimmel S.E. Stabilization of mood from below versus above baseline in bipolar rapid cycling. Submitted for publication.

3.2
Same Data, Different Interpretations
Paul Grof[1]

There is a pressing need to improve the treatment of bipolar disorders as currently diagnosed. The prevalence estimates in the population have expanded from a lifetime risk of 1% up to 5%, even up to 8%, partly due to the broadened approach of DSM-IV which allows other diagnoses in parallel. The enlarged potential market for new mood stabilizers has understandably been a strong incentive for the pharmaceutical industry, and pharmacological treatment of bipolar disorders has become one of the most frequently presented subjects. Charles Bowden's comprehensive review reflects well the impressive expansion of new, experimental treatments in bipolar disorder.

[1] *Royal Ottawa Hospital, 1145 Carling Avenue, Ottawa, Ontario K17 7K4, Canada*

I have in recent years heard a number of review lectures given by other leading experts in this area, and whereas the data presented were largely similar to those of Bowden's chapter, their interpretation and conclusions have varied considerably. There is clearly dissent in what are considered definitions and proofs. While Bowden is leaning to an extreme, which is liberal in the definition of a mood stabilizer and lenient as to the efficacy of medications (valproate is, for example, considered a drug of proven, long-term, prophylactic effect), the interpretation of others move in a different direction.

Guy Goodwin [1, 2], for example, supports a more rigorous definition of mood stabilizers and concludes from a careful meta-analysis that lithium remains the only proven mood stabilizer in bipolar disorder. Based on evidence available to date, Fred Goodwin [3] and Baldessarini and Tondo [4] come to a similar conclusion. Guy Goodwin suggests that the looser definition of mood stabilizers has been made in order to accommodate, for example, antiepileptics. Whereas valproate is undoubtedly effective in the treatment of mania, evidence of its efficacy as a recurrence-preventive mood stabilizer is questionable. As Fred Goodwin points out, with the broader definitions, haloperidol and chlorpromazine would be classified as mood stabilizers as well. Other observations supporting these interpretations include, for example, those of Garnham et al [5], who, in a large naturalistic study, found good support only for the mood-stabilizing efficacy of lithium and to some extent, lamotrigine.

My own experience over the past decades leads to similar comments. As long as one uses lithium in patients with typical, episodic, fully remitting mood disorders—in patients in whom it was proven effective—it remains as effective against manias and depressions as it was in the 1960s and 1970s. Employed in a broadly DSM-IV diagnosed spectrum of bipolar disorders with high comorbidity and poor compliance, lithium's efficacy drops dramatically. Diluted by heterogeneity, the effect of lithium may not even be statistically significant. Undoubtedly, from the 1960s–1970s to the 1980s–1990s, diagnostic practices have clearly shifted [6, 7].

The second major reason for the differences in interpretation is related to the highly capricious course of bipolar disorders. The risk of recurrences is sufficiently high only in patients having had several episodes. At present, patients are started on long-term treatment after a single or a few episodes, and it is then difficult to tell if a patient remains well because of maintenance treatment or spontaneously. While the course of typical, episodic disorders was captured in the 1960s, the natural history of the atypical, nonepisodic illnesses has not been adequately studied. Yet, they probably represent the majority of DSM-IV diagnosed bipolar disorders.

A varied approach to what is considered evidence contributes as well. When, for example, a maintenance study fails to demonstrate significant differences between valproate, lithium and placebo in the primary indicator (recurrence rate), researchers naturally remain reluctant to accept a substitute by secondary indicators and post-hoc analyses.

It is the use of different diagnostic practices, the capriciousness of clinical course and the different requirements for evidence that mainly account for the fact that we encounter such a variety of interpretations of data about the pharmacological treatment of bipolar disorders. And they make it difficult to come to consensus about the value and usefulness of the new, promising pharmacological interventions described in Bowden's article. There are great hopes for efficacy of several new substances—we all share them—but to date the proof is still missing.

REFERENCES

1. Goodwin G.M. (2000) Perspectives for clinical research on bipolar disorders in the new millennium. *Bipolar Disord.*, **2**: 302–304.
2. Goodwin G.M. (2000) Importance of mood stabilization in bipolar disorder. Presented at the Bipolar Global Medical Conference, Amsterdam, 19 September.
3. Goodwin F.K. (2000) Pharmacologic treatment: challenges and controversies. Presented at the American Psychiatric Association 153rd Annual Meeting, Chicago, 13–18 May.
4. Baldessarini R.J., Tondo L. (2000) Does lithium treatment still work? Evidence of stable responses over three decades. *Arch. Gen. Psychiatry*, **57**: 187–190.
5. Garnham J., Munro A., Teehan A., Duffy A., MacDougall M., Passmore M., Slaney C., Alda M. (2001) Bipolar disorder: assessing treatment response in a naturalistic setting. *J. Bipolar Disord.*, **3** (Suppl. 1): 37.
6. Stoll A.L., Tohen M., Baldessarini R.J., Goodwin D.C., Stein S., Katz S., Geenens D., Swinson R.P., Goethe J.W., McGlashan T. (1993) Shifts in diagnostic frequencies of schizophrenia and major affective disorders at six North American psychiatric hospitals, 1972–1988. *Am. J. Psychiatry*, **150**: 1668–1673.
7. Grof P., Alda M., Ahrens B. (1995) Clinical course of affective disorders. Were Emil Kraepelin and Jules Angst wrong? *Psychopathology*, **28** (Suppl. 1): 73–80.

3.3
Treatment as Guided by the Dim Light of Evidence

Gary S. Sachs[1]

At the dawn of the 20th century, Kraepelin coined the term manic-depressive insanity. Cade's 1949 report of the calming effect of lithium spawned a half century of progress which transformed basic aspects of psychiatric

[1] *Partners Bipolar Treatment Center, Massachusetts General Hospital, Harvard Medical School, 50 Staniford St, Boston, MA 02114, USA*

practice. Acceptance of lithium as a therapeutic agent required the invention of the randomized controlled trial. The evidentiary illumination provided by this new technology was sufficient to demonstrate that psychiatric illness was amenable to medical treatment. The science of clinical research also necessitated increased diagnostic rigour. While advancing the entire field of psychiatry, this trend has fostered the paradoxical evolution of manic-depressive illness from an imprecise but narrowly defined condition into operationally defined but more inclusive unipolar and bipolar mood disorders [1]. As the 21st century opens, this nosological paradox is paralleled by a clinical paradox: even as clinical efficacy studies expand our armamentarium of evidence-based treatments, the population of bipolar patients with inadequate response to these treatments seems to grow ever larger.

Bipolar disorder is an incurable common disorder that is frequently disabling and can be deadly. While bipolar disorder usually responds to treatment, its course unfolds in chaotic patterns with irregular phases of depression and mood elevation separated by variable periods of partial or complete euthymia. The extreme variability within and between patients is a hallmark of bipolar illness [2] which complicates the process of clinical management and challenges the processes by which clinical research is conducted and results interpreted.

Charles Bowden meets this challenge first by providing organizing concepts and then uses the conceptual framework to describe the state of evidence for drugs used to treat mania and depression. Finally, he progresses by discussing the application of this evidence in formulating treatment strategies for bipolar patients. This commentary will focus on the organizing concepts.

Bowden's organizing concepts remind us that bipolar research is indeed handicapped by a lack of consistent definitions. Our field has no clear definition of a mood stabilizer, yet this term is used even in professional discourse without qualification. Any reasonable definition that permits an evidence-based determination of whether a treatment meets criteria for inclusion is an acceptable starting point. Bowden's admonition to divide treatment actions into primary and secondary, however, invites us to think more deeply about the evidence by which we determine a drug to be a specific treatment for bipolar disorder rather than a nonspecific tool for reduction of a specific symptom. Determining treatment efficacy on the basis of changes in total rating scale scores leaves us vulnerable to what Bowden characterizes as the fallacy of treating a part of the illness as the whole. Factor analysis might prove useful as a means to determine whether specific symptom clusters respond differentially to any of the mood stabilizing, antimanic, or antidepressant treatments.

Categorizing the evidence into levels of variable strength provides perspective crucial to weighing inputs in an evidence-based approach to treatment. Certainly greatest weight should be assigned to evidence Bowden defines as category 1, "at least one placebo-controlled double-blind study conducted with a sufficient number of patients that at least one of the major planned analyses provided over a 50% likelihood of identifying a significant difference between the groups". Among the 148 references in his chapter there are less than 20 placebo-controlled double-blind trials and not all of these meet the full definition for inclusion as category 1. Category 1 data sufficient to characterize any one treatment as having consistent findings for acute mania, bipolar depression, or prophylaxis varies between scant and nonexistent. Suspending the requirement for placebo control defines category 2, but even combining categories 1 and 2 expands the number of quality studies to no more than 30 studies.

Given the paucity of high-quality data, it may be fair to conclude that all areas of research for treatment of bipolar disorder are still open to research. Such a conclusion does not mean that clinicians are left to make treatment decisions totally in the dark. Quite to the contrary, it seems wise to use the light of available evidence in accordance with the level of illumination it provides. This is to say that when category 1 or category 2 evidence is available, it should be given greater weight than studies that may be flawed by lack of blinding, small sample size, or absence of controls, and relatively little credence should be given to uncontrolled reports and speculative opinion.

Using this perspective can help to minimize potential mistreatment of patients. For instance, uncontrolled case reports described that patients receiving atypical antipsychotics experienced treatment emergent worsening or the apparent induction of mania [3, 4]. These well-intended reports raised concern that this class of medications might frequently cause harm to bipolar patients. Subsequent double-blind placebo-controlled studies provided evidence that such phenomena occur no more frequently during treatment with olanzapine or risperidone than with placebo. Unfortunately, some patients are likely denied these treatments which have demonstrated efficacy out of consideration (however reasonable when first reported) of speculative concerns.

Given the variability in the course of bipolar illness, it is imperative that treatment decisions be based on the best available evidence. Where the brighter light of evidence from double-blind controlled trials is available, reasoned speculation may prompt better study, but should not be allowed to eclipse the controlled data.

REFERENCES

1. Stoll A.L., Tohen M., Baldessarini R.J. Goodwin D.C., Stein S., Katz S., Geenens D., Swinson R.P., Goethe J.W., McGlashan T. (1993) Shifts in diagnostic frequen-

cies of schizophrenia and major affective disorders at six North American psychiatric hospitals, 1972–1988. *Am. J. Psychiatry*, **150**: 1668–1673.
2. Akiskal H.S. (1996) The prevalent clinical spectrum of bipolar disorders: beyond DSM-IV. *J. Clin. Psychopharmacol.*, **16** (Suppl. 1): 4S–14S.
3. Dwight M.M., Keck P.E., Jr., Stanton S.P., Strakowski S.M., McElroy S.L. (1994) Antidepressant activity and mania associated with risperidone treatment of schizoaffective disorder. *Lancet*, **344**: 554–555.
4. Sajatovic M., DiGiovanni S.K., Bastani B., Hattah H., Ramirez L.F. (1996) Risperidone therapy in treatment refractory acute bipolar and schizoaffective mania. *Psychopharmacol. Bull.*, **32**: 55–61.

3.4

The Search for the Holy Grail—The Ideal Mood Stabilizer: Fiction or Future?

Heinz Grunze[1]

Despite all advances and a recent rapid increase of confirmatory controlled trials, the pharmacotherapy of bipolar disorder has still a long way to go to achieve similar success rates as many nonpsychiatric drug treatments. Part of it is due to the fact that bipolar disorder was a long-time neglected orphan in the development of new drugs. Comparing the number of patients in randomized trials between 1988 and 1995, 10 times as many patients had been in controlled trials for atypical antipsychotics in schizophrenia than for all drug treatments of all phases of bipolar disorder [1]. The other part of the story is that the strict definition of Kraepelin's manic-depressive illness has been extended and that bipolar disorder is nowadays considered as a spectrum disorder. However, until very recently, all controlled trials focused on the classical bipolar I patients, with so-called "atypical" features as bipolar II, rapid cycling, mixed states or comorbidity leading to exclusion from systematic studies. This may be a necessity for generating data useful for drug approval, but leaves the clinician alone when treating the routine bipolar patient. It is fair to estimate that probably less than 20% of bipolar patients originally screened are finally eligible for phase III trials and become randomized [2].

Thus, it is always a challenge to review evidence for efficacy of drug treatment of bipolar disorder, as effectiveness may contradict it. Charles Bowden's chapter supplies the reader with an almost complete, as far as space restrictions allow it, and balanced overview on the pharmacological treatment of bipolar disorder. However, it appears that this inherited

[1] *Department of Psychiatry, University of Munich, Nussbaumstrasse 7, 80336 Munich, Germany*

conflict between efficacy and effectiveness, between controlled trial and real-world patient still remains unsolved. Although focusing on randomized, controlled monotherapy trials, the review prefers to use a rather weak definition for the highest level of evidence, that would not withstand criteria of drug approval authorities. On the other hand, especially when considering the effectiveness in bipolar depression and maintenance treatment, the review seems to be slightly hesitant in making use of data from large-scale naturalistic or retrospective analysis. Especially with bipolar depression, a balanced consideration between the risk of a switch into mania and the risk of suicidality is necessary, which, in my opinion, always demands a maximum and usually combination treatment [3].

About 15% of bipolar patients die from suicide [4] and suicidality is an issue in almost 80% of bipolar depressed patients [5]. In a specialized bipolar outpatient setting, more than 25% of the patients had at least one previous suicide attempt [6]. Although an effective agent, lamotrigine monotherapy has not shown so far as much evidence for antisuicidal effects as lithium, although subanalysis of the milestone study of Calabrese et al [7] showed that suicidal idealization is significantly reduced. Furthermore, conclusive head-to-head comparisons of lamotrigine to standard antidepressants concerning efficacy are still missing. Unfortunately, as described in Bowden's review, there is a paucity of controlled studies on the efficacy of antidepressants in bipolar depression. However, the so far largest chart analysis with more than 2000 patients comparing the efficacy of antidepressants in unipolar and bipolar depression showed no statistical difference [3]. This analysis also backed up the observation that mood stabilizers can supply a reasonable, but not absolute protection against a switch [8].

Therefore, treatment recommendations for bipolar depression at this stage should always include initial combination treatment at least for moderate and severe depression [9]. If suicidality has ever played a role in the patient's history, lithium should be considered as first choice until we have more knowledge of antisuicidal properties of other mood stabilizers. Due to their better tolerability compared to tricyclics (TCAs) and lower switch risk, selective serotonin reuptake inhibitors (SSRIs) are natural first choice antidepressants. When the antidepressant has to be switched due to inefficacy or intolerability, it should be kept in mind that a) at least in unipolar depressed males, TCAs seem to be more efficacious than SSRIs [10] and b) not all modern antidepressants have low switch risks. For example, it appears that the switch risk of venlafaxine is of the same magnitude of order as TCAs' [11].

However, lamotrigine should still remain within the primary choice. In acutely unipolar and bipolar depressed patients, it shows antidepressant augmentative properties similar to lithium [12] and may be a first-line choice in continuation and maintenance treatment, alone or together with lithium, as reviewed by Bowden [13, 14].

The general strengths and weaknesses of the different options for maintenance treatment are authoritatively and comprehensively reviewed by Bowden. Two additional aspects should be mentioned. First, almost all so-called controlled maintenance trials lack a most important aspect: duration of study. From the clinicians' view, a true prophylactic effect can only be judged with sufficient observation periods, whereas most controlled trials are for a maximum of 12–18 months. This may be sufficient for rapid cycling, but not for bipolar patients with lower episode frequencies. Effects of discontinuation of previous mood stabilizers, especially lithium [15], will lead to inconclusive results [16]. Furthermore, a true prophylactic effect may only be seen after prolonged exposure, as with lithium [17]. Interestingly, as far as we can say now, lamotrigine seems to have a pattern of responsiveness similar to lithium: in the so far only controlled, 18-month comparison between lamotrigine, lithium and placebo, non-responders in both the lamotrigine and lithium group tended to be early drop outs, with those being stable after one year remaining mostly stable for the rest of the study. In comparison, a recently published controlled milestone study comparing the prophylactic efficacy of carbamazepine with lithium over five years showed a continuous, almost linear decline over time of the number of patients in the carbamazepine arm [18].

These limitations of controlled randomized studies suggest that at least for an estimation of the prophylactic value we should make more use of naturalistic data that may enhance our knowledge of the clinical usefulness of monotherapies (e.g., lithium [19]) or combination treatments (e.g., lithium and valproate [20]), despite all inherited methodological flaws.

Not only in prophylaxis, but in general, skilful polypharmacy is rather the rule than the exception in bipolar disorder [21]. In my opinion, the search for the Holy Grail, the ideal mood stabilizer that cures and prevents all mood deflections in all subtypes of bipolar disorder, will be a never-ending story. Thus, we need right now a trial culture that focuses on other than typical bipolar I patients and on combination treatments, evaluating efficacy, tolerability and simplicity of use, the latter as a most important prerequisite for compliance. Recent trials in acute mania, as the European valproate add-on study [22] or the recent studies on risperidone [23], should warrant more attention from the drug approval authorities, as they are closer to clinical reality.

REFERENCES

1. Ghaemi N., Sachs G., Goodwin F.K. (2000) What is to be done? Controversies in the diagnosis and treatment of manic-depressive illness. *World J. Biol. Psychiatry*, 2: 65–74.

2. Licht R.W., Gouliaev G., Vestergaard P., Frydenberg M. (1997) Generalisability of results from randomised drug trials. A trial on antimanic treatment. *Br. J. Psychiatry*, 170: 264–267.

3. Möller H.-J., Grunze H. (2000) Have some guidelines for the treatment of acute bipolar depression gone too far in the restriction of antidepressants? *Eur. Arch. Psychiatry Clin. Neurosci.*, 250: 57–68.

4. Goodwin F.K., Jamison K.R. (1990) *Manic-Depressive Illness*. Oxford University Press, New York.

5. Dilsaver S.C., Chen Y.W., Swann A.C., Shoaib A.M., Tsai-Dilsaver Y., Krajewski K.J. (1997) Suicidality, panic disorder and psychosis in bipolar depression, depressive-mania and pure-mania. *Psychiatry Res.*, 73: 47–56.

6. Post R.M., Altshuler L.L., Frye M.A., Suppes T., Rush A.J., Keck P.E., Jr., McElroy S.L., Denicoff K.D., Leverich G.S., Kupka R.W. et al (2001) An update on the Stanley Foundation Bipolar Network (SFBN). *Bipolar Disord.*, 3: 13–14.

7. Calabrese J.R., Bowden C.L., Sachs G.S., Ascher J.A., Monaghan E., Rudd G., for the Lamictal 602 Study Group (1999) A double-blind placebo-controlled study of lamotrigine monotherapy in outpatients with bipolar I depression. *J. Clin. Psychiatry*, **60**: 79–88.

8. Bottlender R., Rudolf D., Strauss A., Möller H.-J. (2001) Mood-stabilisers reduce the risk of developing antidepressant-induced maniform states in acute treatment of bipolar I depressed patients. *J. Affect. Disord.*, **63**: 79–83.

9. Walden J., Grunze H. (2000) *Bipolar Affective Disorder. Etiology and Treatment*. Thieme, Stuttgart.

10. Perry P.J. (1996) Pharmacotherapy for major depression with melancholic features: relative efficacy of tricyclic versus selective serotonin reuptake inhibitor antidepressants. *J. Affect. Disord.*, **39**: 1–6.

11. Vieta E., Martínez-Arán A., Colom F., Benabarre A., Reinares M., Gastó C. (2000) Treatment of bipolar depression: paroxetine vs. venlafaxine. *Int. J. Neuropsychopharmacol.*, 3 (Suppl.1): 336–337.

12. Normann C., Schaerer L.O., Hummel B., Grunze H., Walden J. (2001) Lamotrigine as adjunct to paroxetine in the treatment of depression—evaluation of efficacy, safety and drug interaction. *World J. Biol. Psychiatry*, 2: 183.

13. Calabrese J. R., Suppes T., Bowden C. L., Sachs G. S., Swann A., McElroy S. L., Kusamakar V., Ascher J. A., Earl N. L., Greene P. L. et al (2000) A double-blind, placebo-controlled, prophylaxis study of lamotrigine in rapid cycling bipolar disorder. *J. Clin. Psychiatry*, **61**: 841–850.

14. Calabrese J.R., Bowden C.L., DeVeaugh-Geiss J., Earl N.L. (2001) Lamotrigine demonstrates long-term mood stabilization in manic patients. Presented at the American Psychiatric Association 134th Annual Meeting, New Orleans, 13–18 May.

15. Goodwin G. M. (1994) Recurrence of mania after lithium withdrawal. Implications for the use of lithium in the treatment of bipolar affective disorder. *Br. J. Psychiatry*, **164**: 149–152.

16. Bowden C.L., Calabrese J.R., McElroy S.L., Gyulai L., Wassef A., Petty F., Pope H.G., Chou J.C., Keck P.E., Rhodes L.J. et al (2000) A randomized, placebo-controlled 12-month trial of divalproex and lithium in treatment of outpatients with bipolar I disorder. Divalproex Maintenance Study Group. *Arch. Gen. Psychiatry*, **57**: 481–489.

17. Maj M., Pirozzi R., Kemali D. (1991) Long-term outcome of lithium prophylaxis in bipolar patients. *Arch. Gen. Psychiatry*, **48**: 772.

18. Moleman P., Hartong E.G.T.M., Hoogduin C.A.L., Broekman T.G., Nolen W. (2000) Lithium and carbamazepine in bipolar disorder. *Acta Neuropsychiatrica*, **12**: 120–121.
19. Maj M., Pirozzi R., Magliano L., Bartoli L. (1998) Long-term outcome of lithium prophylaxis in bipolar disorder: a 5-year prospective study of 402 patients at a lithium clinic. *Am. J. Psychiatry*, **155**: 30–35.
20. Solomon D.A., Keitner G.I., Ryan C.E., Miller I.W. (1998) Lithium plus valproate as maintenance polypharmacy for patients with bipolar I disorder: a review. *J. Clin. Psychopharmacol.*, **18**: 38–49.
21. Frye M.A., Ketter T.A., Leverich G.S., Huggins T., Lantz C., Denicoff K.D., Post R.M. (2000) The increasing use of polypharmacotherapy for refractory mood disorders: 22 years of study. *J. Clin. Psychiatry*, **61**: 9–15.
22. Müller-Oerlinghausen B., Retzow A., Henn F., Giedke H., Walden J. (2000) Valproate as an adjunct to neuroleptic medication for the treatment of acute episodes of mania. A prospective, randomized, double-blind, placebo-controlled multicenter study. *J. Clin. Psychopharmacol.*, **20**: 195–203.
23. Sachs G., Ghaemi S.N. (2000) Efficacy and tolerability of risperidone versus placebo in combination with lithium or valproate in acute mania. *Eur. Neuropsychopharmacol.*, **10** [Suppl. 3]: S240.

3.5
Novel Mood Stabilizing Strategies and 50 Years of Lithium

Waldemar Greil[1]

Compared to 30 years ago, it has become more difficult to make rational treatment decisions in the management of bipolar disorder. Nowadays, we have many more treatment options and a substantially larger group of patients are diagnosed as bipolar. The review presented by Charles Bowden gives an outstanding orientation for clinical practice by critically discussing the current evidence regarding the available treatment strategies.

For lithium, the classic treatment of choice in bipolar illness, the prophylactic efficacy has been discussed controversially, as most double-blind trials designed to study lithium's preventive efficacy were discontinuation studies, i.e., patients randomized to placebo were withdrawn from stable lithium and compared to patients remaining on the prophylactic drug. Hence, the results might have been biased in favour of lithium by withdrawal reactions in the placebo group [1]. Only when carbamazepine and valproate emerged as putative mood stabilizers did the scientific community pay proper attention to the fact that abrupt lithium withdrawal might trigger psychotic states, although this phenomenon had already been shown in a controlled study in the early 1980s [2, 3]. Since recurrences developing

[1] *Department of Psychiatry, University of Munich, Nussbaumstrasse 7, D-80336 Munich, Germany*

rapidly after discontinuation have mainly been observed in patients not fully stabilized on lithium [2, 3], it might be discussed that the results of the early discontinuation studies on well-selected patients are not essentially falsified by this phenomenon, as has already been carefully discussed by Schou, Thomson and Baastrup in 1970 [4]. Additionally, there are other kinds of prospective studies on prophylactic lithium, and, in sum, the body of evidence clearly shows its efficacy. Furthermore, comparative placebo-controlled studies on novel mood stabilizers including lithium as a standard will clarify lithium's preventive efficacy in accordance with modern methodological standards [5].

It will be significant to see whether rapid withdrawal recurrences are also associated with abrupt discontinuation of other mood stabilizers, such as valproate or lamotrigine, after their long-term use, or whether these drugs are superior in this important regard. Withdrawal effects are best studied in specialized outpatient clinics, e.g. in those joint to the Stanley Foundation [6]. Naturalistic follow-up data will be crucial to study prediction of response, patients' adherence to treatment and development of tolerance. For lithium, it appears that preventive efficacy is maintained over many years [7, 8].

It proved to be rather difficult to establish prophylactic efficacy of the newer mood stabilizers by placebo-controlled randomized trials with adequate power. It is ethically problematic to enrol very ill patients, and when including less ill patients, even large multicentre studies might lack statistic power. In addition, blindness is often difficult to maintain in long-term trials when comparing agents with typical side-effect profiles such as lithium and anticonvulsants [9]. Hence, we often have to rely on second-line evidence such as unblinded randomized trials.

The case of carbamazepine shows how difficult it is to evaluate efficacy from open studies. Although the evidence was rather weak, carbamazepine has officially been approved as antimanic and prophylactic agent by European drug authorities. Accordingly, carbamazepine has been wider used for these indications by European physicians than valproate—which is not yet approved in Europe as a mood stabilizer since the authorities considered the evidence for its long-term efficacy to be insufficient. In our own study, carbamazepine was similarly efficacious as lithium in preventing re-hospitalization in the whole group of bipolar patients broadly diagnosed according to DSM-IV [10]. When applying an outcome criterion closer to clinical practice, which also demands inter-episodic well-being and adherence to treatment, lithium was superior to carbamazepine [10]. Our data were also in favour of lithium regarding suicides and suicide attempts (six suicidal acts under carbamazepine during the study period compared to none under lithium).

As emphasized in Bowden's review, lithium appears to be efficacious in preventing mania, but it seems less sure whether it prevents depression to the same extent. Conversely, lamotrigine appears to be especially useful in preventing bipolar depression but less helpful in preventing mania. Hence, a combination therapy of both, lithium plus lamotrigine, might be a safe and very efficacious mood-stabilizing strategy [11]. Since combinations of mood stabilizers are frequently used but poorly investigated [6, 11], it would be highly interesting to study mood-stabilizer combinations in randomized controlled trials.

The pharmacological treatment options for mood-stabilizing strategies in bipolar disorder have expanded faster than the empirical evidence concerning their effectiveness. Randomized efficacy trials of novel mood stabilizers should be supplemented by naturalistic follow-up studies to clarify the benefit of established and novel prophylactic therapies in clinical practice. Up to now, 50 years of experience with lithium in long-term use as a mood stabilizer faces encouraging research data on an increasing number of modern alternatives.

REFERENCES

1. Suppes T., Baldessarini R.J., Faedda G.L., Tohen M. (1991) Risk of recurrence following discontinuation of lithium treatment in bipolar disorder. *Arch. Gen. Psychiatry*, **48**: 1082–1088.
2. Klein H.E., Broucek B., Greil W. (1981) Lithium withdrawal triggers psychotic states. *Br. J. Psychiatry*, **139**: 255–256.
3. Greil W., Broucek B., Klein H.E., Engel-Sittenfeld P. (1982) Discontinuation of lithium maintenance therapy: reversibility of clinical, psychological and neuroendocrinological changes. In *Basic Mechanisms in the Action of Lithium* (Eds H.R. Emrich, J.B. Aldenhoff, H.D. Lux), pp. 235–248, Excerpta Medica, Amsterdam.
4. Schou M., Thomsen K., Baastrup P.C. (1970) Studies on the course of recurrent endogenous affective disorders. *Int. Pharmacopsychiatry*, **5**: 100–106.
5. Calabrese J.R., Bowden C., DeVeaugh-Geiss J., Earl N., Gyulai L., Sachs G.M., Montgomery P. (2001) Lamotrigine demonstrates long-term mood stabilization in recently manic patients. Presented at the American Psychiatric Association 154th Annual Meeting, New Orleans, 5–10 May.
6. Levine J., Chengappa K.N., Brar J.S., Gershon S., Yablonsky E., Stapf D., Kupfer D.J. (2000) Psychotropic drug prescription patterns among patients with bipolar I disorder. *Bipolar Disord.*, **2**: 120–130.
7. Maj M., Pirozzi R., Kemali D. (1989) Long-term outcome of lithium prophylaxis in patients initially classified as complete responders. *Psychopharmacology*, **98**: 535–538.
8. Kleindienst N., Greil W., Rüger B., Möller H.J. (1999) The prophylactic efficacy of lithium—transient or persistent? *Eur. Arch. Psychiatry Clin. Neurosci.*, **249**: 144–149.
9. Oxtoby A., Jones A., Robinson M. (1989) Is your "double-blind" design truly double-blind? *Br. J. Psychiatry*, **155**: 700–701.
10. Kleindienst N., Greil W. Inter-episodic morbidity and non-completion under carbamazepine and lithium in the maintenance treatment of bipolar disorder. Submitted for publication.

11. Freeman M.P., Stoll A.L. (1998) Mood stabilizer combinations: a review of safety and efficacy. *Am. J. Psychiatry*, **155**: 12–21.

3.6
The Search for an Ideal Mood Stabilizer in the Absence of a Clear Aetiopathogenesis for Bipolar Disorder

K.N. Roy Chengappa[1,2] Lokaranjit Chalasani[1,2] and Joseph Levine[1,3]

Charles Bowden's comprehensive and thoughtful review of the pharmacological treatment of bipolar illness articulates succinctly several fundamental issues and controversies. Not unexpectedly, the issue of "What is a mood stabilizer?" is a central theme. This concept was shaped by lithium and its reported effects for the different phases (acute antimanic, acute antidepressant, and prophylactic against recurrences of mania or depression) of bipolar disorder. However, five decades later, the molecular mechanisms underlying these effects remain incompletely understood, and thus there is no clear knowledge of the biological matrices associated with the processes of mood stabilization. Furthermore, some controlled data and broader clinical experience have questioned lithium's effectiveness in rapid cycling subjects or those with multiple episodes.

If we have only a limited understanding of the underlying aetiopathophysiology of bipolar disorder, we may rightfully question whether the biological mechanisms that underlie the benefits for the acute episodes (mania or depression) or for prophylaxis are the same. If they are not, then agents that are effective for the acute episodes may not be prophylactic agents or vice versa. Examples of this dissociation of therapeutic effect exist in other medical illnesses, such as migraine or asthma or epilepsy. So, it should not be altogether surprising that effective antidepressant or antimanic agents may not be good prophylactic agents. It is also possible that the "switch" or "cycling" biology in bipolar disorder may be different from the biology of the "episode" (either mania or depression). So again, in theory, an "anti-cycling" or "anti-switch" agent may turn out to be a prophylactic agent but with minimal or no benefits for the acute episode.

Given this state of affairs, the heterogeneity of bipolar disorders is equally important to consider. For instance, should we expect agents that are effect-

[1] *Western Psychiatric Institute and Clinic, University of Pittsburgh Medical Center, 3811 O'Hara Street, Pittsburgh, PA 15213–2593, USA*
[2] *Special Studies Center at Mayview State Hospital, 1601 Mayview Road, Bridgeville, PA 15217–1599, USA*
[3] *Bersheeva Mental Health Center, Ben Gurion University in the Negev, Beersheva, Israel*

ive in bipolar II illness to be efficacious in bipolar I disorder? Lamotrigine is illustrative in this respect, with benefits being noted mainly for the rapid cycling subjects with bipolar II but not bipolar I disorder [1].

Polarity in bipolar disorder presents yet another unique challenge that is rare in medicine. The phenomenology (and most likely the underlying biology) of mania is very different from depression, unlike the on-off (or exacerbation and resolution) same phenomenology of recurrent unipolar depression or epilepsy. So, it is important to treat mania without inducing depression or vice versa. However, without a thorough knowledge of the course and the pattern of illness (for instance, depression–mania–euthymia, DME) or mania–depression–euthymia (MDE) or rapid cycling in individual patients, it is very difficult to attribute any "induction" or "exacerbation" or "improvement" to either the natural course of the illness or to the drug in question. First-generation antipsychotic agents were antimanic agents, but their maintenance use was associated with the possible induction of increased depressive episodes (and tardive dyskinesia), so these were not considered mood-stabilizing agents. Robust data exists for the efficacy of olanzapine monotherapy for manic or mixed episodes, and ongoing clinical trials will inform us whether it has efficacy for acute bipolar depression and maintenance treatment. The data for other second-generation antipsychotic agents is weak for monotherapy (except ziprasidone for mania). Heterocyclics, MAO inhibitors, selective serotonin reuptake inhibitors (SSRIs) and the post-SSRI antidepressants would similarly be considered antidepressant agents and not mood stabilizers. Also, they can induce manic switches and possibly accelerate cycling of the illness.

The emerging data for lamotrigine indicate antidepressant efficacy in bipolar I disorder, and evidence for improvement of the rapid cycling course of bipolar II subjects. However, lamotrigine shows no clear evidence as an antimanic agent. To some extent, these properties of lamotrigine inspired the definition of a uniphasic mood stabilizer, i.e. a drug which treats the acute phase (i.e. depression) and does not induce or worsen the opposite pole, and is effective in maintenance treatment in subsets of patients. So, at this point, lamotrigine does not satisfy the lithium inspired definition of a mood stabilizer. Current data regarding divalproex as monotherapy for acute bipolar depression remain scant, and maintenance primary efficacy data have been disappointing as well; so it too does not meet the lithium inspired definition. However, divalproex does appear to have benefits for mixed episode, multiple episode and rapid cycling subjects and does not appear to induce or worsen manic or depressive episodes. Data regarding carbamazepine are mixed, and the data for other anticonvulsants are even less impressive at this time.

Given the complexity and heterogeneity of bipolar disorder, and the fact that several subsets of patients demonstrate partial or lack of adequate response, there is a place for combination pharmacotherapy. Combination or augmentation treatments (two or three mood stabilizers, or mood stabilizers combined with second-generation antipsychotic agents) seem to be effective for manic or mixed episodes, and appear to provide higher response rates than monotherapy. Yet it should be stressed that it is usually monotherapy data that help us distinguish the effects of a specific agent for the acute episodes and/or for prophylaxis. Further, combination treatments trade efficacy for complicated medication regimens, blood and organ system monitoring and eventually impact on adherence to long-term treatment. Also, even though some of the newer definitions of mood stabilizer are articulating patient convenience and/or adherence issues, these are important pragmatic rather than efficacy considerations.

How might we evaluate treatments to answer several treatment issues? Clearly agents that target pathophysiology (if we knew) would be ideal. In the absence of aetiopathological targets, we would suggest well-designed hypothesis-driven small controlled trials (limited to one or a few sites initially) in well-characterized cohorts, to show differences between a candidate agent, either for the acute episode (either mania or depression) or even for prophylaxis. If the results were positive, enlarge the study to a larger number of sites, preferably with sites that can evaluate presumptive aetiopathological mechanisms (biological or imaging studies with "windows" to brain and disease activity) and, if these were positive, then long-term trials with the view to even wider generalizability could be attempted. Alternative designs that have been currently implemented have sought the "effectiveness" model of trying to create a large pool of subjects with bipolar disorder in multiple sites who are treated in a relatively uniform way, and then random-assignment study designs are tested for a particular illness phase or course of illness subtype drawing from this large pool. While this strategy is not without merit, it is less likely to provide definitive answers to the "mood stabilizer" question.

Until then, the lithium inspired definition of a mood stabilizer may be a good goal, even if difficult to achieve in practice (i.e., treatment of depression *and* mania not just either), and also for the agent to demonstrate continued treatment efficacy into the preventative phase (i.e., prophylactic against recurrences of either mania or depression), without inducing or worsening any phase of the illness. This is not to suggest that other drugs are not valuable. In fact, depending on the phase of the illness and patient factors, the drugs described earlier have proved invaluable and even lifesaving. However, the goal of developing one or more monotherapy "cornerstone" mood stabilizers should not be abandoned. To such cornerstone agents, other drugs can be added or subtracted as clinically appropriate.

REFERENCE

1. Calabrese J.R., Suppes T., Bowden C.L., Sachs G.S., Swann A.C., McElroy S.L., Kusumakar V., Ascher J.A., Earl N.L., Greene P.L. *et al* (2000) A double-blind, placebo-controlled, prophylaxis study of lamotrigine in rapid-cycling bipolar disorder. *J. Clin. Psychiatry*, **61**: 841–850.

3.7
Bipolar Disorder: Pharmacological Treatment—Where are We?

Russell T. Joffe[1]

There have been many systematic reviews of the treatment of bipolar disorder (e.g., [1–3]). In this excellent review, Bowden has gone further by imposing a scale to measure study quality. In this way, the review allows for an objective assessment of the quality of the studies and presumably the clinical inferences that may be drawn from them. Bowden's review, however, has to be read within the context of three broad conceptual issues, which do not detract from the scholarly nature of his review, but may influence the interpretation of the studies he considers and the conclusions that are drawn.

First, a rational, commonly accepted approach to the pharmacological treatment of bipolar disorder is based much more on expert opinion and clinical experience than on evidence derived from rigorous clinical trials. Studies of treatment of all phases of bipolar disorder are woefully inadequate in both quality and quantity as compared with the large dossiers of clinical trial data supporting the efficacy of currently used antidepressants and antipsychotics. While the database on randomized controlled trials of treatments for acute mania now approaches respectability, the database for acute treatment of bipolar depression and particularly the longer term prophylactic treatment of all phases of bipolar illness are substantially limited. It makes a review such as Bowden's, I have no doubt, a challenge to write and more particularly difficult to evaluate. In the end, one is struck not so much by the difference in evidence for efficacy of various acute antidepressants or long-term prophylactic agents, but rather by the limitations of the data and the conclusions that can be drawn [1–3].

The second conceptual issue follows directly from the first. In view of the limitations of the data, major caution needs to be expressed in drawing closure on any of the findings to date. This caution should be expressed in

[1] *Department of Psychiatry, New Jersey Medical School, 185 South Orange Avenue, MSB, C-671, Newark, NJ 07103-2714, USA*

both positive and negative terms. From a positive perspective, one should be very cautious about declaring superiority of one treatment over another, particularly for acute depression and prophylactic treatment of bipolar disorder. The increased number of studies of compounds such as divalproex sodium and lamotrigine in all phases of the illness is laudable. These studies [4, 5] confirm our clinical observations that these drugs are of varying efficacy in different stages of the illness. Although confirmation of efficacy using rigorous clinical trial design is highly desirable, this should not imply that other compounds which may be not as extensively studied, due often to lack of commercial interest, have inferior efficacy. Carbamazepine, from clinical experience, clearly has antimanic efficacy and may be useful in other phases of the illness. Lack of systematic investigation makes it difficult to evaluate its comparable efficacy with divalproex sodium. This does not mean that one should conclude that carbamazepine is an inferior compound, particularly for selected patients. Gabapentin was summarily dismissed as an effective agent after one negative study [6]. This has precluded a more comprehensive evaluation of gabapentin and its potential role, even if not as a first-line treatment, for bipolar disorder. The pharmacological armamentarium is so limited for bipolar disorder that one should caution against early discounting of the efficacy of any compound. Future trials should aim for a thorough evaluation of all potentially effective treatments for different phases of bipolar disorder, regardless of commercial interest.

Last, the treatment of bipolar depression has been particularly neglected [2]. Implicit in any treatment decision about acute bipolar depression is weighing the risk of continuing depression versus the risk of a switch into mania or cycle acceleration which is associated with the use of antidepressants in this disorder [7]. All antidepressants will cause mood instability resulting in a switch into mania or an increased frequency of cycling. This risk, probably occurring in 15 to 25% of antidepressant treated bipolar patients, has to be balanced against the continuing risk of bipolar depression, which includes chronicity, episode recurrence, psychosocial morbidity and, of course, suicide. The data on mood stabilizer treatment of bipolar depression remains extremely limited [2] and clinical experience is not always encouraging. Antidepressants are well-established treatment for acute depression including bipolar depression [8]; however, mood stabilizers are not likely to cause a switch into mania which may occur with antidepressants [7, 8]. There is a bias to protecting the bipolar patient from manic switches and cycle acceleration by the preferred use of mood stabilizers over antidepressants. This clinical practice is not necessarily supported by the literature. Carefully and rigorously designed studies will be required to balance and evaluate the risk between switch and cycle acceleration on the one hand and the consequences of depression on the other. In this way, the most seriously debilitating phase of the illness, namely ongoing depression, may be treated in a manner which best fits the patient's needs rather than conforming to any theoretical assumption that to be depressed is less troublesome than to have mood instability and a switch into mania.

Bowden's review is both critical and comprehensive. It explicitly teaches us about the available literature and about state-of-the-art approaches to treatment for acute mania, acute depression and bipolar prophylaxis. It also teaches us, both explicitly and implicitly, about how much more work is needed to provide an objective, comprehensive and scientifically sound database for the pharmacological treatment of bipolar illness.

REFERENCES

1. Bowden C.L. (1997)   Treatment of bipolar disorder. *Curr. Rev. Mood Anxiety Disord,,* **1**: 167–176.
2. Zornberg G.L., Pope H.G. (1993)   Treatment of depression in bipolar disorder: new directions for research. *J. Clin. Psychopharmacol.,* **13**: 397–408.
3. Keck P.E., Jr., McElroy S.L., Strakowski S.M. (1998)   Anticonvulsants and antipsychotics in the treatment of bipolar disorder. *J. Clin. Psychiatry,* **59** (Suppl. 6): 74–81.
4. Bowden C.L., Calabrese J.R., McElroy S.L., Gyulai L., Wassef A., Petty F., Pope H.G., Chou J.C.-Y., Keck P.E., Jr., Rhodes L.J. *et al* (2000)   A randomized, placebo controlled 12-month trial of divalproex and lithium in treatment of outpatients with bipolar disorder. *Arch. Gen. Psychiatry,* **57**: 481–489.
5. Calabrese J.R., Bowden C.L., Sachs G.S, Ascher J.A., Monaghan E., Rudd D.G. (1999). A double-blind placebo-controlled study of lamotrigine monotherapy in outpatients with bipolar I depression. *J. Clin. Psychiatry,* **60**: 79–88.
6. Frye M.A., Ketter T.A., Kimbrell T.A., Dunn R.T., Speer A.M., Osuch E.A., Luckenbaugh D.A., Cora-Locatelli G., Leverich G.S., Post R.M. (2000)   A placebo-controlled study of lamotrigine and gabapentin monotherapy in refractory mood disorders. *J. Clin. Psychopharmacol.,* **20**: 607–614.
7. Altshuler L.I., Post R.M., Leverich G.S., Mikalauskas K., Roseff A., Ackerman L. (1995). Antidepressant-induced mania and cycle acceleration: a controversy revisited. *Am. J. Psychiatry,* **152**: 1130–1138.
8. Nemeroff C.B., Evans D.L., Gyulai L., Sachs G.S., Bowden C.L., Gurgel I.P., Oakes R., Pitts C.D. (2001). Double-blind, placebo-controlled comparison of imipramine and paroxetine in the treatment of bipolar depression. *Am. J. Psychiatry,* **158**: 906–912.

3.8
Long-term Prophylactic Efficacy:
The Most Important Feature of Mood Normalizers

Janusz K. Rybakowski[1]

In his excellent review, Bowden critically updates the main concepts and the evidence for the efficacy of pharmacological treatment in bipolar illness. However, it seems that the relative importance of such "old" drugs as lithium and carbamazepine has been in some aspects underestimated.

Since bipolar disorder is a lifetime illness, the favourable modification of the longitudinal course of the illness over the years is probably the most important feature of mood normalizers. Long-term clinical experiences with drugs which are claimed by Bowden to fulfil the modern criteria for mood normalizers are clearly not equal. It is mostly with lithium that clinical observations of long-term treatment in many patients well exceed 20 years. I am not aware of even naturalistic observations with other drugs (except for carbamazepine) lasting more than five years. Nowadays, in many outpatient clinics (including our clinic in Poznan), a substantial experience has been accumulated with ultra long-term prophylactic treatment (i.e., > 20 years) with lithium, used mostly as a monotherapy. The prophylactic efficacy of lithium has probably not decreased over the recent decades, although so-called excellent lithium responders (those with no recurrences during long-term treatment with lithium alone) may represent no more than one-third of compliant lithium patients. In our recent study, including only bipolar patients who received lithium over a 10-year period, we did not find any difference in the percentage of excellent lithium responders between those entering treatment in the 1970s and in the 1980s (35% vs. 27%) [1].

It is not sufficiently clear why lamotrigine was without hesitation put in the group of proven mood normalizers while carbamazepine was included among those for which evidence is incomplete. This may partly reflect regional differences, i.e. that carbamazepine is for different reasons generally less used than other anticonvulsants in the USA than in Europe. However, carbamazepine has been much more studied than lamotrigine as a prophylactic agent in affective illness and for a longer period of time, as reflected in both older [2] and recent reports [3]. In Europe, carbamazepine is also a drug of first choice for combination with lithium in suboptimal prophylactic lithium responders. It should be noticed that with this combination some side effects of either drug are compensated (e.g., diuretic action of lithium and antidiuretic activity of carbamazepine) and that these drugs exert opposite actions on the hematopoietic system.

[1] Department of Adult Psychiatry, Karol Marcinkowski University of Medical Sciences, 22/27 Szpitalna, Poznan 60–572, Poland

Another question is whether atypical antipsychotics should be included among possible mood-normalizing substances. My answer would be "yes", at least on account of my personal, both acute (antimanic) and long-term, experiences with clozapine in bipolar patients. Our group in Poznan reported the excellent antimanic efficacy of clozapine (although only in an open study) long before this drug was introduced in the USA [4].

There is also the question whether we should vigorously treat hypomanic phases occurring in the course of bipolar II illness. I would agree with Bowden that many patients could profit from such periods and that we should not sedate the patient at all costs.

For the treatment of bipolar depression, there is an increasing tendency to use new generation antidepressants with lesser propensity to induce manic switch. However, a consensus exists that in bipolar I patients they should be combined with mood normalizers. On the other hand, it has been suggested to use new generation antidepressants as a monotherapy in treating depression in bipolar II patients [5, 6]. How long the antidepressant alone should be safely given in such conditions remains unclear. Moreover, whether continuing the antidepressant into the hypomanic phase without a mood normalizer may precipitate subsequent depressive recurrence or rapid cycling remains to be established. In most of such patients, a mood normalizer would be indicated especially as an augmenter in case of non-optimal antidepressant response. Our experience with lithium augmentation shows that this effect is more robust in bipolar than in unipolar depression [7]. Furthermore, in another study, we found that carbamazepine was as effective as lithium for antidepressant augmentation [8], which would further qualify this drug as a mood normalizer.

REFERENCES

1. Rybakowski J.K., Chlopocka-Wozniak M., Suwalska A. (2001)   The prophylactic effect of long-term lithium administration in bipolar patients entering treatment in the 1970s and 1980s. *Bipolar Disord.*, **3**: 63–67.
2. Placidi G.F., Lenzi A., Lazzerini F., Cassano G.B., Akiskal H.S. (1986)   The comparative efficacy and safety of carbamazepine versus lithium: a randomized, double-blind 3-year trial in 83 patients. *J. Clin. Psychiatry*, **47**: 490–494.
3. Kleindienst N., Greil W. (2000)   Differential efficacy of lithium and carbamazepine in the prophylaxis of bipolar disorder: results of the MAP study. *Neuropsychobiology*, **42** (Suppl. 1): 2–10.
4. Strzyzewski W., Rybakowski J., Chlopocka-Wozniak M, Czerwinski A. (1981)   Clozapine in the treatment of manic states (in Polish). *Psychiatr. Pol.*, **15**: 331–332.
5. Amsterdam J.D., Garcia-Espana F., Fawcett J., Quitkin F.M., Reimherr F.W., Rosenbaum J.F., Schweitzer E., Beasley C. (1998)   Efficacy and safety of fluoxetine in treating bipolar II major depressive episode. *J. Clin. Psychopharmacol.*, **18**: 435–440.

6. Amsterdam J.D., Garcia-Espana F. (2000) Venlafaxine monotherapy in women with bipolar II and unipolar major depression. *J. Affect. Disord.*, **59**: 225–229.
7. Rybakowski J., Matkowski K. (1992) Adding lithium to antidepressant therapy: factors related to therapeutic potentiation. *Eur. Neuropsychopharmacol.*, **2**: 161–165.
8. Rybakowski J.K., Suwalska A., Chlopocka-Wozniak M. (1999) Potentiation of antidepressants with lithium or carbamazepine in treatment-resistant depression. *Neuropsychobiology*, **40**: 134–139.

3.9

Choosing Among Antimanic Treatments: Can the Clinician be Guided by the Evidence from Randomized Controlled Trials?

Rasmus W. Licht[1]

During recent years, there have been an increasing number of randomized controlled trials (RCTs) evaluating various drug treatments for mania, as thoroughly reviewed by Charles Bowden. A key issue, which will be briefly touched upon in the following, is to what extent the evidence from these RCTs can guide the clinician in selecting and conducting a proper treatment.

According to Bowden's review, the clinician has several primary antimanic drugs at hand, when facing an acutely manic patient in need of treatment, e.g. lithium, valproate, carbamazepine, various typical and various atypical antipsychotics. Among these options, valproate, lithium (as an internal comparator to valproate), olanzapine, risperidone and ziprasidone have been tested in recent industry driven, rigorously conducted, large multicentre, parallel-group designed RCTs using modern psychometric measures. However, before that, the antimanic potential of lithium, various typical antipsychotics, and to some extent carbamazepine was known from several investigator driven, generally smaller and less sophisticated comparative RCTs [1], open trials and an extended experience from clinical practice. In pharmacoepidemiological surveys from the mid-1990s, typical antipsychotics were the most commonly used antimanics in clinical practice, not only in European samples but also in US samples [2, 3]. In Europe, antipsychotics are still the most commonly used first-line antimanics, since they require no blood sampling (in contrast to lithium and valproate) and since at least some of them can be given intramuscularly in case of severe non-compliance. Based on the available evidence from the more recent

[1] *Mood Disorders Research Unit, Aarhus University Psychiatric Hospital, Skovagervej 2, DK-8240 Risskov, Denmark*

RCTs, Bowden recommends valproate as a first drug of choice for the entire spectrum of acute mania, even for the severe cases. However, due to the potential gap between the highly selected populations approached and enrolled in RCTs and the unselected populations treated in clinical practice, it remains to be investigated to what extent valproate may replace antipsychotics in clinical practice.

In his section on methodology of RCTs in bipolar disorder, Bowden indirectly touches the issue of such potential limitations in generalizability of results from RCTs while mentioning the difficulties in recruitment of subjects for placebo-controlled trials. In trials on acute mania these difficulties seem to be insolubly associated with the illness itself, since moderately or severely ill patients characterized by impaired insight and lack of co-operativeness are not generally approached by researchers and, even when they are, they are not likely to consent to participate in a trial. While conducting an RCT comparing lithium with zuclopenthixol, we compared the randomized patients with the patients who had to be excluded for various reasons, and substantial differences on variables generally related to outcome were found [4]. Large-sized multicentre trials do not overcome this issue. On the contrary, many sites recruit only a very small number of highly selected patients.

Besides limitations in generalizability, the available industry driven RCTs designed for drug approval have other limitations. A drug–placebo difference of 25% in response rates (defined as a 50% or more reduction in a mania rating scale) has been observed for valproate and olanzapine. This implies that four patients have to be treated in order to achieve a modest benefit in one patient, which may not be convincing for the clinician. Hopefully, remission rates will be more commonly reported in future trials. Furthermore, follow-up data on responding and non-responding patients would be very helpful for the clinician, considering the fluctuation of manic and depressive symptoms within each single episode. Given the very high drop-out rates of around 50%, partly due to high requirements for protocol adherence in RCTs conducted for drug approvals, follow-up data of drop outs are also needed.

As pointed out by Bowden, combined treatments are often necessary, but rarely studied. What is also sparsely studied systematically is what to do when first-line treatment fails, although there is some evidence that clozapine or electroconvulsive therapy (ECT) may work in such cases [1].

Predicting individual response is a key issue for the clinician. Until molecular biology eventually facilitates rational drug selection, we must rely on clinical group variables such as diagnostic subtype. Thus, as mentioned by Bowden, post-hoc analyses of results from RCTs have suggested that valproate, in contrast to lithium, is equally effective on manic symptoms in pure manic and in mixed states. However, whether psychotic mania should also give valproate a preference above lithium is still not fully settled.

Besides prediction of acute response, tolerability and patient preference, the prophylactic potential of a given antimanic drug is also important for the clinician when choosing among the various options. In that respect, at least in terms of efficacy, lithium still seems to be the best choice.

Obviously we need RCTs to establish the mood-stabilizing efficacy of new compounds. However, to overcome the gap between results from industry driven RCTs and the needs of clinical practice we also need large-scale pragmatic studies using broad inclusion criteria, comparing the various treatments, alone or in combination, in populations of less selected patients. These studies may be randomized but open and use simple but relevant outcome measures. Large prospective follow-up studies of unselected cohorts treated systematically according to certain algorithms may also lead to reliable results regarding differential response prediction.

Due to the limitations of RCTs as outlined above, the clinician still needs to consider each individual treatment course as a trial in which the various treatments are added and withdrawn in a rational sequence according to a continuing and systematic evaluation of clinical response and side effects.

REFERENCES

1. Licht R.W. (1998) Drug treatment of mania: a critical review. *Acta Psychiatr. Scand.*, **97**: 387–397.
2. Licht R.W., Gouliaev G., Vestergaard P., Lund H., Merinder L., Dybbro J. (1994) Treatment of manic episodes in Scandinavia: the use of neuroleptics in a clinical routine setting. *J. Affect. Disord.*, **32**: 179–185.
3. Chou J.C.Y., Zivkov M., Voldby H., Creelman W.L., Alterman D., Dahl S.G. (1996) Neuroleptics in acute mania: a pharmacoepidemiological study. *Ann. Pharmacother.*, **30**: 1396–1398.
4. Licht R.W., Gouliaev G., Vestergaard P., Frydenberg M. (1997) Generalizability of results from randomized drug trials, exemplified by a trial on antimanic treatment. *Br. J. Psychiatry*, **170**: 264–267.

3.10
Challenges for the Experimental Therapeutics of Bipolar Disorder
Ross J. Baldessarini[1]

In his thoughtful overview of contemporary pharmacological treatments for bipolar manic-depressive illness, Charles Bowden raises points calling for further emphasis. First, reasonable criteria for "mood stabilization" should include more than the short-term antimanic effects for which several agents are FDA-approved with research support. Even lithium, the standard mood stabilizer, is FDA-approved only for mania and its recurrences [1]. Evidence of long-term protection, even against mania, remains strikingly limited for agents other than lithium and perhaps carbamazepine [1]. For mood stabilization, controlled trials lasting more than one year are required, particularly in view of the natural average spontaneous recurrence rate in untreated bipolar disorder of about one new episode/year [2, 3].

A central problem in experimental therapeutics for bipolar disorder is prevention of recurrences of depression. For most proposed alternatives to lithium, evidence for long-term protection against recurrences of bipolar depression remains very limited compared to recurrent unipolar major depression [1, 4]. Indeed, bipolarity, psychosis or mixed states, and suicidality are typical exclusion criteria in antidepressant trials, but are matters of particularly pressing clinical and public health concern [1, 3, 5 ,6]. Lithium appears to be effective long term against recurrent depression in both bipolar I and II disorders [1, 3]. There is also extensive evidence of reduced long-term risks of suicide during lithium maintenance therapy that is unmatched by any other treatment in contemporary psychiatry [5, 6].

Another critical issue for studies of proposed mood-stabilizing treatments in bipolar disorder is the design and interpretation of trials in this inherently unstable and variable condition. Moreover, discontinuing lithium maintenance treatment, particularly rapidly, leads to early excesses not only of mania, but also of mixed states, depression, and suicidal behaviour [5, 7, 8]. It remains unclear how long to gradually discontinue proposed mood-stabilizing agents to minimize this effect, with its substantial clinical risks and potential to increase the duration and cost of trials and complicate their scientific interpretation [7, 9].

Additional important methodological challenges for experimental therapeutics in bipolar disorder include definitions of appropriate clinical outcomes [9]. Many studies have declared success or failure based on the occurrence or latency of even a single new episode of mania or depression. Given the lack of consistent, full protection from new episodes of bipolar

[1] Mailman Research Center, McLean Hospital, 115 Mill Street, Belmont, MA 02478–9106, USA

illness by any available treatment, more appropriate outcome criteria would include the number, frequency, duration, and severity of all illness episodes over prolonged follow-up times, the overall proportion of time ill, and reliable measures of functional status and quality of life [9].

Finally, experimental therapeutics remains strikingly deficient for juvenile and geriatric forms of bipolar disorder [10, 11], and in critically evaluating psychosocial and rehabilitative measures that have proved to be useful adjuncts to medication in recurrent depression and even chronic psychotic disorders [12].

REFERENCES

1. Baldessarini R.J., Tarazi F.I. (2001) Drugs and the treatment of psychiatric disorders. In *Goodman and Gilman's Pharmacological Basis of Therapeutics*, 10th ed. (Eds J.G. Hardman, L.E. Limbird, P.B. Molinoff, R.W. Ruddon, A.G. Gilman), McGraw-Hill, New York (in press).
2. Angst J. (1986) The course of affective disorders. *Psychopathology*, **19** (Suppl. 2): 47–52.
3. Tondo L., Baldessarini R.J., Floris J. (2001) Long-term clinical effectiveness of lithium maintenance treatment in types I and II bipolar manic-depressive disorders. *Br. J. Psychiatry*, **178** (Suppl. 40): S184–S190.
4. Viguera A.C., Baldessarini R.J., Friedberg J. (1998) Risks of interrupting continuation or maintenance treatment with antidepressants in major depressive disorders. *Harvard Rev. Psychiatry*, **5**: 293–306.
5. Tondo L., Baldessarini R.J. (2000) Reduced suicide risk during lithium maintenance treatment. *J. Clin. Psychiatry*, **61** (Suppl. 9): 97–104.
6. Tondo L., Hennen J., Baldessarini R.J. (2001) Reduced suicide risk with long-term lithium treatment in major affective illness: a meta-analysis. *Acta Psychiatr. Scand.* (in press).
7. Baldessarini R.J., Tondo L., Viguera A.C. (1999) Effects of discontinuing lithium maintenance treatment. *Bipolar Disord.*, **1**: 17–24.
8. Viguera A.C., Nonacs R., Cohen L.S., Tondo L., Murray A., Baldessarini R.J. (2000) Risk of discontinuing lithium maintenance in pregnant vs. nonpregnant women with bipolar disorders. *Am. J. Psychiatry*, **157**: 179–184.
9. Baldessarini R.J., Tohen M., Tondo L. (2000) Maintenance treatment in bipolar disorder. *Arch. Gen. Psychiatry*, **57**: 490–492.
10. Faedda G.L., Baldessarini R.J., Suppes T., Tondo L., Becker I., Lipschitz D. (1995) Pediatric-onset bipolar disorder: a neglected clinical and public health problem. *Harvard Rev. Psychiatry*, **3**: 171–195.
11. Baldessarini R.J., Tondo L., Suppes T., Faedda G.L., Tohen M. (1996) Pharmacological treatment of bipolar disorder throughout the life-cycle. In *Mood Disorders Across the Life Span* (Eds K.I. Shulman, M. Tohen, S. Kutcher), pp. 299–338, Wiley, New York.
12. Huxley N.A., Parikh S.V., Baldessarini R.J. (2000) Effectiveness of psychosocial treatments in bipolar disorder: state of the evidence. *Harvard Rev. Psychiatry*, **8**: 126–140.

3.11
Expanding Options to Treat Bipolar Disorder: Science Informs Practice

Alan J. Gelenberg and John Misiaszek[1]

Charles Bowden has done an outstanding job in reviewing a rapidly expanding literature on the treatment of bipolar disorder. Not long ago lithium, advanced by Cade over 50 years ago, was the only medication for this condition. Now, there are many purported pharmacotherapies to alleviate mania, depression, and mixed states, as well as for long-term stabilization of mood. The risk today is that proposed treatments have far outstripped the scientific data underpinning their safe and efficacious use.

Bowden begins by observing that psychiatrists in practice may expect too much from a drug labelled "mood stabilizer". He recommends that the definition of mood stabilizer require benefit from a drug for one "primary aspect of bipolar illness" in acute and maintenance-phase treatment, while not worsening any aspect of the illness. This definition—more modest than an expectation of total long-term mood stabilization—may help set the stage for appropriate polypharmacy, later reviewed by the author. He also emphasizes the importance of separating benefits against *components* of mood episodes, such as sleep disturbances and anxiety, which may be provided by drugs such as clonazepam and gabapentin, and *primary efficacy against mania* or another phase of bipolar disorder.

We appreciate and concur with Bowden's weighing the difficulties of mild hyperthymia versus those of cognitive dulling, which often comes from overmedicating with mood stabilizers. Patients with bipolar disorder can be highly functional, and the long-term goal of protecting life and enhancing its quality must balance mood symptoms against the need for mental clarity.

The author points out many difficulties encountered by the brave souls who labour on clinical research in bipolar disorder. Difficult in any area of clinical research, problems of selection criteria and the placebo response are particularly knotty in this condition. Research criteria for inclusion can result in samples that do not represent the real universe of patients with bipolar disorder. Even the 50% criterion of improvement in baseline mania that Bowden calls "relatively stringent" leaves many patients with life-disrupting symptoms. The upshot is continuing efforts to find enhanced treatment regimens, often involving polypharmacy and inevitable side effects.

Bowden observes a problem in clinical research that cuts across all diagnoses in psychiatry. Eager to enrol subjects in a clinical trial, investigators

[1] *Department of Psychiatry, College of Medicine, University of Arizona, P.O. Box 245002, Tucson, Arizona 85724–5002, USA*

and their staff tend to inflate initial symptom scores on rating scales, only to deflate these once treatment has begun. The result is a higher placebo response rate and number of failed trials. Our proposed remedy would be to borrow a page from the manuals of psychotherapy researchers and sample videotaped interviews from investigators in collaborative studies to assure consistency in rating.

The author touches briefly on an issue important to long-term, maintenance-phase trials in any area of psychiatry (and medicine more broadly): whether a treatment that *induces* remission predicts the best treatment to *maintain* remission. This question must be entertained by any protocol contemplating long-term observations in our field. At the very least, investigators must state clearly the treatment history in the acute phase of an illness and analyse acute-phase data for clues to long-term response.

A new and interesting clue to the use of divalproex for long-term treatment comes in the author's reference to an analysis of maintenance-phase serum-level data. Apparently, higher ($> 125\,\mu g/ml$) levels of valproate were associated with more side effects and less control over mania symptoms.

The author notes the need for systematic studies of antipsychotic drugs for maintenance treatment in bipolar disorder. Particularly for long-term therapy, adverse events and their chronic hazards must be taken into account, both to protect against physical consequences, as well as to diminish non-adherence to medication regimens. Recent concerns with new antipsychotic drugs have included lipid and glucose levels, hyperprolactinemia, and the cardiac QT_c interval.

Carbamazepine is widely used outside of the United States as an alternative to lithium in this disorder. The author aptly notes, however, the dearth of adequately controlled trials to bring science to bear on its clinical application. Available data suggest that carbamazepine may have its best role as an adjunctive therapy. Its congener, oxcarbazepine, has not been studied much in bipolar disorder, but might be equal in efficacy to carbamazepine and appears to have a weaker effect in inducing P450 3A4 isoenzymes.

Recent data on the anti-epileptic drug lamotrigine are encouraging. Lamotrigine, as noted by Bowden, may effectively treat acute depression in bipolar disorder (without worsening the likelihood of a switch into mania) and might extend the interval until the next episode of depression. Treatment of depression in bipolar disorder remains problematic, as evidence on the proper choice of an antidepressant and the duration of its use remains murky. Much of what is employed in practice has been extrapolated from data and experience in treating unipolar depressions. We concur with Bowden's recommendation that an antidepressant be tapered several weeks after recovery. We note, however, a recent retrospective study suggesting that antidepressant discontinuation might increase the risk of depressive relapse in some bipolar patients [1].

We also concur with Bowden's emphasis on the importance of the symptom complex in choosing a treatment for acute mania. Thus, the presence of mixed features, anxiety, psychosis, and rapid cycling are important variables in selecting medication. Divalproex appears to have advantages over lithium for these more complex pictures of mania. Combinations of medications appear more effective than single agents, but, at this stage of knowledge, most experts recommend two failed monotherapy trials before moving on to polypharmacy.

Beyond medications currently considered "mood stabilizers", singly and in combination, physicians often turn to other adjunctive treatments. Clinical experience abounds, but scientific evidence remains scanty. Examples are supplemental thyroxine, benzodiazepines, and natural remedies—most recently, omega 3 fatty acids. In our experience, benzodiazepines are often useful in nipping hypomania in the bud by promoting a return to normal sleep patterns. However, given the greater than 50% likelihood that a patient with bipolar disorder will develop substance abuse during his or her lifetime, where the physician fears a risk of sedative-hypnotic dependency, gabapentin may be an alternative.

Our last piece of advice concerns the need to blend science and clinical experience. Evidence-based medicine requires that we turn first to treatments with well-established safety and efficacy. Evidence in psychiatry is at least equal to that in most other medical specialties. But doctors are confronted daily by problems without scientific answers. In those common instances, the clinician's own wisdom and experience must be balanced against the clinical literature, including controlled trials, case series, and selected anecdotes.

REFERENCE

1. Altshuler L., Kiriakos L., Calcagno J., Goodman R., Gitlin M., Frye M., Mintz J. (2001) The impact of antidepressant discontinuation versus antidepressant continuation on 1-year risk for relapse of bipolar depression: a retrospective chart review. *J. Clin. Psychiatry* (in press).

3.12
The Pharmacological Treatment of Bipolar Disorder: More Questions
Than Answers

Chittaranjan Andrade[1]

More than a century has passed since Kraepelin described manic-depressive psychosis, and more than half a century has passed since Cade ushered in the lithium era; today, despite the availability of lithium, conventional and newer antiepileptic drugs, conventional and atypical antipsychotic drugs, conventional and recent antidepressant drugs, and miscellaneous other drugs for the treatment of bipolar disorder, Bowden correctly identifies fewer than a dozen high quality drug trials which allow evidence-based treatment decisions to be made.

There are many reasons for this dissatisfying state of affairs. For example, Bowden notes that many of the early studies were flawed by the recruitment of patients who were unwittingly predisposed to relapse because of an abrupt withdrawal from lithium. The explosion of new treatment agents, during the last decade, has not had sufficient time for adequate research. All-important long-term maintenance therapy studies have not been conducted, perhaps for ethical reasons, and perhaps for want of patience and funds. Antidepressant drugs and the irregular use of lithium may have impacted adversely upon the long-term course and outcome of the disorder, prejudicing the results of drug therapy. Bipolar disorder presents in varied forms, and the ideal management of each may differ.

Plenty of studies inform us about the efficacy of various drugs in acute phase mania and depression; however, most of these studies examine response rather than remission. This is unfortunate because the goal of therapy is euthymia, and not just improvement. On what evidence do we base treatment decisions when patients respond but are slow to remit?

Moving to a subject of far greater importance, we are woefully ignorant on several subjects related to the maintenance of euthymia. Consider the following:

(a) The use of antipsychotic and antidepressant drugs during continuation and maintenance phases of therapy increases the risk of depression and mania, respectively; accordingly, these drugs are tapered off and withdrawn as early as possible, and the patient is maintained with drugs such as lithium, valproate, carbamazepine, combinations thereof, or alternatives thereto. The timing of withdrawal assumes what has not been proven: that drugs effective in prophylaxis during the maintenance phase are effective in stabilizing mood during the continuation phase.

[1] Department of Psychopharmacology, National Institute of Mental Health and Neurosciences, Bangalore 560 029, India

(b) We still do not have adequately strong and adequately replicated evidence to identify ideal maintenance treatments for bipolar I and bipolar II illness; rapid-cycling and non-rapid-cycling illness; classical and dysphoric/mixed illness; acute phase illness with and without psychotic features.

Furthermore, these four dichotomous groups combine to form no fewer than 16 different presentations; while some are undoubtedly rare, there is no assurance that a management strategy effective for any of the more common presentations will be as effective for any of the others.

Specifically in this context, since an increasing number of patients appear to require polypharmacy for the optimal stabilization of mood, we need to know the best combination of drugs for each presentation of bipolar disorder; at the very least, we need to know the spectrum of efficacy of classical combinations such as lithium and carbamazepine, and lithium and valproate. I also see several rapid-cycling patients to whom other clinicians have prescribed an antipsychotic–antidepressant combination (for maintenance therapy) because of nonresponse to the lithium–carbamazepine–valproate group of drugs; heretical though it may sound, is there a role for an antipsychotic–antidepressant prophylaxis of bipolar disorder?

Treatment schedule optimization of drugs used in maintenance therapy requires better characterization. Consider the following:

(a) With the exception of the case of lithium, we do not have convincing evidence about ideal doses and/or serum levels for effective prophylaxis with different drugs; should we, therefore, best maintain patients at the highest tolerated doses?

(b) Whatever the half-life of the drug (a crude proxy for the duration of its central action), and whatever the apparent half-life of the preparation (as in the case of controlled release formulations), we universally use 12-hour values as the gold standard for estimating serum level relationships with response; is this practice valid, and might this practice be responsible for the failure to establish consistent relationships?

(c) On a subject that has been of interest at our centre: there is an increasing trend to prescribe lithium once daily [1, 2]; although we have ourselves found once-daily lithium dosing as effective as divided dosing in acute [3] and maintenance [4] phases of illness, we realize that neither these nor other studies in world literature [5–10] present sufficiently strong evidence to justify the practice. Once-daily (nighttime) dosing improves compliance, requires lower total daily doses [11] with accompanying benefits such as lower costs and adverse effects [12, 13], and allows peak level adverse effects to dissipate during the hours of sleep [14, 15]; nevertheless, until rigorous studies demonstrate its efficacy as acute and maintenance therapy, the practice should be considered unapproved. Alternate day lithium is still experimental [16–18].

REFERENCES

1. Bramble D. (1992) A survey of lithium use in the elderly. *Int. J. Geriatr. Psychiatry*, **7**: 819–826.
2. Kehoe R.F., Mander A.J. (1992) Lithium treatment. Prescribing and monitoring habits in hospital and general practice. *Br. Med. J.*, **304**: 552–554.
3. Suresh K.P., Prasad K.M.R., Mohan R., Andrade C., Ashok M.V., Chaturvedi S.K., Sreenivas K.N. (1994) Once daily versus divided dosage lithium therapy in acute mania. *Indian J. Psychiatry*, **37**: 9–12.
4. Mohan R., Suresh K.P., Prasad K.M.R., Ashok M.V., Andrade C., Sreenivas K.N., Chaturvedi S.K. (1996) Once daily lithium in the prophylaxis of mood disorders. *Indian J. Psychiatry*, **38**: 104–108.
5. Bech P., Vendsborg P.B., Rafaelsen O.J. (1976) Lithium maintenance treatment of manic-melancholic patients: its role in the daily routine. *Acta Psychiatr. Scand.*, **53**: 70–81.
6. Lokkegaard H., Andersen N.F., Henriksen E., Bartels P.D., Brahm M., Baastrup P.C., Jorgensen H.E., Larsen M., Munck O., Rasmussen K. *et al* (1985) Renal function in 153 manic-depressive patients treated with lithium for more than five years. *Acta Psychiatr. Scand.*, **71**: 347–355.
7. Coppen A., Abou-Saleh M.T., Milln P., Bailey J., Wood K. (1983) Decreasing lithium dosage reduces morbidity and side effects during prophylaxis. *J. Affect. Disord.*, **5**: 353–362.
8. Coppen A., Abou-Saleh M.T. (1988) Lithium therapy: from clinical trials to practical management. *Acta Psychiatr. Scand.*, **78**: 754–762.
9. Muir A., Davidson R., Silverstone T., Dawnay A., Forsling M.L. (1989) Two regimens of lithium prophylaxis and renal function. *Acta Psychiatr. Scand.*, **80**: 579–583.
10. Abraham G., Delva N., Waldron J., Lawson J.S., Owen J. (1992) Lithium treatment: a comparison of once- and twice-daily dosing. *Acta Psychiatr. Scand.*, **85**: 65–69.
11. Lauritsen B.J., Mellerup E.T., Plenge P., Rasmussen S., Vestergaard P., Schou M. (1981) Serum lithium concentrations around the clock with different treatment regimens and diurnal variation of the renal lithium clearance. *Acta Psychiatr. Scand.*, **64**: 314–319.
12. Bowen R.C., Grof P., Grof E. (1991) Less frequent lithium administration and lower urine volume. *Am. J. Psychiatry*, **148**: 189–192.
13. O'Donovan C., Hawkes J., Bowen R. (1993) Effect of lithium dosing schedule on urinary output. *Acta Psychiatr. Scand.*, **87**: 92–95.
14. Plenge P., Mellerup E.T. (1986) Lithium and the kidney: is one daily dose better than two? *Compr. Psychiatry*, **27**: 336–342.
15. Mellerup E.T., Plenge P. (1990) The side effects of lithium. *Biol. Psychiatry*, **28**: 464–466.
16. Jensen H.V., Plenge P., Mellerup E.T., Davidsen K., Toftegaard L., Aggernaes H., Bjorum N. (1995) Lithium prophylaxis of manic-depressive disorder: daily lithium dosing schedule versus every second day. *Acta Psychiatr. Scand.*, **92**: 69–74.

17. Andrade C. (1996) Is alternate day lithium really ineffective? *Acta Psychiatr. Scand.*, **94**: 281–282.
18. Plenge P., Amin M., Agarwal A.K., Greil W., Kim M.-J., Panteleyeva G., Park J.-M., Prilipko L., Rayushkin V., Sharma M. *et al* (1999) Prophylactic efficacy of lithium administered every second day: a WHO multicentre study. *Bipolar Disord.*, **2**: 109–116.

3.13
Efficacy and Effectiveness of Long-term Pharmacological Treatment of Bipolar Disorder

Per Vestergaard[1]

Short-term treatment of manic and depressive episodes may prove a cumbersome task, but eventually the majority of patients will experience a full or partial response. Long-term prophylactic treatment presents both patients and doctors with additional problems which I shall deal with briefly.

In his review, Charles Bowden competently and in great detail examines the evidence for treatment efficacy of various drugs and drug combinations, and it is quite clear that long-term treatment efficacy is far from ideal. In long-term studies of mood stabilizers, the majority of which have been conducted with lithium, efficacy figures for patients responding to lithium only reach levels between 60 and 70% [1, 2]. Figures for treatment effectiveness obtained from so-called naturalistic follow-up studies of bipolar patients in long-term treatment with lithium are even more disappointing, seldomly reaching levels above 30–40% [3].

Regarding treatment efficacy, it is most likely that the potentials are exhausted of such traditional psychotropic drugs which predominantly influence monoamino-transmitter systems by manipulating presynaptic or postsynaptic receptor complexes. The scientific community may in the future direct its attention to other treatment interventions and targets. Further development of electroconvulsive therapy also for long-term application is one option, another is the exploitation of transcranial magnetic stimulation or yet another experimental neurophysiological intervention such as vagus nerve stimulation. Another line of development is the use of nerve signal modulators such as substance P, corticotropin releasing factor analogues and other peptides and protein fractions. Finally, molecular biology may provide more precise information on intracellular signalling cascades during normal and pathological circumstances which may invite yet unknown experimental interventions.

[1] *Aarhus University Psychiatric Hospital, Department A, Skovagervej 2, DK-8240 Risskov, Denmark*

Even when efficacy figures for long-term treatment of bipolar disorder are improved, the everlasting question of treatment effectiveness remains a challenge [3]. Many factors prevent effectiveness figures from reaching the ideals of treatment efficacy. These factors include uncertain diagnostic subgrouping of bipolar patients, non-compliance among patients and non-compliance among health professionals, the latter subject being heavily understudied [4].

Non-compliance among patients probably is the most serious hindrance for improvement of treatment effectiveness. Compliance may be improved through proper selection of bipolar candidates for long-term treatment, through early and aggressive institution of effective pharmacological treatments and vigorous treatment of comorbid substance abuse and somatic illnesses and, finally, through attention to side effects of lithium and other putative mood stabilizers and respect for the attitudes and the (lack of) knowledge of the illness and the treatment exhibited by both patients and their relatives.

Improved compliance and treatment response furthermore depends upon an ideal organization of the treatment package, which should also include psychological assistance and psychosocial interventions. This organizational framework may be a multi-professionally staffed lithium clinic or mood disorders unit. Successful long-term treatment of bipolar patients is definitely a complex and resource-consuming task.

REFERENCES

1. Goodwin F., Jamison K.R. (1990). *Manic-Depressive Illness*. Oxford University Press, New York.
2. Davis J.M., Janicak P.G., Hogan D.M. (1999). Mood stabilizers in the prevention of recurrent affective disorders: a meta-analysis. *Acta Psychiatr. Scand.*, **100**: 406–417.
3. Vestergaard P., Licht R.W. (2001). 50 years with lithium treatment in affective disorders: present problems and priorities. *World Biol. Psychiatry*, **2**: 18–26.
4. Guscott R., Taylor L. (1994) Lithium prophylaxis in recurrent affective illness. Efficacy, effectiveness and efficiency. *Br. J. Psychiatry*, **164**: 741–746.

3.14
Pharmacological Treatment of Bipolar Disorder: The State of the Art
Allan Young[1]

Bipolar affective disorder has been described for most of recorded history and ranked high amongst psychiatric disorders in the global burden of disease study [1]. However, it is arguably still under-recognized. Classical epidemiological studies indicate a lifetime prevalence rate of approximately 1% for bipolar I disorder. However, a wider "bipolar spectrum" also exists. This includes bipolar II disorder or major depression with a history of hypomanic episodes and less commonly recognized subsyndromes combining hypomania and minor depression or manic symptoms alone. Jules Angst's longitudinal studies in Zurich recorded high lifetime prevalence rates of this bipolar spectrum [2]. Although the dangers of widening the concept of the bipolar spectrum are clear, it is likely that many cases of bipolar disorder are not recognized as such but may well be diagnosed as unipolar depressive disorder. Many psychiatric researchers have argued for a "continuum" approach to unipolar major depression and this argument may be valid if unipolar disorders are considered in isolation. However, when one considers the whole range of mood disorders, it is clear that unipolar and bipolar disorders do differ in terms of demography, treatment response and potentially neurobiology. Fuller understanding of the differences and similarities between bipolar and unipolar disorders is likely to advance our understanding of both illnesses and the treatment that we give our patients. Charles Bowden's systematic review provides a masterly overview of the current state of a crucial area of evidence—the pharmacological treatment of bipolar disorder.

The psychopharmacological revolution was initiated by John Cade's discovery of the therapeutic effects of lithium in 1949. This was followed in the 1950s by the advent of both antipsychotics and antidepressants and all three classes of drugs continue to be used frequently in bipolar disorder. The efficacy of lithium was established in clinical trials from the 1960s onwards, but doubts about its effectiveness in clinical practice have recently been raised due in part to the occurrence of rebound manic symptoms upon rapid discontinuation [3]. Lest we too hurriedly dismiss this venerable medication, however, Charles Bowden reminds us that lithium, alone amongst mood stabilizers, has been shown to have a beneficial effect upon suicide. Further understanding of the pharmacological basis of lithium's preventative effect on suicide would help us both to develop new treatments and understand the neurobiology of this tragic phenomenon.

[1] Department of Psychiatry, Leazes Wing, Royal Victoria Infirmary, Newcastle upon Tyne, NE1 4LP, United Kingdom

The introduction of the anticonvulsant drugs, initially carbamazepine and subsequently sodium valproate and lamotrigine (with other candidates waiting in the wings), has given a renewed impetus to research in the field. Antipsychotics are widely used in bipolar disorder and the introduction of novel atypical antipsychotics has extended the range of treatments for bipolar disorder even more. Researchers and clinicians must remain cautious about using the term "mood stabilizer" too loosely and the conceptual and scientific arguments around this topic are fully rehearsed by Bowden. The most demanding criteria for mood stabilizer status demand that a single agent treat mania and bipolar depression, be effective in maintenance treatment and do not promote switching. The gap between these criteria and what is attainable with current monotherapy is illustrated by the common use of multiple drug combinations, which are frequently needed to treat all manifestations of this complex disorder.

A full understanding of the relevant methodological issues is necessary to understand the research evidence summarized by Bowden. These are often highly pertinent to the clinician. A good example is the high "placebo response" rates evident in many studies. It is clear that placebo is not an inert treatment and indeed usually includes medication such as benzodiazepines as well as nursing and medical care. These factors may have powerfully beneficial effects, suggesting that in future we should be broadening our scope to examine all factors in treatment response. In common with much of the rest of clinical medicine, techniques from clinical epidemiology are now being widely utilized to collate research findings and thus guide clinicians in treatment choices for bipolar disorder. However, the current system for ranking evidence frequently used in the United States does differ from that used in other parts of the world [4], and it would clearly be desirable for these tools to be standardized over the near future. Research will advance more quickly if an apparently common language does not separate us.

Recent developments in treatments in bipolar disorder give hope for the future. Bipolar depression and rapid cycling are two of the most difficult complications to treat in this condition. The anticonvulsant lamotrigine has recently been shown not only to have convincing antidepressant properties for bipolar depression (without switching) but also to be efficacious for rapid cycling. The pharmacological basis of the mechanism of action of lamotrigine and indeed all mood stabilizing drugs, including lithium, remains obscure. It is to be hoped, however, that the demonstration of a novel efficacy profile for drugs such as lamotrigine will stimulate the discovery of a new class of related therapeutic agents. At some point we will truly understand how these drugs work and how best to use them in combination with non-pharmacological strategies. Until that point is reached, there will be much art, as well as science, in the treatment of bipolar disorder.

REFERENCES

1. Murray C.J., Lopez A.D. (1997) Global mortality, disability and the contribution of risk factors: Global Burden of Disease Study. *Lancet*, **349**: 1436–1442.
2. Angst J. (1998) The emerging epidemiology of hypomania and bipolar disorder. *J. Affect. Disord.*, **50**: 143–151.
3. Goodwin G.M. (1994) Recurrence of mania after lithium withdrawal. Implications for the use of lithium in the treatment of bipolar affective disorder. *Br. J. Psychiatry*, **164**: 149–152.
4. Shekelle P.G., Woolf S.H., Eccles M., Grimshaw J. (1999) Developing guidelines. *Br. Med. J.*, **318**: 593–596.

3.15
Many Borrowed Drugs, But Still No New Treatments Developed Specifically for Bipolar Disorder

Carlos A. Zarate, Jr[1]

The pharmacological treatment of bipolar disorder has significantly advanced since the publication in 1990 of the textbook titled *Manic-Depressive Illness* by Goodwin and Jamison [1]. In this classic textbook, the somatic treatments that were available then for the treatment of bipolar disorder and reviewed included lithium, carbamazepine, neuroleptics, antidepressants (tricyclic antidepressants, monoamine oxidase inhibitors) and benzodiazepines. Much of the textbook focused on the many studies that were conducted on lithium, describing it as a major treatment for manic-depressive illness. Little information was available at the time on valproate and other anticonvulsants. No one had envisioned back then the major role that the next generation anticonvulsants and the atypical antipsychotic drugs would have in the treatment of bipolar disorder. However, in spite of that, clearly, the discovery of lithium's efficacy as a mood-stabilizing agent has since revolutionized the treatment of patients with bipolar disorder. After nearly 50 years, lithium continues to be the mainstay of treatment for this disorder, both for the acute manic phase, and as prophylaxis for recurrent manic and depressive episodes [2]. Adequate lithium treatment, particularly in the context of a lithium clinic, is also reported to reduce the excessive mortality observed in the illness [3]. However, despite its role as one of psychiatry's most important treatments [1], increasing evidence suggests that a significant number of patients respond poorly to lithium therapy, with recent

[1] *Mood and Anxiety Disorders Program, National Institute of Mental Health, 9000 Rockville Pike, Bethesda, MD 20892, USA*

reviews noting failure rates of lithium to be 50% or higher [4]. Several studies have suggested that particularly low rates of responsiveness to lithium occur in mixed or dysphoric mania, rapid cycling, and substance abuse comorbidity (see [1, 5] for reviews). There is mounting evidence that recurrent mood disorders—once considered "good prognosis diseases"—are, in fact, often very severe and life-threatening illnesses [6]. It is now recognized that, for many patients, the long-term outcome is often much less favourable than previously thought, with incomplete interepisode recovery, and a progressive decline in overall functioning observed [6]. Thus, bipolar disorder patients are likely to be exposed to multiple medications with increased risk of side effects, and may be at increased risk of suicide attempts and early mortality [7].

The recognition of the significant morbidity and mortality of patients with severe mood disorders, as well as the growing appreciation that a significant percentage of patients respond poorly to existing treatments, has made the task of discovering new therapeutic agents that are efficacious and with few side effects increasingly more important. In recent years, there has been an explosion in the number of options available for the treatment of recurrent mood disorders, with a parallel and unprecedented increase in the interest in the treatment of manic-depressive illness by pharmaceutical companies, clinicians, researchers and the public. The two categories of drugs that have received much attention as putative treatments for bipolar disorder are the anticonvulsant and antipsychotic drugs. Significant advances were achieved with the development of the atypical antipsychotic drugs in that, compared to the typical antipsychotic drugs, they are associated with lower rates of extrapyramidal symptoms and tardive dyskinesia and are more efficacious in the treatment of negative symptoms of schizophrenia and in improving the quality of life. The atypical antipsychotic drugs were also noted to have significant thymoleptic properties early on in their development [8]. Almost as rapidly as the anticonvulsants were being introduced into the market for the management of epilepsy and atypical antipsychotic drugs for the treatment of schizophrenia, these drugs were being used by clinicians for the treatment of bipolar disorder. Perhaps, in part this practice resulted from the lack of marketed drugs approved for the treatment of these disorders.

Summarizing all this information on the multiple drugs being clinically used and tested for the treatment of bipolar disorder, and presenting it to clinicians in a palatable way can be a nightmare. However, Charles Bowden once again has been able to eloquently capture the essence of what these somatic treatments are about, how and in what circumstances they should be used, and at the same time present this information in an orderly and comprehensive way from which all of us can learn. In addition, Bowden describes his view of what are mood stabilizers and the primary and

secondary roles of the different somatic treatments. This is e
ful, as unfortunately the term "mood stabilizer" is often
Presenting his view of the concept of mood stabilizer is imp(
it helps put a perspective on what are, and what should be, tl
pharmacological treatments in the treatment of bipolar disord.

While there appears to be an abundance of pharmacological agents for the
treatment of bipolar disorder, much more work is needed. Few of the newer
treatments have been demonstrated in systematic and in controlled conditions to be efficacious in bipolar disorder and only three of them have
received Food and Drug Administration approval for the treatment of
bipolar disorder. Furthermore, the biochemical basis for lithium's antimanic
and mood-stabilizing actions remains to be fully elucidated [9]. At present,
we are borrowing drugs used in the treatment of other disorders but have
yet to develop a specific treatment for bipolar disorder. It is by understanding the biochemical basis of lithium and other effective treatments that we
will be able to discover new therapeutic agents that will hopefully enhance
compliance; work quickly, potently, specifically, and with few side effects.

REFERENCES

1. Goodwin F.K., Jamison K.R. (1990) *Manic-Depressive Illness*. Oxford University Press, New York.
2. Fieve R.R. (1999) Lithium therapy at the millennium: a revolutionary drug used for 50 years faces competing options and possible demise. *Bipolar Disord.*, **1**: 67–70.
3. Tondo L., Jamison K.R., Baldessarini R.J. (1997) Effect of lithium maintenance on suicidal behavior in major mood disorders. *Ann. N. Y. Acad. Sci.*, **836**: 339–351.
4. Goldberg J.F., Harrow M., Leon A.C. (1996) Lithium treatment of bipolar affective disorders under naturalistic follow-up conditions. *Psychopharmacol. Bull.*, **32**: 47–54.
5. Tohen M., Greenfield S.F., Weiss R.D., Zarate C.A. Jr., Vagge L.M. (1998) The effect of comorbid substance use disorders on the course of bipolar disorder: a review. *Harvard Rev. Psychiatry*, **6**: 133–141.
6. Tohen M., Hennen J., Zarate C.A. Jr., Baldessarini R.J., Strakowski S.M., Stoll A.L., Faedda G.L., Suppes T., Gebre-Medhin P., Cohen B.M. (2000) The McLean First Episode Project: two-year syndromal and functional recovery in 219 cases of major affective disorders with psychotic features. *Am. J. Psychiatry*, **157**: 220–228.
7. Tsuang M.T., Woolson R.F. (1978) Excess mortality in schizophrenia and affect-ive disorders. *Arch. Gen. Psychiatry*, **35**: 1181–1185.
8. Tohen M., Zarate C.A. Jr. (1998) Antipsychotic agents in bipolar disorder. *J. Clin. Psychiatry*, **59** (Suppl. 1): 38–48.
9. Manji H.K., Potter W.Z., Lenox R.H. (1995) Signal transduction pathways. Molecular targets for lithium's actions. *Arch. Gen. Psychiatry*, **52**: 531–543.

3.16
New Frontiers—Old Concepts
Trisha Suppes[1]

In contemporary times, one of the changes has been a re-expansion of the definition of bipolar disorder (BD) to include a broader spectrum of symptoms. An example of this was the lack of inclusion of BD patients with psychotic symptoms as having BD vs. schizophrenia in the 1970s, particularly in the US [1]. The current perspective views psychotic symptoms as more nonspecific, and other features of the illness to be the defining characteristics [2, 3]. This change of diagnostic perspective to include potentially more severely ill patients may provide a partial explanation of the more limited long-term efficacy, in contrast to earlier ideas, of lithium treatment. While clearly still an important and clinically useful medication, as noted by Charles Bowden, lithium is not the hoped for panacea. More recently, Hagop Akiskal, Jules Angst, and others have expostulated and expanded on the concept of bipolar spectrum, wherein "soft" bipolar symptoms are seen as a continuum of illness to more severe illness [4, 5]. This shift to include a broader range of less severe to more severely ill patients as bipolar may in part explain the poor functional recovery, despite syndromal recovery, observed in recent studies [6, 7].

One of the outcomes of a focus on more dimensional diagnostic approaches is an increased appreciation of potential implications of a given symptom. For example, the prognostic impact of psychotic symptoms or treatment management considerations when depression symptoms are observed during mania have been considered [8–10]. One of the implications would also be a redefined approach to the concept of mood stabilizer. While it is recognized that mania and depression each have many components unrelated to mood, the principal focus for mood stabilizers continues to be antimanic vs. antidepressant. But as we move both into greater exploration of dimensional approaches, as well as greater knowledge of the physiological basis of different aspects of BD, older concepts of mood stabilizers will be less useful or interesting. Indeed, already in use is the type of definition suggested by Bowden which utilizes the practical use definition of a medication.

As reviewed by Bowden, the newer atypical antipsychotics clearly have a role in the treatment of patients with BD. This class of medications has been clinically beneficial and important for patients. Virtually all treatment and consensus guidelines suggest use of atypical antipsychotics on line 1 or 2. In most settings, clozapine, the first of the atypical antipsychotics, is not considered a first-line treatment. However, despite continued new drug development, clozapine remains an important second-line agent for patients

---

[1] UT Southwestern Medical Center, 5323 Harry Hines Blvd., Dallas, TX 75390–9070, USA

with treatment-resistant forms of the illness [11–13]. Efficacy for clozapine has been demonstrated in one open acute mania study and for open maintenance treatment in two studies (one with a randomized comparison group) and numerous clinical case series [12, 14–16]. Additionally, in smaller case series clozapine has been helpful for patients with rapid cycling and was clinically effective regardless of the presence or history of psychotic symptoms [16, 17].

Little has been published on more specific applications of clozapine as attention has shifted to newer medications. However, clinical observations with clozapine include a more rapid response in patients with more mood lability and the possible combination use of antidepressants where previously mood switches were observed. One of the paradoxes of clozapine is that for patients in need of this medication, and who respond well to it, there is often a willingness to tolerate significant side effects because symptoms of their illness and ability to concentrate and function are so markedly improved. As further evaluation of newer drugs continues and new medications emerge, it is to be hoped additional medications with such robust effects will emerge with fewer side effects.

One area in which we can anticipate informative controlled trials is in the use of combination medications and appropriate maintenance treatments. With multiple approaches to managing acute mania, juxtaposed to the limitations of any one medication in long-term use, and increased appreciation of the limited research on managing depression, emphasis in National Institute of Mental Health (NIMH)-funded studies and within industry is moving to address these issues.

The need to provide treatment guidelines in the absence of controlled studies is reflected in the increasing dissemination of treatment algorithms, pathways, or guidelines—in the NIMH Systematic Treatment Enhancement Program for Bipolar Disorder (STEP-BD) [18, 19] targeting 5000 patients, and in public mental health systems across numerous states following the Texas Medication Algorithm Project (TMAP) [20] results and the Expert Consensus Guidelines [21]. Developers of these efforts are the first to agree that too few data exist addressing each set of recommendations. These efforts rely on clinical consensus and the importance of continued efforts in research addressing best practices cannot be overemphasized.

REFERENCES

1. Cooper J.E., Kendell R.E., Garland B.J., Sharpe L., Copeland J.R.M., Simon R. (1972). *Psychiatric Diagnosis in New York and London: A Comparative Study of Mental Hospital Admissions.* Maudsley Monograph No. 20, Oxford University Press, London.

2. Taylor M.A., Abrams R., Gaztanaga P. (1975) Manic-depressive illness and schizophrenia: a partial validation of research diagnostic criteria utilizing neuropsychological testing. *Compr. Psychiatry*, **16**: 91–96.

3. Pope H.G., Jr., Lipinski J.S., Jr. (1978) Diagnosis in schizophrenia and manic-depressive illness: a reassessment of the specificity of "schizophrenic" symptoms in light of current research. *Arch. Gen. Psychiatry*, **35**: 811–828.

4. Angst J. (1998) The emerging epidemiology of hypomania and bipolar II disorder. *J. Affect. Disord.*, **50**: 143–151.

5. Akiskal H.S. (1996) The prevalent clinical spectrum of bipolar disorders: beyond DSM-IV. *J. Clin. Psychopharmacol.*, **17** (Suppl. 3): 117S–122S.

6. Keck P.E., Jr., McElroy S.L., Strakowski S.M., West S.A., Sax K.W., Hawkins J.M., Bourne M.L., Haggard P. (1998) 12-month outcome of patients with bipolar disorder following hospitalization for a manic or mixed episode. *Am. J. Psychiatry*, **155**: 646–652.

7. Tohen M., Hennen J., Zarate C.M., Baldessarini R.J., Strakowski S.M., Stoll A.L., Faedda G.L., Suppes T., Gebre-Medhin P., Cohen B.M. (2000) Two-year syndromal and functional recovery in 219 cases of first-episode major affective disorder with psychotic features. *Am. J. Psychiatry*, **157**: 220–228.

8. Keck P.E., Jr., McElroy S.L., Strakowski S.M., Balistreri T.M., Kizer D.L., West S.A. (1996) Factors associated with maintenance antipsychotic treatment of patients with bipolar disorder. *J. Clin. Psychiatry*, **57**: 147–151.

9. Tohen M., Waternaux C.M., Tsuang M.T., Hunt A.T. (1990) Four-year follow-up of twenty-four first-episode manic patients. *J. Affect. Disord.*, **18**: 79–86.

10. Swann A.C., Bowden C.L., Morris D., Calabrese J.R., Petty F., Small J., Dilsaver S.C., Davis J.M. (1997) Depression during mania treatment response to lithium or divalproex. *Arch. Gen. Psychiatry*, **54**: 37–42.

11. McElroy S.L., Dessain E.C., Pope H.G., Jr., Cole J.O., Keck P.E., Jr., Frankenberg F., Aizley H.G., O'Brien S. (1991) Clozapine in the treatment of psychotic mood disorders, schizoaffective disorder, and schizophrenia. *J. Clin. Psychiatry*, **52**: 411–414.

12. Calabrese J.R., Kimmel S.E., Woyshville M.J., Rapport D.J., Faust C.J., Thompson P.A., Meltzer H.Y. (1996) Clozapine for treatment-refractory mania. *Am. J. Psychiatry*, **153**: 759–764.

13. Frye M.A., Ketter T.A., Altshuler L.L., Denicoff K.D., Dunn R.T., Kimbrell T.A., Cora-Locatelli G., Post R.M. (1998) Clozapine in bipolar disorder: treatment implications for other atypical antipsychotics. *J. Affect. Disord.*, **42**: 91–104.

14. Kowatch R.A., Suppes T., Gilfillan S.K., Fuentes R.M., Grannemann B.D., Emslie G.J. (1995) Clozapine treatment for children and adolescents with schizophrenia and bipolar disorder: a clinical case series. *J. Child Adolesc. Psychopharmacol.*, **5**: 241–253.

15. Zarate C.A., Tohen M., Hanov M., Weiss M.K., Cole J.O. (1995) Is clozapine a mood stabilizer? *J. Clin. Psychiatry*, **56**: 108–112.

16. Suppes T., Webb A., Paul B., Carmody T., Kraemer H., Rush A.J. (1999) Clinical outcome in a randomized one-year trial of clozapine versus treatment as usual for patients with treatment-resistant illness and a history of mania. *Am. J. Psychiatry*, **156**: 1164–1169.

17. Suppes T., Phillips K., Judd C. (1994) Clozapine treatment of nonpsychotic rapid cycling bipolar disorder: a report of three cases. *Biol. Psychiatry*, **36**: 338–340.

18. Sachs G.S., Thase M.E., Wisniewski S., Leahy L.F., Conley J. (2001) Systematic treatment enhancement program for bipolar disorder (STEP-BD) study design

and sample characteristics. Presented at the 154th Annual Meeting of the American Psychiatric Association, New Orleans, 5–10 May.

19. Sachs G.S., Thase M.E., Wisniewski S., Leahy L.F., Conley J., Nierenberg A.A., Lavori P., Allen M.H. (2001) The systematic treatment enhancement program for bipolar disorder. Presented at the 154th Annual Meeting of the American Psychiatric Association, New Orleans, 5–10 May.

20. Suppes T., Swann A., Dennehy E.B., Habermacher E., Mason M., Crismon L., Toprac M., Rush A.J., Shon S., Altshuler K.Z. (2001) Texas Medication Algorithm Project—development and feasibility testing of a treatment algorithm for patients with bipolar disorder. *J. Clin. Psychiatry*, **62**: 439–447.

21. Sachs G.S., Printz D.J., Kahn D.A., Carpenter D., Docherty J.P. (2000) The Expert Consensus Guidelines Series: medication treatment of bipolar disorder 2000. *Postgrad. Med.*, Special Report, April.

3.17
Perspectives on the Pharmacological Treatment of Bipolar Disorder
Jair C. Soares[1]

The chapter by Charles Bowden provides a very comprehensive and updated overview of currently available evidence on pharmacological treatments of bipolar disorder. In my commentary, I would like to touch on a few points that I feel are particularly relevant, with emphasis on specific areas of need and priorities for future development.

Treatment of refractory mania. For the pharmacological management of treatment-refractory mania, we often have to resort to combination strategies with two mood stabilizers, or combination regimens that would include antipsychotic agents, or other agents currently in investigation for the treatment of bipolar disorder [1]. Few controlled studies have directly compared the various alternatives that are commonly utilized in these clinical situations [2]. Among other agents, calcium channel blockers have been examined, but there is very limited evidence in support of their efficacy, although some potentially promising agents in this group have not yet been adequately tested in double-blind studies [3]. However, with the advent of atypical antipsychotic agents, and their proven efficacy in the treatment of mania [4], either as monotherapies or, most commonly, in combination with mood stabilizers, there is considerable promise for the development of more efficacious strategies for management of refractory mania. Nonetheless, there is still a substantial need for further examination of these agents in the context of properly

[1] *Neurochemical Brain Imaging Laboratory, Western Psychiatric Institute and Clinic, University of Pittsburgh Medical Center, 3811 O'Hara Street, Pittsburgh, PA 15213, USA*

controlled studies in refractory manic patients [1]. Moreover, prior history of non-response to either lithium or valproate does not seem to affect the likelihood that such patients will respond to atypical antipsychotic agents.

Bipolar depression. Recent studies have provided an improved understanding of how challenging the treatment of bipolar depression generally is [5]. Longitudinal studies that have looked at functional recovery suggest that the majority of the impairment resulting from the illness relates to the depressive phase, which often has long-lasting residual symptoms, and those are often impairing and difficult to treat [5]. Recent developments with the anticonvulsant lamotrigine indicate good efficacy in the treatment of this phase of the illness [6]. Lithium is known to have modest antidepressant effects, and valproate and carbamazepine appear to have such effects even to a lesser extent [7]. For this reason, even though maximizing the benefits from ongoing therapy with mood stabilizers is generally the most appropriate initial step in the management of bipolar depression, the introduction of antidepressant agents, most commonly as adjunctive treatments, is often required. Another interesting possibility that deserves further investigation is the suggestion that atypical antipsychotics have antidepressant properties, and could eventually be useful in the management of depressive symptoms in bipolar disorder [8]. However, the evidence available to this date is anecdotal, and controlled studies with these agents in bipolar depression are still not available. Despite evidence that some specific antidepressant agents may induce mania to a lesser extent [9], further investigation that would systematically characterize the comparative risk with the various medications currently available is still needed. For this reason, strategies that will include mood-stabilizing agents that seem to have more pronounced antidepressant properties, e.g. lamotrigine, could be particularly helpful for the management of bipolar depression.

Rapid cyclers. This particular patient subgroup, as we all know, is generally the most difficult to treat among bipolar patients. For this reason, it is a subgroup of special relevance for potential new drug development [1]. Some of the newer treatments seem to benefit these patients to a larger extent than more traditional ones [10], but still, this is a group of patients where polypharmacy is often necessary, with results that are often disappointing. As it currently stands, combination of mood stabilizers that would include some of the newer agents, e.g. valproate or lamotrigine, may often be the most appropriate treatment, even though controlled studies that would specifically examine this question are still needed.

Future drug development. Clearly, despite recent progress in this area, bipolar disorder is still an illness for which further drug development that will result in improved treatments is highly needed. In particular, medications that would work faster, with fewer side effects, and that would be more effective for the most challenging subgroups, e.g. rapid cyclers, refractory mania, refractory depression, mixed states, and patients with other comorbid psychiatric illnesses, would certainly be very important new developments. Because comorbidity with substance abuse and axis II disorders is commonly found in this patient population, it is important that new treatments also be examined in the context of their efficacy for these specific comorbid conditions, and treatments that would also be beneficial in these difficult cases would be specially helpful. It is very gratifying to see the increased interest in this area, which brings hope that improved treatment modalities will become available in the next few years.

Towards a pathophysiology. The pathophysiological mechanisms underlying this severe mental illness are still largely unknown [11]. With further developments in this area of research, it is expected that specific progress in our understanding of the pathophysiology of this illness will occur. Specific development in clinical neurosciences, with improved tools in genetics, brain imaging, cognitive neuropsychology, and neuropharmacology, have raised our hopes that a better understanding of causation of this illness will be achieved. In particular, the elucidation of the specific mechanisms by which an inherited biological vulnerability interacts with specific environmental and developmental factors to result in such a complex and inherently fascinating illness is the ultimate goal, which appears increasingly likely to be attainable. When these mechanisms are elucidated, more meaningful diagnostic classifications are likely to be developed, and more specific and improved targets for drug development in this field will become available.

ACKNOWLEDGEMENTS

This work was partially supported by grants MH 01736, MH 29618 and MH 30915 from NIMH, the Theodore and Vada Stanley Foundation, the National Alliance for Research in Schizophrenia and Affective Disorders (NARSAD), and the American Foundation for Suicide Prevention. Dr. Soares was the 1999–2001 NARSAD Selo Investigator.

REFERENCES

1. Soares J.C. (2000) Recent advances in the treatment of bipolar mania, depression, mixed states, and rapid cycling. *Int. Clin. Psychopharmacol.*, **15**: 183–196.

2. Keck P.E., Jr., Mendlewicz J., Calabrese J.R., Fawcett J., Suppes T., Vestergaard P.A., Carbonell C. (2000) A review of randomized, controlled clinical trials in acute mania. *J. Affect. Disord.*, **59** (Suppl. 1): S31–S37.
3. Goodnick P.J. (2000) The use of nimodipine in the treatment of mood disorders. *Bipolar Disord.*, **2**: 165–173.
4. Ghaemi S.N., Goodwin F.K. (1999) Use of atypical antipsychotic agents in bipolar and schizoaffective disorders: review of the empirical literature. *J. Clin. Psychopharmacol.*, **19**: 354–361.
5. Sachs G.S., Koslow C.L., Ghaemi S.N. (2000) The treatment of bipolar depression. *Bipolar Disord.*, **2**: 256–260.
6. Calabrese J.R., Bowden C.L., Sachs G.S., Ascher J.A., Monaghan E., Rudd G.D. (1999) A double-blind placebo-controlled study of lamotrigine monotherapy in outpatients with bipolar I depression. *J. Clin. Psychiatry*, **60**: 79–88.
7. Soares J.C., Gershon S. (1998) The lithium ion: a foundation for psychopharmacological specificity. *Neuropsychopharmacology*, **19**: 167–182.
8. Ghaemi S.N., Cherry E.L., Katzow J.A., Goodwin F.K. (2000) Does olanzapine have antidepressant properties? A retrospective preliminary study. *Bipolar Disord.*, **2**: 196–199.
9. Sachs G.S., Lafer B., Stoll A.L., Banov M., Thibault A.B., Tohen M., Rosenbaum J.F. (1994) A double-blind trial of bupropion versus desipramine for bipolar depression. *J. Clin. Psychiatry*, **55**: 391–393.
10. Calabrese J.R., Suppes T., Bowden C.L., Sachs G.S., Swann A.C., McElroy S.L., Kusumakar V., Ascher J.A., Earl N.L., Greene P.L. *et al* (2000) A double-blind, placebo-controlled, prophylaxis study of lamotrigine in rapid-cycling bipolar disorder. *J. Clin. Psychiatry*, **61**: 841–850.
11. Neumaier J.F., Dunner D.L. (2000) Toward a pathophysiology of bipolar disorder. In *Bipolar Disorders—Basic Mechanisms and Therapeutic Implications* (Eds J.C. Soares, G. Gershon), pp. 545–553, Dekker, New York.

3.18

Biochemical Changes Elicited by Mood Stabilizers

Brian E. Leonard[1]

It is estimated that the lifetime prevalence of bipolar disorder is 0.6% in the United States and similar figures have been quoted for Europe and Australasia. It is also known that the risk of acquiring the disorder is increased in first-degree relatives of affected individuals. Genetic linkage analyses have led to the identification of several regions in the human genome that may contain genes conferring susceptibility to the disorder. Nevertheless, specific genes that are highly associated with the acquisition of the disease have not so far been unequivocally identified [1]. The complex nature of the genetics of bipolar disorder might thus be explained by the interaction of

[1] *Pharmacology Department, National University of Ireland, Galway, Ireland*

multiple genes with environmental factors [2]. The link between a genetic predisposition to bipolar disorder and specific neurotransmitter malfunction has arisen from the analyses of patients carrying associated RNA transcripts within the frontal cortex [3]. The RNA transcripts which encode the serotonin transporter and components of the NK-kB transcription factor complex were shown to be increased in bipolar illness and also in some patients with schizophrenia. Such findings could be of relevance to our understanding of the mechanisms whereby mood-stabilizing drugs act.

Despite the many advantages of the recently introduced mood stabilizers, such as valproate and carbamazepine, with regard to their reduced side-effect profile, lithium still remains the most widely used drug in this category, because of its proven efficacy [4]. Thus, after over 30 years of use in North America, and even longer in Europe, it continues to be the mainstay of treatment for bipolar disorder, both for the treatment of the acute manic phase and for the prophylactic treatment of the disorder [4]. In addition to its ability to reduce the intensity and frequency of episodes of the illness, lithium has also been shown to reduce the excessive mortality that commonly occurs in patients with bipolar disorder [5]. This may be of relevance to the observed effect of lithium and some other mood stabilizers on aspects of the immune system which are grossly disturbed in bipolar disorder [6].

Despite the importance of lithium in the treatment of bipolar disorder, the cellular and molecular basis for its therapeutic effects remains uncertain. There have been innumerable studies of the effects of lithium in animals and *in vitro* systems, but the relevance in these studies to the pharmacological activity of the drug in man remains an enigma. As with most drugs used in psychiatric practice, lithium usually requires several weeks of treatment before it achieves optimum therapeutic efficacy. This precludes any simple mechanistic interpretation based on its acute biochemical effects. Indeed, it can be argued that the probable explanation for the mechanisms of action of all mood stabilizers is related to their effects on numerous biochemical pathways involved in the regulation of mood rather than on one or more specific neurotransmitter processes. For this reason, much recent research has focused on the second messenger systems and gene expression which occur distal to the changes in post-synaptic receptor function [7].

The mechanisms whereby the various neurotransmitters can be modulated by mood stabilizers to cause secondary changes in the signalling systems may be summarized as follows. Following the activation of the neuronal membrane bound receptor by the appropriate neurotransmitter, the intramembrane G protein, which links the receptor to the second messenger systems, is activated and stimulates phospholipase C located within the neuron. This stimulates a cascade of changes involving the synthesis of inositol trisphosphate (IP3) and diacylglycerol (DAG). IP3 then stimulates the mobilization of calcium ions, which together with DAG activates protein kinase C (PKC). Within the neuron there is a constant cycling of inositol phosphates and DAG. The concentration of myo-inositol in the neuron is critical for the efficiency of the second signalling system, as it acts as the precursor of the phosphoinositides. At therapeutically relevant concentrations, lithium has been shown to interfere with the inositol cycle by inhibiting inositol monophosphatase and inositol polyphosphate 1-phosphatase, key enzymes involved in the recycling of inositol and inositol polyphosphates [8–10]. However, despite the attractive nature of this hypothesis, it is uncertain whether lithium treatment results in a reduction in the synthesis of intermediates in the phosphoinositide cycle which are the substrates for agonist-induced phosphatidyl inositide turnover [11]. Furthermore, there is no evidence, despite the clinical observation that lithium reduces the concentration of myo-inositol in the brains of patients with bipolar disorder, that this action is associated with the therapeutic response to treatment [11].

The PKC pathway has also been the subject of recent investigation, as it is known to play a vital role in regulating pre- and post-synaptic neurotransmission [12]. Quantitative autoradiography has demonstrated that chronic lithium administration results in a significant decrease in membrane associated PKC in the hippocampus, and also in myrisolated alanine rich C kinase substrate (MARCKS) protein, both of which have been implicated in regulating long-term neuroplasticity [13]. The precise clinical relevance of these changes is uncertain, but it is known that PKC isozymes are involved in the regulation of neuronal excitability and neurotransmitter release. As valproate produces similar effects to lithium [14], it can be hypothesized that mood stabilizing drugs ultimately produce similar subcellular changes, which may be relevant to their therapeutic actions. However, the precise sites of action of these drugs on the PKC pathway may differ, which may be reflected in the clinical observation that some patients show a preferential response to one mood stabilizer over another. If so, it may be possible to develop a new generation of mood stabilizers based on their ability to selectively inhibit PKC isozymes. In this respect, it is of interest to note that the anti-oestrogen tamoxifen acts as a potent PKC inhibitor and that preliminary studies show that it has antimanic properties [15].

The reason for the lag period in the therapeutic response and the slow reversal of the therapeutic response when a mood stabilizer is abruptly stopped has been the subject of much speculation. Despite the diverse nature of mood stabilizers now available, there is no evidence that any of them acts more rapidly than lithium. However, at least a consensus appears to be emerging that the prolonged administration of such drugs is necessary for facilitating changes in gene expression. In this regard, the effects of lithium and valproate on the DNA binding activity of some important transcription factors (in particular the activator protein-1 transcription factor family (AP-1)) have been studied. The AP-1 transcription factor is known to activate gene transcription in response to PKC activators, growth factors and cytokines, while the genes known to be regulated by the AP-1 family of transcription factors in the brain include those regulating neuropeptides, neurotrophins, neurotransmitter receptors and the enzymes involved in the synthesis of neurotransmitters [16]. Experimental studies have shown that both lithium and valproate, at therapeutically relevant concentrations, increase the activity of AP-1 transcription factors in rat brain *ex vivo* [17]. In addition, *in vivo* studies have shown that chronically administered lithium increases the synthesis of tyroxine hydroxylase, the rate-limiting step in the synthesis of the catecholamines, in the frontal cortex, hippocampus and striatum [18]. Thus, it may be hypothesized that, following their chronic administration, mood stabilizers, by increasing the expression of nuclear transcription regulating factors, change the plasticity of critical neuronal circuits, changes which underlie the clinical response to treatment. By their very nature, such changes can only occur following prolonged treatment.

Regulation of signal transduction and gene expression within critical regions of the brain can have profound effects on the biochemical events triggered by a range of different transmitters. In the future, it is possible that drugs may be developed that target specific signalling systems (for example, the PKC isozymes) and either directly or indirectly increase the expression of neurotrophic factors.

In conclusion, Bowden's review usefully summarizes the present situation regarding the therapeutic strategies available to treat bipolar illness. However, appraisal of the possible mechanisms whereby the conventional therapeutic agents are thought to act now opens the possibility for developing novel drugs which directly target secondary and tertiary signalling systems. By their neuroprotective and neurotrophic actions, such drugs may assist in the remodelling of the neuronal structure of the brain and in this way improve the efficacy of treatment.

REFERENCES

1. Stine O.C., McMahon F.J., Chen L. (1997) Initial genome screen for bipolar disorder in the NIMH genetics initiative pedigrees: chromosomes 2,11,13,14 and X. *Am. J. Med. Genet.*, 74: 263–269.
2. Gershon E.S. (1989) Recent developments in genetics of manic-depressive illness. *J. Clin. Psychol.*, 50 (Suppl.): 4–7.
3. Sun Y., Zhang L., Johnston E.F., Yolken R.H. (2001) Serial analysis of gene expression in the frontal cortex of patients with bipolar disorder. *Br. J. Psychiatry*, 178 (Suppl. 41): s137–s141.
4. Baldessarini R.J., Tondo L. (2000) Does lithium still work? Evidence of stable responses over three decades. *Arch. Gen. Psychiatry*, 57: 187–190.
5. Nilsson A. (1999) Lithium therapy and suicide risk. *J. Clin. Psychiatry*, 60 (Suppl. 2): 85–88.

6. McAdams C., Leonard B.E. (1993) Neutrophil and monocyte phagocytosis in depressed patients. *Progr. Neuropsychopharmacol. Biol. Psychiatry*, **17**: 971–984.
7. Manji H.K, Lennox R.H. (1999) Protein kinase C signalling in the brain: molecular transduction of mood stabilisation in the treatment of manic depressive illness. *Biol. Psychiatry*, **46**: 1328–1351.
8. Berridge M.J., Downes C.P., Hanley M.R. (1982) Lithium amplifies agonist-dependent phosphatidylinositol response in brain and salivary glands. *Biochem. J.*, **206**: 587–595.
9. Berridge M.J., Downes C.P., Hanley M.R. (1989) Neural and developmental actions of lithium: a unifying hypothesis. *Cell*, **59**: 411–419.
10. Nahorski S.R., Ragan C.I., Challiso R.A.T. (1991) Lithium and phosphoinositide cycle: an example of uncompetitive inhibition and its pharmacological consequences. *Trends Pharmacol. Sci.*, **12**: 297–303.
11. Jope R.S., Williams M.B. (1994) Lithium and brain signal transduction systems. *Biochem. Pharmacol.*, **77**: 429–441.
12. Manji H.K, Lennox R.H. (2000) Signalling: cellular insights into the pathophysiology of bipolar disorder. *Biol. Psychiatry*, **48**: 518–530.
13. Lennox R.H., Williams M.B. (1994) Chronic lithium administration alters a prominent PKC substrate in rat hippocampus. *Brain Res.*, **570**: 333–340.
14. Watson D.G., Watterson J.M., Lennox R.H. (1998) Sodium valproate down regulates the myrisolated alanine rich C kinase substrate (MARCKS) in immortalised hippocampal cells: a property of protein kinase C mediated mood stabilisers. *J. Pharmacol. Exp. Ther.*, **285**: 307–316.
15. Bebchuk J.M., Arfken C.L., Dolan-Manji S. (2000) A preliminary investigation of a protein kinase C inhibitor (tamoxifen) in the treatment of acute mania. *Arch. Gen. Psychiatry*, **57**: 95–97.
16. Hughes P., Dragunow M. (1995) Induction of immediate early genes and the control of neurotransmitter-regulated gene expression within the nervous system. *Pharmacol. Rev.*, **47**: 113–178.
17. Manji H.K., Moore G.K., Chen G. (2001) Bipolar disorder: leads from the molecular and cellular mechanisms of action of mood stabilisers. *Br. J. Psychiatry*, **178** (Suppl. 41): s107–s119.
18. Chen G., Yuan P.X., Jiang Y. (1998) Lithium increases tyrosine hydroxylase levels both in vivo and in vitro. *J. Neurochem.*, **70**: 1768–1771.

3.19
Status and Directions in Drug Treatment of Bipolar Disorder

Michael Berk[1] and Gin S. Malhi[2]

The review of the pharmacological treatment of bipolar disorder by Bowden is an excellent and sober account of an important topic with increasing clinical relevance. Reviews of this kind are of particular gravity in bipolar

[1] *Barwon Health and Geelong Clinic, University of Melbourne, Swanston Centre, P.O. Box 281, Geelong, Victoria 3220, Australia*
[2] *University of New South Wales Mood Disorders Unit, Prince of Wales Hospital, Randwick, Sydney NSW 2031, Australia*

disorder, for a number of important reasons. Firstly, the pool of available high quality, well-designed (randomized and controlled) trials using sufficiently large numbers of subjects is vanishingly small for a condition of such prevalence and impact that it ranks in the top 10 of the WHO global disability list. Secondly, it is a condition without a cure whose outcome is frequently sub-optimal. It is thus essential that the most judicious reviews of the available data be allowed to assist in the development of therapeutic guidelines.

The point raised in the first section regarding the concept of mood stabilization is a critical one. The review highlights the lack of clear consensus regarding the meaning of the term, which differs among interest groups. It is correct that most clinicians regard mood stabilization as a function of preventing cycling and hence maintenance therapy. There are, however, vested interests, particularly in industry, that are keen to embrace the cachet of mood stabilization for agents that have demonstrable efficacy in only one phase of the illness. Thus Bowden's insistence on efficacy in maintenance is supported and should be commended.

A substantial limitation of the field is the absence of a coherent theory of the pathophysiology of this disorder. This is reflected in the array of candidate agents for this disorder with few common pharmacological properties and a wide diversity of mechanisms of action. For instance, with the exception of the serendipitous discovery of lithium, all agents currently in use in the management of bipolar disorder are "borrowed" from other indications. Greater insight into the pathophysiology of this disorder is therefore essential in order to facilitate rational drug development for the future.

A related issue is the assumption that antidepressants trialled in unipolar disorder would necessarily have an equivalent role in the treatment of bipolar depression. Bowden highlights this folly and emphasizes the necessity for antidepressant trials in bipolar depression. This need is doubly pressing as the bulk of the morbidity in bipolar disorder is in the depressive phase of the illness.

Methodological issues have conspired to reduce lithium's perceived benefit. The review appropriately emphasizes the difficulty of discontinuation designs, as well as the impact of other agents, including antidepressants and typical neuroleptics, on the course of the illness. It may be useful, albeit practically difficult, to attempt to study first-episode patients where these issues, as well as the confound of enrolling lithium-refractory patients, could be reduced.

This review correctly emphasizes the propensity of antidepressants to "roughen mood" and increase cycle frequency. However, disproportionate attention is given to switching "up" (above euthymia), whereas switching "down" (below euthymia) may also be a consequence of antidepressant therapy. A possible hypothesis is that antidepressant "poop out" may represent antidepressant induced cycling, particularly if the offset of antidepressant efficacy is abrupt. This is less likely in bipolar I disorder, where the diagnosis is more clear-cut, but may be of particular salience in bipolar II disorder, where a prior episode of mild mania may have been forgotten or overlooked or a bipolar family history is not sufficiently weighed, leading to antidepressant monotherapy in a "pseudo-unipolar" population.

Bipolar II disorder is a condition that is not only more common than bipolar I disorder but is associated with comparable morbidity and mortality. Given that there are only a handful of treatment trials in this disorder, it is one of the most neglected conditions in contemporary psychiatry. Given this paucity of trials and the consequent absence of credible treatment guidelines, treatment in these patients is inconsistent with the application of both unipolar and/or bipolar I protocols. Clearly, it is unlikely that such an approach will do justice to this group. Interestingly, intriguing new data is emerging that suggests treatment response in bipolar II may differ from bipolar I disorder. A post-hoc analysis of data from a recent trial of lamotrigine in rapid cycling patients showed specific advantage in bipolar II patients. The necessity for prospective data in this population is pressing. Indeed, there is an urgent need for much further research on all aspects of bipolar disorder. However, we should proceed with caution incorporating the lessons we have learnt, as this review has been at pains to point out, and only do research that is methodologically sound. In essence, it is critical that we remain critical if we are to advance our understanding of this complex disorder.

REFERENCES

1. Kessler R.C., McGonagle K.A., Zhao S., Nelson C.B., Hughes M., Eshleman S., Wittchen H.U., Kendler K.S. (1994) Lifetime and 12 month prevalence of DSM-III-R psychiatric disorders in the United States. Results from the national comorbidity study. *Arch. Gen. Psychiatry*, **51**: 8–19.
2. Tohen M., Waternaux C.M., Tsuang M.T. (1990) Outcome in mania. A 4-year prospective follow-up of 75 patients utilizing survival analysis. *Arch. Gen. Psychiatry*, **47**: 1106–1111.
3. Keck P.E., Jr., McElroy S.L., Strakowski S.M., West S.A., Sax K.W., Hawkins J.M., Bourne M.L., Haggard P. (1998) 12-month outcome of patients with bipolar disorder following hospitalization for a manic or mixed episode. *Am. J. Psychiatry*, **155**: 646–652.
4. Calabrese J.R., Suppes T., Bowden C.L., Sachs G.S., Swann A.C., McElroy S.L., Kusumakar V., Ascher J.A., Earl N.L., Greene P.L. *et al* (2000) A double-blind, placebo-controlled, prophylaxis study of lamotrigine in rapid-cycling bipolar disorder. *J. Clin. Psychiatry*, **61**: 841–850.

3.20
Bipolar Disorder: A New Field for Rational Polypharmacy
Siegfried Kasper[1]

The review provided by Charles Bowden, one of the world's leading experts in the field, is timely and concisely written and summarizes current evidence concerning mood stabilizers as well as antipsychotic medications available for treatment of different states of bipolar disorder. Furthermore, the role of antidepressants in both acute and long-term treatment is critically reviewed.

Whereas psychopathologically oriented psychiatrists carefully describe different forms of bipolar disorder, there was a lack of such a description with regard to pharmacotherapy in the past 30 years. One of the main reasons was that only lithium and high-potency or low-potency typical neuroleptics were used for treatment of bipolar disorder. However, with the introduction of new atypical antipsychotics as well as second- and third-generation mood stabilizers, the situation changed and doctors now have different pharma-cotherapeutic options for treatment of pure mania, mixed states and psychotic mania/depression. Concerning the long-term approach, the prevention of depression, the prevention of mania and the treatment of rapid, ultra-rapid and ultradian cyclers are addressed on a different level of evidence. Whereas randomized controlled trials are available for a few of those clinical situations, a number of level B and C evidence reports are available for most of them.

Based on the available studies and clinical observations, it is evident that the treatment of mania, depression and mixed states, as well as the prevention of these states, is not possible to achieve with only one medication with a single mechanism of action, e.g. influencing a specific neurotransmitter system. Contrary to this, a medication or a group of medications with a multi-pronged mechanism of action needs to be considered.

There seems to be a transatlantic gap concerning the treatment of bipolar depression between colleagues from North America and Europe. Whereas European psychiatrists tend to use antidepressants more frequently in the depressive state and to continue this medication on a long-term basis, North American colleagues favour the use of mood stabilizers over the latter practice. One of the reasons that might explain this difference is that opinion leaders from North America primarily base their sound clinical knowledge on patient samples largely consisting of rapid, ultrarapid and ultradian cyclers. In these patients it is evident that antidepressants are able to provoke mania and mixed states. Nevertheless, European psychiatrists are well advised to look carefully to their everyday practice when prescribing antidepressant medication to their patients. If there is a sign of drug-induced

[1] *Department of General Psychiatry, University of Vienna, Währinger Gürtel 18–20, A-1090 Wien, Austria*

hypomania, mania or mixed states, future treatment with this regimen should be avoided.

Unfortunately patients with mania are treated quite often with typical neuroleptics, e.g. haloperidol. Randomized controlled trials have clearly indicated that atypical antipsychotics are significantly better for treating affective symptoms, cognitive symptoms, aggression and hostility in schizophrenia as well as bipolar disorder. The different clinical response between these medications can be explained by their different activity on specific pathways (e.g., atypical antipsychotics act more selectively on the mesolinbic system as well as on pathways connecting the brain stem with the prefrontal cortex), as well by their different pharmacodynamic properties (e.g. blocking of serotonin 5-HT2A receptor by atypical antipsychotics). Furthermore, novel antipsychotics have a better side-effect profile, e.g. they are less likely to induce initial extrapyramidal symptoms (EPS) and therefore are also at significantly lower risk to induce tardive dyskinesia (TD). This is particularly important since patients with bipolar disorder have a higher risk of developing EPS and TD. Whereas in the 1970s only clozapine was available as an atypical antipsychotic, we now have several compounds belonging to this category and therefore the everyday practice should be reconsidered with the aim of a more acceptable side-effect profile for our patients, in addition to the individually tailored efficacy in bipolar disorder.

The development of mood stabilizers, starting with lithium (first-generation mood stabilizer) and thereafter carbamazepine and valproic acid (second-generation mood stabilizers) towards lamotrigine, topiramate, gabapentin (third-generation mood stabilizers) also enriched our therapeutic armamentarium. Like neuroleptics/antipsychotics, these medications are different in their mechanism of action and clinical applicability. Lithium seems to work better in patients at an early stage of illness and has the disadvantage, if stopped, that patients may fall back to an even worse clinical situation than before. Furthermore, patients may not respond to lithium if this medication is stopped by themselves or by the doctor and then resumed. Valproic acid and carbamazepine are widely used, however with a geographical difference: valproic acid more in the USA and carbamazepine more in Europe. Valproic acid has specifically shown to be effective in mixed states and rapid-cycling bipolar illness. Third-generation anticonvulsants like lamotrigine and topiramate are now under investigation; they not only offer a better side-effect profile but also a more specific mechanism of action including newly discovered neuroprotective factors that have also been shown for lithium.

The next 10 years of psychopharmacological research will bring new achievements for better understanding of the diagnosis and treatment of bipolar patients. Bowden's review is a valuable step for rationalized medication that for bipolar disorder is very likely to be a rational polypharmacy.

3.21
Whatever Happened to the Calcium Channel Blockers?
Shirley A. Walton[1]

There have been many publications over the last 20 years regarding the role of calcium channel blockers (CCBs) in mood disorders and particularly in mania. However, in a recent review of treatment guidelines for bipolar disorder, they are mentioned in just one out of five guidelines and even then are listed only as late options for euphoric or mixed mania [1]. Charles Bowden's practical review does not mention them at all. What explains the slide into obscurity of these once promising agents?

To answer this, I would like to venture briefly into the history of the use of these drugs in psychiatry. CCBs, including verapamil, nimodipine, nifedipine, diltiazem and flunarizine, are indicated primarily for the treatment of cardiovascular disease. Interest in their role in mood disorders started in the early 1980s. Two independent groups of investigators began to examine their efficacy at more or less the same time [2].

The interest arose from research evidence linking abnormalities in calcium metabolism to mood disorders. It has long been recorded that disorders of calcium metabolism are associated with psychiatric symptoms. Delirium, anxiety, irritability, psychosis, depression and mania may be caused by hypocalcaemia. Hypercalcaemia is commonly associated with depression and stupor [3].

Intracellular calcium ions play an essential role in the regulation of certain physiological processes. These include neural signal propagation and synthesis and release of several neurotransmitters, including serotonin and noradrenaline, which are implicated in the aetiology of mood disorders [4, 5]. A role for dysregulated calcium metabolism in bipolar disorder is also suggested by studies of peripheral cells. Significant elevations of intracellular calcium have been found in resting and stimulated platelets or lymphocytes of manic or bipolar depressed patients. These changes were not found in those of normal controls or unipolar depressed patients, or those made euthymic by various medications or electroconvulsive therapy [5].

Early case reports suggested the efficacy of oral verapamil in mania. This led to several further trials. It appeared that there was a great deal of potential for an inexpensive, well-tolerated agent, which had been well tested in the field of cardiovascular medicine, had few drug–drug interactions, no need for serum level monitoring and low teratogenicity compared to existing options.

———————————
[1] *Department of Psychiatry, University of the Witwatersrand, Chris Hani Baragwanath Hospital, Johannesburg, South Africa*

Most information available on the use of these drugs in bipolar disorder is for the treatment of mania. Verapamil has been the most studied. Early studies reported good antimanic efficacy. These included two open trials, five partially controlled studies and two small placebo-controlled trials. The more recent, larger, better-controlled trials looking at verapamil in acute mania have shown disappointing results and have not supported these findings. These include two open trials, two partially controlled studies and one placebo-controlled trial [6]. The two largest of the above trials showed a significantly superior efficacy of lithium compared to verapamil and no difference between verapamil and placebo, respectively [7, 8]. These discrepancies could perhaps be explained by certain methodological problems of earlier trials. They mostly involved small patient numbers, were of short duration and many patients were not seriously ill. Concomitant medication (including antipsychotics) was used frequently and often obscured the results.

The data regarding the use of verapamil for maintenance or prophylactic therapy are scanty and mainly derive from case studies. This is also true for depressive episodes in bipolar disorder, although one large, well-controlled and well-designed study showed no difference between verapamil and placebo in "depression of various types" [3]. The question of the use of verapamil as an add-on drug to augment existing therapy has not been satisfactorily addressed.

Little is known about the role of other CCBs in mood disorders. Nimodipine has better penetration of the blood-brain barrier than verapamil and has been found to be effective in early controlled studies. No controlled studies have been published regarding the efficacy of diltiazem, nifedipine or flunarizine in bipolar disorder, although there have been open studies and case reports [6].

The history of the use of verapamil for mania highlights many of the problems in bipolar research as discussed by Bowden. It illustrates the caution that must be employed when interpreting the results of clinical trials with multiple methodological limitations. The problems include the often falsely encouraging results observed in open trials and the difficulty of enrolling severely ill patients in trials, which restricts sample size.

Looking back, it is notable that, although there is a long time period during which there has been interest in these agents, they have never been widely used in clinical practice. Many of the newer anticonvulsants (for example, lamotrigine and topiramate) and the newer antipsychotics such as olanzapine and risperidone are already being used extensively by my colleagues and myself. This is in spite of the relatively short time period that they have been considered as options for bipolar disorder. Why the disparity? Certainly, the pharmaceutical companies are not as interested in selling older drugs as they are in promoting newer ones and this affects funding for clinical trials. Nonetheless, it is probable that a perceived lack of efficacy has been a major factor in determining these prescribing practices. The authors of a recent review on calcium channel blockers in psychiatry note that the number of reports has been rather small and that the number published yearly does not seem to be increasing as one would expect with an effective treatment [9].

There are strong links between calcium and bipolar disorder, yet existing data on the use of verapamil is not compelling. Nevertheless, the CCBs vary in terms of their structure and physiological effects [6], and CCBs other than verapamil may differ in their psychotropic profile and clinical potential. There is little information regarding their use in bipolar disorder and further studies into their role may be warranted. Although most of the CCBs are safe, tolerable and inexpensive, there is at present no convincing evidence for their use either as alternatives or as adjuncts to the existing array of medications for bipolar disorder.

REFERENCES

1. Goldberg J.F. (2000) Treatment guidelines: current and future management of bipolar disorder. *J. Clin. Psychiatry*, **61** (Suppl. 13): 12–18.
2. Höschl C. (1991) Do calcium antagonists have a place in the treatment of mood disorders? *Drugs*, **42**: 721–729.
3. Dubovsky S.L., Franks R.D. (1983) Intracellular calcium ions in affective disorders: a review and a hypothesis. *Biol. Psychiatry*, **18**: 781–797.
4. Höschl C., Kozeny J. (1989) Verapamil in affective disorders: a controlled double blind study. *Biol. Psychiatry*, **25**: 128–140.
5. Dubovsky S.L. (1993) Calcium antagonists in manic depressive illness. *Neuropsychobiology*, **27**: 184–192.
6. Levy N.A., Janicak P.G. (2000) Calcium channel antagonists for the treatment of bipolar disorder. *Bipolar Disord.*, **2**: 108–119.
7. Walton S.A., Berk M., Brook S. (1996) Superiority of lithium over verapamil in mania: a randomised, controlled, single-blind trial. *J. Clin. Psychiatry*, **57**: 543–546.
8. Janicak P.G., Sharma R.P., Pandey G, David J.M. (1998) Verapamil for the treatment of acute mania: a double-blind, placebo-controlled trial. *Am. J. Psychiatry*, **155**: 972–973.
9. Hollister L.E., Garza Trevino E.S.G. (1999) Calcium channel blockers in psychiatric disorders, a review of the literature. *Can. J. Psychiatry*, **44**: 658–664.

Psychosocial Interventions for Bipolar Disorder: A Review

Mark S. Bauer

Veterans Affairs Medical Center, Brown University Department of Psychiatry and Human Behavior, 830 Chalkstone Avenue, Providence, RI 02908-4799, USA

INTRODUCTION

As outlined elsewhere in this volume, numerous somatic interventions have been documented to be efficacious in the treatment of various phases of bipolar disorder. These include pharmacologic agents such as mood stabilizers, antidepressants and antipsychotics, as well as non-pharmacologic treatments such as electroconvulsive therapy and bright light. The efficacy of such modalities has, not surprisingly, led to a strongly medical-model view of treatment for this illness. This is seen perhaps most clearly in some of the early descriptions of lithium clinics, which vividly document the emergence of medical model treatment from what had previously been a predominantly psychotherapeutic approach to the illness.

However, as we enter the fourth decade of predominantly medically based treatment for bipolar disorder, there are several reasons to increase attention to psychosocial interventions as adjuncts to medical model treatment. In doing so, we do not move away from the medical model, but actually move in concert with cutting-edge thinking in the management of chronic medical illnesses, which includes a key role for psychosocial as well as medical treatment (e.g., [1–5]).

With regard specifically to bipolar disorder, there are five main reasons for attention to psychosocial adjunctive treatments. First, despite the substantial efficacy of available somatic treatments, nonresponse and breakthrough episodes remain a major problem, with as many as 35–60% remaining chronically ill or having poor outcome (e.g., [6–8]). Thus, it is reasonable to consider whether other modalities, specifically combining

Bipolar Disorder. Edited by Mario Maj, Hagop S. Akiskal, Juan José López-Ibor and Norman Sartorius.
© 2002 John Wiley & Sons Ltd.

medication with psychotherapy, may improve clinical outcome where predominantly medical management alone may not.

Second, lack of treatment adherence makes delivery of efficacious medications difficult. Current evidence indicates that as much as 20–55% of patients with bipolar disorder have major lapses in adherence (e.g., [9–12]).

Third, evidence indicates that both life stressors (e.g., [13, 14]) and social support (e.g., [15]) may impact the course of bipolar disorder. Thus, modulation of these factors, not directly amenable to medication treatment, may improve outcome (reviewed in [16]).

Fourth, social, family, and occupational dysfunction are the rule rather than the exception in bipolar disorder (e.g., [7, 17–23]). Functional deficits may persist in the absence of major affective episodes [7, 8, 17, 18] and even subsyndromal levels of depression appear to be a strong predictor of ongoing functional deficits [24].

Fifth, bipolar disorder is a costly illness, and it is possible that psychosocial interventions in addition to medical model treatment may reduce costs. The overall societal costs of mental illness are substantial, exceeding $148 billion per annum in 1990 dollars, including $67 billion for direct treatment costs—about 10% of all direct treatment costs nationally [25]. Greenberg et al [26] used the approach of Stoudemire et al. [27] to estimate societal costs of affective disorders, including bipolar disorder. They found that costs exceeded $43 billion in 1990 dollars, including over $12 billion in direct treatment costs, and over $7 billion due to lost productivity from premature death and $23 billion from morbidity. Given the above studies on functional impairment, this last estimate is certainly an underestimate, as "only the limited period of the episode itself was assumed to be of concern in calculating morbidity costs" [26]. Wyatt and Hentner [28] estimated that the annual societal costs of bipolar disorder alone exceed $45 billion in 1990 dollars, exceeded only by $64 billion spent on schizophrenia. These costs for bipolar disorder include over $7 billion in indirect treatment costs and over $38 billion in indirect costs. Of direct treatment costs, $2.4 billion are spent on inpatient treatment, $0.3 billion on outpatient treatment, $3.0 billion on nursing home and other extended care, and $2.3 billion on the correctional system. On the positive side, early data from Riefman and Wyatt [29] indicate that treatment innovations can result in societal cost savings. Specifically, they estimated that the introduction of lithium reduced societal expenditures to 53% of pre-lithium levels. Without adequate treatment, a person with bipolar disorder from age 25 can expect to lose 14 years of effective major activity (e.g., work, school, family role function) and nine years of life [30]. Fifteen percent of persons with bipolar disorder are unemployed for at least five consecutive years, and over 25% of those under age 65 receive disability payments [31]. Many individuals with bipolar disorder reside in costly institutional settings. In the book length report of the Epidemiologic Catchment Area Study, Robins and Regier [32] found that 42% of institutionalized manics were in prisons while 58% were in acute or chronic care hospitals. Improving treatment delivery may allow such patients to resume community living.

In this review, we will consider two broad groups of psychosocial interventions: psychotherapy and what the US National Institute of Mental Health has called the "context of care" [25]. "Psychotherapy" refers to verbal and behavioural interaction between a clinician and a patient (or group of patients or patient with support system) in order to relieve the patient's suffering or dysfunction [33]. This review covers a wide range of psychotherapies, including several that are highly structured and supported by manuals that specify explicitly how the therapy is to be implemented, as well as interventions that are more free-form. It is important to keep this distinction in mind as one contemplates using a particular approach for clinical or research purposes or evaluates study data.

By contexts of care we mean the organization of clinical resources to deliver care to patients with bipolar disorder who present for treatment. There are multiple determinants of the context of care, including for example available clinical resources, legislative constraints and stimuli, insurance, other financial concerns, patient resources. In many cases these determinants are fixed and only minimally amenable to manipulation by patients or caregivers, e.g., reimbursement systems. However, several context of care interventions for bipolar disorder have been meticulously described, and a few are being subjected to controlled clinical trials. It is therefore important to review these contexts of care—psychosocial interventions in their own right—in particular with regard to their impact on outcome.

This review is divided into several subsequent sections. Types of psychotherapeutic approaches are briefly described. Quantitative studies of the various modalities are then reviewed. A series of "how-to" references are identified for clinicians and researchers to help them implement particular approaches. Context of care interventions are reviewed next, including both early, qualitative descriptions of lithium clinics and recent state-of-the-art controlled trials. Then common themes across psychosocial modalities are identified. Finally, trends in the evidence are summarized, and based on these, directions for further research are suggested.

RATIONALE FOR PSYCHOTHERAPY INTERVENTIONS

Several psychotherapeutic approaches to bipolar disorder have been used, including (in historical order of development) psychoanalytic, family, interpersonal, cognitive-behavioural, and illness management/psychoeducational. Rationale for each of these is summarized below.

Psychoanalysis and Psychodynamic Psychotherapy

Bipolar disorder attracted the attention of psychoanalysts since the early days of that treatment. Perhaps the most comprehensive review of psychoanalytic thought on bipolar disorder is summarized by Frieda Fromm-Reichmann's group, which undertook extensive study of several cases in an ongoing case supervision seminar [34, 35], and by the more recent work of Jackson [36]. The common threads through much of psychoanalytic thought about bipolar disorder are the contrast of bipolar disorder with schizophrenia, and the conceptualization of mania as an alternate expression of the basic conflicts that produce depression under other circumstances. As with much psychoanalytic thought, the emphasis is placed on mechanisms related to unconscious conflicts that have their origin in early childhood development, the resolution of which will ameliorate present-day affective symptoms.

Family Interventions

Family treatment was another early focus of psychosocial treatment for bipolar disorder (e.g., [37–39]), as it was readily apparent that the illness often caused substantial stress in the marriage (an anecdotal impression that has been borne out quantitatively in studies of functional outcome, as noted above). More recently, quantitative research has also identified family interactions as predictor of course in bipolar disorder. In particular, levels of "expressed emotion" (EE) in these interactions have been shown to be associated with relapse in schizophrenia (e.g., [40]). Miklowitz and coworkers have extended these findings, demonstrating that high EE predicts relapse after hospitalization for bipolar disorder (e.g., [41, 42]).

Interpersonal Interventions

Related to intra-family stress as a potential modulator of bipolar disorder, several investigators have focused more broadly on interpersonal interactions in bipolar disorder from one of two perspectives. Frank and coworkers (e.g., [43]) have written extensively on interpersonal interactions as a key stressor and/or remediating factor in bipolar disorder. Accordingly, they took the approach of adapting Interpersonal Therapy (IPT; [44]) for depression to bipolar disorder and adding elements to stabilize the pattern or rhythm of social interactions.

The second interpersonal approach has focused on the potential therapeutic impact of interpersonal group therapy interventions for individuals with bipolar disorder. Although some authors have cautioned about the negative impact of group interventions on such patients (e.g., [45]), or about the negative impact of patients with bipolar disorder on groups (e.g., [46]), others have utilized primarily interpersonal here-and-now approaches in group format to address interpersonal difficulties (e.g., [47–49]). In addition, others have addressed interpersonal issues of stigma and social isolation by incorporating interpersonal elements into psychoeducational groups (e.g., [50, 51]).

Cognitive-Behavioural Techniques

Cognitive-behavioural techniques, originally outlined by Beck (e.g., [52]) have been elaborated by a number of clinicians and investigators as summarized below. Principally, the cognitive-behavioural conceptualization and treatment of depressive episodes in bipolar disorder is very similar to that for unipolar disorder [53–55]. There is less certainty, and few data, regarding how to conceptualize mania, although in some respects mania may share the same (rather than opposite) negative attributional style regarding negative events as is found in depression [56]. Further, since it appears that life stressors play a modulatory role in the course of bipolar disorder (see above), benefit may derive from helping the individual to deal with cognitive distortions that could worsen the impact of such stressors. Thus the basic cognitive-behavioural approach and techniques of addressing dysfunctional attitudes and cognitive schemata in depression have been applied to bipolar disorder. Further, as Scott [53] points out, educational techniques often draw on cognitive-behaviour therapy's "collaborative, educational style, the use of a step-by-step approach and of guided discovery".

Psychoeducation

Finally, the need for better education regarding the illness and its treatment (often called "psychoeducation" when applied to mental disorders) has been evident as long as compliance and stigma have been recognized as problems in this illness. These techniques were incorporated into various aspects of lithium clinics as early as the 1970s, as described below. In addition, aspects of patient education have been incorporated more or less explicitly into most psychotherapeutic modalities (except perhaps the classic psychoanalytic). However, recently psychoeducation techniques have received growing attention, leading to the development of formal manual-based interventions (e.g., [51, 57]). As noted above, much of this attention has been stimulated by the increasing recognition of the patient as co-manager of his/her illness in both psychiatric (e.g., [58]) and medical (e.g., [1–5]) settings.

AN EVIDENCE-BASED REVIEW OF PSYCHOTHERAPY STUDIES

Evaluating the Literature

Several techniques have been developed to improve the ability to review and summarize scientific literature and draw overall conclusions from often divergent types of data. For instance, quantitative techniques such as meta-analysis provide numeric conclusions with regard to significance of similar interventions in diverse studies (e.g., [59]).

More qualitative techniques of "evidence-based medicine" (e.g., [60–62]) have been used in reviewing and summarizing treatment interventions in medicine and more recently in mental health. Briefly, these techniques consist of comprehensively identifying relevant data-based articles, summarizing their methods and conclusions, and then in a standardized fashion rating the scientific quality of the evidence based on the rigour of their methodology.

For instance, the US Agency for Healthcare Research and Quality (AHRQ, formerly Agency for Health Care Policy and Research, AHCPR), developed guidelines for the identification and treatment of depression in primary care using techniques of evidence-based medicine [63]. This basic system was adapted by the US Department of Veterans Affairs (VA) for developing their treatment guidelines for a wide variety of medical, surgical, and psychiatric disorders (e.g., [64]). Similar evidence-rating schemes have been used, including to address the quality of evidence for psychotherapy for bipolar disorder (e.g., [65, 66]), although the basis of these classification systems has not always been made explicit.

For this review we follow the AHRQ methods as adapted by the VA in delineating three main classes of evidence. These are summarized in Table 4.1. There is no attempt to "weigh" or "integrate" evidence across studies as there would be in meta-analysis. Rather, these techniques of evidence-based medicine provide a "short-hand" method and a common language to categorize studies and facilitate comparison and communication around them.

TABLE 4.1   US Agency for Health Care Policy and Research (AHCPR)/ Agency for Healthcare Research and Quality (AHRQ) evidence classification system

Class A:	Randomized or other controlled trials *Examples*: Randomized controlled trials of intervention vs. waiting list control or no added treatment; other controlled trials with treatment assignment independent of subject characteristic, time of presentation, etc.
Class B:	Well-designed clinical studies *Examples*: Open studies with *a priori* design and follow-up period of designated endpoint; pre/post mirror-image studies with "post" period designed *a priori*.
Class C:	Case series, case reports, retrospective chart reviews. *Examples*: Prospectively gathered data on a series of patients followed in treatment; retrospective chart review after implementation of an intervention.

Review Methodology

This review sought to locate all studies on psychotherapy for bipolar disorder that filled the following criteria: a) published in peer-reviewed journals; b) investigated an intervention in a sample of patients with bipolar disorder, or reported separately results for bipolar subsamples from a diagnostically heterogeneous group; c) specified quantitative outcome variables; d) written in English (an unfortunate, but recognized, limitation of the author).

Literature databases including MedLine, PsychLit and the Cochrane Collaboration were searched. Articles were reviewed by title, abstract, and text as relevant. Authors known to be actively working in the field in the US and Europe were contacted regarding further work in print or in press. The bibliography of each located article was scanned for additional articles. This step was repeated iteratively until no further references were found. The search was completed by December 2000.

The results of the literature search are reviewed below and summarized in Table 4.2. Studies are categorized as Class A, B, or C. In Table 4.2 outcomes are categorized as positive (+), negative (−), or equivocal (+/−) based on results reported in each study. A result is reported as (+) if at least some parameters in the group of outcome variables were positive (e.g., improvement of manic but not depressive symptoms; improvement of some but not all measures of substance abuse). If no statistical analyses are presented (e.g., for Class C and some Class B studies), then the author's qualitative conclusions serve as the basis for the rating.

In all studies located, psychotherapy interventions were used as adjuncts to standard medication management rather than as alternatives to psychopharmacologic agents. Studies are presented chronologically below.

TABLE 4.2 Evidence table for psychotherapy interventions for bipolar disorder

Study	N	Intervention	Study duration	Outcome variables	Study type	Evidence class
Benson, 1975 [67]	31 outpatients	Various modalities including individual, group, or couples group	3–41 months (mean 13)	Emotional or social deterioration (+) or treatment drop-out (+)	Retrospective review	C
Davenport, 1977 [39]	65 former inpatients	Couples group post-discharge	2–10 years (mean 3.9)	Occupational (+/−), social (+), family (+), clinical (+) function	Retrospective review	C
Volkmar, 1981 [68]	20 outpatients	Interpersonal group	2 years	Weeks in hospital (+), occupational status (+)	Retrospective review	C
Cochran, 1984 [69]	28 outpatients	Individual cognitive-behavioural intervention focusing on adherence	6 months	Medication adherence (+/−)	Randomized controlled trial vs. no added treatment	A
Kripke and Robinson, 1985 [50]	14 outpatients	Group focusing on education and problem-solving	10 years	Clinical (+) and occupational (+) status	Retrospective review	C
van Gent et al, 1988 [48], van Gent and Zwart, 1993 [70]	26 outpatients	Group using combination of psychoeducation, interpersonal, and behavioural techniques	5 years	SCL-90 scores (+), admissions (+), lithium discontinuation (+)	Pre/post	C
Clarkin et al, 1990 [71]	21 inpatients	Inpatient Family Intervention (IFI), a family treatment emphasizing education and reduction in stress including maladaptive family interactions. Manual-based	18 months	Global status (+), symptoms (+), social role function (+), family attitudes (+)	Randomized controlled trial vs. no added intervention, with blinded assessments	A
van Gent and Zwart, 1991 [72]	39 partners of patients	Psychoeducational group emphasizing diagnosis, treatment, genetics, social interactions, and partner function	6 months	Knowledge about illness and treatment (+), patient and partner interaction ratings (−), patient mood (−), compliance (−)	Randomized controlled trial vs. no added intervention	A

Study	Patients	Intervention	Duration	Outcome	Design	Grade
Peet and Harvey, 1991 [73]	60 outpatients	Videotape/handout of lithium information followed by in-home visit for further information	24 weeks	Knowledge about (+) and attitudes toward (–) lithium	Randomized controlled trial vs. waiting list control	A
Retzer et al, 1991 [74]	20 outpatients	Family therapy focusing on seven domains of system function	6 sessions (mean) over 14.4 months (mean)	Hospitalization rates (+)	Retrospective review of records pre/post therapy; some interviews	C
Cerbone et al, 1992 [75]	43 outpatients	Group interpersonal, focusing on "here-and-now" and "counselling, education and support"	1 year retrospective, 1 year prospective	Affective episodes (+), hospital days (+), medication adherence (–), neuroleptic use (–), social and interpersonal function (+)	Pre/post	C
Palmer and Williams, 1995 [76]	4 outpatients	Group cognitive-behavioural	9 months	Clinical outcome, social function (+/–)	Prospective open trial	B
Honig et al, 1997 [77]	52 outpatient couples	Multi-couple psychoeducational group	12 weeks	Expressed emotion (+)	Controlled trial vs. waiting list control	A/B
Hlastala et al, 1997 [78]	42 outpatients	Social Rhythms plus Interpersonal Therapy (IPSRT), individual therapy focusing on stabilizing social rhythms and interpersonal stress in an acute mood episode. Manual-based	1 year	Clinical symptoms (–)	Randomized controlled trial vs. no added intervention	A
Clarkin et al, 1998 [84]	33 in- and outpatients	Couples psychoeducation. Manual-based	11 months	Clinical (–) and functional (+) outcome, medication adherence (–)	Randomized controlled trial vs. no added intervention	A

(continues overleaf)

T ABLE 4.2 (*Continued*)

Study	N	Intervention	Study duration	Outcome variables	Study type	Evidence class
Bauer et al, 1998 [85]	29 outpatients, 4 therapists	Life Goals Program, a psychoeducation and behavioural-cognitive group. Manual-based.	18 months (mean)	Therapist adherence (+), patient knowledge base (+), patient functional goal attainment (+)	Open trial	B
Perry et al, 1999 [87]	69 outpatients	Psychoeducation to teach patients to identify early warning signs of relapse and implement action plan for treatment	18 months	Time to relapse (+), social function (+)	Randomized controlled trial vs. no added intervention	A
Frank et al, 1999 [86]	82 outpatients	Relapse-prevention application of IPSRT (see [78])	1 year	Clinical symptoms (−)	Randomized controlled trial vs. no added intervention	A
Zaretsky et al, 1999 [88]	11 outpatients	Cognitive-behaviour with Basco-Rush adaptation for bipolar disorder. Manual-based	20 weeks	Clinical symptoms (+), automatic thoughts (+), dysfunctional attitudes (−)	Open trial	B
Lam et al, 2000 [57]	25 outpatients	Cognitive-behavioural and psychoeducation. Manual-based	1 year	Episodes (+), social function (+)	Randomized controlled trial vs. no added intervention	A
Miklowitz et al, 2000 [89]	101 in- and outpatients	Family-Focused Treatment (FFT), family/couples in-home sessions focused on psychoeducation, response to symptoms, adherence. Manual-based	1 year	Clinical outcome (+), medication compliance (−), expressed emotion (+)	Randomized controlled trial vs. no added intervention	A

| Weiss et al, 2000 [92] | 45 outpatients with comorbid substance dependence | Integrated Group Therapy (IGT), relapse-prevention strategies for both disorders utilizing cognitive-behavioural techniques. Manual-based | 9 months | Substance use and impact (+), mood symptoms (+), compliance (−), hospitalization rates (−) | Open trial with patients assigned to IGT or none in sequential blocks | B |

Outcomes are categorized as positive (+), negative (−), or equivocal (+/−) based on results reported in each study. A result is reported as (+) if at least some parameters in the group of outcome variables were positive (e.g., improvement of manic but not depressive symptoms; improvement of some but not all measures of substance abuse). If no statistical analyses are presented (e.g., for Class C and some Class B studies), then the author's qualitative conclusions serve as the basis for the rating.
SCL-90—Hopkins Symptom Check List 90.

Quantitative Studies of Psychotherapy for Bipolar Disorder

In the early days of lithium treatment, Benson [67] reported a retrospective series of 31 bipolar patients treated in his private practice with individual, group, or couples group interventions. Patients were in almost all cases seen at least bimonthly and several were seen multiple times per week. He followed patients for 3–41 months, and defined treatment "failure" as "emotional and/or social deterioration or dropping out of the study". He did not consider symptomatic worsening since he felt that when this occurred in his series it was associated with drop in lithium level, and symptoms remitted with increase of lithium dose. He reports a failure rate of 14%, "markedly lower than lithium prophylaxis alone", and makes the point that psychotherapy should not be neglected in the context of medication treatment.

Davenport et al [39] reported on a retrospective analysis of follow-up data on a cohort of bipolar patients 2–10 years after discharge from the US National Institute of Mental Health (NIMH). Sixty-five patients were assigned at discharge to attend a weekly couples group based on geographic availability and space in the couples group. Patients living at a geographic distance were referred to community care. Patients who lived near the NIMH but for whom there was no room in the couples group were referred to a lithium maintenance group. The couples group content was not well described in their report, but it appears that Davenport et al emphasized optimizing marital interactions plus addressing issues around fear of episode recurrence. They assessed outcome with a questionnaire covering social, occupational, and clinical function and marital interactions. It appears from responses that the couples group patients did better than the community care group in terms of social function and family interaction and better than the lithium group in terms of family interaction. No note is made of differences in occupational function. The couples group suffered no marital failures or rehospitalizations, despite recurrence of substantial symptoms, while several occurred in each of the other groups.

Volkmar et al [68] retrospectively summarized experience with an interpersonal group based on the approach of Yalom [46]. Twenty patients, highly screened for motivation for group therapy, met weekly with two therapists in 75-minute sessions. Compared to the two years prior to group, hospital days during two years of group decreased from 17 to four weeks on average. They also noted that the number of patients fully employed or full-time students increased from six to 16. Shakir et al [47] published preliminary data on this cohort. It is unclear whether patients had been prescribed lithium during the baseline period, although their data indicate that patients did better with the combination of lithium plus group treatment than prior to the study.

Cochran [69] studied an individual cognitive-behavioural intervention of six weekly groups aimed at improving compliance. Twenty-eight patients newly admitted to an outpatient lithium clinic were randomized to receive either the intervention or no added treatment and were assessed post-treatment, at three months, and at six months on several indices of medication adherence. Immediately post-treatment, intervention patients scored better than control patients on some but not all adherence measures. However, these differences disappeared by three months. By six months intervention patients again scored better than control patients on several indices of compliance. Additionally, control patients were more likely to have had an affective episode precipitated by lithium non-adherence. While intervention patients did not differ from controls in terms of any form of non-adherence, they did have a lower incidence of breaches of treatment that were judged to be major.

Kripke and Robinson [50] summarized retrospectively 10 years of experience with a group of 14 outpatients with bipolar disorder treated in a group that initially focused on medication issues during lithium treatment. The group eventually included psychoeducation around medications and impending symptoms, feedback on status from group members, and problem solving. They report that hospitalization rates were lower than before group and that five improved employment status during treatment.

Van Gent et al [48] studied an initial 10-session group psychotherapy intervention in bipolar patients taking lithium, followed by a five-year ongoing maintenance protocol [70]. Their intervention consisted of an eclectic group led by a social worker and a psychiatrist that met weekly for 90 minutes over 10–13 sessions. The group combined psychoeducation with interpersonal and behavioural interventions. Their pre/post analysis found initially that the group reduced "insufficiency in thinking and behaving" according to the Hopkins Symptom Check List 90 (SCL-90), and this was confirmed in their longer term study, although no other subscale scores changed. They also found that, compared to lithium treatment without group intervention, admissions per year reduced as did the number of lithium discontinuations.

Clarkin et al [71] conducted a study of Intensive Family Intervention (IFI) in a mixed group of inpatients with mood or schizophrenic spectrum disorders, including 21 with bipolar disorder, in a randomized controlled trial of IFI vs. no added intervention. IFI is an individual family intervention that seeks to educate patients and their families about the illness, identify and resolve current and future stresses, and minimize stressful family interactions characterized by high EE. Patients received at least six sessions during their hospital admission. The authors measured symptoms, social role function, global function, and family attitudes using blinded ratings at six and 18 months. The analysis in this report also included results for patients with major depression. While depressive patients did worse with the intervention by 18 months, bipolar patients were better with IFI in terms of global ratings, symptoms, social role function, and family attitudes. Interestingly, the beneficial effects in bipolar patients were solely due to improvement in female patients, while no differences were seen across treatments among male bipolar patients.

Van Gent and Zwart [72] also conducted a randomized controlled trial of a psychoeducation group for 39 partners of patients with bipolar vs. no added treatment controls. Their intervention consisted of five educational sessions covering the disorder, medications, genetics, interpersonal interactions, and the partner's own functioning. They found that knowledge about several aspects of the illness improved in the intervention group compared to controls, although there was no change in measures of interactions in either partner or patient, no change in patient mood, and no change in compliance.

Peet and Harvey [73] studied a videotape lecture, handout, and home visit to convey information regarding lithium to patients attending a lithium clinic. Thirty were randomly assigned to the videotape/handout intervention followed by a home visit to answer questions. Thirty served as waiting-list controls and then received the videotape/handout but no home visit. Pre-test using standardized questionnaires to measure lithium knowledge was followed by post-test six weeks after the intervention. At six weeks the intervention group had greater improvement in scores than the waiting list control group, and their gains in knowledge were maintained until the end of the 24-week study. The waiting-list control group later received the videotape/handout intervention (without home visit); their scores then significantly improved and remained high and indistinguishable from the earlier intervention group. While there were overall improvements in attitude toward lithium, there were no effects of the intervention.

Retzer et al [74] report on the impact of family therapy intervention aimed at seven aspects of systemic function: flexibility of world/family view ("relational reality"), ability to simultaneously consider opposing aspects of reality ("softening/hardening of relational reality"), tendency toward "either/or" thinking ("system logic"), "individuation in the family" among all members' roles, attempts at relational monitoring among family members, interview atmosphere during assessment, and degree to which the index patient was seen as a "victim" vs. an "agent" (the latter taking more responsibility for their own actions). Bipolar patients received a mean of six sessions (range 1–14) over a mean of 14 months (range 0–35). The authors retrospectively reviewed records of 20 patients with bipolar disorder as well as 10 with schizoaffective disorder, and supplemented where possible with follow-up interviews a mean of three years post-therapy. Their quantitative analyses focused on rehospitalization rates compared pre- vs. post-therapy and they found significant improvements in both groups. Qualitatively they also investigated changes in the above seven dimensions across high- and low-relapse groups. They found that movement away from "either/or" toward "both-and" logic was characteristic of both groups. However, the low-relapse group was distinguished by more movement away from seeing the patient as "victim" and more as "agent". Description of medication prescription indicated that patients had a tendency to receive fewer medications after family therapy. It is impossible in such uncontrolled studies to determine whether the view of the patient less as "victim" and more as "agent" was due to actual clinical improvement (i.e., in reality being less of a victim of the illness and more able to take responsibility), or due to a change in willingness to take responsibility leading to or supporting clinical improvement, or both.

Cerbone et al [75] conducted an open trial of open-ended group treatment emphasizing "here-and-now" techniques focusing on "counselling, education, and support". They reviewed charts for one year prior to group and one year during group treatment and extracted scores for rating affective episodes and measuring social and interpersonal adjustment. Although ratings were not blinded, they included extraneous chart notes to reduce bias. Compared to the baseline year, patients had shorter or less severe affective episodes during group, shorter hospital stays among those admitted, and higher social and interpersonal adjustment scores. There were no differences in medication adherence or need for neuroleptics.

Palmer and Williams [76] conducted an open trial feasibility study of cognitive-behavioural techniques adapted for group treatment of bipolar disorder, entering six and studying four patients over nine months. Their closed-group intervention consisted of seventeen 90-minute weekly sessions and six monthly follow-up sessions. The intervention focuses on psychoeducation and development of an "action plan"—i.e., a patient-specific cognitive-behavioural plan for illness management. Results of this pilot study indicated that the treatment package was effective for at least some participants, with 2–3 participants improving on several clinical and/or functional measures.

Honig et al [77] investigated the impact of a multi-couple psychoeducational group in patients with bipolar disorder, with a particular focus on its impact on EE. Their intervention consisted of six 2-hour sessions with the patient and one or more significant other given biweekly. They conducted a controlled trial investigating 29 couples in the intervention group and 23 on a waiting list, although it is not clear whether the couples were assigned randomly or through some other method (e.g., a post-hoc control group). They investigated EE and symptom status at baseline and then report on EE, but do not mention symptom status, at 12-week follow-up. They found more changes from high EE to low EE in the intervention than the control group. However, they also found that EE was relatively stable over the course of the study, with more than 75% of ratings unchanged. Consistent with the hypothesis that high EE is associated with worse course in bipolar disorder, they found that those with consistently low EE during the study, compared to those with consistently high EE, had had fewer admissions prior to the study.

Hlastala *et al* [78] reported initial results with an eclectic intervention developed by Frank *et al* [43]. Their multi-modal manual-based intervention aimed at minimizing the impact of interpersonal and chronobiological stressors on the course of bipolar disorder. Some data indicate that psycho-social stressors can be associated with affective relapse in established bipo-lar disorder (reviewed in [14]). Additional theoretical [79] and empirical (e.g., [80–82]) work indicate that chronobiologic factors may play a role in the course of bipolar disorder. Thus this group's manual-based intervention employs techniques that analyse and stabilize the daily routine of patients with bipolar disorder (Social Rhythms Therapy, SRT), while directly ad-dressing interpersonal stressors using Interpersonal Therapy (IPT), which had been shown to be efficacious in treating and preventing episodes in major depressive disorder (e.g., [83]). The weekly, IPSRT intervention con-sists of four phases. An Initial Phase of weekly sessions lasting several weeks to months focuses on assessment of illness and social rhythms, and on psychoeducation. A several-month Intermediate Phase then includes weekly sessions that focus on developing SRT- and IPT-based strategies to deal with stressors. A Preventive Phase of monthly sessions continues for at least two years, and a Termination Phase concludes treatment with 4–6 monthly sessions. An initial report on a randomized controlled trial of IPSRT vs. no added intervention on 42 subjects [78] found that there was no effect of treatment compared to control. However, it indicated that manic patients were likely to reach remission more quickly than depressed or cycling subjects, who were similar in time to remission.

Clarkin *et al* [84] conducted a randomized controlled trial of a 25-session psychoeducational intervention for patients and their spouses vs. no added treatment in a sample of 33 in- or outpatients. Treatments were given weekly or biweekly to individual couples by experienced social workers using a formalized manual. Clinical outcome, functional outcome, and medication adherence were measured at baseline and after 11 months. Symptom ratings did not change over time between the groups, while functional outcome showed significant improvement for the sample treated with the group intervention. Adherence levels were high in both groups, but were rated higher in the sample treated with the group intervention.

Our group [85] conducted an open trial of the Life Goals Program, a two-phase manual-based [51] group program. Phase 1 contains five weekly highly structured psychoeducational sessions focused on identifying patient illness patterns and developing an "action plan" for response to symptoms. Phase 2 focuses on attainment of functional goals (e.g., social or occupational tasks); it is weekly and open-ended, with patients identifying and working toward specific goals until attainment, and then repeating the process for additional goals. The approach to Phase 2 is eclectic, utilizing mainly cognitive-behavioural tools with interpersonal group elements to support, destigmatization, and problem-solving assistance. We found that the programme could be effectively taught to therapists ($n = 4$) across two sites with good adherence to the manual. Patients ($n = 29$) significantly increased their knowledge base in Phase 1, and 69% successfully completed Phase 1. During a mean treatment time of 18 months in Phase 2, 70% reached their first self-identified goal and did so by a mean of seven months (range 2–17 months). Clinical symptoms were not measured.

A follow-up analysis of IPSRT [86] investigated time to relapse in 82 remitted subjects who entered the Preventive Phase. They found no difference in recurrence rate with IPSRT over one year of follow-up. Interestingly, however, they found that subjects who changed treatment between the Initial and Preventive Phases (either IPSRT to control or vice versa) did worse in a number of analyses than those who remained either in IPSRT or the control condition. Of further interest is that these findings are true both for relapses close to the time of potential change and for relapses more than 12 weeks after the time of potential change, and that only the treatment modality and not the therapist changed. The authors also reported that changing therapist due to job change or maternity leave did not appear to be associated with relapse. They hypothesize that changing from any treatment that worked (by definition the patients in the Preventive Phase had remitted) is a stress that can negatively impact the course of their illness.

Perry et al [87] conducted a randomized controlled trial of a psychoeducation programme vs. no added intervention in a group of 69 outpatients with bipolar disorder. Their intervention consists of two stages: training the patient to identify prodromal symptoms of an affective episode and developing an action plan for response. The intervention was given individually by a psychologist and a median of nine sessions was delivered (range 0–12). They assessed symptomatic relapses and social function at three, six, and 18 months. Time to manic relapse and overall days manic, but not time to depressive relapse or overall days depressed, was significantly better in the experimental group. The experimental group also had better social and occupational function at 18 months, but not earlier.

Zaretsky et al [88] applied the cognitive-behavioural techniques outlined in the manual by Basco and Rush [55] in an open trial of 11 bipolar patients currently depressed. They delivered 20 weekly individual sessions and tracked symptom levels and dysfunctional attitudes. Three of the 11 dropped out and their data were deleted from the analysis rather than using the more typical last-value-carried-forward method. They report significant reductions compared to baseline in several measures of depression and automatic thoughts, but not in dysfunctional attitudes. In a case-control post-hoc comparison, a sample of unipolar depressed patients showed both symptomatic and attitudinal improvement compared to baseline.

Lam et al [57] implemented a randomized controlled trial of cognitive therapy adapted for bipolar disorder in 25 outpatients who received either the intervention or no added treatment. Their manual-based intervention consisted of 12–20 individual sessions over six months focusing on standard cognitive approaches plus psychoeducation specifically about bipolar disorder, behavioural skills to cope with prodromal symptoms, and coping with functional sequelae of the illness. They found that, compared to the control group, those treated with cognitive therapy had fewer total and hypomanic episodes without difference in depressive episodes, and higher social function. The intervention group also showed better scores at coping with prodromal manic symptoms at six and 12 months and with prodromal depressive symptoms by 12 months.

Miklowitz et al [89] report a randomized controlled trial of Family-Focused Therapy (FFT) vs. no additional treatment in 101 bipolar in- or outpatients. FFT is manual-based and consists of three modules of one-hour family or couples sessions given weekly to monthly in the patient's home over nine months, and is an outgrowth of Behavioral Family Management developed by Miklowitz and Goldstein [90]. The first module consists of psychoeducation about the disorder, including identification and management of prodromal symptoms and development of a management plan. The second module focuses on improving intrafamilial communication to reduce stress. The third module focuses on continued problem solving during ongoing treatment. They found that over one year FFT patients had fewer relapses and greater time to relapse than controls, as well as greater improvement of depressive but not manic symptoms. There was no effect on medication adherence. Although high EE did not in itself predict relapse or symptoms scores over time, patients with high-EE families showed the greatest improvement in symptom scores under FFT, consistent with the theoretical underpinnings of the treatment. Further, additional analyses [91] indicated that families of patients treated with FFT showed more positive nonverbal interactions than did control families, although no reduction in negative nonverbal interactions was seen.

Weiss et al [92] developed Integrated Group Treatment (IGT) to address the needs of patients with comorbid bipolar disorder and substance dependence. IGT focuses on the commonalities in recovery and relapse across the two disorders and implements a set of cognitive-behavioural relapse prevention strategies. The intervention is manual-based and is given in 12 and subsequently 20 weekly hour-long sessions. They conducted an open study that enrolled sequential blocks of patients either in IGT ($n = 21$) or no added treatment ($n = 24$) and investigated effects on substance use and its impact, mood symptoms, and compliance. They measured outcome over six months and then three months post-treatment. In terms of substance use outcome, patients showed improvement in most (but not all) formal ratings of drug and alcohol use, including months abstinent. In terms of mood symptoms, they found improvement in mania ratings but not depression ratings. Reported medication compliance was high but not different across the groups. Hospitalization rates did not differ across the groups.

One additional study, not published at the time of this writing but may be by the time of publication, deserves specific mention. In a recent randomized controlled trial of family therapy developed by I.W. Miller and colleagues (presented in scientific meetings, as summarized in [93]), single-family and multi-family group interventions produced better recovery rates than no added intervention, and the two family treatments did not differ. Patients with poor family function prior to treatment were reported to benefit from the family interventions while those with good function showed no difference in outcome.

ADDITIONAL PSYCHOTHERAPY STUDIES AND "HOW-TO" PSYCHOTHERAPY RESOURCES

To complement the above quantitative studies, a wealth of anecdotal or qualitative literature exists on the psychotherapy of bipolar disorder. These studies are often valuable for the detailed descriptions and/or case vignettes they contain of particular types of interventions. As such they may serve as "how-to" references to aid investigators and clinicians seeking to implement a particular modality. Table 4.3 includes a select list of references that seemed particularly valuable in this regard. Some of these refer to interventions reviewed above, while others are chosen as examples that illustrate application of a particular general approach (e.g., psychodynamic, psychoeducational) in bipolar disorder.

CONTEXTS OF CARE

Lithium Clinics

As noted above, psychotherapeutic interventions primarily utilize individual or team therapists to address issues with individual patients or groups who receive care together. An additional type of psychosocial

TABLE 4.3 "How-to" references for psychosocial interventions in bipolar disorder

Area	Suggested references
A. Psychotherapy	
Psychodynamic-Psychoanalytic	Cohen et al [35]; Teixeira [94]; Kahn [95]; Jackson [36]
Marital	Fitzgerald [37]; Greene et al [38]; Lesser [96]; van Gent and Zwart [72]
Family	Miklowitz and Goldstein [97]; Weber et al [98]
Cognitive-Behavioural	Basco and Rush [55]; Scott [53, 54]; Lam et al [99]
Interpersonal (Individual)	Frank et al [100]
Interpersonal (Interactive Group)	Volkmar et al [68]; Pollack [49]; Graves [101]; Wuslin et al [102]
Psychoeducation	Powell et al [103]; Kripke and Robinson [50]; Foelker et al [104]; Bauer and McBride [51]; Bauer and McBride [105]
Patient education for chronic medical conditions	Lorig et al [2]
Useful psychotherapy reviews	Goodwin and Jamison [79]; Colom et al [106]; Craighead et al [93]; Swartz and Frank [65]; Huxley et al [107]
B. Contexts of care	
Lithium clinics	Fieve [108]; Gitlin and Jamison [108]; Seeger et al [110]
Multi-modal care delivery systems	Shea et al [111]; Bauer et al [112]

intervention is the organization of the care-giving system itself. The recent burgeoning of interest in manipulating contexts of care to optimize treatment for bipolar disorder actually has its roots as far back as the 1970s.

With the dissemination of lithium for the treatment of bipolar disorder in that decade, the conceptual approach to treatment shifted from a predominantly psychotherapeutic to a medical model approach, as outlined in the introduction. The impact of this shift can be seen from contrasting some of the pre-lithium psychoanalytic references cited (e.g., [34, 35]) to traditional psychotherapeutic references from early in the lithium era (e.g., [37, 38]). The earlier references treated bipolar disorder as psychological in origin and in need of solely psychological treatment. However, the latter psychoanalytic references, although employing a strong psychotherapeutic emphasis, work from a perspective that assumes that integrated psychotherapeutic and medical model treatment is necessary. Thus virtually all psychotherapeutic interventions for bipolar disorder, even psychoanalytic (e.g., [95]), embrace to some degree a bio- as well as psychosocial model for treatment of bipolar disorder.

The issue of how to organize medical model treatment was explored by clinicians treating large numbers of patients with bipolar disorder. There seemed to be potential efficiencies and opportunities for standardization of care if patients were treated in specialty clinics staffed by physicians and support staff who were comfortable with dealing with the disorder. In turn, concentration of patients with the same staff allowed development of further expertise. Additionally, in community mental health systems, financial limitations made it advantageous for psychiatrists to work in teams with non-physician providers to implement care for this group (e.g., [112]).

Information about lithium clinics comes both from early description of programs (e.g., [104, 107, 109, 110]) and from a survey of programs by Gitlin and Jamison [108]. Typically, lithium clinics use a team approach including psychiatrist, nurse or other medical paraprofessional, and sometimes social worker or other counsellor. Standardized patient and family information comprise part of the assessment for all patients in most clinics. Importantly for quality of care, a standardized battery of baseline and follow-up labs are implemented. Follow-up appointments are provided at regular intervals. All of the standardization not only supports high-quality care but also the conduct of research as a common database evolved on all patients. Unfortunately, there are to our knowledge no quantitative data on the impact of lithium clinics.

This emphasis on medical model efficiency did not, however, mean that psychotherapy was neglected. On the contrary, it was recognized from the earliest days of these clinics that psychotherapeutic interventions were necessary to optimize medical model management. Most notable is that several types of psychotherapeutic interventions (e.g., psychoeducation, interpersonal process groups) evolved as part of lithium clinics (e.g., [50, 103, 104, 113, 114]).

More Recently Developed Contexts of Care: Manual-Based Interventions and Controlled Clinical Trials

Neither lithium nor the plethora of more recently developed medications have proven to be the panacea for bipolar disorder. As the availability of treatment of proven efficacy for bipolar disorder has grown, so has the complexity of treatment. Further, the problems of adherence and patient knowledge deficit continue, and provider knowledge deficit regarding the ever-widening range of available treatments also becomes an issue. All these contribute to what has been called the "efficacy-effectiveness gap" for bipolar disorder [111], as has been recognized for other illnesses as well [115]. This term refers to the difference between the performance of an intervention in highly controlled trials (efficacy) and its performance in real-world clinical practice (effectiveness). At least two randomized controlled trials are underway currently that investigate care organization interventions specifically designed to improve effectiveness—i.e., improved delivery and acceptance by patients of optimal medication management—of treatment for bipolar disorder.

The first such intervention is a randomized controlled trial of a tripartite intervention for patients treated in the VA health care system. This study randomly assigns patients hospitalized for bipolar disorder at the point of discharge either to continue usual care or to enter the Bipolar Disorders Program (BDP; study described in detail in [111]). The BDP addresses three aspects of treatment: patient education, provider education, and access and continuity to a consistent team of caregivers. Patient education is administered through the psychoeducational component (Phase 1) of Bauer and McBride [51, 105] reviewed above. Provider education is supplied through an adaptation of the VA treatment guidelines for bipolar disorder (reviewed in [64]). Access and continuity are provided by a primary mental health nurse who implements manual-based procedures to ensure timely access to care for the patient (described in [111, 112, 116]). Preliminary data from an open pre/post design indicated reductions in service utilization and cost of almost 50% with the BDP compared to pre-BDP, as well as improvement in several process measures thought to be markers for quality of care [117]. Of additional relevance to the issue of psychotherapy for bipolar disorder, one of the major predictors of service utilization in this cohort was a history of childhood physical or sexual abuse [118]. This suggests that psychotherapeutic interventions aimed at these issues may improve outcome and reduce costs for bipolar disorder. The current randomized controlled trial of the BDP vs. usual VA care is tracking clinical outcome, functional outcome, and health care costs over three years of prospective follow-up in 330 subjects across 11 hospitals coast- to-coast. It is due to finish in 2003.

Similarly, in another staff model health care organization, the Group Health Cooperative (GHC) of Puget Sound, Greg Simon and coworkers are funded by the US NIMH to test a similar programme designed to provide patient education, patient-level feedback to providers, and improved access to patients with bipolar disorder [119]. This programme has enrolled 441 outpatients with bipolar disorder in various phases of their illness and randomized them either to receive a multi-modal program to optimize treatment, or to no added care. Their programme, implemented across three sites in the greater Seattle area, consists of both phases of the Life Goals Program summarized above [51, 105] to address both psychoeducational and functional needs of patients plus computer-guided medication treatment algorithm recommendations that are provided for treating psychiatrists. A nurse clinician provides telephone outreach to the patient and liaison for the treating psychiatrists involved. Clinical and functional outcome and healthcare costs are being tracked over two years.

The GHC intervention provides an interesting comparison with the VA BDP in several respects. Both interventions are being tested in samples designed to reflect the populations from which they are being drawn, rather than using highly selected patients. Both interventions address the same triad of aspects of care: access, patient education, and provider guidance. Both approach patients as important collaborators in the management of their illness.

On the other hand, there are several ways in which the GHC study will be complementary to the VA study. First, it studies outpatients rather than patients who are sufficiently ill as to require acute hospitalization. Second, there are several demographic differences between the samples, with the GHC sample being of generally higher socioeconomic status and of fairly even gender distribution. Third, the GHC intervention does not control all aspects of treatment, but rather provides information and feedback to treating psychiatrists who are not trained in the research intervention. To do so it uses sophisticated computer technology to convey algorithm recommendations through nurse facilitators to treating psychiatrists. In contrast, the VA BDP takes over responsibility for outpatient treatment of bipolar disorder, but emphasizes collaboration with other clinicians on an as-needed basis for management of medical and psychiatric comorbidities.

SUMMARY

Common Themes Across Psychosocial Modalities

Qualitative inspection of the studies reviewed above reveals certain themes and consistencies that appear in multiple interventions. First, and by definition, psychotherapy presupposes a collaborative practice approach to managing bipolar disorder. This collaboration includes patient, provider, and where possible partner or family members. Rather than a paternalistic, order-following approach to treatment, all interventions expect the patient and significant others to become educated regarding the illness and to become partners in managing it. Although the specific methods and priorities may differ somewhat (e.g., work with couples, group work with patients, individual cognitive interventions), this theme is perhaps most evident across all modalities. The care organization interventions of Bauer *et al* [111, 116] and Simon and coworkers [119] also build upon this basic collaborative approach.

Second, few interventions manage the patient in isolation. Family or couples interventions have been tested in those whose social network has not unravelled. In those interventions that work with a less select group, the individual is often seen as part of a group, to enhance social support, reinforce teaching, and combat stigma and demoralization.

Third, the degree of convergent validity regarding agenda for disease management information and skills to be imparted is impressive. Specifically, imparting education, focusing on early warning symptoms and triggers of episodes, and developing detailed and patient-specific action plans are an important part of such diverse approaches as the cognitive-behavioural interventions of Palmer and Williams [76] and Lam et al [57]; the psychoeducational interventions of Bauer et al [85], Perry et al [87], and Weiss et al [92]; the IPSRT intervention of Frank et al [43]; and the family intervention of Miklowitz et al [97].

Thus, given the positive results most of these interventions with explicit disease management components—patient education, collaborative management strategies with the patient, inclusion of as wide a social support system as is available—have produced, it is likely that this basic approach will be critical. It will, perhaps, be more critical even than the specific type of intervention in which these disease management components are embedded.

Consistent Evidence

Table 4.4 reanalyses the studies summarized in Table 4.2 in order to identify patterns of efficacy across interventions and across three outcome domains. Interventions have been grouped into roughly similar categories based on the target group or type of intervention, and the class of evidence is noted for each study. Outcome domains include indices of clinical outcome (e.g., symptom ratings, hospitalization rates), functional outcome (e.g., social, occupational, or family function), and disease management skills (e.g., adherence to treatment, knowledge about illness). Studies are categorized, as in Table 4.2, as positive, negative, or equivocal for each outcome domain, with studies listed as positive if any of multiple measures within that domain were positive.

Such lumping of studies and data can be questioned (e.g., How similar are Davenport and Clarkin's interventions? Can one really consider as similar lithium adherence and a paper and pencil test of disease knowledge?). However, it is also a useful method with which to look for general patterns so that general recommendations for researchers and clinicians can be formulated.

From this retabulation we can first of all see that most of the published studies have reported at least some positive results. There is no evidence that the more rigorous studies (Class A) are less frequently positive than less

TABLE 4.4 Patterns of efficacy across psychotherapy type and outcome domain

Intervention	Clinical outcome	Functional outcome	Disease management skills
Couples/Partners	+ Davenport et al [39] (C) − Clarkin et al [84] (A)	+ Davenport et al [39] (C) + Honig et al [77] (A/B) + Clarkin et al [84] (A)	+ van Gent and Zwart [72] (A) − Clarkin et al [84] (A)
Group, interpersonal and/or psychoeducational	+ Volkmar et al [68] (C) + Kripke and Robinson [50] (C) + van Gent et al [48]; van Gent and Zwart [70] (C) + Cerbone et al [75] (C) + Weiss et al [92] (B)	+ Volkmar et al [68] (C) + Kripke and Robinson [50] (C) + Cerbone et al [75] (C) + Bauer et al [85] (B)	+ van Gent et al [48]; van Gent and Zwart [70] (C) + Cerbone et al [75] (C) + Bauer et al [85] (B) − Weiss et al [92] (B)
Cognitive-behavioural	+/− Palmer and Williams [76] (B) + Zaretsky et al [88] (B) + Lam et al [57] (A)	+/− Palmer and Williams [76] (B) + Lam et al [57] (A)	+/− Cochran [69] (A)
Family	+ Clarkin et al [71] (A) + Retzer et al [74] (C) + Miklowitz et al [89] (A)	+ Clarkin et al [71] (A)	− Miklowitz et al [89] (A)
Interpersonal/Social rhythms	− Hlastala et al [78] (A) − Frank et al [86] (A)		
Individual psychoeducation	+ Perry et al [87] (A)	+ Perry et al [87] (A)	+ Peet and Harvey [73] (A)
Other/Eclectic	+ Benson [67] (C)		

Studies from Table 4.2, reanalysed by type of intervention, positive (+), negative (−), or equivocal (+/−) impact on the outcome domain noted, and quality of evidence (A, B, or C). See text for details.

rigorous studies (Classes B and C). This overall high rate of positive results is not surprising given the bias against submitting (and/or accepting by peer-reviewed journals) negative studies in the peer-reviewed literature.

Perhaps the most surprising exception to overall positive results across interventions is the case of IPSRT, which showed no difference between the intervention and the control arm of no intervention added to clinical management either acutely [78] or in terms of relapse prevention [43]. This may say more about the efficacy of the control arm's good clinical management at this centre of expertise (which no doubt includes many of the disease management characteristics noted in the preceding section) than it does about the lack of utility of IPSRT in improving outcome of the disorder.

Second, there appears to be no type of intervention that is more typically positive in its results. This may either be a nonspecific finding (e.g., due to bias in publication) or due to the fact that most or all of these programmes contain the same core of sensible disease management components outlined in the preceding section.

Third, it appears that psychotherapeutic interventions may be able to improve not only clinical outcome, but functional outcome as well. Interventions to improve functional outcome in bipolar disorder are sorely needed, as available data indicate substantial functional impairment even in the absence of clinical symptoms (see the introduction). Thus, the fact that clinical and functional outcome are to some degree orthogonal [24] highlights the need to develop treatments specifically targeted at functional outcome.

Incomplete Evidence

Clearly it will be advantageous to move several of the studies with positive results in Class B and C studies into testing at the Class A level. Individual areas for future research are outlined below.

Areas Still Open to Research

If, as proposed above, all of the major psychosocial approaches include the common core of disease management components outlined above—education, collaboration, social support inclusion—the critical issue becomes whether benefit derives from these core disease management components, or from the specific aspects of the intervention (e.g., working with families, group work, cognitive techniques). It will be interesting to see whether the US NIMH's Systematic Treatment Enhancement Program (STEP, Principal

Investigators: Gary Sachs, Michael Thase), which is studying various types of psychotherapies in conjunction with various types of medications, is able to address this issue.

Further, this drive to isolate the active components of these interventions should always look toward issues of parsimony, since the most cost-effective interventions are likely to be the most widely disseminated. Specifically, cost-utility analyses (from the patient's and society's perspectives) and cost-minimization studies (which will be the primary concern of the payor), will both be of great importance.

Finally, there are as yet no Class A data on the efficacy or cost-effectiveness (broadly defined) of specific contexts of care. However, data are in the pipeline from studies funded by the US VA Department and NIMH. Results from these staff-model health maintenance organizations (HMOs) will likely be useful in identifying principles for organizing care in other types of care delivery systems for bipolar disorder and perhaps for other types of serious mental illness.

ACKNOWLEDGEMENTS

Portions of this chapter are reprinted from Bauer M., McBride L. (2002) *Structured Group Psychotherapy for Bipolar Disorder: The Life Goals Program*, 2nd Ed. Springer, New York. This work was supported in part by US Department of Veterans Affairs Cooperative Study Program #430.

REFERENCES

1. Kaplan S.H., Greenfield S., Ware J.E. (1989) Assessing the effects of physician–patient interactions on the outcomes of chronic disease. *Med. Care*, **27**: S110–S127 and 679.
2. Lorig K., Holman H., Sobel D., Laurent D., Gonzalez V., Minor M. (1994) *Living a Health Life with Chronic Conditions*. Bull Publishing Company, Palo Alto.
3. Wagner E.H., Austin B.T., von Korff M. (1996) Organizing care for patients with chronic illness. *Milbank Quarterly*, **74**: 511–544.
4. Von Korff M., Gruman J., Schaefer J., Curry S.J., Wagner E.H. (1997) Collaborative management of chronic illness. *Ann. Intern. Med.*, **127**: 1097–1102.
5. Ciechanowski P.S., Katon W.J., Russo J.E., Walker E.A. (2001) The patient–provider relationship: attachment theory and adherence to treatment in diabetes. *Am. J. Psychiatry*, **158**: 29–35.
6. Keller M., Lavori P., Coryell W., Andreasen N., Endicott J., Clayton P., Klerman G., Hirschfeld R. (1986) Differential outcome of episodes of illness in bipolar patients. Pure manic, mixed/cycling, and pure depressive. *JAMA*, **255**: 3138–3142.
7. Harrow M., Goldberg J., Grossman L., Meltzer H. (1990) Outcome in manic disorders. A naturalistic follow-up study. *Arch. Gen. Psychiatry*, **47**: 665–671.

8. O'Connell R., Mayo J., Flatow L., Cuthbertson B., O'Brien B. (1991) Outcome of bipolar disorder on long-term treatment with lithium. *Br. J. Psychiatry*, **159**: 123–129.
9. Gitlin M.J., Cochran S.D., Jamison K.R. (1989) Maintenance lithium treatment: side effects and compliance. *J. Clin. Psychiatry*, **50**: 127–131.
10. Harvey N.S., Peet M. (1991) Lithium maintenance. 2. Effects of personality and attitude on health information acquisition and compliance. *Br. J. Psychiatry*, **158**: 200–204.
11. Lee S., Wing Y.K., Wong K.C. (1992) Knowledge and compliance towards lithium therapy among Chinese psychiatric patients in Hong Kong. *Aust. N.Z. J. Psychiatry*, **26**: 444–448.
12. Keck P., McElroy S., Strakowski S., Bourne M., West S. (1997) Compliance with maintenance treatment in bipolar disorder. *Psychopharmacol. Bull.*, **33**: 87–91.
13. Ellicott A., Hammen C., Gitlin M., Brown G., Jamison K. (1990) Life events and the course of bipolar disorder. *Am. J. Psychiatry*, **147**: 1194–1198.
14. Johnson S., Roberts J.R. (1995) Life events and bipolar disorder: implications from biological theories. *Psychol. Bull.*, **117**: 434–449.
15. Johnson S.L., Winett C.A., Meyer B., Miller I. (1999) Social support and the course of bipolar disorder. *J. Abnorm. Psychol.*, **108**: 558–566.
16. Johnson S., Greenhouse W., Bauer M. (1999) Psychosocial approaches to the treatment of bipolar disorder. *Curr. Opin. Psychiatry*, **13**: 69–72.
17. Winokur G., Clayton P., Reich T. (1969) *Manic-Depressive Illness*. Mosby, St Louis.
18. Carlson G., Kotin J., Davenport Y., Adland M. (1974) Follow-up of 53 bipolar manic depressive patients. *Br. J. Psychiatry*, **124**: 134–139.
19. Dion G., Tohen M., Anthony W., Waternaux C. (1988) Symptoms and functioning of patients with bipolar disorder six months after hospitalization. *Hosp. Commun. Psychiatry*, **39**: 652–657.
20. Coryell W., Keller M., Endicott J., Andreasen N.C., Clayton P., Hirschfeld R. (1989) Bipolar II illness: course and outcome over a five-year period. *Psychol. Med.*, **19**: 129–141.
21. Tohen M., Waternaux C., Tsuang M. (1990) Outcome in mania. A 4-year prospective follow-up of 75 patients utilizing survival analysis. *Arch. Gen. Psychiatry*, **47**: 1106–1111.
22. Keck P.E. Jr., McElroy S.L., Strakowski S.M., West S.A., Sax K.W., Hawkins J.M., Bourne M.L., Haggard P. (1998) 12-month outcome of patients with bipolar disorder following hospitalization for a manic or mixed episode. *Am. J. Psychiatry*, **155**: 646–652.
23. Strakowski S.M., Keck P.E. Jr., McElroy S.L., West S.A., Sax K.W., Hawkins J.M., Kmetz G.F., Upadhyaya V.H., Tugrul K.C., Bourne M.L. (1998) Twelve-month outcome after a first hospitalization for affective psychosis. *Arch. Gen. Psychiatry*, **55**: 49–55.
24. Bauer M.S., Kirk G., Gavin C., Williford W. (2001) Correlates of functional and economic outcome in bipolar disorder. a prospective study. *J. Affect. Disord.* (in press).
25. National Advisory Mental Health Council (NAMC) (1993) Health care reform for Americans with severe mental illness: report of the National Advisory Mental Health Council. *Am. J. Psychiatry*, **150**: 1445–1465.
26. Greenberg P.E., Stiglin L.E., Finkelstein S.N., Berndt E.R. (1990) The economic burden of depression in 1990. *J. Clin. Psychiatry*, **54**: 405–418.

27. Stoudemire A., Frank R., Hedemark N., Kamlet M., Blazer D. (1986) The economic burden of depression. *Gen. Hosp. Psychiatry*, **8**: 387–394.
28. Wyatt R.J., Hentner I. (1995) An economic evaluation of manic-depressive illness—1991. *Soc. Psychiatry Psychiatr. Epidemiol.*, **30**: 213–219.
29. Riefman A., Wyatt R.J. (1980) Lithium: a brake in the rising cost of mental illness. *Arch. Gen. Psychiatry*, **37**: 385–388.
30. Department of Health, Education and Welfare Medical Practice Project (1979) *A State-of-the-Science Report for the Office of the Assistant Secretary for the US Department of Health, Education, and Welfare*. Policy Research, Baltimore.
31. Klerman G., Olfson M., Leon A., Weissman M. (1992) Measuring the need for mental health care. *Health Affairs*, **11**: 23–33.
32. Robins L., Regier D. (1990) *Psychiatric Disorders in America. The Epidemiologic Catchment Area Study*. Free Press, New York.
33. Beahrs J.O., Gutheil T. (2001) Informed consent in psychotherapy. *Am. J. Psychiatry*, **158**: 4–10.
34. Fromm-Reichmann F. (1949) Intensive psychotherapy of manic-depressives: a preliminary report. *Confinia Neurologica*, **9**: 158–165.
35. Cohen M.B., Baker G., Cohen R.A., Fromm-Reichmann F., Weigert E.V. (1954) An intensive study of twelve cases of manic-depressive psychosis. *Psychiatry*, **17**: 103–137.
36. Jackson M. (1993) Manic-depressive psychosis: psychopathology and individual psychotherapy within a psychodynamic milieu. *Psychoanal. Psychother.*, **7**: 103–133.
37. Fitzgerald R.G. (1972) Treatment with family therapy and lithium carbonate. *Am. J. Psychother.*, **26**: 547–553.
38. Greene B.L., Lee R.R., Lustig N. (1975) Treatment of marital disharmony where one spouse has a primary affective disorder (manic depressive illness): I. General overview—100 couples. *J. Marriage Family Counseling*, **1**: 39–50.
39. Davenport Y.B., Ebert M., Adland M.L., Goodwin F.K. (1977) Couples group therapy as an adjunct to lithium maintenance of the manic patient. *Am. J. Orthopsychiatry*, **47**: 495–502.
40. Vaughan C.E., Leff J.P. (1976) The influences of family and social factors on the course of psychiatric illness. *Br. J. Psychiatry*, **129**: 125–137.
41. Miklowitz D.J., Goldstein M.J. (1988) Family factors and the course of bipolar affective disorder. *Arch. Gen. Psychiatry*, **45**: 225–231.
42. Simoneau T.L., Miklowitz D.J., Richards J.A., Saleem R. (1998) Expressed emotion and interactional patterns in the families of bipolar patients. *J. Abnorm. Psychol.*, **107**: 497–507.
43. Frank E., Swartz H., Kupfer D. (2000) Interpersonal and social rhythm therapy: managing the chaos of bipolar disorder. *Biol. Psychiatry*, **48**: 593–604.
44. Klerman G.L., Weissmann M.M., Rounsaville B.J. (1984) *Interpersonal Psychotherapy of Depression*. Basic Books, New York.
45. Kufferle B. (1988) Group dynamics as an emotional turmoil precipitating psychotic manifestations. *Psychopathology*, **21**: 111–115.
46. Yalom I.D. (1975) *The Theory and Practice of Group Psychotherapy*. Basic Books, New York.
47. Shakir S.A., Volkmar F.R., Bacon S., Pfefferbaum A. (1979) Group psychotherapy as an adjunct to lithium maintenance. *Am. J. Psychiatry*, **136**: 455–456.
48. Van Gent E.M., Vida S.L., Zwart F.M. (1988) Group therapy in addition to lithium therapy in patients with bipolar disorders. *Acta Psychiatr. Belg.*, **88**: 405–418.

49. Pollack L.E. (1990) Improving relationships: groups for inpatients with bipolar disorder. *J. Psychiatr. Nursing*, **28**: 17–22.
50. Kripke D.F., Robinson D. (1985) Ten years with a lithium group. *McLean Hosp. J.*, **10**: 1–11.
51. Bauer M.S., McBride L. (1996) *Structured Group Psychotherapy for Bipolar Disorder: The Life Goals Program*. Springer, New York.
52. Beck A.T., Rush A.J., Shaw B.F., Emery G. (1979) *Cognitive Therapy of Depression*. Guilford, New York.
53. Scott J. (1996) The role of cognitive behavior therapy in bipolar disorder. *Behav. Cogn. Psychother.*, **24**: 195–208.
54. Scott J. (1996) Cognitive therapy for clients with bipolar disorder. *Cogn. Behav. Pract.*, **3**: 29–51.
55. Basco M., Rush A.J. (1996) *Cognitive Behavioral Therapy for Bipolar Disorder*. Guilford, New York.
56. Reilly-Harrington N.A., Alloy L.B., Fresco D.M., Whitehouse W.G. (1999) Cognitive styles and life events interact to predict bipolar and unipolar symptomatology. *J. Abnorm. Psychol.*, **108**: 567–578.
57. Lam D.H., Bright J., Jones S., Hayward P., Schuck N., Chisolm D., Sham P. (2000) Cognitive therapy for bipolar illness—a pilot study of relapse prevention. *Cogn. Ther. Res.*, **24**: 503–520.
58. Hastings D. (1989) Self-management in bipolar affective disorder. *Can. J. Psychiatry Nursing*, **30**: 20–22.
59. Irwig L., Tosteson A.N., Gatsonis C., Lau J., Colditz G., Chalmers T.C., Mosteller F. (1994) Guidelines for meta-analyses evaluating diagnostic tests. *Ann. Intern. Med.*, **120**: 667–676.
60. Evidence-Based Working Group (EBMG) (1997) A new approach to teaching the practice of medicine. *JAMA*, **268**: 2420–2425.
61. Chalmers I. (1993) The Cochrane Collaboration: preparing, maintaining, and disseminating systematic reviews of the effects of health care. *Ann. N.Y. Acad. Sci.*, **703**: 156–163.
62. American College of Cardiology/American Heart Association (ACC/AHA) Task Force on Practice Guidelines (1996) ACC/AHA guidelines for the management of patients with acute myocardial infarction. *J. Am. Coll. Cardiol.*, **28**: 1328–1428.
63. DHHS PHS Agency for Health Care Policy and Research (1993) *Depression in Primary Care*, Volume 1. *Detection and Diagnosis*, USGPO Publication #93–0550. USGPO, Washington.
64. Bauer M.S., Callahan A., Jampala C., Petty F., Sajatovic M., Schaefer V., Wittlin B., Powell B. (1999) Clinical practice guidelines for bipolar disorder from the Department of Veterans Affairs. *J. Clin. Psychiatry*, **60**: 9–21.
65. Swartz H.A., Frank E. (2001) Psychotherapy for bipolar depression: a phase-specific treatment strategy? *Bipolar Disord.*, **3**: 11–22.
66. Craighead W.E., Miklowitz D.J., Vajc F.C., Frank E. (1998) Psychosocial treatments for bipolar disorder. In *A Guide to Treatments that Work* (Eds P.E. Nathan, J.M. Gorman) pp. 240–248, Oxford University Press, New York.
67. Benson R. (1975) The forgotten treatment modality in bipolar illness: psychotherapy. *Dis. Nerv. Syst.*, **36**: 634–638.
68. Volkmar F.R., Bacon S., Shakir S., Pfefferbaum A. (1981) Group therapy in the management of manic-depressive illness. *Am. J. Psychother.*, **35**: 226–234.
69. Cochran S. (1984) Preventing medical noncompliance in the outpatient treatment of bipolar affective disorders. *J. Consult. Clin. Psychol.*, **52**: 873–878.

70. Van Gent E.M., Zwart F.M. (1993) Five year follow-up after educational group therapy added to lithium prophylaxis: five years after group added to lithium. *Depression*, **1**: 225–226.
71. Clarkin J.F., Glick I., Haas G., Spencer J., Lewis A., Peyser J., DeMane N., Good-Ellis M., Harris E., Lestell V. (1990) A randomized clinical trial of inpatient family intervention. V. Results for affective disorder. *J. Affect. Disord.*, **18**: 17–28.
72. Van Gent E.M., Zwart F.M. (1991) Psychoeducation of partners of bipolar-manic patients. *J. Affect. Disord.*, **21**: 15–18.
73. Peet M., Harvey N.S. (1991) Lithium maintenance: 1. A standard education programme for patients. *Br. J. Psychiatry*, **158**: 197–200.
74. Retzer A., Simon F.B., Weber G., Stierlin H., Schmidt G. (1991) A followup study of manic-depressive and schizoaffective psychoses after systemic family therapy. *Family Process*, **30**: 139–153.
75. Cerbone M., Mayo J., Cuthbertson B., O'Connell R.A. (1992) Group therapy as an adjunct to medication in the management of bipolar affective disorder. *Group*, **16**: 174–187.
76. Palmer A.G., Williams H. (1995) CBT in a group format for bipolar affective disorder. *Behav. Cogn. Psychother.*, **23**: 153–168.
77. Honig A., Hofman A., Rozendaal N., Dingemans P. (1997) Psycho-education in bipolar disorder: effect on expressed emotion. *Psychiatry Res.*, **72**: 17–22.
78. Hlastala S.A., Frank E., Mallinger A.G., Thase M.E., Ritenour A.M., Kupfer D.J. (1997) Bipolar depression: an underestimated treatment challenge. *Depress. Anxiety*, **5**: 73–83.
79. Goodwin F.K., Jamison K. (1990) *Manic-Depressive Illness*, Oxford University Press, New York.
80. Wehr T.A., Sack D.A., Rosenthal N.E. (1987) Sleep reduction as a final common pathway in the genesis of mania. *Am. J. Psychiatry*, **144**: 201–204.
81. Carney P.A., Fitzgerald C.T., Monaghan C.E. (1988) Influence of climate on the prevalence of mania. *Br. J. Psychiatry*, **152**: 820–823.
82. Gottschalk A., Bauer M., Whybrow P. (1995) Evidence for chaotic mood variation in bipolar disorder. *Arch. Gen. Psychiatry*, **53**: 947–959.
83. Klerman G.L., DiMascio A., Weissman M., Prusoff B., Paykel E.S. (1974) Treatment of depression by drugs and psychotherapy. *Am. J. Psychiatry*, **131**: 186–191.
84. Clarkin J.F., Carpenter D., Hull J., Wilner P., Glick I. (1998) Effects of psychoeducational intervention for married patients with bipolar disorder and their spouses. *Psychiatr. Serv.*, **49**: 531–533.
85. Bauer M.S., McBride L., Chase C., Sachs G., Shea N. (1998) Manual-based group psychotherapy for bipolar disorder: a feasibility study. *J. Clin. Psychiatry*, **59**: 449–455.
86. Frank E., Swartz H., Mallinger A.G., Thase M.E., Weaver E.V., Kupfer D.J. (1999) Adjunctive psychotherapy for bipolar disorder: effects of changing treatment modality. *J. Abnorm. Psychol.*, **108**: 579–587.
87. Perry A., Tarrier N., Morriss R., McCarthy E., Limb K. (1999) Randomised controlled trial of efficacy of teaching patients with bipolar disorder to identify early symptoms of relapse and obtain treatment. *Br. Med. J.*, **318**: 149–153.
88. Zaretsky A.E., Segal Z.V., Gemar M. (1999) Cognitive therapy for bipolar depression: a pilot study. *Can. J. Psychiatry*, **44**: 491–494.
89. Miklowitz D.J., Simoneau T.L., George E.L., Richards J.A., Kalbag A., Sachs-Ericsson N., Suddath R. (2000) Family-focused treatment of bipolar disorder: 1-year effects of a psychoeducational program in conjunction with pharmacotherapy. *Biol. Psychiatry*, **48**: 582–592.

90. Miklowitz D.J., Goldstein M.J. (1990) Behavioral family treatment for patients with bipolar affective disorder. *Behav. Modif.*, **14**: 457–489.

91. Simoneau T.L., Miklowitz D.J., Richards J.A., Saleem R., George E.L. (2000) Bipolar disorder and family communication: effects of a psychoeducational treatment program. *J. Abnorm. Psychol.*, **108**: 588–597.

92. Weiss R.D., Griffin M.L., Greenfield S.F., Najavits L.M., Wyner D., Soto J.A., Hennen J.A. (2000) Group therapy for patients with bipolar disorder and substance dependence: results of a pilot study. *J. Clin. Psychiatry*, **61**: 361–367.

93. Craighead W.E., Miklowitz D.J., Vajc F.C., Frank E. (2000) Psychosocial interventions for bipolar disorder. *J. Clin. Psychiatry*, **61** (Suppl. 13): 58–64.

94. Teixeira M.A. (1992) Psychoanalytic theory and therapy in the treatment of manic-depressive disorders. *Psychoanal. Psychother.*, **11**: 162–177.

95. Kahn D.A. (1993) The use of psychodynamic psychotherapy in manic-depressive illness. *J. Am. Acad. Psychoanal.*, **21**: 441–455.

96. Lesser A.L. (1983) Hypomania and marital conflict. *Can. J. Psychiatry*, **28**: 362–366.

97. Miklowitz D.J., Goldstein M.J. (1997) *Bipolar Disorder: A Family-Focused Treatment Approach*. Guilford, New York.

98. Weber G., Simon F.B., Stierlin H., Schmidt G. (1988) Therapy for families manifesting manic-depressive behavior. *Family Process*, **27**: 33–49.

99. Lam D.H., Jones S.H., Hayward P., Bright J.A. (1999) *Cognitive Therapy for Bipolar Disorder. A Therapist's Guide to Concepts, Methods, and Practice*. Wiley, New York.

100. Frank E., Kupfer D.J., Ehlers C.L., Monk T.H., Cornes C., Carter S., Frankel D. (1994) Interpersonal and social rhythm therapy for bipolar disorder: integrating interpersonal and behavioral approaches. *Behav. Ther.*, **17**: 143–149.

101. Graves J.S. (1993) Living with mania: a study of outpatient group psychotherapy for bipolar patients. *Am. J. Psychother.*, **47**: 113–126.

102. Wulsin L., Bachop M., Hoffman D. (1988) Group therapy in manic-depressive illness. *Am. J. Psychother.*, **42**: 263–271.

103. Powell B.J., Othmer E., Sinkhorn C. (1977) Pharmacological aftercare for homogeneous groups of patients. *Hosp. Commun. Psychiatry*, **28**: 125–127.

104. Foelker G.A. Jr., Molinari V., Marmion J.J., Chacko R.C. (1986) Lithium groups and elderly bipolar outpatients. *Clin. Gerontol.*, **5**: 297–307.

105. Bauer M.S., McBride L. (1997) Psychoeducation: conceptual framework and practical considerations. *J. Pract. Psychiatry Behav. Health*, **3**: 18–27.

106. Colom F., Vieta E., Martinez A., Jorquera A., Gasto C. (1998) What is the role of psychotherapy in the treatment of bipolar disorder? *Psychother. Psychosom.*, **67**: 3–9.

107. Huxley N.A., Parikh S.V., Baldessarini R.J. (2000) Effectiveness of psychosocial treatments in bipolar disorder: state of the evidence. *Harvard Rev. Psychiatry*, **8**: 126–140.

108. Fieve R.R. (1975) The lithium clinic: a new model for the delivery of psychiatric services. *Am. J. Psychiatry*, **132**: 1018–1022.

109. Gitlin M.J., Jamison K.R. (1984) Lithium clinics: theory and practice. *Hosp. Commun. Psychiatry*, **35**: 363–368.

110. Seeger P.A., Stern S.L., Dennert J.W. (1989) A combined group and individual approach to outpatient lithium treatment. *Ohio Med.*, **85**: 300–302.

111. Shea N., McBride L., Gavin C., Bauer M.S. (1997) Effects of an ambulatory collaborative practice model on process and outcome of care for bipolar disorder. *J. Am. Psychiatr. Nurses Assoc.*, **3**: 49–57.

112. Bauer M.S., Williford W., Dawson E., Akiskal H., Altshuler L., Fye C., Gelenberg A., Glick H., Kinosian B., Sajatovic M. (2002) Principles of effectiveness trials and their implementation in VA Cooperative Study #430, "Reducing the Efficacy-Effectiveness Gap in Bipolar Disorder." *J. Affect. Disord.* (in press).
113. Shelley E.M., Fieve R.R. (1974) The use of nonphysicians in a health maintenance program for affective disorders. *Hosp. Commun. Psychiatry*, **25**: 303–305.
114. Ellenberg J., Salamon I., Meaney C. (1980) A lithium clinic in a community mental health center. *Hosp. Commun. Psychiatry*, **31**: 834–836.
115. Institute of Medicine (IOM) (1985) *Assessing Medical Technologies.* National Academy Press, Washington.
116. Bauer M.S. (2001) The collaborative practice model in bipolar disorder: design and implementation in a multi-site randomized controlled trial. *Bipolar Disord.*, **3**: 233–244.
117. Bauer M.S., McBride L., Shea N., Gavin C., Holden F., Kendall S. (1997) Impact of an easy-access clinic-based program for bipolar disorder: quantitative analysis of a demonstration project. *Psychiatr. Serv.*, **48**: 491–496.
118. Bauer M.S., Shea N., McBride L., Gavin C. (1997) Predictors of service utilization in veterans with bipolar disorder: a prospective study. *J. Affect. Disord.*, **44**: 159–168.
119. Simon G.E., Lundman E.J., Unutzer J., Bauer M.S. (2002) Design and implementation of a randomized trial evaluating systematic care for bipolar disorder. *Bipolar Disord.* (in press).

Commentaries

4.1
Uncharted Waters: Bipolar Disorder and Psychosocial Treatment

David J. Miklowitz[1]

Although psychosocial interventions for bipolar disorder have long existed, only recently have they been systematically evaluated in randomized controlled trials. Mark Bauer's thoughtful review provides relatively objective criteria for judging the current status of this field. His overall conclusion is that manual-based psychosocial interventions—and systems of care that include psychosocial components—are effective in combination with pharmacotherapy in decreasing illness morbidity. A key point is that various investigators, despite having designed psychosocial interventions from widely different theoretical perspectives, have come to similar conclusions about the necessary ingredients: collaborations between patients, families, and mental health providers; education about bipolar disorder; inclusion of family and social supports in ongoing preventative maintenance; and illness management strategies such as early identification and treatment of prodromal symptoms.

Several issues stand out as domains for future research. First, no psychosocial treatment studies have been undertaken that target early-onset or geriatric bipolar populations. The early-onset form of the disorder is associated with a highly pernicious course, high rates of suicide, multiple comorbidities, drug and alcohol abuse, and severe psychosocial impairments [1]. Likewise, older bipolar patients are often treatment refractory and may require complex combinations of anticonvulsants, atypical antipsychotics, and other agents [2]. Both of these populations have distinct psychosocial problems associated with their stages of life, yet few efforts have been undertaken to design interventions to address these problems.

Second, existing psychosocial studies have done little to identify treatment moderators or mediators. Whereas studies often report that an experimental treatment works better than a control condition, few are adequately powered in sample size or sample diversity to determine the subpopulations who benefit most. Even less is known about treatment mechanisms,

[1] *Department of Psychology, University of Colorado at Boulder, Muenzinger Bldg., Boulder, CO 80309–0345, USA*

which is critical to determining why treatments work for some patients and not others, why treatments often do not produce the degree of improvement (or the longevity of improvement) that we would predict, or whether more cost-effective treatments could accomplish the same objectives. Can we assume, for example, that when a cognitive-behavioural treatment has positive effects on patients' outcomes, the avenue of change includes modifying dysfunctional attitudes or core dysfunctional beliefs? When a family treatment leads to reduced relapse rates, are correlated changes in family affect, relationships, and interaction patterns observed? Alternatively, do any of these interventions operate through less specific means, such as increasing patients' acceptance of the disorder, adherence with medication regimes, or consistency of medical follow-up?

Third, it is unclear whether manic versus depressive episodes have different psychosocial correlates or should be addressed by different psychosocial interventions. Johnson *et al* [3] found that patients' levels of social support predicted their improvements in depressive but not manic symptoms during a follow-up. In contrast, Malkoff-Schwartz *et al* [4] found that a certain type of life stressor—events that were likely to disrupt patients' social rhythms—occurred more frequently prior to manic than depressive episodes. Miklowitz *et al*'s [5] family-focused psychoeducational treatment had a stronger impact on depressive symptoms than on manic symptoms. Perry *et al*'s [6] psychoeducational approach achieved the reverse. Large-scale effectiveness trials such as the Systematic Treatment Enhancement Program for Bipolar Disorder [7] may help to address questions regarding illness polarity and treatment choice.

Fourth, future studies need to address the large issue of *access to care*. Most psychosocial interventions are time-intensive and their costs exceed the allotments for outpatient treatment in community health clinics. Community therapists often voice frustration that they cannot get access to training materials for these treatments. Thus, briefer psychosocial treatments need to be developed which are easily learned by practitioners and contain some of the active ingredients of the more intensive treatments, in abbreviated form (for example, self-instruction on how to stabilize sleep/wake rhythms or implement behavioural activation strategies). Another possibility is to develop non-traditional methods of treatment delivery, such as the World Wide Web, Internet, cable television, and telemedicine [8, 9]. For example, teaching patients to identify early warning signs of mania and choose among various treatment options may be accomplished with the aid of computer-based instruction. These options have the potential to reach larger, more remote, and more diverse populations of patients.

Finally, the psychosocial treatment literature has neglected the important area of prevention. Many children, adolescents, and young adults present for treatment with subsyndromal manifestations of bipolar disorder, which may or may not progress into the fully syndromal adult forms [10]. We know relatively little about why some children with early warning signs develop the disorder and some do not. Identifying environmental factors that moderate the expression of genetic risk—perhaps through longitudinal high-risk paradigms—will contribute to our understanding of who to target in early-stage interventions. In turn, preventative interventions that educate at-risk individuals about bipolar disorder and enhance their ability to cope with provocative stress agents may improve the long-term outcome of the disorder.

REFERENCES

1. Geller B., Luby J. (1997)   Child and adolescent bipolar disorder: a review of the past 10 years. *J. Am. Acad. Child Adolesc. Psychiatry*, **36**: 1168–1176.
2. McDonald W.M. (2000)   Epidemiology, etiology, and treatment of geriatric mania. *J. Clin. Psychiatry*, **61** (Suppl. 13): 3–11.
3. Johnson S.L., Winett C.A., Meyer B., Greenhouse W.J., Miller I. (1999)   Social support and the course of bipolar disorder. *J. Abnorm. Psychol.*, **108**: 558–566.
4. Malkoff-Schwartz S., Frank E., Anderson B., Sherrill J.T., Siegel L., Patterson D., Kupfer D.J. (1998)   Stressful life events and social rhythm disruption in the onset of manic and depressive bipolar episodes: a preliminary investigation. *Arch. Gen. Psychiatry*, **55**: 702–707.
5. Miklowitz D.J., Simoneau T.L., George E.A., Richards J.A., Kalbag A., Sachs-Ericsson N., Suddath R. (2000)   Family-focused treatment of bipolar disorder: one-year effects of a psychoeducational program in conjunction with pharma-cotherapy. *Biol. Psychiatry*, **48**: 582–592.
6. Perry A., Tarrier N., Morriss R., McCarthy E., Limb K. (1999)   Randomised controlled trial of efficacy of teaching patients with bipolar disorder to identify early symptoms of relapse and obtain treatment. *Br. Med. J.*, **16**: 149–153.
7. Sachs G. (1998)   Treatments for bipolar disorder. Unpublished grant proposal (NIMH Contract No. N01MH80001).
8. Christensen A., Miller W.R., Muñoz R.F. (1978)   Paraprofessionals, partners, peers, paraphernalia, and print: a model for the use of therapeutic adjuncts to prevention, treatment, and maintenance. *Prof. Psychol.*, **9**: 249–270.
9. Muñoz R.F., Glish M., Soo-Hoo T., Robertson J. (1982)   The San Francisco Mood Survey Project: Preliminary work toward the prevention of depression. *Am. J. Commun. Psychol.*, **10**: 317–329.
10. Lewinsohn P.M., Klein D.N., Seeley J.R. (2000)   Bipolar disorder during adolescence and young adulthood in a community sample. *Bipolar Disord.*, **2**: 281–293.

4.2
Psychosocial Treatments in Bipolar Disorder: Their Time is Approaching

Eugene S. Paykel[1]

The comparatively small number of published controlled trials of psychosocial therapies in bipolar affective disorder included in Mark Bauer's excellent and comprehensive review contrasts with what is now a large literature on unipolar disorder. One of the reasons is the prevalent view that bipolar disorder has mainly biological causes. This is probably true: for instance the literature suggests stronger genetic effects than in unipolar disorder [1]. However, it is not entirely relevant, since psychosocial therapies can have profound effects irrespective of causes. Neurologists do not need convincing of the value of rehabilitation for stroke: rehabilitation is an essential component in modern stroke units. Educational measures are the standard method to improve organically caused mental retardation. Even when biological causes become fully understood, and bipolar disorder still has a very long way to go in this regard, they may not be curable, and where they are, other forms of management may still have a role in ameliorating secondary disabilities and interpersonal consequences. Good treatment in psychiatry is usually eclectic and multimodal.

The *prima facie* case for employment of psychosocial treatments in bipolar disorder is good. It depends on several rationales, as Bauer notes. First, although outcome with lithium, other mood stabilizers and other somatic therapies in many people is excellent, in an important minority of at least one-third it is not, and in some it is poor. Something in addition is needed.

Secondly, the difficulties which many people with bipolar disorder have in coming to terms with their illness have been well documented, particularly by Kay Jamison [2, 3]. Patients feel controlled by lithium, by psychiatric professionals, and by recurrent illness, and seek to shed them. This produces real difficulties in medication taking and in recognition of periods of illness, particularly when combined with the lack of insight characteristic of mania.

Third, long and recurrent illness, irrespective of causes, can produce secondary psychosocial consequences which then impede recovery. In the author's clinical practice in treatment-resistant unipolar disorder, problems in interpersonal relationships and in resumption of lost roles secondary to long illness are almost universal, and tackling them psychotherapeutically is often the key to converting a temporary remission to a sustained one. This applies particularly to the readjustments in family constellations which

[1] *Department of Psychiatry, University of Cambridge, Douglas House, 18c Trumpington Road, Cambridge CB2 2A11, United Kingdom*

have occurred as the patient's roles are taken over by others, so that there is no gap to resume them.

For bipolar disorder the evidence is still somewhat sparse and there are some notable gaps which need to be filled. For psychosocial therapies to be used more there need to be clearer indications as to when they should be applied: when are they effective, when is outcome good even without them? The place of medication in bipolar disorder is undisputed and it is in combination with medication that psychosocial approaches need to be evaluated. Comparative trials of different psychological and psychothera-peutic modalities are also required. It may be, as evidence in this review so far suggests, that there are not major differences in effects of different therapies. On the other hand, it may require more studies and larger ones, with direct comparisons. In the earlier literature on unipolar depression, there were hints that interpersonal therapy provided particular benefit in improving interpersonal relationships [4]. Recent evidence points strongly to a particular effect of cognitive approaches in preventing relapse and recurrence [5–8].

This is a rapidly moving field. Psychoeducational group approaches, although not fully evaluated, are now being offered to bipolar patients in many UK centres. Shortly after Bauer's literature search was completed, Scott et al [9] published the results of a pilot controlled trial in which 42 bipolar subjects were randomly assigned either to treatment as usual alone or with the addition of six months' cognitive therapy. At six months cogni-tive therapy subjects showed lower symptoms and better functioning. Over 18 months there were suggestive changes in relapse rates.

A large multi-centre controlled trial is now under way in the UK, funded by the Medical Research Council [10]. Among five centres (Cambridge, Glasgow, Liverpool, Manchester, Preston), 250 recurrent bipolar subjects have been randomized to receive either cognitive therapy for six months plus treatment as usual or treatment as usual alone, with a further one year follow-up. The manualized cognitive therapy approach is broad, incorpor-ating standard cognitive therapy of depression, modification of attitudes to medication and illness, relapse prevention and early relapse recognition derived from Perry et al [11].

After a slow start, the pace is accelerating. It appears likely that in the next five years the available evidence will increase considerably. Psychosocial therapies are more costly than medications, and in cost-conscious mental health services evidence of efficacy and effectiveness is required, together with cost-benefit evidence which should include the very high societal costs for bipolar disorder. We should before long be able to look forward to standard deployment of psychosocial therapies in combination with medi-cation secured by a good evidence base.

REFERENCES

1. Nurnberger J.I., Gershon E.S. (1992) Genetics. In *Handbook of Affective Disorders*, 2nd ed. (Ed. E.S. Paykel), pp. 131–148, Churchill Livingstone, Edinburgh.
2. Jamison K.R. (1995) *An Unquiet Mind.* Knopf, New York.
3. Jamison K.R., Gerner R.H., Goodwin F.K. (1979) Patient and physician attitudes toward lithium: relationship to compliance. *Arch. Gen. Psychiatry*, **36**: 866–869.
4. Paykel E.S., DiMascio A., Klerman G.L., Prusoff B.A,. Weissman M.M. (1976) Maintenance therapy of depression. *Pharmakopsychiat. Neuro-Psychopharmacol.*, **9**: 127–136.
5. Fava G.A., Rafanelli C., Grandi S., Canestrari R., Morphy M.A. (1998) Six year outcome for cognitive behavioural treatment of residual symptoms in major depression. *Am. J. Psychiatry*, **155**: 1443–1445.
6. Fava G.A., Rafanelli C., Grandi S., Conti S., Belluardo P. (1998) Prevention of recurrent depression with cognitive behavioural therapy: preliminary findings. *Arch. Gen. Psychiatry*, **55**: 816–820.
7. Paykel E.S., Scott J., Teasdale J.D., Johnson A.L., Garland A., Moore R., Jenaway A., Cornwall P.L., Hayhurst H., Abbott R. *et al* (1999) Prevention of relapse in residual depression by cognitive therapy. A controlled trial. *Arch. Gen. Psychiatry*, **56**: 829–835.
8. Teasdale J.T., Segal Z.V., Williams J.M.G., Ridgeway V.A., Soulsby J.M., Lau M.A. (2000) Prevention of relapse/recurrence in major depression by mindfulness-based cognitive therapy. *J. Consult. Clin. Psychol.*, **68**: 615–623.
9. Scott J., Garland A. Moorhead S. (2001) A pilot study of cognitive therapy in bipolar disorders. *Psychol. Med.*, **31**: 459–467.
10. Scott J., Paykel E.S., Kinderman P., Bentall R.P., Morriss R. (1999) Randomised controlled trial of cognitive behavioural therapy for bipolar affective disorders. Medical Research Council Grant.
11. Perry A., Tarrier A., Morriss R., McCarthy E., Limb K. (1999) Randomised controlled trial of efficacy of teaching patients with bipolar disorder to identify early symptoms of relapse and obtain treatment. *Br. Med. J.*, **318**: 149–153.

4.3

Some Unanswered Questions Regarding Psychosocial Treatments for Bipolar Disorder

Sheri L. Johnson[1]

As reviewed by Mark Bauer, the results of a multitude of outcome studies are relatively uniform in indicating that adjunctive psychotherapy for bipolar disorder provides important benefits. Available approaches are diverse,

[1] *Department of Psychology, University of Miami, Merrick 209f, Coral Gables, FL 33124–2010, USA*

as the field has grown to encompass psychoeducational, cognitive-behavioural, interpersonal, family, and marital approaches. The outcomes measured are also quite varied, including symptoms, treatment adherence, functioning, and interpersonal consequences. The psychotherapy literature mirrors the complexity embodied within this disorder, in that a broad range of strategies have evolved to target different aspects of the illness.

What are the next steps for research? One goal would be to examine more specific aspects of symptoms and functioning. For example, symptom outcomes could be divided more finely, such that depression and mania are considered as separate targets. Many of the current treatments were originally developed for unipolar depression, and so focus on interpersonal conflict, negative maladaptive cognitions, and stress. As several dozen studies suggest that the psychosocial triggers for unipolar and bipolar depression are similar [1], this application of strategies from unipolar depression appears to be a reasonable approach for treating the depressive side of bipolar disorder. Indeed, evidence suggests that strategies to reduce family conflict, interpersonal stress, and negative cognitions have more effectiveness in relieving depression than mania [2–4].

On the other hand, there may be quite different biopsychosocial factors that trigger manic symptoms. For example, sleep deprivation may provoke manic episodes [5, 6]. Mania has also been theorized to reflect dysregulation in the brain system moderating responses to reward [7]. In support of this model, achievement-striving traits, self-report reward responsiveness scores, and life events involving goal attainment have each been found to predict increases in manic symptoms over time [8, 9]. Given unique triggers for manic symptoms, it appears important to consider distinct psychosocial treatment strategies for the prevention of these symptoms. So far, treatments that appear to reduce manic symptoms involve symptom monitoring [e.g., 10, 11]. It may also be fruitful to consider interventions to alleviate manic-specific triggers. For example, recent case studies suggest that sleep regulation strategies may help reduce manic symptoms [12, 13].

Beyond symptom-focused interventions, functioning deficits are strikingly complex. For example, social and occupational functioning appear to be relatively orthogonal within bipolar disorder [14], and even within social functioning, one could differentiate goals of establishing a broad social network, forming a circle of close friends, maintaining family relationships, helping others understand the illness, reducing expressed emotion, and increasing prosocial interactions. Indeed, it is not uncommon for a person who experiences a manic episode to experience profound deteriorations in each of these areas. Given the breadth of problems, rehabilitation models comparable in intensity to those used within the schizophrenia field may merit consideration for individuals who have just experienced extreme losses in social and employment areas.

There is good cause for optimism, as techniques for addressing many different symptom and functioning goals are available in the current set of psychotherapy manuals, and outcomes relevant to each of these areas have been positive. These strategies, however, remain components of specific approaches, rather than a more integrated approach to the disorder. That is, there has been little consideration of which strategies to choose for particular individuals (see [15] for an exception). For example, early in the illness, psychoeducation, treatment acceptance, and symptom monitoring may be critical to the ability to achieve any other type of intervention. As treatment and symptoms become more stabilized, individuals may vary in their need for conflict resolution, occupational accomplishments, or other goals. Similarly, the relative history of manic versus depressive symptoms may help guide choice of treatment approach. In treatments such as the Life Goals Program and Interpersonal Psychotherapy, the therapist and individual choose among goals clinically. Nonetheless, there is very little known on the match between patients and their treatment goals. Similarly, there is a dearth of research that dismantles interventions to identify the key components.

In sum, a great deal has been accomplished in understanding the role of psychotherapy in bipolar disorder. It is this richness that provides an opportunity for the next wave of research.

REFERENCES

1. Johnson S.L., Kizer A. (2001) Psychosocial factors in the course of unipolar and bipolar depression. In. *Handbook of Depression and Its Treatment* (Eds I. Gotlib, C. Hammen), Guilford, New York (in press).
2. Miklowitz D.J., Simoneau T.L., Richards J.A. (1997) Family-focused psychoeducation in the outpatient treatment of bipolar disorder. Presented at the Association for the Advancement of Behavior Therapy 31st Annual Convention, Miami, 14 November.
3. Frank E., Kupfer D.J., Gibbons R., Houck P., Kostelnik B., Mallinger A., Swartz H.A., Thase M.E. (2000) Interpersonal psychotherapy. Presented at the 15th Annual Meeting of the Society for Research in Psychopathology, 2 December.
4. Zaretzky A.E., Segal Z.V., Gemar M. (1999) Cognitive therapy for bipolar depression: a pilot study. *Can. J. Psychiatry*, **44**: 491–494.
5. Leibenluft E., Albert P.S., Rosenthal N.E., Wehr T.A. (1996) Relationship between sleep and mood in patients with rapid-cycling bipolar disorder. *Psychiatry Res.*, **63**: 161–168.
6. Wehr T.A. (1991) Sleep-loss as a possible mediator of diverse causes of mania. *Br. J Psychiatry*, **159**: 576–578.
7. Depue R.A., Krauss S.P., Spoont M.R. (1987) A two-dimensional threshold model of seasonal bipolar affective disorder. In *Psychopathology: An Interactional Perspective* (Eds D. Magnuson, A. Ohman), pp. 95–123, Academic Press, San Diego.

8. Johnson S.L., Sandrow D., Meyer B., Winters R., Miller I., Keitner G., Solomon D. (2000) Increases in manic symptoms following life events involving goal-attainment. *J. Abnorm. Psychol.*, **109**: 721–727.
9. Lozano B., Johnson S.L. (2001) Do personality traits predict depressive and manic symptoms? *J. Affect. Disord.*, **63**: 103–111.
10. Lam D.H.., Bright J., Jones S., Hayward P., Schuck N., Chisolm D., Sham P. (2000) Cognitive therapy for bipolar illness—a pilot study of relapse prevention. *Cogn. Ther. Res.*, **24**: 503–520.
11. Perry A., Tarrier N., Morriss R., McCarthy E., Limb K. (1999) Randomised controlled trial of efficacy of teaching patients with bipolar disorder to identify early symptoms of relapse and obtain treatment. *Br. Med. J.*, **318**: 149–153.
12. Wehr T.A., Turner E.H., Shimada J.M., Lowe C.H., Barker C., Leibenluft E. (1998) Treatment of rapidly cycling bipolar patient by using extended bed rest and darkness to stabilize the timing and duration of sleep. *Biol. Psychiatry*, **43**: 822–828.
13. Wirz-Justice A., Quinto C., Cajochen C., Werth E., Hock C. (1999) A rapid-cycling bipolar patient treated with long nights, bedrest, and light. *Biol. Psychiatry*, **45**: 1075–1077.
14. Greenhouse W. (2001) Social and occupational functioning in bipolar disorder: a theoretical model. Unpublished doctoral dissertation, University of Miami.
15. Miller I. (1992) *Family Treatment of Bipolar Disorder.* National Institute of Mental Health Grant No. 1R01MH048171.

4.4

Convergent Strategies or Phase-Specific Interventions?

Holly A. Swartz[1]

In his comprehensive review of psychosocial interventions for bipolar disorder, Mark Bauer observes: "The degree of convergent validity regarding agenda for disease management information and skills to be imparted is impressive." He notes that most—if not all—of the described treatment strategies include psychoeducation, identification of early warning signs of relapse, and identification of a patient-specific action plan. Bauer challenges us to consider the notion that the active ingredients of these disparate treatments may be more alike than they are different.

Historically, it has been difficult to demonstrate a difference between two (or more) active psychotherapy conditions [1]. It is often suggested that the non-specific factors common to all psychotherapies outweigh the treatment-specific effects [2]. If this assertion were true of treatments for bipolar disorder, one would expect to see consistent outcomes across interventions. Indeed, Bauer notes that most of the authors report positive effects on diverse outcome measures. A closer reading of the text, however, suggests

[1] *University of Pittsburgh School of Medicine, 3811 O'Hara Street, Pittsburgh, PA 15213, USA*

that, with respect to manic and depressive symptoms, different treatments may produce different results.

Bauer identifies seven Class A (i.e., randomized, controlled) studies that report information on clinical and/or symptom outcomes. These treatments can be categorized as family therapy [3, 4], couples therapy [5], interpersonal therapy [6, 7], psychoeducation [8], or cognitive-behavioural therapy (CBT) [9]. With two exceptions, all of these rigorously designed studies reported differential treatment effects on manic and depressive symptoms. Of the two that do not, one used as its primary clinical outcome measure a composite global functioning and symptom score that did not differentiate depressive and manic symptoms. It therefore would be impossible to determine whether or not there were differential effects on these outcomes [3]. The other report found that a marital intervention led to improved patient functioning but had no impact on symptoms over an 11–month period [5].

The remaining five studies, however, reported significant or trend level differences on outcome measures of mania and depression. Miklowitz *et al* found that subjects assigned to family-focused therapy showed significantly greater improvement than control subjects in depressive (but not manic) symptoms [4]. Trend level findings from the acute phase of our ongoing study of interpersonal and social rhythm therapy (IPSRT) suggest that depressed (but not manic) subjects assigned to IPSRT recover twice as quickly as those assigned to the control condition [6]. Preliminary findings from the maintenance phase of this study further suggest that IPSRT confers protection against subsyndromal depressive (but not manic) symptoms [10]. In contrast, Perry *et al* observed that a group assigned to a psychoeducational relapse prevention intervention differed significantly from control subjects for time to first manic (but not depressive) relapse. They also observed a significant reduction in the total number of manic (but not depressive) relapses over 18 months [8]. Similarly, Lam *et al* reported that, compared to controls, those assigned to CBT experienced significant reductions in manic (but not depressive) symptoms at 12-month follow-up [9].

Collectively, these results suggest that the relational treatments (family therapy and interpersonal therapy) may have selectively positive effects on the depressive phase of the disorder, while the cognitive-behavioural treatments (psychoeducation and CBT) may have selectively positive effects on the manic phase. Interestingly, Johnson *et al* recently demonstrated that, among patients with bipolar disorder, low social support predicts a longer time to recovery from depression (but not mania) and a greater chance of a depressive (but not manic) recurrence [11]. We could speculate that relational treatments for bipolar disorder may, in part, exert their antidepressant effects by increasing interpersonal effectiveness and social support. By contrast, the cognitive-behavioural strategies may do little to enhance social support and instead exert their effects by helping patients to track carefully the behaviours and cognitions that herald mania.

As Bauer suggests, we may be able to identify some common themes critical to the success of any adjunctive psychosocial intervention for bipolar disorder. But we may also need to attend to the distinct effects of dissimilar treatments in order to find strategies that are effective across the phases of the disorder. Given the complexity of bipolar disorder, we may need to design "polytherapy" approaches that combine common denominator strategies to promote global mood stability with phase-specific interventions to manage the particular problems of mania, depression, and mixed states.

REFERENCES

1. Elkin I., Shea M.T., Watkins J.T., Imber S.D., Sotsky S.M., Collins J.F., Glass D.R., Pilkonis P.A., Leber W.R., Docherty J.P. *et al* (1989) National Institute of Mental Health Treatment of Depression Collaborative Research Program: general effectiveness of treatments. *Arch. Gen. Psychiatry*, **46**: 971–982.
2. Frank J. (1971) Therapeutic factors in psychotherapy. *Am. J. Psychother.*, **25**: 350–361.
3. Clarkin J.F., Glick I.D., Haas G.L., Spencer J.H., Lewis A.B., Peyser J., DeMane N., Good-Ellis M., Harris E., Lestelle V. (1990) A randomized clinical trial of inpatient family intervention: V. Results for affective disorders. *J. Affect. Disord.*, **18**: 17–28.
4. Miklowitz D.J., Simoneau T.L., George E.A., Richards J.A., Kalbag A., Sachs-Ericsson N., Suddath R. (2000) Family-focused treatment of bipolar disorder: one year effects of a psychoeducational program in conjunction with pharmacotherapy. *Biol. Psychiatry*, **48**: 582–592.
5. Clarkin J.F., Carpenter D., Hull J., Wilner P., Glick I. (1998) Effects of psychoeducational intervention for married patients with bipolar disorder and their spouses. *Psychiatr. Serv.*, **49**: 531–533.
6. Hlastala S.A., Frank E., Mallinger A.G., Thase M.E., Ritenour A.M., Kupfer D.J. (1997) Bipolar depression: an underestimated treatment challenge. *Depress. Anxiety*, **5**: 73–83.
7. Frank E., Swartz H.A., Mallinger A.G., Thase M.E., Weaver E.V., Kupfer D.J. (1999) Adjunctive psychotherapy for bipolar disorder: effects of changing treatment modality. *J. Abnorm. Psychol.*, **108**: 579–587.
8. Perry A., Tarrier N., Morriss R., McCarthy E., Limb K. (1999) Randomised controlled trial of efficacy of teaching patients with bipolar disorder to identify early symptoms of relapse and obtain treatment. *Br. Med. J.*, **318**: 149–153.
9. Lam D.H., Bright J., Jones S., Hayward P., Schuck N., Chisholm D., Sham P. (2000) Cognitive therapy for bipolar illness—a pilot study of relapse prevention. *Cogn. Ther. Res.*, **24**: 503–520.
10. Frank E. (1999) Interpersonal and social rhythm therapy prevents depressive symptomatology in bipolar 1 patients. *Bipolar Disord.*, **1**: 13.
11. Johnson S.L., Meyer B., Winett C., Small J. (2000) Social support and self-esteem predict changes in bipolar depression but not mania. *J. Affect. Disord.*, **58**: 79–86.

4.5
Some Comments on Recent Developments in Psychosocial Treatments for Bipolar Disorder

Michael E. Thase[1]

By the early 1990s it was clear that a majority of patients with bipolar disorder will experience multiple episodes and that a significant minority will suffer from prolonged periods of psychosocial disability. Kraepelin's "good prognosis illness" has not fared too well in the post-modern world. Patients with polyepisodic or chronic bipolar disorders, who are almost always either resistant to or nonadherent with lithium therapy, are usually not well managed by a strict medical-model or medication-clinic approach. The combination of psychotherapy and pharmacotherapy has been suggested to be the best approach for treatment of these challenging patients [1] and, indeed, a survey of people with bipolar disorder confirmed that psychotherapy receives high marks for consumer satisfaction [2]. Yet, until recently, there has been virtually no evidence from well-controlled studies to confirm that adding individual, group, or family forms of psychotherapy actually improves the outcomes of patients with bipolar disorder. Now, after a decade of research, the results of a first wave of randomized clinical trials are available. Mark Bauer carefully reviews the findings of these studies and concludes that the weight of the evidence supports the value of a variety of adjunctive psychotherapies for people with bipolar disorder.

Bauer suggests that a core group of relatively straightforward therapeutic elements may account for a large portion of the success of psychological interventions for bipolar disorder. These "trans-theoretical" factors include: a) education about, and explicit collaboration on development of, an illness management plan; b) repair, stabilization, and (if possible) enhancement of social support networks; and c) content-based interventions dealing with symptom management, recognition of early warning signs, and problem solving. Bauer challenges the field to design and deliver interventions that cover these basic elements in the most efficient and least costly manner possible.

I share Bauer's optimism that this type of approach could quickly define a new state of the art for the collaborative care of people with bipolar disorder. I further support Bauer's conviction that these elements can be incorporated, in a cost-effective way, within the context of a disease management plan. Hopefully, the results of the ongoing projects of Bauer's group and Simon and colleagues will confirm that such streamlined efforts make a valuable difference.

[1] *Department of Psychiatry, University of Pittsburgh School of Medicine, Western Psychiatric Institute and Clinic, 3811 O'Hara Street, Pittsburgh, PA 15213–2593, USA*

Nevertheless, despite considerable progress from research evaluating the role of psychotherapy for bipolar disorder, a number of critical questions still must be answered. For example, can the positive results of demonstration studies such as Bauer's project actually be transported to everyday practice without some form of oversight and contingency management? This question is especially pertinent to the quality of care provided in chronically underfunded community mental health clinics and other related public care facilities. Moreover, once confirmed, how quickly will these research findings be incorporated within the required curricula of psychiatric residents, clinical and counselling psychology graduate students, social workers, and other mental health professionals?

Another question concerns the indications for more labour-intensive, and costly, interventions tailored for individuals who relapse or remain chronically impaired despite participation in a state-of-the-art, disease management programme. For example, Bauer is correct to point out that in preliminary analysis of the Pittsburgh Maintenance Therapy of Bipolar Disorder (MTBD) study, an individually tailored, Interpersonal Social Rhythms Therapy (IPSRT) did not improve time to stabilization or simple relapse risk relative to a comprehensive clinical management programme [3]. However, in more recent analyses of time spent ill or euthymic, a strong advantage emerged favouring the maintenance interpersonal psychotherapy group during the latter months of the first year of treatment [4]. Moreover, among the patients treated in the clinical management arms of the MTBD study, approximately 30% failed to stabilize and another 25% suffered at least one recurrent episode of mania or depression during the first 12 months after stabilization of the index episode [3]. This higher risk group, despite receiving excellent overall care, still appears to have required something more. Could they have obtained greater benefit if an alternative individual or family-based intervention had been added to the treatment plan? And, if so, are there ways to identify which patients would gain the most benefit from an individual intervention and which patients would get the most benefit from couples/family interventions?

Another topical issue concerns the use of problem-focused psychotherapies to prescriptively treat episodes of bipolar depression in lieu of antidepressant medications. The very preliminary report by Zaretsky et al. [5] illustrates the potential promise of this approach. But, what confidence can be placed in the generalizability of the outcomes of eight (possibly handpicked) patients? Given the likelihood of side effects associated with antidepressant therapy (e.g., sexual dysfunction, weight gain, or insomnia), and the possibility of antidepressant-induced mania or rapid cycling, it is remarkable that this topic still has not been addressed more systematically in the research literature. It is especially puzzling that the role of psychotherapy has not been evaluated in bipolar II depression, for which there is little consensus about the relative merits of antidepressants or mood stabilizers.

The studies reviewed by Bauer by and large fail to establish causal or mediative relationships between the methods that define a type of psychotherapy and clinical benefits. I would not be too nihilistic about the relative lack of evidence, to date, linking the syndromal effects to a specific aspect of a psychotherapy. One only needs to recall the difficulty establishing plasma level/clinical response relationships for tricyclic antidepressants or, for that matter, between divalproex blood levels and mania outcomes, as examples of how hard it is to establish mediating effects. And, we do not measure constructs such as social support, expressed emotion, or even treatment adherence nearly as reliably as we measure medication concentrations! Effect sizes are going to be modest and some amalgam of nonspecific (trans-theoretical) therapeutic factors is bound to account for a large portion of the explained variance.

The methods of randomized controlled clinical trials, the complexities of bipolar disorder and the intricacies of psychotherapy research have not led to an easy "mix". Most of the psychotherapy research reviewed by Bauer would be considered as examples of "early phase II" research [6] using the terminology of the US Food and Drug Administration. Generally speaking, it is difficult to complete a well-designed psychotherapy trial of bipolar disorder at a single site within three to five years. Moreover, meaningful outcomes in the real world, such as reducing rates of suicide attempts, rehospitalization, or unemployment by 10% to 15%, cannot be confirmed with confidence until we conduct studies that enrol hundreds of patients. There is no economic force behind psychotherapy development that even approaches the financial support marshalled to enable a single promising new medication to move from an early Phase II level through Phase III, regulatory approval and widespread clinical use.

The solution to these problems will necessitate multicentre research networks, and infrastructural support, unlike never before devoted to the scientific study of psychosocial treatments. Now, for the first time, there is evidence that psychotherapeutic approaches offer enough chance of extra benefit to justify investment of scarce research funds. One such research network, the US NIMH-funded Systematic Treatment Enhancement Program for Bipolar Disorder (STEP-BD) is off the ground and, as of 28 August, 2001, has enrolled more than 1400 (about 28%) of a planned base of 5000 patients. There is much work to be done!

REFERENCES

1. American Psychiatric Association (1994) Practice guideline for the treatment of patients with bipolar disorder. *Am. J. Psychiatry*, **151** (Suppl. 12): 1–35.
2. Lish J.D., Dime-Meenan S., Whybrow P.C., Price R.A., Hirschfeld R.M.A. (1994) The National Depressive and Manic-Depressive Association (NDMDA) survey of bipolar members. *J. Affect. Disord.*, **31**: 281–294.
3. Frank E., Swartz H.A., Kupfer D.J. (2000) Interpersonal and social rhythm therapy: managing the chaos of bipolar disorder. *Biol. Psychiatry*, **48**: 593–604.
4. Frank E. (2001) Interpersonal and social rhythm therapy. Presented at the Fourth International Conference on Bipolar Disorder, Pittsburgh, 16 June.
5. Zaretsky A.E., Segal Z.V., Gemar M. (1999) Cognitive therapy for bipolar depression: a pilot study. *Can. J. Psychiatry*, **44**: 491–494.
6. Rush A.J. (1984) A phase III study of cognitive therapy of depression. In: *Psychotherapy Research. Where Are We and Where Should We Go?* (Eds J.B.W. Williams, R.L. Spitzer), pp. 216–233, Guilford, New York.

4.6

Beyond Pharmacotherapy: Integrating Psychosocial Treatments and Health Services Innovations for Bipolar Disorder

Sagar V. Parikh[1]

Is biology destiny? Does bipolar disorder, the most biological of psychiatric disorders, merit treatment only through somatic interventions? As Mark Bauer, in his evidence-based review, tells us, the answer is clear: a wealth of techniques—psychotherapeutic, educational, and health system innovations—offer clear benefit in the overall management of bipolar illness.

Bauer begins by reminding us of the many limitations of pharmacotherapy alone: incomplete symptom control, problems with compliance, and increasing evidence about broader risk factors for poor outcome, including life stressors and social support. Additional factors include the reciprocal and complex relationship between poor symptom outcome and family and occupational dysfunction, and the enormous financial costs of managing the disorder. In looking at efforts to improve outcome, a broader perspective on interventions is employed—those that might be traditionally termed psychotherapeutic, and those that look at the context of care strategies largely derived from chronic disease management principles.

Psychotherapy studies prior to 1990 were few and generally did not employ adequate control groups; since then, major advances in study meth-

[1] *Centre for Addiction and Mental Health (Clarke Institute site), 250 College St., Toronto, Ontario, M5T 1R8, Canada*

odology have included the almost mandatory use of a formal therapy manual, frequent use of random assignment, and in some studies, the use of proper controls [1]. These studies generally fall into three somewhat overlapping areas: primarily brief psychoeducational, primarily lengthy family/couple, and lengthy cognitive-behavioural therapy (CBT)/interpersonal therapy (IPT) interventions. The strength of the psychoeducational studies is the attention to relapse prevention, mediated largely through increased medication compliance and to the fact that such psychoeducational strategies are easy and economical to implement and use, both for clinicians and for patients. For treatments to be generalizable, an intervention must be potent, clear, and marketable: the intervention proposed by Perry *et al*, consisting of 7–12 sessions of individual psychoeducation with striking efficacy in the prevention of relapse into mania, meets the mark [2]. Coupled with the results of other psychoeducational intervention studies, we should feel comfortable in asserting that explicit, brief psychoeducation with attention to a relapse drill should be as routine at the outset of bipolar treatment, as doing lab work prior to initiation of mood stabilizers [3]. Indeed, such interventions should be seen as vital from a quality assurance perspective.

The lessons from family/couple interventions are more ambiguous, and much less generalizable. The biggest strength of these studies is that they address more recently identified risk factors (expressed emotion, social support) correlated to outcome. Key studies employ formal manuals, but the process of either family therapy or couple therapy is much more complex, and much less controllable, than individual therapy. Study methodologies are weaker, controls are usually "treatment as usual", and clinical outcomes are less consistent. Most striking, though, is the complexity and length of the interventions. Clarkin *et al*'s study [4] utilized 25 sessions of couple therapy; Miklowitz's family focused therapy [5] requires 21 sessions. The success of these interventions is gratifying, and in addition to providing a treatment modality, such studies may identify the key mechanisms and ingredients necessary for success. However, the intensity of service and the training required for these highly specific therapies belies widespread applicability. Epidemiologic data consistently show patterns of limited service use for all mental disorders, even in countries with (free) universal health care; clinical data and experience suggest many patients will not comply with complex treatment regimens involving many visits [6, 7]. Extended family/couple treatments may be like the Concorde—effective, impressive, but destined to be available only for a few locations.

The small but rapidly growing number of individual CBT-based studies, and the limited work with IPT, suggest more promise. Two of the key psychoeducational intervention studies [2, 8] relied on CBT principles; Zaretsky *et al*'s application of CBT [9] relied on Beck's traditional CBT of depression, with promising pilot results. Two studies have presented encouraging pilot results on CBT developed explicitly for bipolar disorder in the maintenance phase [10, 11]. Lam developed a specific manual for the CBT of bipolar disorder, tested it in a pilot study, and most recently presented preliminary results of a large ($n = 103$) randomized controlled trial, pitting up to 20 sessions of CBT against treatment as usual [12, 13]. Initial results show not only reductions in relapse and hospitalization, but particular protection against depression as well as hypomania (in contrast to psychoeducation, which largely protects against manic relapse rather than depression) and the suggestion of overall reduced mood lability. Results with IPT are less promising, with a single trial failing to show efficacy beyond the already high-quality "treatment as usual" given at that academic centre. The strength of the CBT interventions, in contrast to family/couple treatments, is that they are already widely available, training is relatively easy, and they have a long tradition of evolution into more practical modalities, i.e. group interventions, shortened (significantly fewer than 20 sessions) courses, and even self-help and computer-aided versions.

In addition to traditional psychotherapeutic treatments, evidence about the utility of disease management strategies is just emerging, as Bauer notes describing two large American trials. Both these randomized controlled trials use elements of patient education, physician guidance, and improved access, to see if such approaches are superior to treatment as usual. But then, how do we choose among treatments? The answer, in part, will lie in looking at the potential benefits of each component and matching the intervention with local resources and treatment structure [14]. A brief psychoeducational intervention, coupled with a "care-manager" nurse who aids patients in understanding and complying with treatment, for instance, might be equal to a 20-session individual CBT intervention added onto usual medical care. The 4th International Conference on Bipolar Disorder, in 2001, featured many research poster presentations on psychosocial treatments and disease management strategies, suggesting a plethora of new data. Studies included enhanced psychoeducation methods (21 group sessions), with positive results in a randomized controlled trial [15], telemedicine interventions [16], our novel treatment optimization programme involving simultaneous interventions for the patient and the patient's family physician [17], and a variety of techniques to optimize treatment compliance, such as Motivational Interviewing [18]. Beyond the specific interventions, issues such as "dosing" of psychosocial interventions, based both on cost considerations as well as burden to the patient, must be considered. New research approaches must be tried; for instance, in Toronto, our group has nearly completed a study looking at brief (seven psychoeducational sessions) versus standard (same seven plus another 13 CBT sessions) treatment derived from the Basco and Rush manual for CBT in bipolar disorder [19, 20]. Crossing modalities, in a study just funded by the Stanley Foundation, we are about to begin a comparison of five sessions of group psychoeducation against 20 sessions of individual CBT. Will such a brief group intervention give say 50% of the benefit of the 20-session CBT, at much less cost and with a much higher likelihood of attracting patients and completing the treatment? Such aspects of effectiveness must be considered along with more traditional efficacy studies. The complexity of treating bipolar disorder invites new theoretical approaches to the treatment of mental disorders, by requiring the ability to blend psychosocial interventions, sophisticated pharmacotherapy, and health services innovations together in order to achieve optimal results.

REFERENCES

1. Huxley N.A., Parikh S.V., Baldessarini R.J. (2000) Effectiveness of psychosocial treatments in bipolar disorder: state of the evidence. *Harvard Rev. Psychiatry*, **8**: 126–140.
2. Perry A., Tarrier N., Morriss R, McCarthy E, Limb K. (1999) Randomized controlled trial of efficacy of teaching patients with bipolar disorder to identify early symptoms of relapse and obtain treatment. *Br. Med. J.*, **318**: 149–153.
3. Parikh S.V. (2000) Practical management of bipolar disorder: key steps to implement psychosocial interventions. *Can. Psychiatr. Assoc. Bull.*, **32**: 114–116.
4. Clarkin J.F., Carpenter D., Hull J., Wilner P., Glick I. (1998) Effects of psychoeducational intervention for married patients with bipolar disorder and their spouses. *Psychiatr. Serv.*, **49**: 531–533.
5. Miklowitz D.J., Simoneau T.L., George E.L., Richards J.A., Kalbag A., Sachs-Ericsson N., Suddath R. (2000) Family-focused treatment of bipolar disorder: 1-year effects of a psychoeducational program in conjunction with pharmacotherapy. *Biol. Psychiatry*, **48**: 582–592.
6. Parikh S.V., Lin E., Lesage A.D. (1997) Mental health treatment in Ontario: selected comparisons between the primary care and specialty sectors. *Can. J. Psychiatry*, **42**: 929–934.
7. Tohen M., Goodwin F.K. (1995) Epidemiology of bipolar disorder. In *Textbook in Psychiatric Epidemiology* (Eds M.T. Tsuang, M. Tohen, G.E.P. Zahner), pp. 301–315, Wiley-Liss, New York.
8. Cochran S. (1984) Preventing medical noncompliance in the outpatient treatment of bipolar affective disorders. *J. Consult. Clin. Psychol.*, **52**: 873–878.
9. Zaretsky A.E., Segal Z.V., Gemar M. (1999) Cognitive therapy for bipolar depression: a pilot study. *Can. J. Psychiatry*, **44**: 491–494.
10. Lam D.H., Bright J., Jones S., Hayward P., Schuck N., Chisolm D., Sham P. (2000) Cognitive therapy for bipolar illness—a pilot study of relapse prevention. *Cogn. Ther. Res.*, **24**: 503–520.
11. Scott J. (2001) Pilot study of cognitive therapy in bipolar disorders. *Bipolar Disord.*, **3** (Suppl. 1): 56.
12. Lam D.H., Jones S.H., Hayward P., Bright J.A. (1999) *Cognitive Therapy for Bipolar Disorder. A Therapist's Guide to Concepts, Methods, and Practice.* Wiley, New York.

13. Lam D., Watkins E., Hayward P., Bright J., Sham P. (2001) *Bipolar Disord.*, **3** (Suppl. 1): 19.
14. Holloway F. (2001) Balancing clinical values and finite resources. In *Textbook of Community Psychiatry* (Eds G. Thornicroft, G. Szmukler), pp. 167–178, Oxford University Press, New York.
15. Colom F., Martinez-Aran A., Reinares M., Benabarre A., Corbella B., Vieta E. (2001) Psychoeducation and prevention of relapse in bipolar disorders: preliminary results. *Bipolar Disord.*, **3** (Suppl. 1): 32.
16. D'Souza R., Hustig H. (2001) A case control study in the use of telemedicine for treatment adherence in remote and rural bipolar patients. *Bipolar Disord.*, **3** (Suppl. 1): 33.
17. Parikh S.V., Goering P.N., Kennedy S.H., Kusznir A., Parker C., Chopra E., Norton L. (2001) The bipolar treatment optimization program: a novel simultaneous patient and provider intervention. *Bipolar Disord.*, **3** (Suppl. 1): 50–51.
18. Taylor R.I, Mallinger A.G., Thase M.E., Zuckoff A., Swartz H.A., Frank E. (2001) Pharmacotherapy treatment adherence in patients with bipolar disorder: can motivational interviewing strategies make a difference? *Bipolar Disord.*, **3** (Suppl. 1): 59.
19. Basco M., Rush A.J. (1996) *Cognitive Behavioral Therapy for Bipolar Disorder.* Guilford, New York.
20. Zaretsky A.E., Parikh S.V., Lancee W.E. (2001) A randomized controlled trial of adjunctive CBT in the maintenance treatment of bipolar disorder. *Bipolar Disord.*, **3** (Suppl. 1): 63.

4.7

Closing the Circle: The Use of Adjunctive Psychotherapies to Improve Treatment Outcomes for Bipolar Patients

Barbara O. Rothbaum and Millie C. Astin[1]

In a sense, our understanding and treatment of bipolar disorders have almost come full circle over the last half century. Before the introduction of lithium, bipolar disorder was treated largely as a psychodynamic illness related to early childhood experiences and familial environment. The discovery that lithium could stabilize the excessive mood states of mania and depression in the bipolar patient revolutionized the way bipolar illness was conceptualized, and treated, as well as the questions being asked about the nature of bipolar disorders.

Essentially, a purely biological and medical model replaced the earlier psychodynamic views of the disorder. This in turn stimulated research into the biochemistry and genetics of the disorder. Risk rates for developing bipolar disorder from twin studies, identification in chromosome 18 of a

[1] *Trauma and Anxiety Recovery Program, Emory University School of Medicine, 1365 Clifton Road, NE, Atlanta, GA 30322, USA*

site of risk for development of bipolar disorder, the successful use of anti-seizure medications such as valproate and carbamazepine, followed by newer generation medications, have further delineated bipolar disorder as a primarily biological and genetic phenomenon rather than a psychosocial one [1].

As Mark Bauer points out, adjunctive psychotherapy was included from the beginning in the lithium clinics that developed in the 1970s. However, its use was not applied systematically and was primarily valued solely in terms of increasing medication adherence. Other than the use of mixed-diagnosis group therapy during hospitalization or the minimal supportive and education components of medication management, systematic and consistent use of psychosocial interventions were all but abandoned in the treatment of bipolar patients. Furthermore, research investigating their usefulness was sparse until the last decade.

Without doubt, pharmacotherapy is the primary treatment of choice for bipolar disorder. In fact, psychotherapy with unmedicated bipolar patients is usually considered fruitless given both the difficulties with managing manic patients and the efficacy of antimanic medications. Nevertheless, a growing body of literature, as indicated in Bauer's review, suggests that psychotherapy in combination with medication can increase treatment response across several domains [2–4].

When treating a patient for any disorder, it would be ideal to use treatments or treatment packages that result in the greatest and broadest levels of improvement. Too often, however, we focus on symptom reduction alone, ignoring the impact the illness has had on other areas of functioning. Bipolar disorder is a case in point. Reducing symptoms of mania and depression, of course, is crucial. However, clinicians and researchers have increasingly considered whether symptoms really can be managed if other areas of functioning are ignored. Bipolar disorder generally takes a huge toll on interpersonal, social, and occupational functioning both in terms of disruptions and consequences resulting from mood episodes as well as in terms of residual dysfunction. Naturally, as with any individual, disruption in any of these domains is stressful for bipolar patients. What sets bipolar patients apart is that these problems can be exacerbated by their illness and their illness can be exacerbated by these problems. As Bauer documents, stress is associated with increased mood episodes and hospitalizations. This is true despite effective medications even in compliant clients. Thus, a broader perspective which addresses domains other than symptom reduction and medication adherence is essential for comprehensive treatment of bipolar patients.

The good news is that the evidence that psychotherapies used as adjuncts to pharmacotherapy can address these broader domains is increasing. Not all studies have been randomized or well controlled, and little repetition of findings exists for the well-designed studies which do exist. Nevertheless, the current empirical data generally have found positive results for the use of psychotherapy with bipolar patients. There is also little evidence to date that one treatment is superior to another for bipolar patients as controlled comparative studies are nonexistent to date. As evidence grows that bipolar patients who receive adjunctive therapy fare better than those who receive medication only, comparison studies of treatment modalities will be needed.

While all of this is encouraging for the treatment of bipolar patients, outside of the research setting, widespread use of adjunctive therapies for bipolar patients has yet to occur. Most inpatient treatment includes some form of group therapy for patients. These may be psychoeducational in nature or process-oriented, and usually include all patients on the ward irrespective of diagnosis. Thus, addressing issues that pertain particularly to bipolar patients is limited. In outpatient treatment, bipolar patients rarely receive any form of adjunctive therapy specifically to address issues related to bipolar illness. When psychotherapies become a regular component of the treatment of bipolar patients, we will have indeed come full circle.

REFERENCES

1. Tohen M. (1997) Mania. In *Acute Care Psychiatry: Diagnosis and Treatment* (Eds. L.I. Sederer, A.J., Rothschild), pp. 141–165, Williams and Wilkins, Baltimore.
2. Craighead W.E., Miklowitz D.J., Vajik F.C., Frank E. (1999) Psychosocial treatments for bipolar disorder. In *A Guide to Treatments that Work* (Eds P.E. Nathan, J.M. Gorman), pp. 240–248, Oxford University Press, New York.
3. Parikh S.V., Kusumakar V., Haslam D.R., Matte R., Sharma V., Yatham L.N. (1997) Psychosocial interventions as an adjunct to pharmacotherapy in bipolar disorders. *Can. J. Psychiatry*, **42** (Suppl. 2): 74S–78S.
4. Rothbaum B.O., Astin M.C. (2000) Integration of pharmacotherapy and psychotherapy for bipolar disorder. *J. Clin. Psychiatry*, **61** (Suppl. 9): 68–75.

4.8
Psychosocial Approaches for Bipolar Disorder: Is There Room for Change in Addition to Coping?

Yiannis G. Papakostas, Iannis M. Zervas and George N. Christodoulou[1]

Mark Bauer's meticulous review leaves us with an inescapable impression: consistent themes with striking similarities run across the existing psychosocial treatments of bipolar disorder (BD). First, most of these approaches have developed as adjuncts, rather than alternatives, to pharmacological therapy. Second, alongside the specific aspects of each intervention, they all include, and appear to rely heavily on, what Bauer refers to as the "common core of disease management components". Finally, the displayed favourable outcome of these treatments is, interestingly, uniformly equal. This finding is interpreted by the author to represent either a publication bias or to reflect the fact that almost all of these interventions share features that deal with "sensible disease management". Following the same line of reasoning we expect that, in the future, efforts to empirically identify this optimum "common core" (i.e. to help the patient better *cope* with the illness) and to estimate the magnitude of the therapeutic outcome, will be continued and intensified.

However, current thinking on psychosocial interventions for BD is plagued by certain conceptual limitations. Current therapeutic methods represent merely "symptom"-driven (data-driven or "bottom-up") approaches, as opposed to the plethora of theory-driven ("top-down") approaches in use for unipolar depression. A theory-driven approach encompasses both proximal (precipitation, maintenance) and distal causes (e.g. the vulnerability issue) of an illness, thus providing principles and guidelines or, at the very least, cues for intervention. The lack of such approaches in BD is understandable, in view of the prevailing conceptualization of BD as a biologically based illness, its bi-directionality in clinical phenomenology and its frequent switching of mood states, all significant obstacles to psychological explanations [1]. However, no matter how difficult or remote this possibility may seem to be, the development of such theories, together with their biological counterparts, will increase our understanding of the course and treatment of this devastating mental illness. Furthermore, they may be used to design more specific therapy approaches based on psychological and neuropsychological models of BD, in addition to the approaches currently in use, which are based primarily on sound clinical management and psychoeducation.

_____

[1] *Department of Psychiatry, Athens University Medical School, 74 Vasilissis Sophias Avenue, Athens, GR 115 28, Greece*

Psychoanalysis, of course, was a forerunner in proposing such theories, although the validity and/or clinical utility of such an approach have not been established in large-scale and/or controlled studies. There are, however, indications that psychological formulations derived from the two main contemporary psychotherapeutic approaches to affective illness, interpersonal and cognitive, albeit at an infantile stage, are starting to appear. In addition, there is an effort for these to be linked to the biological and neuropsychological knowledge acquired on BD.

For example, interpersonal and social rhythm therapy (IPSRT) is an attempt to link standard interpersonal therapy with the psycho-chronobiological theory of affective illness [2]. According to this theory, individuals with BD have a genetic predisposition to circadian rhythm and sleep–wake abnormalities, that may be responsible in part for the clinical picture of the illness [3]. Hence IPSRT consists of strategies aimed at directly addressing interpersonal stressors, in accordance with the premises of interpersonal therapy, and strategies promoting rhythm integrity during the daily routine of patients. Despite some preliminary negative results, the proponents of this approach argue in its favour, hoping that this conceptualization will improve the outcome in BD [2].

On the other hand, hypotheses about the psychological vulnerability to BD are already starting to be formulated in cognitive terms. Reilly-Harrington et al. [1] found that the bipolar patients' attributional style for negative events, dysfunctional attitudes and negative self-referent information processing interacted with stressful life events to increase the severity of both manic and depressive symptoms over a one-month period. Regarding the type of episode a BD patient will experience at a particular time, these authors speculate that this might depend on the particular type of stressful events, for example depression following a loss event and mania a stressful event that disrupts the sleep–wake cycle. It has also been demonstrated, in accordance with Beck's theory, that self-schemata in the interpersonal domain (sociotropy)—but not self-schemata in the autonomous domain—interact with interpersonal life events to predict subsequent symptom severity among bipolar patients [4]. It might be possible then that cognitive-behavioural interventions aiming at modifying maladaptive cognitive styles and schemata may be of value in treating BD. In addition, emerging neuropsychological information about BD may be utilized to design cognitive-behavioural or psychotherapeutic approaches specifically tailored to the individual's clinical presentation, aiming at rehabilitation [5].

In conclusion, our argument, and comment, is not meant to support the clinical application of the particular experimental therapies proposed in the examples above, but rather to expand our thinking about the promising future perspective of psychosocial intervention. It is important to allow for the possibility of *specific* psychosocial approaches, to develop in association with theoretically driven and scientifically based concepts and models of BD. So, in addition to existing methods, a new generation of more specific therapies may become available, focused more on promoting *change* rather than teaching *coping*.

REFERENCES

1. Reilly-Harrington N.A., Alloy L.B., Fresco D.M., Whitehouse W.G. (1999) Cognitive styles and life events interact to predict bipolar and unipolar symptomatology. *J. Abnorm. Psychol.*, **108**: 567–578.
2. Frank E., Swartz H.A., Kupfer D.J. (2000) Interpersonal and social rhythm therapy: managing the chaos of bipolar disorder. *Biol. Psychiatry*, **48**: 593–604.
3. Wehr T.A., Sack D.A., Rosenthal N.E. (1987) Sleep reduction as a final common pathway in the genesis of mania. *Am. J. Psychiatry*, **144**: 201–204.
4. Hammen C., Ellicott A., Gitlin M. (1992) Stressors and sociotropy/autonomy: a longitudinal study of their relationship to the course of bipolar disorder. *Cogn. Ther. Res.*, **16**: 409–418.
5. Post R.M., Denicoff K.D., Leverich G.S., Huggins T., Post S.W., Luckenbaugh D. (2000) Neuropsychological deficits of primary affective illness: implications for therapy. *Psychiatr. Ann.*, **30**: 485–494.

4.9
Psychosocial Treatments for Bipolar Disorder: Is There Evidence That They Work?

Paul J. Goodnick[1]

In the current scenario in which biological origins of bipolar disorder continue to be elucidated, and advances in pharmacological treatment are reported on a regular basis, it is not surprising that results of investigations of psychosocial treatments are not generally known, even in academic centres. Therefore, the review provided by Mark Bauer is quite welcome and timely. It is important to learn if these techniques have any role in this day of biological pre-eminence. For many years, it was simply assumed by proponents of psychodynamic psychotherapy that it must be helpful in all situations, including bipolar disorder, leading to development of methods for treatment without proven benefit [1]. Unfortunately, as in other arenas of psychopathology, its usefulness remains to be proven. However, at the same time, others with views originating from laboratory work deride any

[1] *Department of Psychiatry and Behavioral Sciences, University of Miami School of Medicine, D79, 1400 NW 10 Avenue, Miami, FL 33136, USA*

usefulness for psychosocial techniques. It becomes apparent in looking at current evidence that the type of results that might meet those of USA registration studies for pharmacological interventions are not available.

Despite that fact, there are at least controlled studies with positive results in the domain of family interventions. Two different studies with a total sample size of over 100 patients were conducted in randomized trials. The results of both studies indicated the presence of clinical symptom benefits for a period over one year. However, neither one showed that the intervention had any impact on the degree of adherence to treatment plan [2, 3]. Here there are specific benefits for the clinician in that each study was based on a specific manual that might be obtained for application. In contrast, although there have been five different studies of group or psychoeducational interventions, none were performed in randomized, controlled conditions. Therefore, the positive results of these programmes cannot be generalized. Despite the presence of a manual, excellent studies with interpersonal/social rhythms failed to show benefit [4].

Yet, practically all published studies have at least *some* positive results. This is not surprising, because of the reluctance to submit or accept for publication manuscripts with negative results. Not only that, but studies with more rigorous designs were equally likely to have positive results as those that were less stringent. Actually, in one way the negative results of the interpersonal rhythms trials [4, 5] may actually have useful clinical applications. As many manuals are available for conducting various interventions, the clinician needs to know how to choose a modality. However, with most showing benefits, confusion may reign as to where to place a focus of training. The key focus may very well be on the clinician's personal abilities to adhere and follow competently and empathically a particular mode of intervention. And above all, the clinician should not change modes of treatment due to wish to experiment, frustration, etc. Frank *et al.*'s research [4] clearly indicated that patients who did worse in maintenance treatment were those who were *switched* from one modality to another. Therefore, it would appear that individual psychotherapy, family-focused psychoeducational therapy [6], as well as cognitive-behavioural therapy even in challenging rapid-cycling bipolar patients [7], can all be beneficial. However, it is most important to be consistent for the patient.

Where should treatment take place for bipolar patients has never been fully resolved. Initially, the development of lithium clinics by Fieve [8], which was based on a medical model, enhanced assessments and regular follow-up. However, it was not adopted nationally in the USA, nor, in that model, was the role for psychoeducation or process groups clearly defined. In the USA at the current time, there are two large-scale studies underway, one in the US Department of Veterans Affairs health care system and one at the Group Health Cooperative (Puget Sound), a more private treatment environment, studying benefits of combinations of "access, patient education, and provider guidance". The results of these two studies will be more applicable to the generally found treatment environment.

As the results of psychosocial investigations involving both technique and environment as reported have been positive, it is yet to be determined as to the source of benefit. This result, when available, will help physicians, therapists, and patients, as well as administrators of health care, to know whether and which psychosocial approach to adopt and under what circumstances to pursue it.

REFERENCES

1. Cohen M.B., Baker G., Cohen R.A., Fromm-Reichmann F., Weigert E.V. (1954) An intensive study of twelve cases of manic-depressive psychosis. *Psychiatry*, **17**: 103–137.
2. Clarkin J.F., Glick I., Haas G., Spencer J., Lewis A., Peyser A., DeMane N., Good-Ellis M., Harris E., Lestell V. (1990) A randomized clinical trial of inpatient family intervention. V. Results for affective disorder. *J. Affect. Disord.*, **18**: 17–28.
3. Miklowitz D.J., Simoneau T.L., George E.L., Richards J.A., Kalbag A., Sachs-Ericsson N., Suddath R. (2000) Family-focused treatment of bipolar disorder: 1-year effects of a psychoeducational program in conjunction with pharmacotherapy. *Biol. Psychiatry*, **48**: 582–592.
4. Frank E., Swartz H.A., Mallinger A.G., Thase M.E., Weaver E.V., Kupfer D.J. (1999) Adjunctive psychotherapy for bipolar disorder: Effects of changing treatment modality. *J. Abnorm. Psychol.*, **108**: 579–587.
5. Frank E., Swartz H.A., Kupfer D.J. (2000) Interpersonal and social rhythm therapy: managing the chaos of bipolar disorder. *Biol. Psychiatry*, **48**: 593–604.
6. Weiss R.D., Griffin M.L., Greenfield S.F., Najavits L.M., Wyner D., Soto J.A., Hennen J.A. (2000) Group therapy for patients with bipolar disorder and substance dependence: results of a pilot study. *J. Clin. Psychiatry*, **61**: 361–367.
7. Satterfield J.M. (1999) Adjunctive cognitive-behavioral therapy for rapid-cycling bipolar disorder: an empirical case study. *Psychiatry*, **62**: 357–369.
8. Fieve R.R. (1975) The lithium clinic: a new model for the delivery of psychiatric services. *Am. J. Psychiatry*, **132**: 1018–1022.

4.10
The Impact of Adjunctive Psychosocial Treatments in Bipolar Disorder and the Need for a Theoretical Framework

Andrés Heerlein[1]

Despite the strong development of pharmacological strategies for the acute and prophylactic treatment of bipolar disorder (BD), several studies have shown that the incidence, frequency of relapses, comorbidity, complications and functional impairment of patients with BD have increased in recent decades [1]. Subjects with BD are prone to recurrences even when they are regularly maintained on lithium or anticonvulsant regimens. 90% of bipolar patients have thought about stopping medication several times. 50% of lithium responders stop taking the drug against medical instructions at least once in their life, and one-third try several times. 69% of individuals relapse within two years, and in five years only 23.4% of patients remain on lithium and free from episodes [1]. BD is also associated with significant problems in personal management, family and marital dysfunction, and occupational problems.

Mark Bauer's accurate presentation of two main psychosocial interventions in patients with BD, namely psychotherapy and "context of care", shows us the significant role of an adequate psychosocial approach in this field. Five main reasons are mentioned supporting psychosocial adjunctive treatments: the high prevalence of pharmacological treatment-resistant cases, the frequently poor compliance, the evidence that life events may influence the course of BD, the high prevalence of social, family and occupational dysfunction, and the overall costs of BD.

We would like to add another reason: according to several studies, the mortality of patients with BD is significantly higher than in the general population, not only as a consequence of the higher rates of suicide and accidents but also for cardiovascular or other diseases—for instance, hypothyroidism and hyperthyroidism [2, 3]. Long-term medication treatments can reduce by two-thirds suicides among bipolar patients [3]. With efficient psychotherapeutic support, an even better outcome should be expected, due to improved compliance, medical monitoring and psychosocial functioning.

In the past years there has been a substantial increase in the number and quality of studies demonstrating the gains of adding psychosocial treatments to the medication management of BD [1, 4].

Several authors agree that family and marital psychoeducational interventions and individual interpersonal and social rhythm therapy can enhance patients' adherence to medications, ability to cope with environ-

---

[1] *Departamento de Psiquiatría, Facultad de Medicina, Universidad de Chile, Av. La Paz 1003, Santiago de Chile, Chile*

mental stress triggers and social-occupational functioning [5]. A recent study concluded that family-focused psychoeducational treatment appears to be an efficacious adjunct to pharmacotherapy for BD [6]. It may also help to reduce the high prevalence of marital and familiar dysfunction associated with bipolarity.

Interpersonal and social rhythm therapy (IPSRT) assumes that life events may cause disruptions in patients' social rhythms, which can perturb circadian rhythms and sleep–wake cycles, leading to the development of bipolar symptoms. Administered in combination with medications, IPSRT may help to regularize daily routines, diminish interpersonal problems, adhere to medication regimens and improve overall functioning. An initial report could not demonstrate a significant effect of IPSRT on medication treatment of BD [7]. However, a recent study suggests that interpersonal and social rhythm therapy may be particularly useful for bipolar depression [8]. A new approach has recently been proposed for the treatment of BD including "the use of phase-specific sequenced psychotherapies delivered in variable patterns and linked to fluctuating mood states" [7].

Preliminary data on cognitive-behavioural therapy (CBT) for BD suggest that it may be helpful by increasing compliance, improving quality of life and functioning, facilitating recognition of early symptoms, decreasing relapses and depressive symptomatology [9]. CBT is the only non-pharmacological therapeutic strategy that has been tested for the treatment of bipolar depression, and recent data suggests that it may be particularly useful for this kind of depression.

Since the retrospective study of Rennie [10], several reports have indicated the importance of psychosocial factors for the onset, clinical course and outcome of BD. Personality variables have also been identified as important factors affecting pathogenesis, diagnosis, treatment response, outcome and mortality of these patients [11–13]. It has been suggested that the integrated consideration of life events and personality traits or disorders in specific psychosocial strategies for BD could improve significantly the clinical course and be very helpful in reducing relapses and mortality. Some preliminary studies have demonstrated specific personality traits associated with a poor long-term outcome in BD [12]. Nevertheless, till now life event and personality research have gone separate ways. An integrative view of the interaction between personality patterns and life events in the emergency of bipolar symptoms is needed. An interesting contribution has been provided by the school of Heidelberg, describing two opposed personality structures called *typus melancholicus* and *typus manicus* [14, 15]. According to this model, bipolars often have opposite traits or develop tendencies contrary to unipolars in their social, occupational and family roles. Based on phenomenological assumptions, this model provides an integration of personality patterns and life events in a comprehensive approach to bipolarity.

Kraus proposed an identity theory which considers the importance of social roles and other identity variables in BD [16]. Future research in the field of psychotherapy of BD should also consider outcome studies that go beyond simple pre-post comparisons, including a detailed model of the underlying pathogenetic mechanism which is addressed by a therapeutic technique. No consensus has yet been found regarding the best psychotherapeutic strategies in BD and results are still rather inconsistent [17]. We therefore emphasize the necessity not only for systematic clinical research but also for a theoretical framework considering the integration of symptoms, personality patterns and life events.

REFERENCES

1. Johnson S.L., Greenhouse W., Bauer M. (2000) Psychosocial approaches to the treatment of bipolar disorder. *Curr. Opin. Psychiatry*, **13**: 69–72.
2. Rorsman B. (1974) Mortality among psychiatric patients. *Acta Psychiatr. Scand.*, **50**: 354–375.
3. Angst J., Sellaro R., Angst F. (1998) Long-term outcome and mortality of treated versus untreated bipolar and depressed patients: a preliminary report. *Int. J. Psychiatry Clin. Pract.*, **2**: 115–119.
4. Craighead W.E., Miklowitz D.J., Vajc F.C., Frank E. (2000) Psychosocial interventions for bipolar disorder. *J. Clin. Psychiatry*, **61** (Suppl. 13): 58–64.
5. Clarkin J.F., Carpenter D., Hull J., Wilner P., Glick I. (1998) Effects of psychoeducational intervention for married patients with bipolar disorder and their spouses. *Psychiatr. Serv.*, **49**: 531–533.
6. Miklowitz D.J., Simoneau T.L., George E.L., Richards J.A., Kalbag A., Sachs-Ericsson N., Suddath R. (2000) Family-focused treatment of bipolar disorder: 1-year effects of a psychoeducational program in conjunction with pharmacotherapy. *Biol. Psychiatry*, **48**: 582–592.
7. Frank E., Swartz H.A., Kupfer D.J. (2000) Interpersonal and social rhythm therapy: managing the chaos of bipolar disorder. *Biol. Psychiatry*, **48**: 430–432.
8. Swartz H.A., Frank E. (2001) Psychotherapy for bipolar depression: a phase-specific treatment strategy? *Bipolar Disord.*, **3**: 11–22.
9. Patelis-Siotis I. (2001) Cognitive-behavioral therapy: applications for the management of bipolar disorder. *Bipolar Disord.*, **3**: 1–10.
10. Rennie T.A.C. (1942) Prognosis in manic-depressive psychoses. *Am. J. Psychiatry*, **98**: 801–814.
11. Heerlein A., Santander J., Richter P. (1996) Premorbid personality aspects in mood and schizophrenic disorders. *Compr. Psychiatry*, **37**: 430–434.
12. Heerlein A., Richter P., González M., Santander J. (1998) Personality patterns and outcome in depressive and bipolar disorders. *Psychopathology*, **31**: 15–22.
13. Angst J., Clayton P. (1986) Premorbid personality of depressive, bipolar, and schizophrenic patients with special reference to suicidal issues. *Compr. Psychiatry*, **27**: 511–532.
14. Tellenbach H. (1983) *Melancholie, Problemgeschichte, Endogenität, Typologie, Pathogenese, Klinik*. Springer, Berlin.
15. Von Zerssen D., Pössl J. (1990) The premorbid personality of patients with different subtypes of an affective illness. *J. Affect. Disord.*, **18**: 39–50.

16. Kraus A. (1995) Psychotherapy based on identity problems of depressives. *Am. J. Psychother.*, **49**: 197–212.
17. Vieta C.F., Martinez A., Jorquera A., Gasto C. (1998) What is the role of psychotherapy in the treatment of bipolar disorder? *Psychother. Psychosom.*, **67**: 3–9.

4.11
The Role of Psychotherapy for Treating Residual Symptoms in Bipolar Disorder

Giovanni A. Fava[1]

The role of psychosocial treatments is attracting increasing interest in bipolar disorder. Bauer's review analyses the very promising literature already available. At the same time, he calls for further research in the area, which has been relatively neglected compared to unipolar depression. A large body of evidence—reviewed in detail elsewhere [1]—has identified a substantial residual symptomatology in patients with both unipolar and bipolar disorders. In bipolar illness, this residual symptomatology encompasses subclinical mood and anxiety symptoms, irritable mood, impaired psychological well-being and social adjustment. Keitner *et al* [2] have estimated that, in patients who appear to have recovered, residual mania is present in 70% of cases and residual depression in about 60%. Subsyndromal fluctuations were found to increase risk of relapse [3, 4]. Benazzi [4] suggested that residual symptoms in bipolar II patients may have a kindling effect and lead to new acute episodes.

Also in unipolar depression, residual symptoms were found to be one of the strongest risk factors for relapse. In two randomized controlled trials [5, 6], cognitive-behavioural treatment of residual symptoms was found to significantly improve long-term outcome of recurrent depression, by acting on those residual symptoms that progress to become prodromes of relapse [5] or by improving psychological well-being and coping skills [5, 6]. This has led to the development of a sequential strategy based on the use of pharmacotherapy in the acute phase of illness and of cognitive behavioural therapy (CBT) in its residual phase [7].

This sequential approach was recently applied to 15 patients with bipolar I disorder who relapsed while on lithium prophylaxis [8], despite initial response and adequate compliance. The residual symptoms of these patients were treated by cognitive-behavioural methods in an open trial. A two

[1] *Affective Disorders Program, Department of Psychology, University of Bologna, Viale Berti Pichat 5, 40127 Bologna, Italy*

to nine year follow-up was performed. Only five of the 15 patients had a new affective episode during follow-up. These preliminary results suggest that a trial of CBT addressed to residual symptomatology may enhance lithium prophylaxis and improve long-term outcome of bipolar disorder. They are supported by another recent trial [9], which found that CBT was associated with statistically significant greater improvements in symptoms and functioning than allocation to a waiting-list control group.

The two studies [8, 9] thus indicate that CBT may enhance the level of recovery in patients undergoing pharmacological prophylaxis and this may result in an improved outcome. Reduction of residual symptomatology may become a target for psychosocial efforts in bipolar disorder, together with psychoeducation and lifestyle changes, leading to a more enduring recovery than that entailed by current purely pharmacological strategies [10].

REFERENCES

1. Fava G.A. (1999) Subclinical symptoms in mood disorders. *Psychol. Med.*, **29**: 47–61.
2. Keitner G.I., Solomon D.A., Ryan C.E., Miller I.W., Mallinger A., Kupfer D.J., Frank E. (1996) Prodromal and residual symptoms in bipolar I disorder. *Compr. Psychiatry*, **37**: 362–367.
3. Keller M.B., Lavori P.W., Kane J.M., Gelenberg A.J., Rosenbaum J.F., Walzer E.A., Baker L.A. (1992) Subsyndromal symptoms in bipolar disorder. *Arch. Gen. Psychiatry*, **49**: 371–376.
4. Benazzi F. (2001) Prevalence and clinical correlates of residual depressive symptoms in bipolar II disorder. *Psychother. Psychosom.* (in press).
5. Fava G.A., Rafanelli C., Grandi S., Conti S., Belluardo P. (1998) Prevention of recurrent depression with cognitive behavioral therapy. *Arch. Gen. Psychiatry*, **55**: 816–820.
6. Paykel E.S., Scott J., Teasdale J.D., Johnson A.L., Garland A., Moore R., Jenaway A., Cornwall P.L., Hayhurst H., Abbott R., Pope M. (1999) Prevention of relapse in residual depression by cognitive therapy. *Arch. Gen. Psychiatry*, **56**: 829–835.
7. Fava G.A. (1999) Sequential use of pharmacotherapy and psychotherapy in depressive disorders. In *Depressive Disorders* (Eds M. Maj, N. Sartorius), pp. 226–228, Wiley, Chichester.
8. Fava G.A., Bartolucci G., Rafanelli C., Mangelli L. (2001) Cognitive behavioral management of patients with bipolar disorder relapsing while on lithium prophylaxis. *J. Clin. Psychiatry* (in press).
9. Scott J., Garland A., Moorhead S. (2001) A pilot study of cognitive therapy in bipolar disorders. *Psychol. Med.* (in press).
10. Vestergaard P., Licht R.W. (2001) 50 years with lithium treatment in affective disorders. *World J. Biol. Psychiatry*, **2**: 18–26.

4.12
Information Processing and Self-Related Models in Bipolar Disorder
Anne Palmer and Malcolm Adams[1]

An important feature of Mark Bauer's paper is a resurgence of interest in the "context of care" being regarded as a psychosocial intervention in its own right. In 1995, we argued for a service-based, rehabilitation model of care for patients with bipolar disorder (BD) [1], in which the emphasis was on disturbances in functioning (disability) rather than on symptomatology (impairment) *per se*.

It has been postulated that the disability and impairment associated with BD depend in part on information-processing biases, with particular emphasis on self-related meaning. However, until recently there were meagre experimental insights to aid our understanding as to whether, and if so, how such biases are related to mood states. While less extensive than research on unipolar depression or schizophrenia, there is an emerging literature indicating that patients with BD clearly process information and self-related meanings in different ways from the normal population, and we are now beginning to understand something about immediate information processing in patients with bipolar disorder. This in turn, has implications for the type of psychosocial intervention offered. An important question is whether these differences are closely related to mood state or persist when patients are in remission.

Recently, a longitudinal study was conducted in which 18 patients with BD were tested on a series of cognitive tasks in manic, depressed and euthymic moods and compared to matched controls [2]. Since each participant acted as their own control, there could be no sampling confound between manic and depressed states as would be the case in a cross-sectional design. Results showed that the ability to sustain attention and inhibit a response to a well-established set was impaired in patients with BD compared to controls, in each of the manic, depressed and euthymic phases. There was evidence that patients with BD had more trouble in manic than in depressed phases when re-engaging with a task following a withhold response. There was also some impairment of sentence memory—but at equivalent levels in manic and depressed states. This finding is consistent with many other previous demonstrations that patients with BD have deficits in non-semantic processing, even when they are technically in remission, as recently reviewed by Murphy and Sahakian [3].

Similarly, a recent study of euthymic BD clients demonstrated that, between episodes of illness, clients show similar patterns of cognitive

[1] *Norfolk Mental Health Care Trust, Kingfisher House, Hellesdon Hospital, Drayton High Road, Drayton, Norwich, NR8 6BH, United Kingdom*

vulnerability to individuals with unipolar depression [4]. In comparison to healthy controls, BD clients had lower levels of self-esteem, higher levels of dysfunctional attitudes (particularly related to need for approval and perfectionism), and poorer problem-solving skills. This is consistent with the findings of Collen [5] that between illness episodes patients experience fluctuating levels of subclinical symptomatology and that increases in the amplitude of these fluctuations act as an early warning sign for onset of an illness episode.

Other results indicate that there are also mood-related biases. O'Curry [6] found that, as in unipolar depression, depressed BD patients recalled fewer specific memories than non-depressed people on an autobiographical memory task. In addition, BD patients in a manic phase recalled fewer negative memories than either depressed BD patients or normal controls. Barnard et al [2] also found differences between processing of meaning in depressed and manic phases. When patients with bipolar disorder were in manic states, discrepancies in propositional meaning [7], be they positive, negative or neutral, were more likely to pass unnoticed in the flow of ideation and more attention was paid to more general, abstract meanings or schema. This is consistent with the observation that rapid ideation, creative and "dendritic" thought patterns [8] are common, along with impulsive or disinhibited behaviours whose consequences are either not scrutinized or appraised as important in the prevailing context.

Newman et al [9] observe that patients with BD demonstrate information-processing biases that look like traits (long-standing predispositions) and states (respond to environmental triggers and biological activation). Insofar as some of these biases in information processing are relatively stable, then returns to normal levels of symptomatology, and therefore to functioning, may not be realistic, and thus a context of care, rehabilitation approach will be an important part of the treatment package.

REFERENCES

1. Palmer A.G., Williams H., Adams M. (1995) Cognitive behavioural therapy for bipolar affective disorder in a group format. *Behav. Cogn. Psychother.*, **23**: 153–168.
2. Barnard P., Palmer A., Scott S., Knightly W. Immediate processing of schema discrepant meaning in bipolar disorders. Submitted for publication.
3. Murphy F.C., Sahakian B.J. (2001) Neuropsychology of bipolar disorder. *Br. J. Psychiatry* (in press).
4. Scott J., Stanton B., Garland A., Ferrier I.N. (2000) Cognitive vulnerability in patients with bipolar disorder. *Psychol. Med.*, **30**: 467–472.
5. Collen A. (1995) Early warning signs in manic-depression: a prospective longitudinal study of four single cases. Unpublished ClinPsyD thesis, University of East Anglia.

6. O'Curry S. (1999) Is mania a defence against depression? Unpublished Clin-PsyD thesis, University of East Anglia.
7. Barnard P.J., Teasdale J.D. (1991) Interacting cognitive subsystems: a systemic approach to cognitive-affective interaction and change. *Cognition and Emotion*, 5: 1–39.
8. Jamison K.R. (1993) *Touched with Fire: Manic-Depressive Illness and the Artistic Temperament.* Simon & Schuster, New York.
9. Newman C.F., Leahy R.L., Beck A.T., Reilly-Harrington N., Gyulai L. (2001). *Bipolar Disorder: A Cognitive Therapy Approach.* American Psychological Association, Washington (in press).

4.13
Beyond Medications: Taking a New Look at
Psychosocial Treatments for Bipolar Disorder

Nancy A. Huxley[1]

Bipolar disorder is a severe, recurring or chronic group of illnesses. Its symptoms can be ameliorated by pharmacological treatments with varying success, and with highly variable types and levels of sustained disability, associated with both non-adherence and incomplete effectiveness of long-term pharmacotherapy. Such limitations of pharmacological treatments at both symptomatic and functional levels, combined with emerging support for the role of environmental factors as contributors to the expression of the disorder, highlight the need for additional interventions to optimize comprehensive programmes of treatment and rehabilitation. As noted by Mark Bauer, individual, group, and family psychosocial treatments are increasingly being studied for their contributions to relapse prevention, medication adherence, functional improvement, modulation of the impact of life stressors, and reducing overall costs to society, and increasingly applied empirically, even without definitive research support.

In evaluating what we know about these treatments, it is important to emphasize the very limited number of studies published on the topic of psychosocial interventions in bipolar disorder, which stands in marked contrast to the much more extensive research in depression [1], schizophrenia [2] and anxiety disorders [3]. To a large extent, this disparity may derive from the false, though evidently common, belief that bipolar disorder is a contraindication for psychotherapy [4]. Most of the few available studies of psychosocial interventions in bipolar disorder report positive outcomes, so far at least, regardless of the specific form of the intervention or the theory

[1] *Intensive Outpatient Program for Bipolar Disorders, McLean Hospital, 115 Mill Street, Belmont, MA 02478, USA*

behind it. However, there are no reports of studies that compared randomly the potential benefits of multiple types of interventions, some of which have been initiated for schizophrenia, for instance [5]. Moreover, it will be essential to define which components of therapy are necessary or sufficient for positive outcomes.

Mark Bauer notes common elements among the interventions studied, including educational and illness-management efforts. Although it seems intuitive that illness education and management skills are likely to be important to limiting risk of illness recurrence and disability, such information is not consistently imparted to patients in clinical practice in the United States. This status of psychosocial efforts for bipolar disorder may reflect a failure to appreciate its importance, as well as current fragmentation in the organization and financing of medical care in this country. Many practising mental health clinicians are not well informed about bipolar disorder, and the design of many care delivery systems currently concentrates on medication as the primary therapeutic intervention in bipolar disorder. Mark Bauer considers several ways of addressing these shortcomings in the development of comprehensive and continuous systems of care for bipolar disorder patients. Continued development of empirically tested and reproducible methods of providing psychological and rehabilitative care for bipolar disorder patients, their families, and primary care providers will certainly contribute to minimizing risks of symptomatic relapse, long-term disability, and the high indirect costs associated with this disorder.

At McLean Hospital, we have developed a comprehensive group therapy programme for the treatment of bipolar disorder patients. Various types of group therapy are available, each designed specifically for bipolar disorder patients, with attention to illness education, relapse prevention, cognitive and behavioural skills, interpersonal stressors, treatment adherence, and vocational problems. Interventions are tailored to the evolving needs of specific patients. With a first-episode patient, we might focus primarily on illness education, relapse prevention, and discussion of reactions to having the illness. Later groups, instead, might focus on challenges of returning to work and social relations. Individual differences in patient knowledge and mastery of skills call for a high degree of flexibility in the design and implementation of treatment programmes. Moreover, there are many serious, often limiting, challenges in securing financial support for such interventions.

Finally, there are still very few, if any, studies of rehabilitative or vocational interventions with bipolar disorder patients. Given the high functional disability associated with the disorder, such interventions may be particularly important for limiting disability, enhancing self-efficacy, improving other dimensions of outcome, and reducing indirect costs related to disability. Rehabilitative interventions have established efficacy with other psychiatric disorders, including schizophrenia [6]. My own experience in leading vocational groups for bipolar disorder patients supports their value in increasing ability to manage workplace stress and deal with fluctuating moods, fears, and concerns about competency. In my opinion, a high priority should be given to developing and evaluating such rehabilitation-oriented programmes as a component of comprehensive care of this group of common and often severe disorders, following the lead of advances in care for other major neuropsychiatric conditions.

REFERENCES

1. Frank E. (1991) Interpersonal psychotherapy as a maintenance treatment for patients with recurrent depression. *Psychotherapy*, **28**: 259–266.
2. Huxley N.A., Rendall M., Sederer L. (2000) Psychosocial treatments in schizophrenia: a review of the literature. *J. Nerv. Ment. Dis.*, **188**: 187–201.
3. Power K.G., Simpson R.J., Swanson V., Wallace L.A. (1990) Controlled comparison of pharmacological and psychological treatment of generalized anxiety disorder in primary care. *Br. J. Gen. Pract.*, **40**: 289–294.
4. Yalom I.D. (1985) *The Theory and Practice of Group Psychotherapy*. Basic Books, New York.
5. Falloon I.R.H., McGill C.W., Boyd J.L., Pederson J. (1987) Family management in the prevention of morbidity of schizophrenia: social outcome of a two-year longitudinal study. *Psychol. Med.*, **17**: 59–66.
6. Lehman A.F. (1995) Vocational rehabilitation in schizophrenia. *Schizophr. Bull.*, **21**: 645–656.

4.14
Adjunctive Family Treatment in Bipolar Disorder:
Is it Useful? Is it Feasible?

Gabor I. Keitner[1]

The pendulum is still swinging. From Kraepelin's biologically determined framework for the etiology and course of manic-depressive psychosis [1] to Frieda Fromm-Reichman's analytic assumptions about its etiology [2], to recent emphasis on neurotransmitter dysregulation and the primacy of pharmacotherapy, there is again a recognition for the important role that psychosocial variables play in the evolution of bipolar disorder. Psychosocial treatments (individual, couples, family, group) have become more

[1] *Department of Psychiatry, Rhode Island Hospital and Mood Disorders Program, 593 Eddy Street, Providence, RI 02903, USA*

refined and more clearly explicated in manuals that allow for more uniform and reproducible applications. A number of these psychosocial treatments have been tested for efficacy in carefully designed studies using methodology borrowed from clinical trials of pharmaceutical agents.

This is clearly for the good, as the pharmacotherapy of mania, and particularly of depression, leaves a large percentage of patients with significant residual psychopathology. It should not be a surprise to find that a chronic relapsing/remitting illness that undermines a patient's security in his/her emotional and cognitive stability should also cause major disruptions in the patient's and their significant other's lives. If we really accept the biopsychosocial model of illness, then combining pharmacotherapy with individual and family treatment should be the norm rather than the exception.

Mark Bauer's comprehensive review of the literature confirms that there is good evidence for the usefulness of adjunctive psychosocial treatments in bipolar disorder. A wide range of treatments in different settings, using somewhat different methods, have been found to be helpful. Our research group in the Mood Disorders Program and the Family Research Program at Brown University has also been studying the impact that mood disorders (major depression, bipolar disorders) have on family functioning for over 25 years [3].

The conceptual framework that we use for understanding the role of the family in psychiatric disorders, including bipolar disorder, is the McMaster Model of Family Functioning (MCMFF) [4]. The MCMFF attempts to understand families along six dimensions of functioning, including problem solving, communication, roles, affective responsiveness, affective involvement and behaviour control. In addition to this multidimensional perspective of family functioning, the model has significant research applicability in that it has a variety of assessment instruments that allow for quantitative evaluation of these family dimensions from a number of different perspectives.

The Family Assessment Device (FAD) is a self-report questionnaire filled out by family members that evaluates their perception of their functioning along the six dimensions of the McMaster Model as well as on a general functioning scale which assesses the overall level of family functioning [5]. The FAD provides an internal perspective of the families' functioning. The McMaster Clinical Rating Scale (MCRS) is a seven-item rating scale of the six dimensions of the MCMFF as well as an overall health pathology rating designed to be completed by an external rater, providing a more external view of the families' functioning [6]. The MCRS rating can be made using the McMaster Structured Interview for Family Functioning (McSIFF), a structured interview of family functioning designed to provide necessary information about the full range of family dimensions to arrive at a reliable and valid rating of the family [7]. All of the above instruments have been psychometrically tested and validated.

Finally, a family treatment approach, the Problem Centered Systems Therapy of the Family (PCSTF), has also been developed and detailed in a treatment manual [8]. The PCSTF is a highly structured, multidimensional short-term and systems oriented treatment. The integration of assessment instruments and a treatment programme lends this model to systematic clinical application, training, and research.

In a recently completed study of the value of adjunctive family treatment in bipolar disorder, we randomly assigned 92 patients to receive either standard treatment (medications plus clinical management), or family therapy (the PCSTF) plus standard treatment, or a multi-family psychoeducation group plus standard treatment. We wanted to know not only whether adjunctive family treatment was helpful in bipolar disorder but also if the particular format of the family intervention was important. Would families benefit from a form of family therapy geared to their particular concerns or would a more generic multi-family psychoeducational group provide similar benefits [9]?

Preliminary analyses of the results from this study suggest that adjunctive family interventions led to an increased rate of recovery from the bipolar episode at four and 10 months follow-up in contrast to those patients who received pharmacotherapy alone, although the difference was not statistically significant. Patients receiving the PCSTF therapy had a recovery rate of around 42%, those receiving the multi-family psychoeducation group of 38%, and those receiving pharmacotherapy alone of 20%. It is noteworthy that even with the adjunctive psychosocial intervention there was only a 40% recovery rate in this severely ill population. The very low recovery rate on pharmacotherapy alone is similarly poor to results from patients with severe unipolar depression treated with pharmacotherapy alone.

There is both good and bad news here. The good news is that the evidence does support the added benefit of psychosocial interventions in bipolar disorder. The availability and delivery of these treatments, however, remain very problematic. There are not enough well-trained therapists to provide tested psychosocial treatments. There is a tendency for therapists to pick up components of various treatment packages at brief workshops and seminars and then to modify them according to their belief systems and personalities. The treatments consequently used are not the ones tested. We have to make a greater effort to educate our profession about the availability of effective treatment models and the importance of receiving adequate training in them.

An additional problem is the need for coordination between therapists. The psychiatrist, the psychotherapist and the family therapist all need to communicate with each other about their formulation of the patient's problems and their particular approach to it. This integration across treatment modalities is difficult because of the timing and energy involved, particularly when the time is not reimbursed.

A broader socio-economic and political problem is the lack of sufficient reimbursement for the kind of comprehensive treatment approach that is advocated by Bauer's review. Health insurance companies, at least in North America, are disinclined to provide sufficient resources to enable patients to receive combined biological and psychosocial treatments from the best trained practitioners. More studies highlighting the cost effectiveness of this approach will be necessary before insurers become convinced that the greater upfront cost will be worthwhile in the long-term management of this chronic illness.

REFERENCES

1. Kraepelin E. (1921) *Manic Depressive Insanity and Paranoia*. Livingstone, Edinburgh.
2. Fromm-Reichman F. (1949) Intensive psychotherapy of manic-depressives: a preliminary report. *Confinia Neurologica*, **9**: 158–165.
3. Miller I.W., Ryan C.E., Keitner G.I., Bishop D.S., Epstein N.B. (2000) The McMaster approach to families: theory, assessment, treatment and research. *J. Family Therapy*, **22**: 168–189.
4. Epstein N., Bishop D., Levin S. (1978) The McMaster model of family functioning. *J. Marriage Family Counseling*, **4**: 19–31.
5. Epstein N., Baldwin L., Bishop D. (1983) The McMaster Family Assessment Device. *J. Marital Family Therapy*, **9**: 171–180.
6. Miller I.W., Kabacoff R.I., Epstein N.B., Bishop D.S., Keitner G.I., Baldwin L., van der Spuy H.I.J. (1994) The development of a clinical rating scale for the McMaster Model of Family Functioning. *Family Process*, **33**: 53–69.
7. Bishop D., Epstein N., Keitner G., Miller I., Zlotnick C. (1980) *The McMaster Structured Interview for Family Functioning*. Brown University Family Research Program, Providence.
8. Epstein N., Bishop D., Keitner G., Miller I. (1988) *Treatment Manual—Problem Centered Systems Therapy of the Family*. Brown University Family Research Program, Providence.
9. Miller I.W., Norman W.H., Keitner G.I. (1999) Combined treatment for patients with double depression. *Psychother. Psychosom.*, **68**: 180–185.

4.15
Interpersonal Problems in Bipolar Disorder and Their Psychotherapeutic Treatment

Carl Salzman[1]

All too often clinicians who treat patients with bipolar disorder are provided with expert information regarding psychotropic drugs, but little information on the non-pharmacologic aspects of treatment of this complicated disorder. Mark Bauer provides in lucid and comprehensive fashion a scholarly review of published studies and clinical reports regarding the efficacy and importance of various psychosocial techniques that have been used as part of the treatment of bipolar disorder. These techniques include psychodynamic and psychoanalytically oriented psychotherapy, family and interpersonal interventions, cognitive and behavioural techniques, and psychoeducation. Each of these has demonstrated efficacy so that clinicians should be aware of their usefulness and importance.

I would like to add yet another therapeutic approach that is based on clinical experience treating seriously ill bipolar patients, described in a clinical case report [1]. It has long been apparent to clinicians that bipolar disorder produces considerable stress in the marital partner, who needs to be aware of mood shifts, be able to identify them in their early phases, and assure proper treatment of the spouse if they become severe.

The clinical dilemma facing a marital partner can be summarized as follows: the patient gradually becomes manic with displays of inappropriate and occasionally dangerous behaviour. The marital partner, recognizing these behaviours from previous episodes, suggests that it is time to visit the psychiatrist, restart medication, raise the dose, or some such therapeutic intervention. The manic patient denies that there is a problem, and an argument ensues in which the patient accuses the partner of misunderstanding his/her newly increased energy, optimism, enthusiasm, etc. The partner, on the other hand, tries to convince the patient that the elevated affect is really a developing manic process that needs treatment.

This difference in perspective regarding the patient's symptoms and the partner's response commonly leads to significant marital stress and sometimes separation and divorce. If the patient has received prior treatment, or if the behaviour is so disordered that the patient comes to medical attention, the marital partner may be called upon to provide a description of the pathologic affect and behaviour. At this point the patient often accuses the partner of colluding with the medical establishment, trying to control or undermine his or her creativity/exuberance/grandiosity. It is not unusual

[1] *Harvard Medical School, Massachusetts Mental Health Center, 74 Fenwood Road, Boston, MA 02115, USA*

at this juncture for the patient to express a wish to separate from the partner who is considered to be controlling, not understanding, and "a drag on the system". It is also not unusual for the partner to express a wish to separate from the patient out of exhaustion, frustration, or anger.

But the problems between patient and partner have only just begun. Assuming the patient is stabilized on medication, there comes the necessity for maintenance psychotropic drug treatment, and monitoring of this treatment. Since noncompliance is not unusual in bipolar patients, clinicians sometimes ask the partner to provide information regarding the patient's medication-taking behaviour. As illustrated in the reference, the patient may come to believe that the clinician and marital partner are then in collusion against him/her. If the patient is a woman and the clinician a man, there is the additional accusation that both men are trying to control the woman, suppress her assertiveness and creativity, and interfere with her drive towards independence and autonomy [1]. Female bipolar patients, while hypomanic, may leave their husbands and therapy declaring freedom at last from male domination. Unfortunately these flights into "freedom" are often short-lived as the patient's manic behaviour continues to escalate, often with unfortunate results.

In order to deal with this dilemma, an additional therapeutic strategy that could be added to Bauer's excellent summary is the use of a couples intervention technique. The clinician openly acknowledges these dilemmas in the three-way setting (patient–partner–clinician), and attempts to discuss them before the illness escalates. This requires an acknowledgement on the clinician's part that, indeed, there may be times when information from the marital partner may be sought. It must be emphasized to the patient, however, that this is not a collusive attempt to control behaviour, but simply to provide an early-warning mechanism which is ultimately in the patient's best interest. In some cases in which the patient is a woman, it may be necessary for the clinician to be a woman as well in order to avoid the concern of control by two men.

Couples therapy techniques commonly employ many of the suggestions that are included in Bauer's review of other psychosocial therapeutic approaches. There is certainly a strong element of educational input to the couple regarding the nature of bipolar illness. There may also be psychodynamic aspects that need to be explored (as in any marriage) in order to determine why there are misinterpretations by the patient of the spouse's behaviour (or, if the spouse is, indeed, attempting to exert inappropriate behavioural control). Cognitive-behavioural techniques regarding irritability, sleep schedules, and inappropriate behaviours may also need to be employed.

In summary, the psychosocial treatments so eloquently described by Bauer inform an additional common therapeutic strategy for the bipolar patient: couples work with patient and marital or significant partner. It has been my experience that without couples work, treatment of the seriously and recurrently ill bipolar patient may be seriously impaired by treatment noncompliance, distortions, and misunderstanding of each person's communication and behaviour, and ultimately a prolongation of symptomatic distress. The use of couples therapy in conjunction with pharmacologic treatment and the other psychosocial measures described by Bauer can be a powerful therapeutic tool.

REFERENCE

Salzman C. (1988) Integrating pharmacotherapy and psychotherapy in the treatment of a bipolar patient. *Am. J. Psychiatry*, **155**: 686–688.

4.16
Culture Matters Too in Bipolar Disorder

Driss Moussaoui and Nadia Kadri[1]

The biological component of bipolar disorder is unquestionable, as it is the case in most, if not all, mental disorders. Psychosocial aspects are, however, important, although usually neglected, especially in their cultural component. This component is clearly missing in the excellent review of Mark Bauer. It is true that very few studies exist in this field, and this is difficult to understand. As a matter of fact, bipolar disorder is a frequently encountered condition, with a rich behavioural expression. It would be improbable that it does not have an important relationship to culture. This is what we will try to show through two examples.

The first study we would like to mention was conducted in a sample of bipolar female patients in Casablanca, Morocco [1]. Forty patients hospitalized for a manic episode were interviewed, as well as some of their significant others. The surprising result was that about 14% of the patients recognized that they made their living out of prostitution. The significant others gave information which indicated that at least double this figure had in one way or another activities related to prostitution.

In a country like Morocco, where sexuality is socially highly monitored and controlled, this result was a surprise to us. But the significance of the finding is easy to understand. In a morally strict cultural environment, it is

[1] *University Psychiatric Center Ibn Rushd, Rue Tarik Ibn Ziad, Casablanca, Morocco*

unacceptable for the family to see female manic patients having extra-marital sexual relationships, or "liberated" behaviour such as smoking or going out at night. After a period of severe repression, and despite psychiatrists' explaination that this is in fact a pathological behaviour, the family gives up, and excludes the patient. It also happens that the patient leaves the family because of the constant conflict his/her behaviour induces. The only remaining survival alternative then of unskilled and often illiterate girls is prostitution. With this result in hand, we paid more attention to the issue of sexual behaviour of female manic patients, in order to work with the families to avoid such social consequences of the illness.

Another research conducted in Casablanca studied relapses during the fasting month of Ramadan in bipolar patients under lithium therapy [2]. Twenty patients were enrolled during the month of Ramadan after having given their informed consent. The patients were assessed four times: one week before Ramadan, the second and the fourth week of the fasting month and the first week after its end. Females represented 55% of the sample. The mean age was 32.1 ± 7.7 years (range 21–57); the mean duration of illness was 7.9 ± 4.0 years (range 3–16 years). The mean duration of lithium therapy was 26 ± 20 months (range 3–60 months).

The main results of the study were:

- 45% of the sample relapsed (70% of them during the second week and the remaining at the end of Ramadan). These relapses had no positive association with plasma levels of lithium. Most of the patients developed a manic episode (71.4%).
- Patients who did not relapse showed symptoms such as insomnia and anxiety during the second and third week of the study.
- Side effects of lithium increased in frequency, and were observed in 48% of the sample, mostly mouth dryness, thirst sensation and tremor.

Knowing that about 1 billion people in the world fast or will fast during their adult life, these preliminary results are of utmost importance, and more studies should be conducted in this field. The proposed explanation for such a high rate of relapse is that, most probably, the abrupt switch in social rhythms (e.g. in sleep, food intake, professional activity) is involved. As a matter of fact, fasting people usually sleep less, wake up in the night to eat before sunrise, eat more during the night, and have shifted working hours.

In order to prevent relapses, according to the current state of knowledge, bipolar patients should avoid fasting during the Ramadan month. Although Mark Bauer showed that the interpersonal and social rhythm therapy (IPSRT) has not yet proven its efficacy [3], we advise patients who fast to try not to change their daily rhythms (i.e., to keep the usual pattern of sleep and if possible daily activities).

These two examples show how culture could influence the illness, and how a better understanding of the mechanisms involved might be of help in its management. Even in the most "biological" of mental disorders, psychosocial aspects are of great importance to help understanding and treatment.

REFERENCES

1. Kadri N. (1995) Unpublished data.
2. Kadri N., Mouchtaq N., Hakkou F., Moussaoui D. (2000) Relapses in bipolar patients: changes in social rhythm? *Int. J. Neuropsychopharmacol.*, **3**: 45–49.
3. Frank E., Kupfer D., Ehlers C.L., Monk T.H., Cornes C., Carter S., Frankel D. (1994) Interpersonal and social rhythm therapy for bipolar disorder: integrating interpersonal and behavioral approaches. *Behav. Ther.*, **17**: 143–148.

5

Effects of Gender and Age on Phenomenology and Management of Bipolar Disorder: A Review

Kenneth I. Shulman, Ayal Schaffer, Anthony Levitt and Nathan Herrmann

Department of Psychiatry, Sunnybrook & Women's College Health Sciences Centre, 2075 Bayview Avenue, Toronto, Ontario, M5P 3C6, Canada

INTRODUCTION

Age and gender are increasingly identified as important variables in understanding the nature and management of bipolar disorder (BD). In this review, we focus on the similarities and differences among the full age range from youth to geriatrics. Similarly, we try to identify gender differences that may influence our understanding of phenomenology and management.

We provide a critical analysis of the available data, highlighting the importance of these variables and weighing the strength of the evidence. The final section summarizes the highlights of the review and the state of our current knowledge.

PHENOMENOLOGY

Gender

Prevalence Rates

A number of studies have found similar lifetime prevalence rates of BD in men and women. Epidemiological surveys have provided the most unbiased data, given that selection bias is less of a factor than it would be with clinical samples. Lifetime prevalence rates of BD derived from

Bipolar Disorder. Edited by Mario Maj, Hagop S. Akiskal, Juan José López-Ibor and Norman Sartorius.
© 2002 John Wiley & Sons Ltd.

epidemiological surveys completed in the United States, Canada, Germany, and New Zealand did not find an overall effect of sex on lifetime rates of BD [1]. Lifetime prevalence rates in the individual countries were as follows: 0.8% in males, 1.0% in females in the United States; 0.7% in males, 0.6% in females in Edmonton, Canada; and 1.1% in males, 1.0% in females in New Zealand. The German site had an insufficient number of subjects to complete meaningful comparison. The National Comorbidity Survey, an American epidemiological study involving 8098 respondents, also found similar lifetime prevalence rates of BD in men (0.42%) and women (0.47%) [2].

Preliminary evidence suggests that women may be more likely than men to be diagnosed with BD type II. Hendrick *et al* [3] reviewed the medical charts of 131 bipolar patients seen at a specialized Mood Disorders Clinic in Los Angeles [3], and found that 48% of their clinic population were women, but that women accounted for 60% of the cases of BD type II. Although these differences did not reach statistical significance, they do raise the possibility that women may be more likely than men to suffer from BD type II. Contradictory evidence was reported by Szádóczky *et al* [4], who obtained data from a Hungarian epidemiological survey of 2953 adults, and found similar rates of BD type II in men and women.

Age of Onset

There has been some suggestion in the literature that women with BD may have a later onset of illness than men with BD [5]. For instance, Robb *et al.* [6], in a review of 69 euthymic bipolar patients, found that women were significantly older than men at the time of first depression (mean age 27.2 versus 22.4 years) and first mania (25.9 versus 21.8 years). Such studies are hampered by their retrospective design, which cannot identify possible sex differences in paths of entering the medical system, or in attribution of behaviours or symptoms to a bipolar illness. For instance, subsyndromal depressive symptoms may be considered more normative in young women than in young men, leading to a delay in diagnosing women. As well, the higher prevalence rates of substance use disorders in men with BD as compared to women with BD may lead to a Berkson's bias, whereby patients (in this case men) with more than one disorder are more likely to come to the attention of a medical professional, and thus have any future symptoms or behaviours attributed to a bipolar illness.

An increasing number of studies, although also retrospective, have not found an effect of sex on age of onset of BD [3, 7–10]. Unfortunately, most of these studies did not provide age at the time of first mania and first depression. Hendrick *et al* [3] did provide this information, and failed to show an effect of sex on age at the time of first manic or depressive episode. In their study, the mean age at onset of first mania was 24.4 years in men and 24.8 years in women. The mean age at onset of first depression was 22.5 years in men and 21.4 years in women, a non-significant difference. Further evidence for a lack of sex effect on age of onset was provided by Taylor and Abrams [11], who subdivided patients into early- and late-onset BD based on a cutoff of age 30. In this group of 134 bipolar inpatients, females accounted for 35% of subjects in the early-onset group versus 22% of subjects in the late-onset group, a non-significant difference.

Hospitalizations and Episodes of Illness

Studies have retrospectively [3, 6, 8] and prospectively [9] compared the course of illness in men and women with BD. Attempts have been made at identifying sex differences in number of hospital admissions and episodes of bipolar illness. Table 5.1 summarizes the results of a number of these studies. Results are inconsistent, reflecting either the different methodologies used or, more likely, evidence that sex does not appear to significantly impact the course of bipolar illness in terms of number of hospitalizations or mood episodes. The striking fact that studies do not consistently find more depressive episodes in women must be reconciled with the well-known evidence that major depressive disorder is approximately twice as common in women as in men [1, 12].

Mixed Mania

There are a variety of definitions of mixed mania, ranging from the presence of one depressive symptom to a full depressive syndrome in an individual with a current hypomania or mania [13]. These different definitions have hindered comparison across studies, but a number of investigators have found that mixed episodes may be more common in women than men with BD. Using a dimensional model of number of depressive symptoms, Arnold et al [13], in a review of sex effects in mixed mania, suggested that as the definition of mixed mania involves an increasing number of depressive symptoms, the ratio of women to men with mixed mania increases. This was supported by the findings of Akiskal et al [14], who evaluated sex differences in pure mania (defined by an absence of depressive symptoms), probable dysphoric mania (defined by the presence of two depressive symptoms), and definite dysphoric mania (defined by the presence of ≥ 3 depressive symptoms) in a French multisite study involving 104 bipolar patients. In this study, females accounted for 58% of subjects with pure

TABLE 5.1 Effect of sex on number of hospitalizations and mood episodes

	Total number of hospitalizations	Number of hospitalizations for mania	Number of hospitalizations for depression	Total number of mood episodes	Total number of manic episodes	Total number of depressive episodes
Roy-Byrne et al [8]	M = F	M > F	F > M		M = F	M = F
Winokur et al [9]					M > F	F > M
Robb et al [6]				M = F	M = F	M = F
Hendrick et al [3]	F > M	F > M	M = F			

M = males, F = females

mania ($n = 66$), 63% of subjects with probable dysphoric mania ($n = 16$), and 91% of subjects with definite dysphoric mania ($n = 22$). Despite no significant differences in "depressive temperament" between men and women, the authors of this study felt that these findings may be accounted for by a greater likelihood of women having a baseline depressive temperament.

Other studies have taken a more categorical approach to examining the role of sex in mixed mania. A comprehensive review of 17 mixed mania studies by McElroy et al [15] identified five studies in which women were more likely than men to experience mixed episodes. In these five studies, female patients accounted for 57–90% of subjects with mixed mania; however, in two of these studies, females also accounted for a larger proportion of the total number of patients. One study in the review found that male patients accounted for 59% of the subjects with dysphoric mania. The other 11 studies did not report on the sex of subjects. In a more recent study, Robb et al [6] identified a trend towards females experiencing more mixed episodes during the year prior to entry into the study; however, this study involved a relatively small number of subjects. Overall, there is some evidence that women with BD may be more likely than men to experience mixed episodes, but this finding has not been consistent across all studies.

Rapid Cycling

There has been remarkable consistency to the finding that women are more likely than men to experience a rapid-cycling phase to their bipolar illness. This consistency across studies may be due, in part, to the consistency in defining rapid-cycling BD. Rapid cycling is said to occur when a patient experiences at least four distinct mood episodes during a 12-month period. Tondo and Baldessarini [16] pooled the data from 10 studies that reported the sex distribution of patients with rapid-cycling and non-rapid-cycling BD. Among the 2057 patients included, women on average accounted for 71.7% of the cases of rapid cycling, representing a 2.5-fold difference over men. Of interest, rapid cycling occurred in 29.6% of all female BD patients, and in 16.5% of all male BD patients. Taking into account the greater number of female subjects in the studies produced a smaller 1.8-fold difference. Although only six of the 10 studies found statistically significant differences between the percentage of women and men with rapid-cycling BD, nine of the 10 studies found that women numerically accounted for a larger proportion of rapid-cycling patients, and the only study in which men were over-represented only involved a total of 17 subjects.

Two studies that were not included in the Tondo and Baldessarini [16] analysis both supported a sex difference in rapid-cycling BD. Wehr et al

[17], in evaluating 70 inpatients at the United States National Institute of Mental Health (NIMH), found that women accounted for 92% of the 51 patients with a history of rapid cycling, and only 44% of the 19 patients without a history of rapid cycling, a significant difference. Similarly, in another small study, Robb et al [6] found that women accounted for 7/8 (88%) of the cases of rapid cycling among a group of 69 bipolar patients.

Several different explanations for the effect of sex on rapid cycling have been proposed. These have included higher rates of hypothyroidism in women, more frequent use of antidepressants in women, and the effects of the menstrual cycle on mood fluctuations [5]. Leibenluft [5] summarized the results from eight studies (total $n = 204$) which examined whether hypothyroidism was more common among rapid-cycling than non-rapid cycling BD patients. The studies were split evenly, with only four of the eight studies documenting a greater prevalence of hypothyroidism in rapid-cycling BD patients. Interpretation of the results was complicated by the fact that not all studies took into account relevant differences in age and duration of lithium treatment. If hypothyroidism were a risk factor for the development of rapid cycling, this would likely have a greater impact on women, given the higher rates of hypothyroidism in females with BD as compared to males with BD [7]. However, since the results are inconclusive, using hypothyroidism to explain the greater prevalence of rapid cycling in female bipolar patients remains speculative.

As described earlier in this paper, some studies have suggested that women with BD may experience more depressions than men with BD. If true, this could potentially lead to greater use of antidepressants in women with bipolar depression. Furthermore, since antidepressant medications have been implicated in the induction and maintenance of rapid cycling [17–19], greater use of antidepressants in women with BD has been proposed as an explanation for higher rates of rapid cycling. No studies have yet tested this hypothesis, and therefore the possibility that greater use of antidepressants by women can explain higher rates of rapid cycling remains an interesting, but untested theory.

In a further attempt to understand sex differences in rapid cycling, Wehr et al [17] evaluated whether the menstrual cycle or menopause had any effect on rapid cycling. Among 47 women with rapid cycling, only five (11%) experienced mood cycles which were similar in duration to their menstrual cycle. Three of these subjects were followed prospectively. In two, the similarity between mood and menstrual cycles was not sustained, and the third subject continued to cycle during pregnancy. In 23/47 (49%) subjects, the rapid-cycling course of illness began or continued during menopause. Overall, these preliminary results do not support the notion that rapid cycling in women is related to hormonal fluctuations.

Bipolar Disorder across the Reproductive Life Cycle

Pregnancy. Pregnancy, the postpartum period, and menopause are each stages of the reproductive life cycle that may impact bipolar illness. Some have suggested that pregnancy may be a time in which women with BD experience a relief from their mood symptoms. However, this opinion has not been conclusively supported by the available evidence. Most notably, Blehar *et al.* [7] closely examined the timing of pregnancy and emotional problems in 51 women with BD type I, and found that 19/51 (37%) reported mood episodes during their pregnancy, and 7/51 (14%) reported mood episodes during both pregnancy and the postpartum period. During their pregnancy, 7/51 (14%) of the women reported a manic episode, and 3/51 (6%) were hospitalized. Although preliminary, these results suggest that pregnancy may not be protective in terms of mood episodes in women with BD.

Postpartum. The postpartum period has been well established as a time of high risk for women with BD. Nonacs and Cohen [20] reviewed a number of studies, and found that women with BD had a 20–50% risk of relapse during the postpartum period. The risk of postpartum relapse appears to be even higher in women with a past history of postpartum psychosis. The strongest evidence for these findings comes from a well-designed study, in which Kendell *et al* [21] linked the Edinburgh Psychiatric Case Register to the Scottish maternity discharge database. This study encompassed 54 087 child-births over an 11-year period, and also obtained information about prior psychiatric admissions. Among all women, a psychiatric admission with psychosis during the first 90 days after childbirth was 14.3% more likely than before childbirth. The most striking finding of this study was the degree to which a diagnosis of manic-depressive illness increased the risk of post-partum psychosis. Among the 486 women who had a prior psychiatric admission for manic-depressive illness, manic or circular type, 21.4% required an admission in the first 90 days postpartum. This was significantly greater than the risk in women with a history of schizophrenia (3.4% risk) or depressive neurosis (1.9% risk).

In an interesting study, Davenport and Adland [22] found that men with BD whose wives were pregnant or recently gave birth, are also at high risk of relapse. Fifty percent of the 40 male subjects experienced mood episodes during this time, raising explanatory models involving sleep changes or psychological stress.

Menopause. The effect of menopause on the course of BD has not received much research attention, and what has been reported has been contradict-ory [5]. In a recent study by Blehar *et al* [7], the effect of menopause on 56 postmenopausal women with BD type I was evaluated. Eleven women (19%) reported emotional problems in relation to menopause, most commonly depression (13%), followed by mania (4%) and anxiety/agitation (4%). No control groups were involved in the study, which makes the interpretation of these results difficult. Ideally, studies of the effect of menopause on women with BD should involve longitudinal evaluations, spanning the years prior to, during, and after menopause.

Children and Adolescents

Prevalence Rates

Many patients with BD experience their first symptoms during childhood or adolescence. In a survey of members of the National Depressive and Manic-Depressive Association in the United States, 59% endorsed experiencing "signs of the illness" prior to the age of 20 [23]. Reviewing the charts of 200 patients with manic-depressive illness, Loranger and Levine [24] found that 20% of the patients had experienced their first symptoms by age 20, and 12.5% had already been hospitalized by that age. Supporting these findings, Lewinsohn *et al* [25] identified a 0.94% lifetime prevalence rate of BD among a community sample of 1709 older adolescents. Overall, the data suggests that, for a large number of bipolar patients, the illness will onset during their youth.

Rates of BD among clinical populations of youth vary greatly across studies, most of which may be accounted for by methodological differences. A study using the Danish national psychiatric case register found that only 1.2% of child psychiatry inpatients had manic-depressive psychosis [26]. In contrast, among 262 consecutive referrals to a pediatric psychopharmacology clinic in Boston, 16% met DSM-III-R criteria for mania [27]. Overall, despite a difference in reported prevalence rates, there is general consensus that BD can and does exist in children and adolescents, and furthermore, that it leads to marked impairment in functioning.

Effect of Bipolar Disorder on Psychosocial Functioning

The onset of a bipolar illness can have a devastating effect on the overall functioning of a child or adolescent. Two Canadian studies, both reported by Kutcher and colleagues, examined the premorbid functioning of 44 adolescents with BD type I, and found that 90% had average or excellent peer relationships, 64% had good to excellent secondary school achievement, and 72% had good to excellent academic work effort [28]. A post-onset of illness assessment of functioning in these same subjects found a marked deterioration in academic achievement, work effort, peer relationships and extracurricular involvement [29]. Similar results have been shown in prepubertal and early adolescent bipolar populations. Geller *et al* found that 93 prepubertal and early adolescents with BD had significantly poorer psychosocial functioning in a variety of spheres, including maternal, paternal and peer relationships, as compared with 81 children with attention deficit hyperactivity disorder (ADHD) or 94 community controls [30].

Bipolar Symptoms in Youth versus Adults

Differences in the symptomatic expression of BD in youth versus adults have not been consistent across studies. For instance, Ballenger *et al* [31] found psychotic symptoms to be more common among manic patients under the age of 21 as compared to manic patients over the age of 30, yet McElroy *et al* [32] in a larger, more recent study, found that adolescents had fewer psychotic features during mania than adults. There has been more consistency in the findings that youth with BD appear to have higher rates of mixed mania [32–34] and rapid or ultra-rapid cycling [33]. Of interest, an Indian study found that 21 youth with DSM-III-R diagnosed BD had presentations that were very similar to adults with the illness. The most common symptoms among the youth with mania were psychomotor agitation (100%), reduced sleep duration (90%), and pressure of speech (90%). Rapid cycling was only evident in 19% of the youth, and none had a comorbid diagnosis of ADHD [35].

Fewer studies have examined differences in the symptomatic expression of bipolar depression. Goodwin and Jamison [36] summarized the results of several studies, and showed that youth with bipolar depression were significantly less likely to experience anhedonia, morning worsening, fatigue, anorexia, hopelessness, agitation, psychomotor retardation, and definite delusions as compared with adults. On the other hand, youth with bipolar depression were significantly more likely than adults to have a depressed appearance, poor self-esteem, somatic complaints, and hallucinations.

Phenomenology of Early-onset versus Late-onset Bipolar Disorder

In an attempt to identify subtypes of BD, a number of investigators have compared phenomenology based on different age of onset. Complicating the interpretation of results is the lack of an agreed upon definition of early versus late age of onset. A French study compared 58 bipolar patients with an early onset of illness (before age 18) to 39 bipolar patients with a late onset (after age 40). The early-onset patients were more likely to have psychotic symptoms (47% vs. 26%), mixed episodes (30% vs. 6%) and comorbid panic disorder (21% vs. 3%), and were less likely to respond to lithium (43% vs. 64%) [37]. Using data from the Suffolk County Mental Health Project, Carlson et al [38] completed a two-year prospective study of patients admitted with an index episode of psychotic mania. They compared patients whose BD began prior to age 21 ($N = 23$) to those whose BD began after age 30 ($N = 30$). Patients with an early onset were more likely to be male (70% vs. 27%), and have greater psychopathology as evident by higher rates of substance use disorders (70% vs. 30%), paranoia (100% vs. 80%), childhood behavioural problems (61% vs. 10%), and lower likelihood of achieving remission (10% vs. 41%). In contrast, a long-term follow-up study of bipolar patients discharged from a residential treatment facility [39] found a similar outcome in 35 adolescent-onset patients (current mean age of 45 years) as compared with 31 adult-onset patients (current mean age of 56 years).

An early age of onset has also been linked with greater psychosocial impairment. The previously mentioned survey of the United States National Depressive and Manic-Depressive Association found that participants whose illness began prior to age 20 had a significantly higher likelihood of school dropout (55% vs. 23%), financial difficulties (70% vs. 54%) or of not being married (58% vs. 47%) [23]. The differences in illness characteristics between youth- versus adult-onset BD can be attributed either to the possibility that an earlier age of onset signifies a more severe biological form of the illness, or that an earlier onset interrupts psychosocial development. Deciphering the relative contribution of each of these possibilities will be difficult. However, both factors are likely involved in explaining the consistent findings that an earlier age of onset tends to be associated with greater overall psychopathology and impairment. These findings make it even more important that youth with BD receive appropriate treatment for their illness, both in terms of psychopharmacological management, as well as non-pharmacological treatments that promote psychosocial development.

Predicting the Switch from Unipolar to Bipolar Disorder

Several prospective studies have attempted to identify risk factors that can be used to predict the development of BD in youth with depression. Strober and Carlson [40] examined 60 adolescents prospectively for 3–4 years following a hospitalization for depression, and compared characteristics of the 12 patients who developed BD to the 48 patients who did not. Adolescents who developed BD were more likely to have a shorter duration of onset of symptoms, severe depressed mood, self-reproach, bodily concerns, diminished concentration, psychomotor retardation, mood-congruent delusions, hallucinations, a positive family history of BD, and pharmacologically precipitated hypomania. The cluster of psychomotor retardation, psychosis, and a rapid onset of symptoms characterized 67% of adolescents who developed BD, but only 4% of adolescents who did not. A 2–5 year prospective study by Geller *et al* [41], involving 79 children with major depression, supported the finding that a strong family history of major affective disorder (defined as either ≥ 3 first or second degree relatives, or three generations with a major affective disorder) predicted subsequent switching to BD. A small Japanese study prospectively examined youth that experienced their first depressive episode between the ages of 10 and 15. Twelve youth subsequently developed BD. Psychotic symptoms were present during the depression in 10/12 of these subjects, and 6/12 had a positive family history of mental illness [42]. Overall, accumulating evidence has identified several risk factors that increase the likelihood of switching from depression to mania. These include a positive family history of mood disorders, antidepressant-induced hypomania, and the depression being characterized by a rapid onset, with accompanying psychosis and psychomotor retardation.

Medication-induced Mania

A number of psychotropic medications have been linked to induction of manic symptoms in youth with or without BD. Table 5.2 lists the medications that have been associated with precipitating or worsening of manic symptoms. Caution should be used when prescribing these medications to youth, and patients should be closely observed for evidence of possible induction of mania [43–54].

Prognosis

A number of long-term, prospective studies have now been published which help to elucidate the prognosis for youth with BD. Each of these

TABLE 5.2   Medications associated with induction of manic symptoms

Medications	Reference
Tricyclic antidepressants	43–46
Selective serotonin reuptake inhibitors	47–49
Monoamine oxidase inhibitors	50
Carbamazepine	51, 52
Guanfacine (an α-2 adrenergic agonist)	53
Methylphenidate	54

studies has yielded important data, yet results continue to vary greatly. In a naturalistic, five-year follow-up of 54 consecutively admitted adolescents with BD, Strober *et al* [55] observed that the pattern of outcome for these patients was compatible with a remitting illness, and was similar to the outcome of adult patients with BD. Table 5.3 summarizes the results of this study. Overall, only 4% of subjects did not achieve recovery from the index episode at any time during follow-up. Forty-four percent of subjects who recovered went on to relapse at some point during the five years of follow-up. Suicide attempts that required medical attention occurred in 20% of the adolescents. The notion that recovery from an episode of BD is the rule rather than the exception is supported by the findings of an Indian study which prospectively examined 30 youth with bipolar disorder over a period of 4–5 years [56]. All 30 of the subjects recovered from their index episode. However, 20/30 (67%) relapsed during the period of follow-up.

A very different assessment of prognosis is provided by Geller *et al* [57], who evaluated 93 prepubertal and early adolescents (mean age 10.9 years) with current mania or hypomania over the course of six months. At six months, only 13/91 (14%) of patients had recovered from the index episode of mania, and half of these "recovered" patients (6/13) were experiencing a depression. At one-year follow-up, only 37% recovered from the index episodes, and of those that did recover, 38% relapsed [58]. Only 51% of these subjects were receiving an anti-manic medication; therefore, these results do not necessarily reflect response to treatment. The different findings across studies may be the result of differences in age groups and length of follow-up. However, it is also likely that BD in youth is a heterogeneous phenomenon, resulting in varying degrees of chronicity or relapse.

Youth with BD appear to be at high risk of suicide. In a comparison of adolescent suicide victims ($n = 27$) to adolescent suicidal inpatients ($n = 56$), Brent *et al* [59] found that the rate of BD was disproportionately higher in the suicide victims (22%) as compared to suicidal inpatients (5.4%). Strober *et al* [55], in the previously described study, found that

TABLE 5.3   Outcome of adolescent bipolar disorder

Type of mood episode at time of entry	N (% of total study population)	Median time to recovery from index episode	Cumulative probability of recovery through the first 20 weeks	Cumulative probability of relapse during course of study
Manic	20 (37%)	9 weeks	90%	42%
Mixed	10 (19%)	11 weeks	80%	40%
Depressed	14 (26%)	26 weeks	43%	38%
Rapid cycling	10 (19%)	15 weeks	60%	60%

Adapted from Strober *et al* [55].

20% of adolescents with BD attempted suicide within a five-year period. A study by Lewinsohn *et al* [25] found a history of suicide attempts to be much more common among adolescents with BD (44%) than among adolescents with major depressive disorder (22%) or healthy controls (1%). These studies show that adolescents suffering from BD are at considerable risk of suicide, and therefore clearly require ongoing close clinical observation for suicide risk.

Comorbidity

Children and adolescents with BD frequently present with additional or comorbid psychiatric syndromes that may impact on treatment or outcome. Whether the presence of a comorbid syndrome represents a true second clinical entity, rather than a variation of the "phenotype" of the underlying bipolar illness remains unclear.

In a group of 34 adolescents hospitalized for mania, West *et al* [60] found that 86% met criteria for an additional psychiatric disorder. The most common comorbidity was attention deficit hyperactivity disorder (ADHD) (69%), followed by substance use disorders (39%), anxiety disorders (31%), Tourette's syndrome (8%), and bulimia nervosa (3%). Focusing on personality disorders, Kutcher *et al.* [61] determined that among 20 euthymic adolescents with BD, 35% met DSM-III-R criteria for a personality disorder. Borderline and narcissistic personality disorders accounted for the majority of the diagnosis, each being present in 15% of the adolescents. There is limited available data on the presence and significance of other comorbid diagnoses in youth with BD. Various reports have identified elevated rates of pervasive developmental delay [62] and Tourette's syndrome [63] in bipolar youth. Replication is required to validate the findings of these preliminary studies. The following sections will focus on comorbidity of two conditions that have received the most attention in the literature: ADHD and conduct disorder.

Attention Deficit Hyperactivity Disorder (ADHD)

A growing body of literature has examined the comorbidity of ADHD in children and adolescents with BD, yet many questions remain unanswered. First and foremost, the question whether children with ADHD are being misdiagnosed with mania remains a topic of ongoing debate. Two large studies of children with mania found rates of comorbid ADHD above 90% [64, 65]. Among adolescents with BD, rates of comorbid ADHD have ranged from 22 to 88% [66]. The distinction between these two syndromes is made difficult by the overlap in symptoms such as hyperactivity, distractibility, rapid speech, and overall functional impairment that often accompanies both diagnoses.

Biederman and colleagues in Boston have argued that many children who are diagnosed with ADHD may in fact be suffering from an early form of BD [67]. This view is indirectly supported by the recent finding that adult BD patients with a childhood history of ADHD retrospectively appear to have an earlier age of onset of affective episodes (mean age = 12.1 years), as compared to adult BD patients without a childhood history of ADHD (mean age = 20.0 years) [68]. Others have argued that manic symptoms represent a non-specific measure of psychopathology and that children and early adolescents with manic symptoms should not necessarily be diagnosed with BD [69]. Carlson *et al* [66] have proposed that manic symptoms in youth be viewed in a similar manner to psychotic symptoms and schizophrenia. That is, that manic symptoms may be evidence of BD in some individuals, but that there may be other etiologies of the manic syndrome. Despite the debate over nosology, there is general agreement that the magnitude of the comorbidity is staggering.

Conduct Disorder

Prevalence rates of conduct disorder among bipolar youth have been reported as 41–69% [70–72]. The study by Kovacs and Pollock [71] found that, among 8–13-year-old bipolar youth, the presence of conduct disorder was associated with fewer number of mood episodes, but more time spent symptomatic. This study, and a separate one by Biederman [73], both found higher rates of parental substance abuse amongst bipolar youth with comorbid conduct disorder, an interesting finding which suggests some degree of overlap across different diagnostic entities. Similar to the debate as to the relationship between BD and ADHD, questions remain as to whether conduct disorder in bipolar youth represents a separate illness, or a manifestation of the BD itself.

Elderly

The clinical presentation of BD in old age is influenced by its close association with a heterogeneous group of neurologic disorders, especially cerebrovascular disease [74, 75]. Hence, cognitive dysfunction is also a prominent feature in most descriptive studies of mania in the elderly [76]. Even when compared to age-matched depressives, elderly manic patients demonstrate greater cognitive impairment [77]. The higher Hachinski scores found in this subgroup also reflect the high prevalence of underlying cerebrovascular pathology. Moreover, the cognitive dysfunction associated with manic syndromes in old age does not tend to remit with treatment as in depressive pseudodementia [78, 79]. This suggests that cognitive dysfunction in this group is more than a deficit in attention and concentration. In a follow-up study of five to seven years, Dhingra and Rabins [79] reported scores of less than 24 on the Mini-Mental State Examination (MMSE) in almost one-third of their elderly manic subjects. Despite the high prevalence of cognitive impairment and the original observation of high first admission rates for mania in old age, the original speculation that this syndrome heralded the onset of a degenerative dementia [80] has not been borne out by outcome studies. Nonetheless, since Alexopoulos *et al* [81] found a high prevalence of irreversible dementia in longer term follow-up of depressive pseudodementia patients, this suggests that longer term prospective follow-up in manic patients may be necessary.

The neurologic literature running parallel to studies of bipolarity in psychiatric journals has focused on the clinical phenomenon of "disinhibition" [82]. Disinhibition syndromes include criteria virtually identical to those of a manic episode described in DSM-IV [83]. The signs and symptoms include the same features of irritability, euphoria, grandiosity, hyperactivity, pressure of speech as well as perceptual abnormalities including hallucinations with paranoia [74]. However, the evidence for this is based exclusively on individual case reports and case series.

Except for the extent of cognitive dysfunction, the type and range of manic symptoms in the elderly is very similar to mixed age samples but tends towards lower severity and intensity [84–86]. Using the Mania Rating Scale, Young [86] found a low association between age and factors such as activity-energy, libido and motivation. An earlier impression that elderly bipolars present with more mixed episodes [87] has not been substantiated in recent studies. Because of the treatment implications, especially for the use of divalproex [88], this is an important phenomenologic issue that remains to be pursued. While etiological factors may differ, the phenomenology of mania in older subjects remains similar to adults, but attenuated.

MANAGEMENT

Gender

Efficacy of Mood Stabilizers

Possible sex differences in response to treatment with mood stabilizers have been an understudied area, especially with regards to the anticonvulsant medications. Recent large efficacy studies of divalproex [89, 90] and lamotrigine [91] did not report efficacy data based on the participant's sex. In contrast, possible sex differences in response to treatment with lithium have been more extensively described. Viguera et al [92] reviewed 17 lithium studies (total $n = 1548$ patients) which reported efficacy data for both women and men. Most, but not all studies exclusively involved subjects with BD. Response to treatment with lithium was reported in 684/1043 (65.6%) women and 308/505 (61.0%) men, a non-significant difference. Similar results were found in studies involving only bipolar patients, with response rates of 64.1% for women and 61.5% for men. This review provides quite strong evidence that response rates to lithium do not appear to be altered by sex.

Mood Stabilizers in Pregnancy

Decisions regarding treatment of BD during pregnancy must balance the risks associated with untreated depression or mania versus possible terato-genic effects of mood-stabilizing medications. To complicate matters fur-ther, the considerable ethical and clinical challenges of conducting prospective, randomized medication trials during pregnancy have meant that clinicians must rely on non-randomized, often retrospective data to inform clinical decision making. Studies in this area have tended to focus on determining the potential risks of treatment with mood stabilizers, but little data is available on the potential efficacy of these medications during pregnancy. The little available information has focused on lithium. Viguera et al [93] retrospectively determined the risk of recurrence after lithium discontinuation in 42 pregnant and 59 non-pregnant women. This study also included nine women who chose to continue lithium during the course of their pregnancy and postpartum period. During the first 40 weeks of follow-up after lithium discontinuation, a recurrence occurred in 22/42 (52.4%) of pregnant women and 34/59 (57.6%) of non-pregnant women. None of the nine women who continued lithium treatment had a recurrence during pregnancy. Among the women who discontinued lithium and did not experience a recurrence during the first 40 weeks of follow-up, a recur-rence occurred during weeks 41–64 in 14/20 (70%) of the postpartum women and in 6/25 (24%) of the women who had not been pregnant. Of importance, 3/9 women who continued lithium during pregnancy did eventually experience a recurrence during the postpartum period. The authors concluded that pregnancy appeared to be "risk neutral", that is that pregnancy did not provide any protection from relapse following lithium discontinuation. The efficacy of the anticonvulsant medications during pregnancy has not been studied.

The possible teratogenic effects of mood stabilizers have been known for years. Early findings from a voluntary reporting, cross-national database of babies exposed to lithium in utero were critical to alerting clinicians about the possible teratogenic effects of lithium. The greatest concern became the apparent elevated risk of Ebstein's anomaly, a rare cardiac malformation, which occurred in 6/225 (2.7%) of infants exposed to lithium [94]. Although the limitations of a voluntary reporting system were apparent, this reported risk of Ebstein's anomaly became the established risk. In recent years, a number of studies of infants exposed to lithium in utero have not replicated the elevated risk of Ebstein's anomaly, although they do continue to show higher risk of congenital cardiovascular abnormalities, with rates 10–20 times higher than that of the general population [95]. It has been suggested that all mothers who continue to take lithium during pregnancy should have a detailed ultrasound to rule out major congenital abnormalities. Furthermore, lithium levels in the mother should be tested every 1–4 weeks during pregnancy and even more frequently around the time of delivery to limit the risk of maternal, and therefore fetal, lithium toxicity.

In utero exposure to the anticonvulsants valproic acid and carbamazepine has been associated with elevated rates of neural tube defects. These rates are highest if exposure occurs during the first trimester, when the fetal nervous system is developing. In women with epilepsy, the risk following exposure to carbamazepine is 0.5–1.0% [95], and the risk following exposure to valproic acid is 1–2% [96]. These rates may be lowered if women take prophylactic high-dose folic acid prior to conception. It has also been recommended that all women who take valproic acid or carbamazepine during pregnancy be screened for neural tube defects with ultrasound and blood levels of α-fetoprotein [96]. In utero exposure to valproic acid and carbamazepine has also been associated with an increased risk of dysmorphic features and developmental delay [94], although further studies are needed before the extent of this risk can be determined.

Mood Stabilizers during the Postpartum Period

In the area of mood stabilizer use during the postpartum period, most of the research attention has gone to determining the potential risks of using these medications while breastfeeding. The studies of mood stabilizers that have attempted to quantify the potential benefits during the postpartum period have again been focused on lithium. Cohen et al [97] retrospectively determined the postpartum course in 27 women with BD, 14 of whom were taking prophylactic mood stabilizers. All of the women had been diagnosed with recurrent episodes of BD. Among the 14 women receiving medications, nine were taking lithium monotherapy, four were taking lithium in combination with other psychotropics, and one was taking carbamazepine monotherapy. During the three months following delivery, a recurrence of affective instability occurred in 1/14 (7.1%) of the women taking prophylactic mood stabilizers, and in 8/13 (61.5%) of the women not receiving medications. An earlier report by Stewart *et al* [98] also found lithium to have prophylactic effectiveness during the postpartum period. Overall, it has been estimated that treatment with lithium during the final stages of pregnancy and into the postpartum period can reduce by 5-fold the risk of a postpartum relapse [99].

All mood stabilizers, antidepressants, and neuroleptics are passed into breast milk. Therefore, a detailed risk-benefit assessment must be completed prior to nursing mothers receiving any of these medications. This section will focus on what is known about the use of mood stabilizers. Both the psychiatric and neurological literatures provide numerous case reports and case series of mother/infant pairs who have been treated with lithium, valproic acid, carbamazepine, and lamotrigine. Excellent reviews regarding the relevant pharmacokinetic [100] and clinical [101] factors have recently been published. Overall, none of the mood stabilizers have been shown to be uniformly safe for nursing infants, although no adverse effects were found in the majority of reported cases. Specific adverse effects that have been documented include toxicity in infants exposed to lithium [101], thrombocytopenia in an infant exposed to valproic acid [102], and hepatic dysfunction in infants exposed to carbamazepine [103, 104]. Unfortunately, the paucity of data precludes global recommendations: decision making must rely on a detailed risk-benefit evaluation by the clinician and parent. Consideration should be given to alternatives to breast feeding but, if the decision is made to breastfeed, the health of the infant must be closely monitored, with early intervention if he or she appears unwell or develops any adverse effects.

Sexual Side Effects

There is growing literature on the issue of sexual side effects in patients with unipolar depression or anxiety disorders who are treated with antidepressants. Far less is known regarding these side effects in patients treated for BD, and there is little data on sex differences in this regard. Case reports and small studies [105–107] have documented sexual dysfunction in both men and women treated with lithium. Ghadirian *et al* [108] assessed for sexual dysfunction 45 male and 59 female bipolar outpatients receiving treatment with lithium. Overall, 42% of men and 25% of women reported some degree of sexual dysfunction. However, only 14% of the patients on lithium monotherapy reported sexual dysfunction. Patients taking a combination of lithium and benzodiazepine had the highest likelihood of sexual dysfunction (49%).

The possibility of sexual side effects occurring in bipolar patients receiving anticonvulsants has not been studied. The epilepsy literature does provide preliminary evidence that use of anticonvulsants can produce sexual side effects. Carbamazepine, through induction of liver enzymes, may lower levels of testosterone in men, leading to decreased sexual interest [109]. One case report described male infertility presumably caused by treatment with valproic acid [110]. Further studies are needed to confirm these findings.

Weight Gain

Many of the mood stabilizing medications carry a risk of inducing weight gain. This side effect appears to be most prominent in patients taking lithium, valproic acid, carbamazepine, or the atypical antipsychotics. Few studies have examined differences in medication-induced weight gain based on the sex of the patient. Elmslie *et al* [111] evaluated the weight of 445 healthy controls and 89 euthymic bipolar patients on a variety of medications. They found that female patients were less likely than female controls to be at a healthy weight (37% vs. 62%), but that the likelihood of male patients being at a healthy weight was similar to male controls (52% vs. 47%). However, both male and female patients had significantly greater mean waist : hip ratio than their healthy counterparts, signifying greater central obesity in the bipolar patients compared to healthy controls, irrespective of sex. Given that central obesity has been linked to higher risk of cardiovascular disease and diabetes, the side effect of weight gain must be monitored for in all bipolar patients.

Polycystic Ovary Syndrome

Women who receive treatment with valproic acid may be at higher risk of developing polycystic ovary syndrome (PCO). A Finnish study by Isojärvi *et al* [112] evaluated 29 women with epilepsy who were taking valproic acid monotherapy. They found that 13/29 (45%) of the women had some form of menstrual disturbance, and 10/23 (43%) had evidence of PCO on ultrasound. The risk was especially high in women who began treatment with valproic acid prior to age 20, with 80% having polycystic ovaries or elevated serum testosterone, a marker for PCO. Among the 12 women taking a combination of valproic acid and carbamazepine, 3/12 (25%) had some form of menstrual disturbance, and 2/12 (17%) had evidence of PCO. In comparison, menstrual disturbances were less likely to occur in women taking carbamazepine monotherapy (23/120, 19%) or healthy controls (8/51, 16%). A recent study by Rasgon *et al* [113] examined 10 women with BD taking divalproex sodium, and did not identify any women with PCO, although 6/10 (60%) of the women did have some type of menstrual disturbance. Given that both studies involved a small number of women taking valproic acid, and had conflicting results, the true risk of PCO in women taking valproic acid remains unknown. A reasonable suggestion for monitoring of women taking valproic acid has been to obtain a baseline menstrual history and encourage charting of the menstrual cycle, with any significant changes prompting a work-up for possible PCO [114].

Children and Adolescents

As is the case with other mental disorders that occur in both adults and youth, the majority of the evidence used to make treatment decisions for bipolar youth is based on studies of adult bipolar populations [115]. Given this fact, it is not surprising that youth with BD tend to receive similar treatment as adults with BD. This was shown by Carlson et al [66], who found no significant differences in the medications prescribed for psychotic mania in 15–20 year olds, as compared with patients over the age of 30. Of note, they also found similar rates of non-compliance to treatment, with 45% of adolescents and 41% of adults over age 30 discontinuing medications during a four-year follow-up period.

In recent years, a growing body of literature has emerged that informs the treatment of youth with BD. Most of the studies have focused on the treatment of mania, with little attention paid to treatment options for the depressive phase of the illness. This once again parallels the adult literature. The following sections will review the available information on the treatment of bipolar youth with lithium, anticonvulsants, and antipsychotics, as well as the treatment of bipolar depression.

Lithium

Lithium has been prescribed to youth for a variety of reasons since the late 1950s [116]. Dozens of case reports and case series involving the use of lithium in both children and adolescents have been published. In general, these reports lack the rigorous methodology needed to allow for evidence-based treatment decisions to be made. In recent years, several publications have expanded our knowledge about the use of lithium for the treatment of BD in youth.

In a non-blinded study, Kowatch et al [117] randomly assigned 42 outpatients (ages 8–18 years) with BD type I or II in a current manic or mixed episode to six weeks of treatment with lithium, divalproex sodium, or carbamazepine. Using a 50% decrease in the Young Mania Rating Scale (YMRS) as the primary outcome, they found that 5/13 (38%) of those treated with lithium achieved a response. This was not significantly different from the rates of response achieved with divalproex sodium (8/15, 53%) or carbamazepine (5/13, 38%). When improvement of 1 or 2 on the Clinical Global Impression (CGI) scale was used as the outcome, 46% of patients on lithium responded, as did 40% of patients on divalproex sodium, and 31% of patients on carbamazepine.

In the only randomized, double-blind, placebo-controlled study of lithium for the treatment of adolescents with BD, Geller et al [118] evaluated 25 adolescents with BD and secondary substance dependency over the course of six weeks. Mean age was 16.3 years, mean age of illness onset was 9.6 years, and mean age of onset of substance dependency was 15.3 years. Outcome measures included response as defined by a score on the Children's Global Assessment Scale (CGAS) of ≥ 65, as well as positive random weekly urine drug testing. At endpoint, adolescents receiving lithium were found to have a significantly greater improvement on the CGAS, as well as having significantly fewer positive urine drug tests. Using categorical outcomes, 6/13 (46%) of adolescents receiving lithium achieved a positive response on the CGAS, as compared to 1/12 (8%) of those receiving placebo. Limitations of this study included the small sample size, the fact that all subjects had active substance dependency, as well as the broad definition of BD. Subjects could be defined as having BD if their current diagnosis was unipolar major depressive disorder, but they had at least one risk factor for the development of BD, such as delusions, antidepressant-induced switching, marked psychomotor retardation or a first-degree relative with BD.

Two studies by Strober et al [119, 120] attempted to identify predictors of response to lithium in youth with BD. In the first study, 50 adolescent inpatients with BD were treated with lithium, and divided into groups based on whether their illness began prior to age 12. Subjects with adolescent-onset BD were more likely to experience an antimanic effect from treatment with lithium (80%) than were subjects with childhood-onset BD (40%). In the second study, adolescents with mania and a history of early childhood ADHD were compared to adolescents with mania that did not have any premorbid psychiatric illnesses. Both groups responded well to treatment with lithium. However, subjects with a childhood history of ADHD experienced a less robust decrease in the Bech–Rafaelsen Mania Scale (58% vs. 81%), as well as a longer median time to sustained response (23 days vs. 17 days). This finding suggests that comorbidity adversely affects outcome in adolescents, just as it does in adults with BD.

In the only discontinuation study of lithium in bipolar youth, Strober et al [121] evaluated 37 adolescents who had been stabilized on lithium while in hospital and then naturalistically followed them for 18 months. The

13 subjects who chose to discontinue their lithium were compared with the 24 subjects who continued on maintenance lithium throughout the 18-month period. Relapse rates were significantly higher among those who chose to discontinue lithium (92%) versus those who continued on maintenance treatment (38%). Given the non-randomized design of this study, the possibility that factors other than discontinuation of lithium may have accounted for different relapse rates could not be ruled out. Nonetheless, it is likely that prolonged continuation of lithium may lead to dramatically better outcomes in adolescents with BD.

There are few studies examining the safety of long-term use of lithium in youth. An Indian study followed four children who took lithium for 3–5 years and found no evidence of renal impairment [122]. Additional information regarding the long-term implications of treatment with lithium in children and adolescents is clearly needed.

Anticonvulsants

In recent years, on the basis of a number of placebo-controlled trials, anticonvulsant medications have become first or second line treatments for adults with bipolar mania or depression. This has led to their use in youth with BD. However, surprisingly few studies have evaluated the efficacy or safety of anticonvulsants in this population. Furthermore, none of the available reports have been placebo-controlled.

A small number of trials and case reports have shown divalproex sodium to be effective for BD in youth [117, 123–125]. Papatheodorou et al [123] used divalproex sodium (mean dosage 1423 mg/day) in an open fashion to treat 15 adolescents (mean age 17.3 years) with acute mania. Over the course of seven weeks, 8/15 subjects had a ≥ 75% reduction in manic symptoms, 4/15 subjects had a 50–74% reduction in manic symptoms, one subject had a 25–49% reduction in manic symptoms, one subject discontinued treatment due to lack of response, and one subject discontinued treatment due to sedation and dizziness. All 13 completers required the use of other psychotropic medications during the seven-week study period. In a previously described study, Kowatch et al [117] randomly assigned 42 youth with mania to open-label treatment with lithium, divalproex sodium, or carbamazepine. Of the 15 subjects in the divalproex group, eight (53%) had a ≥ 50% improvement in their YMRS scores, and six (40%) had a 1 or 2 score improvement on the CGI. These response rates did not differ significantly from subjects treated with lithium or carbamazepine, suggesting that many bipolar youth treated with a mood stabilizer such as divalproex as monotherapy may not achieve an adequate response. Ideally, future efficacy studies of divalproex in this population of patients should include combinations of treatment.

Other than the above-mentioned study by Kowatch *et al* [117], the use of carbamazepine has been described in only three other reports, involving a total of six adolescents with BD [126–128]. These reports described an antimanic response to treatment with carbamazepine, either as monotherapy or in combination with other psychotropics. Further studies of carbamazepine in this population would be required before any conclusions about efficacy and safety can be drawn. There have been no published studies of the use of other anticonvulsant medications, such as lamotrigine or gabapentin, for the treatment of BD in youth. Reports from the epilepsy literature have documented a paradoxical worsening in behaviours among children treated with gabapentin [129], and an elevated rate of adverse effects to lamotrigine. Therefore, caution is warranted if these medications are being considered.

In most academic centres, anticonvulsant medications are commonly used as first-line treatment for acute mania or hypomania. However, this treatment choice is based on clinical experience and not on a wealth of evidence. Further studies are required to confirm the clinical impression that these medications are helpful for youth with BD.

Antipsychotics

Despite the common use of antipsychotics in the management of youth with BD [66, 130], there have been no controlled studies of either typical or atypical antipsychotics in this population. Furthermore, given that interest in the phenomenon of BD in youth is fairly recent, available studies have focused exclusively on atypical antipsychotics.

Three case series and one case report have found the atypical antipsychotic olanzapine to have antimanic effects in bipolar youth [131–134]. In the largest case series, 23 bipolar youth (ages 5–14) were treated with olanzapine monotherapy for eight weeks in an open-label fashion. All subjects were experiencing a manic or mixed episode at time of entry. Sixty-one percent of the subjects met the modest response criteria of $\geq 30\%$ improvement on the YMRS. Only one patient discontinued treatment due to an adverse event, but there was a mean weight gain of almost 5 kilograms over the course of eight weeks. In a smaller case series, Soutullo *et al* [132] reported that 5/7 manic adolescents had a marked or moderate response to add-on treatment with olanzapine (mean dose 0.146 mg/kg/day) in six of the subjects and as monotherapy in one subject. The other case series reported a rapid antimanic response when olanzapine was added to other psychotropic medications in three children aged 9–12 with mania [133]. The dose of olanzapine in this study ranged from 2.5 to 5 mg/day.

The atypical antipsychotic risperidone was evaluated in a retrospective chart review of 28 youth (mean age of 10.4 years) with BD [135]. Twenty-five subjects were experiencing a mixed episode and three subjects were experiencing a hypomanic episode when treatment with risperidone was initiated. Subjects had an average of 2.6 comorbid diagnoses, 13/28 (46%) were experiencing psychosis, 27/28 (96%) were receiving other medications, and only 1/28 subjects was female. The addition of risperidone at an average dose of 1.7 mg resulted in a robust improvement of manic and aggressive symptoms in 82% of subjects and in psychotic symptoms in 69% of subjects. Although only 18% of subjects in this study experienced weight gain, another report of risperidone in child or adolescent inpatients documented weight gain in 78% of subjects [136].

The literature on the use of other atypical antipsychotic medications such as quetiapine and clozapine for the treatment of youth with BD is limited to case reports [137, 138].

In summary, there is preliminary evidence that atypical antipsychotics may be effective treatments for acute mania, and in many clinical settings these treatments have become first-line therapy for acute mania. The safety and tolerability of long-term use of these medications in adolescents are unknown, and thus no firm conclusions can be drawn regarding maintenance treatment.

Treatment of Bipolar Depression

The management of the depressive component of BD in youth has been understudied. Biederman et al [47] have recently published the only study evaluating the effects of different treatments on depressive symptoms in bipolar youth. In this retrospective chart review of 59 patients with BD (mean age 10.8 years), the effect of different classes of psychotropics on symptomatology in the following visits was examined. Only the selective serotonin reuptake inhibitors (SSRIs) were associated with a decrease in depressive symptoms (relative risk 6.7). Tricyclic antidepressants, stimulants, mood stabilizers, and typical antipsychotics were not associated with improvement in depressive symptoms. Of importance to the overall management of BD, only the SSRIs were also found to significantly increase the likelihood of a worsening of manic symptoms (relative risk 3.0). However, the antimanic effects of mood stabilizers were not significantly diminished by concomitant use of an SSRI. These results suggest that SSRIs may improve the depressive symptoms of youth with BD, but that there is an associated risk of worsening mania, unless there is antimanic coverage. No studies could be identified which evaluated the use of mood stabilizers for the depressive phase of BD in youth.

The use of light therapy (10 000 lux twice a day) to treat subsyndromal depressive symptoms in seven bipolar youth (age 16–22 years) was evaluated by Papatheodorou and Kutcher [139]. Three subjects had a > 70% subjective improvement in depressive symptoms, two subjects had a 40–70% improvement in depressive symptoms, and two subjects had a mild or no response. No adverse effects, including a switch to mania, were noted.

In a noteworthy study, Geller *et al* [140] found lithium to be no better than placebo for the treatment of unipolar depression in youth, 80% of whom had a family history of BD.

Using antidepressant medications for the treatment of bipolar depression carries a risk of induction of mania or rapid cycling. Of course, prolonged depression unresponsive to mood stabilizers is commonly treated with antidepressants, but the choice to institute an antidepressant, even with mood stabilizer coverage, is a clinically weighty decision that should be done after consideration of the risks of mania and only after careful discussion with the patient, and their parents or guardians. Consultation with experts in the field is recommended in this circumstance.

Other Treatments

A number of case reports have demonstrated antimanic effects in youth of a variety of treatments, including electroconvulsive therapy [141, 142], melatonin [143], lecithin [144], and nimodipine [145]. No clinically meaningful conclusions can be drawn about these treatments at present.

Elderly

While numerous clinical guidelines suggest that treatment of BD in the elderly should be different from younger populations, there are actually no randomized controlled treatment trials in elderly bipolars to ground these recommendations in an evidence-based approach [146–148]. Unfortunately, well-documented age-related changes in pharmacokinetics and pharmacodynamics, which will be reviewed next, make the adoption of treatment recommendations from studies of middle-aged patients hazardous. Furthermore, the elderly frequently suffer from chronic medical illnesses and are being treated with numerous concomitant medications which make the risk of adverse drug reactions and drug interactions much greater.

Age-related pharmacokinetic changes involve the absorption, distribution, metabolism and elimination of psychotropic drugs [149]. While absorption of drugs from the gastrointestinal tract might theoretically be impaired due to decreases in acid secretion, mesenteric blood flow, and membrane transport, most orally ingested psychotropics are still well absorbed in the elderly. Conversely, changes in volume and distribution can have profound effects. With ageing, lean body mass and total body water decrease, while total body fat increases. Since most psychotropics, with the exception of lithium carbonate, are lipophilic, the volume of distribution for these drugs will be significantly increased. This results in longer half lives with drugs remaining in the elderly body for a much longer time. Hepatic metabolism may also decline with age, leading to prolonged half life. These changes can have dramatic effects with the elimination half lives of some psychotropics being two to three times longer in the elderly than in younger patients. Drugs that are eliminated by the kidney, such as lithium carbonate, will also be affected by age. Glomerular filtration rate declines 6–10% per decade beginning at age 40, which would reduce renal excretion, leading to significant accumulation of drugs like lithium. Pharmacodynamic changes associated with ageing may affect the biochemical, physiologic and behavioural effects of psychotropics. Changes in the brain, such as neuronal loss, alterations of neurotransmitter receptor density or sensitivity, etc., may increase or decrease response to psychotropics. For example, due to age-related declines in cholinergic function, the elderly are much more sensitive to the anticholinergic effects of many psychotropic drugs. Finally, similar pharmacokinetic and pharmacodynamic alterations may occur in the elderly as a result of medical illnesses such as cardiac, hepatic, and renal disease, or even poor nutritional status. All these factors necessitate cautious prescribing and careful monitoring of psychotropics, leading to the geriatric pharmacology mantra of "start low, go slow".

The basic principles of management for elderly bipolars would be similar to a younger population: clarifying the diagnosis, managing the acute affective episode, instituting prophylactic therapy, and providing ongoing follow-up. For the elderly, clarifying the diagnosis involves a thorough medical and psychiatric assessment to rule out other psychiatric disorders (example: delirium, dementia), medical conditions (example: hypothyroidism, cerebrovascular disease), or drugs (example: anti-parkinsonians) that may present with symptoms that could appear like bipolar disorder. Laboratory investigations are a necessary part of the process to clarify diagnosis, but also provide baseline values for renal, hepatic, cardiac and hematological function that are necessary prior to treatment with any of the currently available mood stabilizing medications. Hospitalization may be necessary to protect the patient against harm, not only from suicide but also from exhaustion and dehydration, given the medical frailty of many elderly patients. There have been no studies of psychotherapy with elderly bipolar patients, though psychotherapy and especially psychoeducational approaches would likely lead to improved medication compliance.

Lithium

Despite many years of clinical use and the suggestion that lithium carbonate may be used more commonly in the elderly compared with younger populations [150], there have been no published randomized controlled trials examining its use in elderly bipolars. Data from uncontrolled and retrospective trials suggest that response rates are similar in this population [151–154]. Due to renal changes mentioned previously, there are important pharmacokinetic changes associated with lithium use in the elderly. Kinetic studies suggest geriatric patients would require one-third to one-half less lithium to achieve similar blood levels, and single daily doses would be appropriate [155]. Given studies which report increased adverse reactions and toxicity at serum levels considered "therapeutic" in younger populations [156–158], clinical recommendations suggest aiming for serum levels of 0.5 to 0.8 mmol/l [146, 147]. Most patients aged 65 to 75 would be able to achieve serum levels of 0.5 mmol/l with doses ranging from 300 to 600 mg/day, while patients $\geq$ 80 years of age or the frail elderly would achieve these levels with doses between 150 and 300 mg/day [159].

The elderly may be more susceptible than younger populations to lithium-induced side effects, such as delirium [151, 152], prolonged neurotoxicity [160], and increased lithium-induced hypothyroidism [150]. Toxicity may also be caused by drug interactions. For example, drugs such as thiazide diuretics, angiotensin converting enzyme inhibitors and indomethacin can all lead to increases of serum lithium and possible toxicity.

Anticonvulsants

Even less data exists for the use of anticonvulsant mood stabilizers in the elderly. There are several case reports and case series which suggest that valproic acid is effective and well tolerated [161–164]. In one study of 21 elderly manics, 90% of patients improved and only two were reported to have experienced significant adverse reactions. Patients in this study were treated with an average of 1400 mg/day, with an average valproate level of 72 mg/l [165]. There was no relationship between serum levels and outcome. In contrast, in a retrospective comparison of elderly bipolars treated with either lithium or valproate, therapeutic serum levels of valproate seemed to be more important [166]. While lithium seemed more effective overall, patients on valproate whose levels were between 65 and 90 mg/l had similar outcomes to patients treated with therapeutic levels of lithium. The authors of this report note that levels of 65 to 90 mg/l would represent the upper range of therapeutic levels for young patients treated with valproate and suggest that for some, yet to be determined, reason the elderly may require higher serum levels of valproate for therapeutic effect.

There are only a few case reports on the use of carbamazepine for elderly bipolars [167, 168]. Recommendations for use in the elderly suggest that serum levels must be relatively low as levels about 9 µg/ml are associated with increased adverse effects [169]. There is also a small amount of preliminary data describing the use of other anticonvulsants such as gabapentin [170, 171] and lamotrigine [172].

Atypical Antipsychotics

While studies of the atypical antipsychotics olanzapine and risperidone suggest they are effective agents for young bipolar patients, there is no data on their use in elderly bipolars. There is one small series of three elderly manics treated successfully with clozapine [153]. Finally, electroconvulsive therapy may also be effective for elderly patients with bipolar disorder [173].

SUMMARY

Consistent Evidence

- Prevalence rates, age of onset and clinical course of BD do not differ on the basis of gender. What is clear is that the rapid-cycling form of BD is indeed more common in females. However, the hypothesis that underlying thyroid abnormalities may explain this phenomenon has yet to be conclusively addressed. We also have strong data showing that the postpartum period is a time of high risk for women with BD, conferring a significant risk of developing a postpartum psychosis.
- The onset of BD at a relatively early stage is now well established, with a mean age at onset of about 20 years. There is strong evidence that almost 60% of bipolar patients report "signs of the illness" prior to the age of 20. Another robust finding is that the onset of bipolarity in adolescence has devastating effects on psychosocial functioning. Thus, early onset confers greater overall psychopathology and impairment as well as an increased risk of suicide.
- Comorbidity is well established in adolescence, involving primarily ADHD, which has been highlighted as a frequent misdiagnosis in early onset bipolar patients. Other relatively common comorbid conditions include conduct disorder, substance use and anxiety disorders. Personality disorders most frequently associated with bipolarity in youth include borderline and narcissistic types.

- In the elderly, the evidence is based largely on case series and case reports. Nonetheless, the multiplicity of sources and frequency of documentation strongly suggest a role for heterogeneous neurologic disorders including cognitive dysfunction. However, this is not necessarily the onset of a degenerative dementia. The type and range of symptoms of BD in the elderly appear to be very similar to mixed age samples except for less severity.

Incomplete Evidence

- Females appear to be more likely to develop mixed manic episodes, but the evidence is still based on limited data. Data on the phenomenologic differences between youth and mixed age samples are inconsistent, but no substantive differences have emerged. Finally, the clinical course of adolescent onset BD shows inconsistencies with respect to recovery and relapse rates.
- The use of mood stabilizers in pregnancy carries a risk of teratogenicity. Lithium has been associated with Ebstein's anomaly, while divalproex and carbamazepine have been associated with neural tube defects. In the postpartum period, mood stabilizers continue to carry certain risks during breastfeeding as they all pass into breast milk. While mood stabilizers appear to confer significant protection from relapse during the postpartum period, the final clinical decision must rest on a detailed risk-benefit evaluation by clinician and parent.
- In the elderly, there are no randomized controlled trials of drug treatment of BD. However, the age-related changes and pharmacokinetics affecting absorption, distribution, metabolism and elimination are well documented, as are pharmacodynamic changes associated with brain sensitivity and medical illness. This has allowed for some extrapolation from mixed age populations. For example, lithium pharmacokinetic studies suggest that approximately one-third the dose is needed to achieve similar serum lithium levels to adult patients. However, for pharmacodynamic reasons, the recommended serum level is somewhat lower, closer to 0.5 mmol/l, which is achieved in the young-old with doses ranging from 300–600 mg of lithium, while in the very old, 150 mg of lithium may be sufficient. The risk of neurotoxicity associated with lithium in the elderly is well established.

Areas Still Open to Research

- More data is needed on children and adolescents to establish whether there are fundamental phenomenologic differences compared to adult and elderly populations.

- Treatment of youth has focused primarily on manic episodes of BD. Much more work is needed to understand bipolar depression in adolescence. The use of lithium is not really evidence-based and there are no placebo-controlled trials in adolescents for any of the anticonvulsants including divalproex and carbamazepine. Moreover, there are no studies reported on the newer anticonvulsant mood stabilizers, namely, gabapentin and lamotrigine. Similarly, concerning the antipsychotic treatment of BD, there are no controlled studies, and current evidence is based on case reports and small case series. Furthermore, depression is grossly understudied in adolescent BD. The evidence is based on a retrospective chart review suggesting that only the SSRIs are effective treatments for bipolar depression as opposed to tricyclic antidepressants and mood stabilizers. However, there is preliminary evidence that the SSRIs also confer increased risk of mania and hence this is an area deeply in need of further research.
- In general, more research is needed into gender differences than currently exists. It would appear that pregnancy is "risk neutral" for protection from relapse following discontinuation of lithium. However, more work is needed in this area. Specifically, concerning sexual side effects, more study related to lithium is needed and there are no studies with the anticonvulsants. For polycystic ovary syndrome, there are only small case series available to determine its relationship to treatment with mood stabilizers.
- In the elderly, longer term outcome studies are needed to determine whether the disinhibition syndromes and BD of old age eventually develop into irreversible dementias. For management in old age, more systematic data is needed about the use of newer mood stabilizers, including divalproex, lamotrigine and gabapentin, and the atypical antipsychotics.

REFERENCES

1. Weissman M.M., Bland R., Joyce P.R., Newman S., Wells J.E., Wittchen H.-U. (1993) Sex differences in rates of depression: cross-national perspectives. *J. Affect. Disord.*, **29**: 77–84.
2. Kessler R.C., Rubinow D.R., Holmes C., Abelson J.M., Zhao S. (1997) The epidemiology of DSM-III-R bipolar I disorder in a general population survey. *Psychol. Med.*, **27**: 1079–1089.
3. Hendrick V., Altshuler L.L., Gitlin M.J., Delrahim S., Hammen C. (2000) Gender and bipolar illness. *J. Clin. Psychiatry*, **61**: 393–396.
4. Szádóczky E., Papp Z., Vitrai J., Ríhmer Z., Füredi J. (1998) The prevalence of major depressive and bipolar disorders in Hungary: results from a national comorbidity survey. *J. Affect. Disord.*, **50**: 153–162.

5. Leibenluft E. (1996) Women with bipolar illness: clinical and research issues. *Am. J. Psychiatry*, **153**: 163–173.
6. Robb J.C., Young L.T., Cooke R.G., Joffe R.T. (1998) Gender differences in patients with bipolar disorder influence outcome in the medical outcomes survey (SF-20) subscale scores. *J. Affect. Disord.*, **49**: 189–193.
7. Blehar M.C., DePaulo J.R., Gershon E.S., Reich T., Simpson S.G., Nurnberger J.I. (1998) Women with bipolar disorder: findings from the NIMH genetics initiative sample. *Psychopharmacol. Bull.*, **34**: 239–243.
8. Roy-Byrne P., Post R.M., Uhde T.W., Porcu T., Davis D. (1985) The longitudinal course of recurrent affective illness: life chart data from research patients at the NIMH. *Acta Psychiatr. Scand.*, **71** (Suppl. 317): 5–34.
9. Winokur G., Coryell W., Akiskal H.S., Endicott J., Keller M., Mueller T. (1994) Manic-depressive (bipolar) disorder: the course in light of a prospective ten-year follow-up of 131 patients. *Acta Psychiatr. Scand.*, **89**: 102–110.
10. Taylor M.A., Abrams R. (1981) Gender differences in bipolar affective disorder. *J. Affect. Disord.*, **3**: 261–277.
11. Taylor M.A., Abrams R. (1981) Early- and late-onset bipolar illness. *Arch. Gen. Psychiatry*, **38**: 58–61.
12. Kessler R.C., McGonagle K.A., Swartz M., Blazer D.G., Nelson C.B. (1993) Sex and depression in the National Comorbidity Survey I: lifetime prevalence, chronicity and recurrence. *J. Affect. Disord.*, **29**: 85–96.
13. Arnold L.M., McElroy S.L., Keck P.E. (2000) The role of gender in mixed mania. *Compr. Psychiatry*, **41**: 83–87.
14. Akiskal H.S., Hantouche E.G., Bourgeois M.L., Azorin J.-M., Sechter D., Allilaire J.-F., Lancrenon S., Fraud J-P., Châtenet-Duchêne L. (1998) Gender, temperament, and the clinical picture in dysphoric mixed mania: findings from a French national study (EPIMAN). *J. Affect. Disord.*, **50**: 175–186.
15. McElroy S.L., Keck P.E., Pope H.G., Hudson J.I., Faedda G.L., Swann A.C. (1992) Clinical and research implications of the diagnosis of dysphoric or mixed mania or hypomania. *Am. J. Psychiatry*, **49**: 1633–1644.
16. Tondo L., Baldessarini R.J. (1998) Rapid cycling in women and men with bipolar manic-depressive disorders. *Am. J. Psychiatry*, **155**: 1434–1436.
17. Wehr T.A., Sack D.A., Rosenthal N.E., Cowdry R.W. (1998) Rapid cycling affective disorder: contributing factors and treatment responses in 51 patients. *Am. J. Psychiatry*, **145**: 179–184.
18. Coryell W., Endicott J., Keller M. (1992) Rapid cycling affective disorder: demographics, diagnosis, family history, and course. *Arch. Gen. Psychiatry*, **49**: 126–131.
19. Bauer M.S., Calabrese J., Dunner D.L., Post R., Whybrow P.C., Gyulai L., Kai Tay L., Younkin S.R., Bynum D., Lavori P., Price R.A. (1994) Multisite data reanalysis of the validity of rapid cycling as a course modifier for bipolar disorder in DSM-IV. *Am. J. Psychiatry*, **151**: 506–515.
20. Nonacs R., Cohen L.S. (1998) Postpartum mood disorders: diagnosis and treatment guidelines. *J. Clin. Psychiatry*, **59** (Suppl. 2): 34–40.
21. Kendell R.E., Chalmers J.C., Platz C. (1987) Epidemiology of puerperal psychoses. *Br. J. Psychiatry*, **150**: 662–673.
22. Davenport Y.B., Adland M.L. (1982) Postpartum psychoses in female and male bipolar manic-depressive patients. *Am. J. Orthopsychiatry*, **52**: 288–297.
23. Lish J.D., Dime-Meenan S., Whybrow P.C., Price R.A., Hirschfeld R.M.A. (1994) The National Depressive and Manic-depressive Association (DMDA) survey of bipolar members. *J. Affect. Disord.*, **31**: 281–294.

24. Loranger A.W., Levine P.M. (1978) Age of onset of bipolar affective illness. *Arch. Gen. Psychiatry*, **35**: 1345–1348.
25. Lewinsohn P.M., Klein D.N., Seeley J.R. (1995) Bipolar disorders in a community sample of older adolescents: prevalence, phenomenology, comorbidity, and course. *J. Am. Acad. Child Adolesc. Psychiatry*, **34**: 454–463.
26. Thomsen P.H., Moller L.L., Dehlholm B., Brask B.H. (1992) Manic-depressive psychosis in children younger than 15 years: a register-based investigation of 39 cases in Denmark. *Acta Psychiatr. Scand.*, **85**: 401–406.
27. Wozniak J., Biederman J., Kiely K., Ablon J.S., Faraone S.V., Mundy E., Mennin D. (1995) Mania-like symptoms suggestive of childhood-onset bipolar disorder in clinically referred children. *J. Am. Acad. Child Adolesc. Psychiatry*, **34**: 867–876.
28. Kutcher S.P., Robertson H.A., Bird D. (1998) Premorbid functioning in adolescent onset bipolar I disorder: a preliminary report from an ongoing study. *J. Affect. Disord.*, **51**: 137–144.
29. Quackenbush D., Kutcher S., Robertson H.A., Boulos C., Chaban P. (1996) Premorbid and postmorbid school functioning in bipolar adolescents: description and suggested academic interventions. *Can. J. Psychiatry*, **41**: 16–22.
30. Geller B., Bolhofner K., Craney J.L., Williams M., DelBello M.P., Gundersen K. (2000) Psychosocial functioning in a prepubertal and early adolescent bipolar disorder phenotype. *J. Am. Acad. Child Adolesc. Psychiatry*, **39**: 1543–1548.
31. Ballenger J.C., Reus V.I., Post R.M. (1982) The "atypical" clinical picture of adolescent mania. *Am. J. Psychiatry*, **139**: 602–606.
32. McElroy S.L., Strakowski S.M., West S.A., Keck P.E. Jr., McConville B.J. (1997) Phenomenology of adolescent and adult mania in hospitalized patients with bipolar disorder. *Am. J. Psychiatry*, **154**: 44–49.
33. Geller B., Sun K., Zimerman B., Luby J., Frazier J., Williams M. (1995) Complex and rapid-cycling in bipolar children and adolescents: a preliminary study. *J. Affect. Disord.*, **34**: 259–268.
34. Krasa N.R., Tolbert H.A. (1994) Adolescent bipolar disorder: a nine-year experience. *J. Affect. Disord.*, **30**: 175–184.
35. Janardhan Reddy Y.C., Girimaji S., Srinath S. (1997) Clinical profile of mania in children and adolescents from the Indian subcontinent. *Can. J. Psychiatry*, **42**: 841–846.
36. Goodwin F.K., Jamison K.R. (1990) *Manic-Depressive Illness*. Oxford University Press, New York.
37. Schürhoff F., Bellivier F., Jouvent R., Mouren-Siméoni M.-C., Bouvard M., Allilaire J.-F., Leboyer M. (2000) Early and late onset bipolar disorders: two different forms of manic-depressive illness? *J. Affect. Disord.*, **58**: 215–221.
38. Carlson G.A., Bromet E.J., Sievers S. (2000) Phenomenology and outcome of subjects with early- and adult-onset psychotic mania. *Am. J. Psychiatry*, **157**: 213–219.
39. McGlashan T.H. (1988) Adolescent versus adult onset of mania. *Am. J. Psychiatry*, **145**: 221–223.
40. Strober M., Carlson G. (1982) Bipolar illness in adolescents with major depression. *Arch. Gen. Psychiatry*, **39**: 549–555.
41. Geller B., Fox L.W., Clark K.A. (1994) Rate and predictors of prepubertal bipolarity during follow-up of 6- to 12-year-old depressed children. *J. Am. Acad. Child Adolesc. Psychiatry*, **33**: 461–468.
42. Shiratsuchi T., Takahashi N., Suzuki T., Abe K. (2000) Depressive episodes of bipolar disorder in early teenage years: changes with increasing age and the significance of IQ. *J. Affect. Disord.*, **58**: 161–166.

43. Geller B., Fox L.W., Fletcher M. (1993) Effect of tricyclic antidepressants on switching to mania and on the onset of bipolarity in depressed 6- to 12-year-olds. *J. Am. Acad. Child Adolesc. Psychiatry*, **32**: 43–50.
44. Strober M. (1998) Mixed mania associated with tricyclic antidepressant therapy in prepubertal delusional depression: three cases. *J. Child Adolesc. Psychopharmacol.*, **8**: 181–185.
45. Biederman J., Mick E., Prince J., Bostic J.Q., Wilens T.E., Spencer T., Wozniak J., Faraone S.V. (1999) Systematic chart review of the pharmacologic treatment of comorbid attention deficit hyperactivity disorder in youth with bipolar disorder. *J. Child Adolesc. Psychopharmacol.*, **9**: 247–256.
46. Kashani J.H., Hodges K.K., Shekim W.O. (1980) Hypomanic reaction to amitriptyline in a depressed child. *Psychosomatics*, **21**: 867–872.
47. Biederman J., Mick E., Spencer T.J., Wilens T.E., Faraone S.V. (2000) Therapeutic dilemmas in the pharmacotherapy of bipolar depression in youth. *J. Child Adolesc. Psychopharmacol.*, **10**: 185–192.
48. Vankataraman S., Naylor M.W., King C.A. (1992) Mania associated with fluoxetine treatment in adolescents. *J. Am. Acad. Child Adolesc. Psychiatry*, **31**: 276–281.
49. Ghaziuddin M. (1994) Mania induced by sertraline in a prepubertal child. *Am. J. Psychiatry*, **151**: 944.
50. Mattsson A., Seltzer R.L. (1981) MAOI-induced rapid cycling bipolar affective disorder in an adolescent. *Am. J. Psychiatry*, **138**: 677–679.
51. Pleak R.R., Birmaher B., Gavrilescu A., Abichandani C., Williams D.T. (1988) Mania and neuropsychiatric excitation following carbamazepine. *J. Am. Acad. Child Adolesc. Psychiatry*, **27**: 500–503.
52. Reiss A.L., O'Donnell D.J. (1984) Carbamazepine-induced mania in two children: case report. *J. Clin. Psychiatry*, **45**: 272–274.
53. Horrigan J.P., Barnhill L.J. (1999) Guanfacine and secondary mania in children. *J. Affect. Disord.*, **54**: 309–314.
54. Koehler-Troy C., Strober M., Malenbaum R. (1986) Methylphenidate-induced mania in a prepubertal child. *J. Clin. Psychiatry*, **47**: 566–567.
55. Strober M., Schmidt-Lackner S., Freeman R., Bower S., Lampert C., DeAntonio M. (1995) Recovery and relapse in adolescents with bipolar affective illness: a five-year naturalistic, prospective follow-up. *J. Am. Acad. Child Adolesc. Psychiatry*, **34**: 724–731.
56. Srinath S., Janardhan Reddy Y.C., Girimaji S.R., Seshadri S.P., Subbakrishna D.K. (1998) A prospective study of bipolar disorder in children and adolescents from India. *Acta Psychiatr. Scand.*, **98**: 437–442.
57. Geller B., Zimerman B., Williams M., Bolhofner K., Craney J.L., DelBello M.P., Soutullo C.A. (2000) Six-month stability and outcome of a prepubertal and early adolescent bipolar disorder phenotype. *J. Child Adolesc. Psychopharmacol.*, **10**: 165–173.
58. Geller B., Craney J.L., Bolhofner K., DelBello M.P., Williams M., Zimerman B. (2001) One-year recovery and relapse rates of children with a prepubertal and early adolescent bipolar disorder phenotype. *Am. J. Psychiatry*, **158**: 303–305.
59. Brent D.A., Perper J.A., Goldstein C.E., Kolko D.J., Allan M.J., Allman C.J., Zelenak J.P. (1988) Risk factors for adolescent suicide. *Arch. Gen. Psychiatry*, **45**: 581–588.
60. West S.A., Strakowski S.M., Sax K.W., McElroy S.L., Keck P.E., McConville B.J. (1996) Phenomenology and comorbidity of adolescents hospitalized for the treatment of acute mania. *Biol. Psychiatry*, **39**: 458–460.
61. Kutcher S.P., Marton P., Korenblum M. (1990) Adolescent bipolar illness and personality disorder. *J. Am. Acad. Child Adolesc. Psychiatry*, **29**: 355–358.

62. Wozniak J., Biederman J., Faraone S.V., Frazier J., Kim J., Millstein R., Gershon J., Thornell A., Cha K., Snyder J.B. (1997) Mania in children with pervasive developmental disorder revisited. *J. Am. Acad. Child Adolesc. Psychiatry*, **36**: 1552–1559.

63. Kerbeshian J., Burd L. (1996) Case study: comorbidity among Tourette's syndrome, autistic disorder, and bipolar disorder. *J. Am. Acad. Child Adolesc. Psychiatry*, **35**: 681–685.

64. Faraone S.V., Biederman J., Wozniak J., Mundy E., Mennin D., O'Donnell D. (1997) Is comorbidity with ADHD a marker for juvenile-onset mania? *J. Am. Acad. Child Adolesc. Psychiatry*, **36**: 1046–1055.

65. Geller B., Williams M., Zimerman B., Frazier J., Beringer L., Warner K.L. (1998) Prepubertal and early adolescent bipolarity differentiate from ADHD by manic symptoms, grandiose delusions, ultra-rapid or ultradian cycling. *J. Affect. Disord.*, **51**: 81–91.

66. Carlson G.A., Lavelle J., Bromet E.J. (1999) Medication treatment in adolescents vs. adults with psychotic mania. *J. Child Adolesc. Psychopharmacol.*, **9**: 221–231.

67. Biederman J. (1998) Resolved: mania is mistaken for ADHD in prepubertal children: affirmative. *J. Am. Acad. Child Adolesc. Psychiatry*, **37**: 1091–1093.

68. Sachs G.S., Baldassano C.F., Truman C.J., Guille C. (2000) Comorbidity of attention deficit hyperactivity disorder with early- and late-onset bipolar disorder. *Am. J. Psychiatry*, **157**: 466–468.

69. Klein R.G., Pine D.S., Klein D.F. (1998) Resolved: mania is mistaken for ADHD in prepubertal children: negative. *J. Am. Acad. Child Adolesc. Psychiatry*, **37**: 1093–1096.

70. Kutcher S.P., Marton P., Korenblum M. (1989) Relationship between psychiatric illness and conduct disorder in adolescents. *Can. J. Psychiatry*, **34**: 526–529.

71. Kovacs M., Pollock M. (1995) Bipolar disorder and comorbid conduct disorder in childhood and adolescence. *J. Am. Acad. Child Adolesc. Psychiatry*, **34**: 715–723.

72. Biederman J., Faraone S.V., Chu M.P., Wozniak J. (1999) Further evidence of a bidirectional overlap between juvenile mania and conduct disorder in children. *J. Am. Acad. Child Adolesc. Psychiatry*, **38**: 468–476.

73. Biederman J., Faraone S.V., Wozniak J., Monuteaux M.C. (2000) Parsing the associations between bipolar, conduct, and substance use disorders: a familial risk analysis. *Biol. Psychiatry*, **48**: 1037–1044.

74. Shulman K.I. (1997) Disinhibition syndromes, secondary mania and bipolar disorder in old age. *J. Affect. Disord.*, **46**: 175–182.

75. Steffens D.C., Krishnan K.R.R. (1998) Structural neuroimaging and mood disorders. Recent findings, implications for classification, and future directions. *Biol. Psychiatry*, **43**: 705–712.

76. Shulman K.I., Herrmann N. (1999) The nature and management of mania in old age. *Psychiatr. Clin. North Am.*, **22**: 649–665.

77. Berrios G.E., Bakshi N (1991) Manic and depressive symptoms in the elderly: their relationships to treatment outcome, cognition and motor symptoms. *Psychopathology*, **24**: 31–38.

78. Savard R.J., Rey A.C., Post R.M. (1980) Halstead-Reitan Category Test in bipolar and unipolar affective disorders: relationship to age and phase of illness. *J. Nerv. Ment. Dis.*, **168**: 297.

79. Dhingra U., Rabins P.V. (1991) Mania in the elderly: a five-to-seven year follow-up. *J. Am. Geriatr. Soc.*, **39**: 582–583.

80. Spicer C.C., Hare E.H., Slater E. (1973) Neurotic and psychotic forms of depressive illness: evidence from age-incidence in a national sample. *Br. J. Psychiatry*, **123**: 535–541.

81. Alexopoulos G.S., Meyers B.S., Young R.C., Mattis S., Kakuma T. (1993) The course of geriatric depression with "reversible dementia": a controlled study. *Am. J. Psychiatry*, **150**: 1693–1699.

82. Starkstein S.E., Robinson R.G. (1997) Mechanism of disinhibition after brain lesions. *J. Nerv. Ment. Dis.*, **185**: 108–114.

83. American Psychiatric Association (1994) *Diagnostic and Statistical Manual of Mental Disorders*, 4th ed. American Psychiatric Association, Washington.

84. Young R.C., Falk J.R. (1989) Age, manic psychopathology, and treatment response. *Int. J. Geriatr. Psychiatry*, **16**: 125–131.

85. Broadhead J., Jacoby R. (1990) Mania in old age: A first prospective study. *Int. J. Geriatr. Psychiatry*, **5**: 215–222.

86. Young R.C. (1997) Bipolar disorder in the elderly. *Psychiatr. Clin. North Am.*, **20**: 121–136.

87. Shulman K., Post F. (1980) Bipolar affective disorder in old age. *Br. J. Psychiatry*, **136**: 26–32.

88. Bowden C.L., Janicak P.G., Orsulak P., Swann A.C., Davis J.M., Calabrese J.R., Goodnick P., Small J.G., Rush A.J., Kimmel S.E. *et al* (1996) Relation of serum valproate concentration to response in mania. *Am. J. Psychiatry*, **153**: 765–770.

89. Bowden C.L., Brugger A.M., Swann A.C., Calabrese J.R., Janicak P.G., Petty F., Dilsaver S.C., Davis J.M., Rush A.J., Small J.G. *et al* (1994) Efficacy of divalproex vs lithium and placebo in the treatment of mania. *JAMA*, **271**: 918–924.

90. Bowden C.L., Calabrese J.R., McElroy S.L., Gyulai L., Wassef A., Petty F., Pope H.G., Chou JC-Y., Peck P.E., Rhodes L.J. *et al* (2000) A randomized, placebo-controlled 12-month trial of divalproex and lithium in treatment of outpatients with bipolar I disorder. *Arch. Gen. Psychiatry*, **57**: 481–489.

91. Calabrese J.R., Bowden C.L., Sachs G.S., Ascher J.A., Monaghan E., Rudd G.D. (1999) A double-blind placebo-controlled study of lamotrigine monotherapy in outpatients with bipolar I depression. *J. Clin. Psychiatry*, **60**: 79–88.

92. Viguera A.C., Tondo L., Baldessarini R.J. (2000) Sex differences in response to lithium treatment. *Am. J. Psychiatry*, **157**: 1509–1511.

93. Viguera A.C., Nonacs R., Cohen L.S., Tondo L., Murray A., Baldessarini R.J. (2000) Risk of recurrence of bipolar disorder in pregnant and nonpregnant women after discontinuing lithium maintenance. *Am. J. Psychiatry*, **157**: 179–184.

94. Schou M. (1998) Treating recurrent affective disorders during and after pregnancy: what can be taken safely? *Drug Safety*, **18**: 143–152.

95. Llewellyn A., Stowe Z.N., Strader J.R. (1998) The use of lithium and management of women with bipolar disorder during pregnancy and lactation. *J. Clin. Psychiatry*, **59** (Suppl. 6): 57–64.

96. Kennedy D., Koren G. (1998) Valproic acid use in psychiatry: issues in treating women of reproductive age. *J. Psychiatry Neurosci.*, **23**: 223–228.

97. Cohen L.S., Sichel D.A., Robertson L.M., Heckscher E., Rosenbaum J.F. (1995) Postpartum prophylaxis for women with bipolar disorder. *Am. J. Psychiatry*, **152**: 1641–1645.

98. Stewart D.E., Klompenhouwer J.L., Kendall R.E., Van Hulst A.M. (1991) Prophylactic lithium in puerperal psychosis: the experience of three centers. *Br. J. Psychiatry*, **158**: 393–397.

99. Viguera A.C., Cohen L.S. (1998) The course and management of bipolar disorder during pregnancy. *Psychopharmacol. Bull.*, **34**: 339–346.

100. Hägg S., Spigset O. (2000) Anticonvulsant use during lactation. *Drug Safety*, **22**: 425–440.

101. Chaudron L.H., Jefferson J.W. (2000) Mood stabilizers during breastfeeding: a review. *J. Clin. Psychiatry*, **61**: 79–90.

102. Stahl M.M.S., Neiderud J., Vinge E. (1997) Thrombocytopenic purpura and anemia in a breast-fed infant whose mother was treated with valproic acid. *J. Pediatrics*, **130**: 1001–1003.

103. Frey B., Schubiger G., Musy J.P. (1990) Transient cholestatic hepatitis in a neonate associated with carbamazepine exposure during pregnancy and breast-feeding. *Eur. J. Pediatrics*, **150**: 136–138.

104. Merlob P., Mor N., Litwin A. (1992) Transient hepatic dysfunction in an infant of an epileptic mother treated with carbamazepine during pregnancy and breastfeeding. *Ann. Pharmacother.*, **26**: 1563–1565.

105. Blay S.L., Ferraz M.P., Calil H.M. (1982) Lithium-induced male sexual impairment: two case reports. *J. Clin. Psychiatry*, **43**: 497–498.

106. Kristensen E., Jorgensen P. (1987) Sexual function in lithium-treated manic-depressive patients. *Pharmacopsychiatry*, **20**: 165–167.

107. Aizenberg D., Sigler M., Zemishlany Z., Weizman A. (1996) Lithium and male sexual function in affective patients. *Clin. Neuropharmacol.*, **19**: 515–519.

108. Ghadirian A.-M., Annable L., Bélanger M.-C. (1992) Lithium, benzodiazepines, and sexual function in bipolar patients. *Am. J. Psychiatry*, **149**: 801–805.

109. Penovich P.E. (2000) The effects of epilepsy and its treatment on sexual and reproductive function. *Epilepsia*, **41** (Suppl. 2): S53–S61.

110. Yerby M.S., McCoy G.B. (1999) Male infertility: possible association with valproate exposure. *Epilepsia*, **40**: 520–521.

111. Elmslie J.L., Silverstone J.T., Mann J.I., Williams S.M., Romans S.E. (2000) Prevalence of overweight and obesity in bipolar patients. *J. Clin. Psychiatry*, **61**: 179–184.

112. Isojärvi J.I.T., Laatikainen T.J., Pakarinen A.J., Juntunen K.T.S., Myllylä V.V. (1993) Polycystic ovaries and hyperandrogenism in women taking valproate for epilepsy. *N. Engl. J. Med.*, **329**: 1383–1388.

113. Rasgon N.L., Altshuler L.L., Gudeman D., Burt V.K., Tanavoli S., Hendrick V., Korenman S. (2000) Medication status and polycystic ovary syndrome in women with bipolar disorder: a preliminary report. *J. Clin. Psychiatry*, **61**: 173–178.

114. Piontek C.M., Wisner K.L. (2000) Appropriate clinical management of women taking valproate. *J. Clin. Psychiatry*, **61**: 161–163.

115. Davanzo P.A., McCracken J.T. (2000) Mood stabilizers in the treatment of juvenile bipolar disorder. *Child Adolesc. Psychiatr. Clin. North Am.*, **9**: 159–182.

116. Jefferson J.W. (1982) The use of lithium in childhood and adolescence: an overview. *J. Clin. Psychiatry*, **43**: 174–177.

117. Kowatch R.A., Suppes T., Carmody T.J., Bucci J.P., Hume J.H., Kromelis M., Emslie G.J., Weinberg W.A., Rush A.J. (2000) Effect size of lithium, divalproex sodium, and carbamazepine in children and adolescents with bipolar disorder. *J. Am. Acad. Child Adolesc. Psychiatry*, **39**: 713–720.

118. Geller B., Cooper T.B., Sun K., Zimerman B., Frazier J., Williams M., Heath J. (1998) Double-blind and placebo-controlled study of lithium for adolescent bipolar disorders with secondary substance dependency. *J. Am. Acad. Child Adolesc. Psychiatry*, **37**: 171–178.

119. Strober M., Morrell W., Burroughs J., Lampert C., Danforth H., Freeman R. (1988) A family study of bipolar I disorder in adolescence. *J. Affect. Disord.*, **15**: 255–268.

120. Strober M., DeAntonio M., Schmidt-Lackner S., Freeman R., Lampert C., Diamond J. (1998) Early childhood attention deficit hyperactivity disorder

predicts poorer response to acute lithium therapy in adolescent mania. *J. Affect. Disord.*, **51**: 145–151.
121. Strober M., Morrell W., Lampert C., Burroughs J. (1990)   Relapse following discontinuation of lithium maintenance therapy in adolescents with bipolar I illness: a naturalistic study. *Am. J. Psychiatry*, **147**: 457–461.
122. Khandelwal S.K., Varma V.K., Murthy R.S. (1984)   Renal function in children receiving long-term lithium prophylaxis. *Am. J. Psychiatry*, **141**: 278–279.
123. Papatheodorou G., Kutcher S.P., Katic M., Szalai J.P. (1995)   The efficacy and safety of divalproex sodium in the treatment of acute mania in adolescents and young adults: an open clinical trial. *J. Clin. Psychopharmacol.*, **15**: 110–116.
124. Whittier M.C., West S.A., Galli V.B., Raute N.J. (1995)   Valproic acid for dysphoric mania in a mentally retarded adolescent. *J. Clin. Psychiatry*, **56**: 590–591.
125. Kastner T., Friedman D.L. (1992)   Verapamil and valproic acid treatment of prolonged mania. *J. Am. Acad. Child Adolesc. Psychiatry*, **31**: 271–275.
126. Hsu L.K.G., Starzynski J.M. (1986)   Mania in adolescence. *J. Clin. Psychiatry*, **47**: 596–599.
127. Woolston J.L. (1999)   Case study: carbamazepine treatment of juvenile-onset bipolar disorder. *J. Am. Acad. Child Adolesc. Psychiatry*, **38**: 335–338.
128. Craven C., Murphy M. (2000)   Carbamazepine treatment of bipolar disorder in an adolescent with cerebral palsy. *J. Am. Acad. Child Adolesc. Psychiatry*, **39**: 680–681.
129. Lee D.O., Steingard R.J., Cesena M., Helmers S.L., Riviello J.J., Mikati M.A. (1996)   Behavioural side effects of gabapentin in children. *Epilepsia*, **37**: 87–90.
130. Biederman J., Mick E., Bostic J.Q., Prince J., Daly J., Wilens T.E., Spencer T., Garcia-Jetton J., Russell R., Wozniak J. et al (1998)   The naturalistic course of pharmacologic treatment of children with maniclike symptoms: a systematic chart review. *J. Clin. Psychiatry*, **59**: 628–637.
131. Khouzam H.R., El-Gabalawi F. (2000)   Treatment of bipolar I disorder in an adolescent with olanzapine. *J. Child Adolesc. Psychopharmacol.*, **10**: 147–151.
132. Soutullo C.A., Sorter M.T., Foster K.D., McElroy S.L., Keck P.E. (1999)   Olanzapine in the treatment of adolescent acute mania: a report of seven cases. *J. Affect. Disord.*, **53**: 279–283.
133. Chang K.D, Ketter T.A. (2000)   Mood stabilizer augmentation with olanzapine in acutely manic children. *J. Child Adolesc. Psychopharmacol.*, **10**: 45–49.
134. Frazier J.A., Biederman J., Jacobs T.G., Tohen M.F., Toma V., Feldman P.D., Rater M.A., Tarazi R.A., Kim G.A., Garfield S.B. et al (2000)   Olanzapine in the treatment of bipolar disorder in juveniles. Presented at the 40th Annual New Clinical Drug Evaluation Unit Meeting, Boca Raton, 30 May–2 June.
135. Frazier J.A., Meyer M.C., Biederman J., Wozniak J., Wilens T.E., Spencer T.J., Kim G.S., Shapiro S. (1999)   Risperidone treatment for juvenile bipolar disorder: a retrospective chart review. *J. Am. Acad. Child Adolesc. Psychiatry*, **38**: 960–965.
136. Martin A., Landau J., Leebens P., Ulizio K., Cicchetti D., Scahill L., Leckman J.F. (2000)   Risperidone-associated weight gain in children and adolescents: a retrospective chart review. *J. Child Adolesc. Psychopharmacol.*, **10**: 259–268.
137. Schaller J.L., Behar D. (1999)   Quetiapine for refractory mania in a child. *J. Am. Acad. Child Adolesc. Psychiatry*, **38**: 498–499.
138. Fuchs D.C. (1994)   Clozapine treatment of bipolar disorder in a young adolescent. *J. Am. Acad. Child Adolesc. Psychiatry*, **33**: 1299–1302.
139. Papatheodorou G., Kutcher S. (1995)   The effect of adjunctive light therapy on ameliorating breakthrough depressive symptoms in adolescent-onset bipolar disorder. *J. Psychiatry Neurosci.*, **20**: 226–232.

140. Geller B., Cooper T.B., Zimerman B., Frazier J., Williams M., Heath J., Warner K. (1998) Lithium for prepubertal depressed children with family history predictors of future bipolarity: a double-blind, placebo-controlled study. *J. Affect. Disord.*, **51**: 165–175.

141. Carr V., Dorrington C., Schrader G., Wale J. (1983) The use of ECT for mania in childhood bipolar disorder. *Br. J. Psychiatry*, **143**: 411–415.

142. Hill M.A., Courvoisie H., Dawkins K., Nofal P., Thomas B. (1997) ECT for the treatment of intractable mania in two prepubertal male children. *Convulsive Ther.*, **13**: 74–82.

143. Robertson J.M., Tanguay P.E. (1997) Case study: the use of melatonin in a boy with refractory bipolar disorder. *J. Am. Acad. Child Adolesc. Psychiatry*, **36**: 822–825.

144. Schreier H.A. (1982) Mania responsive to lecithin in a 13-year-old girl. *Am. J. Psychiatry*, **139**: 108–110.

145. Davanzo P.A., Krah N., Kleiner J., McCracken J. (1999) Nimodipine treatment of an adolescent with ultradian cycling bipolar affective illness. *J. Child Adolesc. Psychopharmacol.*, **9**: 51–61.

146. Shulman K.I., Herrmann N. (1999) The nature and management of mania in old age. *Psychiatry Clin. North Am.*, **22**: 649–665.

147. Shulman K.I., Herrmann N. (1999) Bipolar disorders in old age. *Can. Fam. Physician*, **45**: 1229–1237.

148. Herrmann N., Bremner K., Naranjo C.A. (1997) Pharmacotherapy of mood disorders in late life. *Clin. Neurosci.*, **4**: 41–47.

149. Naranjo C.A., Herrmann N., Mittmann N., Bremner K.E. (1995) Recent advances in geriatric psychopharmacology. *Drugs Aging*, **7**: 184–202.

150. Head L., Dening T. (1998) Lithium in the over-65s: who is taking it and who is monitoring it? *Int. J. Geriatr. Psychiatry*, **13**: 64–171.

151. Himmelhoch J.M., Neil J.F., May S.J., Fuchs C.Z., Licata S.M. (1980) Age, dementia, dyskinesia, and lithium response. *Am. J. Psychiatry*, **137**: 941–945.

152. Schaffer C.B., Garavey M.J. (1984) Use of lithium in acutely manic elderly patients. *Clin. Gerontol.*, **3**: 58–60.

153. Shulman R.W., Singh A., Shulman K.I. (1997) Treatment of elderly institutionalized bipolar patients with clozapine. *Psychopharmacol. Bull.*, **33**: 113–118.

154. Van der Velde C.D. (1970) Effectiveness of lithium carbonate in treatment of manic-depressive illness. *Am. J. Psychiatry*, **127**: 345–351.

155. Hardy B.G., Shulman K.I., Mackenzie S.E., Kutcher S., Silverberg J. (1987) Pharmacokinetics of lithium in the elderly. *J. Clin. Psychopharmacol.*, **7**: 153–158.

156. Murray N., Hopwood S., Balfour D.J.K., Hewick D.S. (1983) The influence of age on lithium efficacy and side effects in out-patients. *Psychol. Med.*, **13**: 53–60.

157. Roose S.P., Bone S., Haidorfer C., Dunner D.L., Fieve R.R. (1979) Lithium treatment in older patients. *Am. J. Psychiatry*, **136**: 843–844.

158. Smith R.E., Helms P.M. (1982) Adverse effects of lithium therapy in the acutely ill elderly patient. *J. Clin. Psychiatry*, **43**: 94–99.

159. Sproule B.A., Hardy B.G., Shulman K.I. (2000) Differential pharmacokinetics of lithium in elderly patients. *Drugs Aging*, **16**: 165–177.

160. Nambudiri D.E., Meyers B.S., Young R.C. (1991) Delayed recovery from lithium neurotoxicity. *J. Geriatr. Psychiatry Neurol.*, **4**: 40–43.

161. McFarland B.H., Miller M.R., Straumfjord A.A. (1990) Valproate use in the older manic patient. *J. Clin. Psychiatry*, **51**: 479–481.

162. Risinger R.C., Risby E.D., Risch S.C. (1994) Safety and efficacy of divalproex sodium in elderly bipolar patients. *J. Clin. Psychiatry*, **55**: 215.

163. Kando J.C., Tohen M., Castillo J., Zarate C.A. (1996)   The use of valproate in an elderly population with affective symptoms. *J. Clin. Psychiatry*, **57**: 238–240.
164. Mordecai D.J., Sheikh J.I., Glick I.D. (1999)   Divalproex for the treatment of geriatric bipolar disorder. *Int. J. Geriatr. Psychiatry*, **14**: 494–496.
165. Noaghiul S., Narayan M., Nelson J.C. (1998)   Divalproex treatment of mania in elderly patients. *Am. J. Geriatr. Psychiatry*, **6**: 257–262.
166. Chen S.T., Altshuler L.L., Melnyk K.A., Erhart S.M., Miller E., Mintz J. (1999)   Efficacy of lithium vs valproate in the treatment of mania in the elderly: a retrospective study. *J. Clin. Psychiatry*, **60**: 181–186.
167. Kellner M.B., Neher F. (1991)   A first episode of mania after age 80. *Can. J. Psychiatry*, **36**: 607–608.
168. Schneier H.A., Kahn D. (1990)   Selective response to carbamazepine in a case of organic mood disorder. *J. Clin. Psychiatry*, **51**: 485.
169. Young R.C. (1996)   Treatment of geriatric mania. In *Mood Disorders Across the Life Span* (Eds. K.I. Shulman, M. Tohen, S.P. Kutcher), pp. 425–441, Wiley-Liss, New York.
170. Sheldon L.F., Ancill R.J., Holliday S.G. (1998)   Gabapentin in geriatric psychiatry patients. *Can. J. Psychiatry*, **43**: 422–423.
171. Ghaemi S.N., Katzow J.J., Desai S.P., Goodwin F.K. (1998)   Gabapentin treatment of mood disorders: a preliminary study. *J. Clin. Psychiatry*, **59**: 426–429.
172. Kusumakar V., Yatham L.N. (1997)   Lamotrigine treatment of rapid cycling bipolar disorder. *Am. J. Psychiatry*, **154**: 1171–1172.
173. Mukherjee S., Sackeim H.A., Schnur D.B. (1994)   Electroconvulsive therapy of acute manic episodes: a review of 50 years' experience. *Am. J. Psychiatry*, **151**: 169–176.

Commentaries

Heterogeneity of Bipolar Disorder: Does Childhood Onset Make a Difference?

Stephen V. Faraone[1]

In their masterful chapter about gender and age in bipolar disorder, Shulman et al have provided us with a comprehensive view of the heterogeneity of bipolar disorder (BD). As they describe, age at onset is a dimension of heterogeneity that has received much attention in recent years. With one report finding that 59% of BD patients had symptom onset prior to the age of 20, it would appear that this seriously disabling mental disorder frequently begins in youth.

Despite such strong evidence for youth onset BD, its existence was ignored for many years. Then, in the 1980s, several case reports and series described children presenting with symptoms suggestive of BD, which responded to lithium carbonate [1–4]. Yet many of these children had never been diagnosed with a mood disorder, which suggested that the pediatric form of BD, rather than being rare, might be difficult to diagnose due to atypical clinical features.

These atypical features have been well characterized in the literature [5, 6]. Among BD children, the most common mood disturbance is not euphoria [2, 7]. Instead, these children present with severe irritability and prolonged and aggressive outbursts of temper [6]. The irritability of childhood BD is severe, persistent, and often violent [8]. Although these severe outbursts are episodic, these children are chronically irritable or angry [2, 7, 9]. In their literature review, Geller and Luby [9] concluded that childhood-onset BD is a non-episodic, chronic, rapid-cycling, mixed manic state. Thus, one reason why pediatric BD is difficult to diagnose is because it presents with an atypical picture characterized by predominantly irritable mood, mixed with symptoms of major depression, and chronic course, as opposed to euphoric, biphasic, and episodic course. With some exceptions, the clinical features of BD are similar in childhood and adolescence [10]. Notably, the atypical features of youth BD are similar to the syndrome of mixed BD, which affects about one-fourth of BD adults [11].

[1] Pediatric Psychopharmacology Unit, Massachusetts General Hospital and Harvard Medical School Department of Psychiatry, 15 Parkman Street, Boston, MA 02114, USA

As Shulman *et al* note, another source of diagnostic dilemma for childhood BD is its frequent comorbidity with attention deficit hyperactivity disorder (ADHD). Most BD youth meet diagnostic criteria for ADHD, with prevalence figures ranging from 60% to 90% [8, 12–14]. Faraone *et al.* [10] found that adolescents with childhood-onset BD had the same rates of comorbid ADHD as manic children (90%) and that both these groups had higher rates of ADHD than adolescents with adolescent-onset BD (60%). Sachs *et al* [15] reported that, among adults with bipolar disorder, a history of comorbid ADHD was only evident in those subjects with onset of BD before 19 years of age. Chang *et al.* [16] reported that the onset of BD in adults with a history of ADHD was 11.3 years of age. These findings suggest that early onset of BD may identify a developmental subtype of the disorder that is frequently comorbid with ADHD [10, 17, 18].

The high levels of comorbidity between BD and ADHD raise a fundamental, nosologic question: do children presenting with BD and ADHD have ADHD, BD, or both? One method to address these uncertainties has been to examine the transmission of comorbid disorders in families [19]. As shown in a meta-analysis by Faraone *et al* [20], studies that examined rates of ADHD (or ADD, hyperactivity) among the offspring of adults with BD found higher rates of ADHD among these children compared with controls. Likewise, the meta-analysis showed that family studies of ADHD children find high rates of BD among relatives.

In three different samples, Faraone *et al* [20–22] found that relatives of children with BD were at high risk for ADHD, that was indistinguishable from the risk in relatives of children with ADHD and no BD. However, BD and the comorbid condition of BD plus ADHD selectively aggregated among relatives of manic youth compared with those with ADHD and comparison children. This pattern of transmission in families suggested that BD in children might be a familially distinct subtype of either BD or ADHD, an idea which is consistent with the work of Strober *et al* [23, 24] and Todd *et al* [25], who proposed that pediatric BD might be a distinct subtype of BD with a high familial loading.

Like ADHD, conduct disorder (CD) is strongly associated with pediatric BD. This has been seen separately in studies of children with CD, ADHD and BD [8, 26–28]. These reports are consistent with the well-documented comorbidity between CD and major depression [29], considering that juvenile depression often leads to BD [30, 31].

Biederman *et al* [32, 33] investigated the overlap between BD and CD in a consecutive sample of referred youth and in a sample of ADHD subjects to clarify its prevalence and correlates. They found a striking similarity in the features of BD regardless of comorbid CD. Both the comorbid and non-comorbid subjects with BD had high rates of major depression, anxiety disorders, oppositional disorder, and psychosis than CD and ADHD children [32, 33]. In addition, BD comorbid with CD was associated with poorer functioning and an increased risk for psychiatric hospitalization [32]. Subjects with both CD and BD also had a higher familial and personal risk for mood disorders than other CD subjects, who had a higher personal risk for antisocial personality disorder [20]. These studies suggest that subjects who receive diagnoses of both CD and BD may have both disorders. Although more research is needed to clarify this issue, it raises the hope that some cases of delinquency may respond to mood stabilizers.

Although clinical lore has long attributed bipolar symptoms in children to trauma, there have been few systematic studies of this issue. Kessler *et al* reported elevated rates of BD among adults and adolescents with post-traumatic stress disorder (PTSD) [34] and Helzer *et al* [35] found high rates of BD among adults with PTSD. Neither of these studies determined if the BD was primary or secondary to the trauma. In a longitudinal study, Wozniak *et al* [36] identified pediatric BD as an important antecedent for, rather than consequence of, traumatic life events. Although these findings need independent replication, they suggest that clinicians treating traumatized children should not dismiss severe irritability and mood lability as consequences of the trauma. These may indicate an underlying BD, and thus have implications for treatment.

Let us hope that Shulman *et al*'s call for more research is heeded. As they suggest, the field needs more data about youth-onset BD to more firmly establish the fundamental phenomenologic differences with adult-onset BD. Ideally, such work would lead to developmentally sensitive diagnostic criteria which take into account differential symptom expression with age. New criteria are needed to better differentiate typical and atypical BD.

Studies of phenomenology will provide a firm nosologic foundation for further work examining the causes and correlates of BD. Ideally, studies from multiple domains (e.g., neuroimaging, genetics, family environment) will eventually clarify if putative clinical subtypes of BD have different causes or pathophysiologic correlates in the brain.

We also need much more treatment research in youth. The outcome measures used in treatment studies of youth BD should attend to the wide range of symptoms of mood dysregulation, aggression and ADHD symptoms. The high levels of comorbidity between BD and other disorders suggest that multiple treatment strategies may be needed. Given the severity of BD, designing such studies in an ethical manner presents a major challenge for clinical researchers.

REFERENCES

1. DeLong G.R., Nieman G.W. (1983) Lithium-induced behavior changes in children with symptoms suggesting manic-depressive illness. *Psychopharmacol. Bull.*, **19**: 258–265.
2. Carlson G.A. (1984) Classification issues of bipolar disorders in childhood. *Psychiatr. Develop.*, **2**: 273–285.
3. Akiskal H.S., Downs J., Jordan P. (1985) Affective disorders in referred children and younger siblings of manic-depressives: mode of onset and prospective course. *Arch. Gen. Psychiatry*, **42**: 996–1003.
4. Weller R.A., Weller E.B., Tucker S.G., Fristad M.A. (1986) Mania in prepubertal children: has it been underdiagnosed? *J. Affect. Disord.*, **11**: 151–154.
5. Weinberg W.A., Brumback R.A. (1976) Mania in childhood. *Am. J. Dis. Children*, **130**: 380–385.
6. Davis R.E. (1979) Manic-depressive variant syndrome of childhood: a preliminary report. *Am. J. Psychiatry*, **136**: 702–706.
7. Carlson G.A. (1983) Bipolar affective disorders in childhood and adolescence. In *Affective Disorders in Childhood and Adolescence* (Eds D.P. Cantwell, G.A. Carlson), pp. 61–83, Spectrum Publications, New York.
8. Wozniak J., Biederman J., Kiely K., Ablon S., Faraone S., Mundy E., Mennin D. (1995) Mania-like symptoms suggestive of childhood onset bipolar disorder in clinically referred children. *J. Am. Acad. Child Adolesc. Psychiatry*, **34**: 867–876.
9. Geller B., Luby J. (1997) Child and adolescent bipolar disorder: a review of the past 10 years. *J. Am. Acad. Child Adolesc. Psychiatry*, **36**: 1168–1176.
10. Faraone S.V., Biederman J., Wozniak J., Mundy E., Mennin D., O'Donnell D. (1997) Is comorbidity with ADHD a marker for juvenile onset mania? *J. Am. Acad. Child Adolesc. Psychiatry*, **36**: 1046–1055.
11. McElroy S.L., Keck P.E., Jr., Pope H.G., Jr., Hudson J.I., Faedda G., Swann A.C. (1992) Clinical and research implications of the diagnosis of dysphoric or mixed mania or hypomania. *Am. J. Psychiatry*, **149**: 1633–1644.
12. Borchardt C.M., Bernstein G.A. (1995) Comorbid disorders in hospitalized bipolar adolescents compared with unipolar depressed adolescents. *Child Psychiatry Hum. Develop.*, **26**: 11–18.
13. Geller B., Sun K., Zimmerman B., Luby J., Frazier J., Williams M. (1995) Complex and rapid-cycling in bipolar children and adolescents: a preliminary study. *J. Affect. Disord.*, **34**: 259–268.
14. West S., McElroy S., Strakowski S., Keck P., McConville B. (1995) Attention deficit hyperactivity disorder in adolescent mania. *Am. J. Psychiatry*, **152**: 271–274.
15. Sachs G.S., Baldassano C.F., Truman C.J., Guille C. (2000) Comorbidity of attention deficit hyperactivity disorder with early- and late-onset bipolar disorder. *Am. J. Psychiatry*, **157**: 466–468.
16. Chang K.D., Steiner H., Ketter T.A. (2000) Psychiatric phenomenology of child and adolescent bipolar offspring. *J. Am. Acad. Child Adolesc. Psychiatry*, **39**: 453–460.
17. Biederman J., Mick E., Faraone S.V., Spencer T., Wilens T.E., Wozniak J. (2000) Pediatric mania: a developmental subtype of bipolar disorder? *Biol. Psychiatry*, **48**: 458–466.
18. Faraone S.V., Biederman J., Mennin D., Wozniak J., Spencer T. (1997) Attention-deficit hyperactivity disorder with bipolar disorder: a familial subtype? *J. Am. Acad. Child Adolesc. Psychiatry*, **36**: 1378–1387.

19. Faraone S.V., Tsuang D., Tsuang M.T. (1999) *Genetics and Mental Disorders: A Guide for Students, Clinicians, and Researchers.* Guilford, New York.

20. Faraone S.V., Biederman J., Mennin D., Russell R.L. (1998) Bipolar and anti-social disorders among relatives of ADHD children: parsing familial subtypes of illness. *Neuropsychiatr. Genet.,* **81**: 108–116.

21. Faraone S.V., Biederman J., Monuteaux M.C. (2001) Attention deficit hyper-activity disorder with bipolar disorder in girls: further evidence for a familial subtype? *J. Affect. Disord.,* **64**: 19–26.

22. Wozniak J., Biederman J., Mundy E., Mennin D., Faraone S.V. (1995) A pilot family study of childhood-onset mania. *J. Am. Acad. Child Adolesc. Psychiatry,* **34**: 1577–1583.

23. Strober M., Morrell W., Burroughs J., Lampert C., Danforth H., Freeman R. (1988) A family study of bipolar I disorder in adolescence: early onset of symptoms linked to increased familial loading and lithium resistance. *J. Affect. Disord.,* **15**: 255–268.

24. Strober M (1992) Relevance of early age-of-onset in genetic studies of bipolar affective disorder. *J. Am. Acad. Child Adolesc. Psychiatry,* **31**: 606–610.

25. Todd R., Neuman R., Geller B., Fox L., Hickok J. (1993) Genetic studies of affective disorders: should we be starting with childhood onset probands? *J. Am. Acad. Child Adolesc. Psychiatry,* **32**: 1164–1171.

26. Kovacs M., Pollock M. (1995) Bipolar disorder and comorbid conduct disorder in childhood and adolescence. *J. Am. Acad. Child Adolesc. Psychiatry,* **34**: 715–723.

27. Kutcher S.P., Marton P., Korenblum M. (1989) Relationship between psychi-atric illness and conduct disorder in adolescents. *Can. J. Psychiatry,* **34**: 526–529.

28. Wicki W., Angst J. (1991) The Zurich study. X. Hypomania in a 28- to 30-year-old cohort. *Eur. Arch. Psychiatry Clin. Neurosci.,* **240**: 339–348.

29. Angold A., Costello E.J. (1993) Depressive comorbidity in children and ado-lescents: empirical, theoretical and methodological issues. *Am. J. Psychiatry,* **150**: 1779–1791.

30. Geller B., Fox L., Clark K. (1994) Rate and predictors of prepubertal bipolarity during follow-up of 6- to 12-year-old depressed children. *J. Am. Acad. Child Adolesc. Psychiatry,* **33**: 461–468.

31. Strober M., Carlson G. (1982) Bipolar illness in adolescents with major depres-sion: clinical, genetic, and psychopharmacologic predictors in a three- to four-year prospective follow-up investigation. *Arch. Gen. Psychiatry,* **39**: 549–555.

32. Biederman J., Faraone S., Hatch M., Mennin D., Taylor A., George P. (1997) Conduct disorder with and without mania in a referred sample of ADHD children. *J. Affect. Disord.,* **44**: 177–188.

33. Biederman J., Faraone S.V., Chu M.P., Wozniak J. (1999) Further evidence of a bidirectional overlap between juvenile mania and conduct disorder in children. *J. Am. Acad. Child Adolesc. Psychiatry,* **38**: 468–476.

34. Kessler R., Sonnega A., Bromet E., Hughes M., Nelson C. (1995) Posttraumatic stress disorder in the national comorbidity survey. *Arch. Gen. Psychiatry,* **52**: 1048–1060.

35. Helzer J., Robins L., McEvoy L. (1987) Post-traumatic stress disorder in the general population. *N. Engl. J. Med.,* **317**: 1630–1634.

36. Wozniak J., Crawford M.H., Biederman J., Faraone S.V., Spencer T.J., Taylor A., Blier H.K. (1999) Antecedents and complications of trauma in boys with ADHD: findings from a longitudinal study. *J. Am. Acad. Child Adolesc. Psychi-atry,* **38**: 48–55.

5.2
Bipolar Disorders in Children and Adolescents: Critical Diagnostic Issues for Clinicians Across the World

Carlos E. Berganza[1]

Due to the lack of pathognomonic biological markers for most of psychopathology, and with the current emphasis on facts rather than theory in defining psychiatric syndromes, phenomenology is of critical importance for the scientific development of psychiatry. The international success of the most visible current diagnostic systems in psychiatry (the DSM-IV and the ICD-10), both based on phenomenology, attest to the great importance researchers and clinicians ascribe to the symptomatic expression of disorders in their daily professional activities across the world.

Child psychiatric disorders are more difficult to characterize than those afflicting adults. Although important advances in diagnosis have been accomplished, many treatments in child psychiatry are still prescribed for rather vaguely defined disorders such as "aggressiveness", "difficult behaviour" or "depression". Many factors contribute to this. Firstly, children have traditionally been neglected in the provision of services, and the very concept of childhood, with a demarcation of the particular characteristics and needs of this developmental stage, is relatively new. Secondly, although the phenomenology of psychiatric disorders in childhood can be conceived in the same dimensions of the adult disorders, "abnormality" in children is influenced by maturation and development, making it more difficult for the diagnostician to interpret indicators of brain dysfunction [1]. Thirdly, the child lacks in richness of behavioural expressions of psychopathology in comparison with the adult, making differential diagnosis a more difficult task, and probably increasing rates of comorbidity. Finally, the child has more difficulties in describing psychological symptoms or associating them within informative factual relationships that would facilitate the development by the clinician of appropriate assumptions of causality and explanation.

Shulman and co-authors offer a good review of the evidence, strongly suggesting not only that bipolar disorders (BD) are present within the child psychiatric population, but also that their prevalence is increasing. They also point to the fact that a good number of children presenting with this disorder for clinical care are misdiagnosed. However, their review offers little solution to the problem of early diagnosis of BD in children and adolescents, which in our opinion is critical for the assessment of the efficacy of various treatments proposed for the disorder in this patient population.

---

[1] *Clinica de Psiquiatria Infantil, Avenida La Reforma 13–70, Zona 9, Guatemala 00109, Guatemala*

The reasons for the misdiagnosis of BD are complex and some of them are only beginning to be clarified in the child psychiatric literature; however, it seems that the lack of a set of diagnostic criteria that allows a clear differentiation of BD from other similar syndromes of childhood, such as attention deficit hyperactivity disorders (ADHD), makes it very difficult for clinicians to resolve this critical diagnostic dilemma.

Arriving at an early diagnosis of BD is a very important clinical objective for the child psychiatrist for several reasons. Firstly, as Shulman and co-authors indicate, this disorder is a source of serious psychosocial dysfunction for children and adolescents with "devastating consequences" for their lives. The behavioural constellation showed by a child or an adolescent with BD is so disturbing to those surrounding the youngster that very frequently they react in ways that compound the emotional problems of the afflicted patient. For instance, many such patients get expelled from school or end up in correctional institutions, long before an appropriate diagnosis is made of their psychobiological condition. Secondly, there is evidence that the longer a psychiatric syndrome evolves—such as BD—the more refractory it becomes to treatment [2]. That could explain, at least partially, why BD of early age presents a worse prognosis than BD of late beginning, as Shulman's review clearly indicates.

In child psychiatry we are still at a stage of theoretical development where we need "to be mindful of the limits of our observations, both research and clinical, and of our need to balance the use of 'judgment' and 'knowledge'..." [3]. Therefore, this commentary must be taken with care, since it is based on clinical experience and the review of written evidence that still—like most of the field—needs further review.

For child psychiatrists around the world, three main diagnostic issues are of great importance to facilitate early diagnosis of BD in children and adolescents. The first one is to identify the symptoms suggestive of mania; the second one is to discriminate between mania and ADHD [4], when no psychotic symptoms are present; and the third one is to discriminate between mania and schizophrenia when psychotic manifestations are evident [5]. Table 5.2.1 summarizes what we consider the most important clinical clues for helping the clinician to arrive at an early diagnosis of BD in children and adolescents who present for assessment and care, by clarifying the differential diagnosis between mania without psychotic symptoms and ADHD.

Departing from the most important criteria proposed by ICD-10, Table 5.2.1 offers some guidelines for judging the clinical data volunteered by the patient or the family as compared with the presentation of BD in the adult population and also in comparison with the way ADHD usually expresses itself in the child psychiatric population. It seems evident that for this process of clinical "judgement" to be effective, the clinician must rely on as many sources of information as possible to ensure reliable observations concerning

TABLE 5.2.1 Main differences between mania without psychotic symptoms and attention deficit hyperactivity disorder (ADHD) in children and adolescents

Mania in adults (ICD-10)	Mania in children and adolescents	ADHD
Mood must be predominantly elevated, expansive or irritable, and definitely abnormal for the individual concerned. The mood change must be prominent and sustained for at least one week (unless it is severe enough to require hospital admission).	The younger the child, the more difficult it is for him/her to describe his/her mood. Irritability and emotional lability tend to be more obvious to parents and this may be more frequently reported by informants. Wide fluctuations in mood (mood swings) are reported if questioned. As the child grows up, the elevated or expansive mood may become more predominant and may be reported by the patient.	Wide fluctuations in mood are infrequent and tend to be present more often after emotional problems complicate the symptomatology of ADHD. Although variations in mood are included in some rating scales of ADHD, these scales do not differentiate ADHD from mania.
Increased activity or physical restlessness	Hyperactivity is usually intense. Children are frequently described as "flying around like a kite". The wide variations in levels of activity are of great diagnostic value. In severe cases the hyperactivity is continuous and the child cannot be calmed down.	Hyperactivity can be intense; however, it tends to show some consistency through the times. The wide variations in levels of activity seen in mania are not as common here.
Increased talkativeness ("pressure of speech")	The amount of speech rather than the "pressure" seems important here. Again, the report of wide variation in talkativeness is quite informative. In severe cases speech is quite pressured, and the child cannot stop speaking.	The child may show some talkativeness as part of the general pattern of hyperactivity, but it tends to be less extreme and more consistent through the times.

(continues overleaf)

TABLE 5.2.1 (*continued*)

Mania in adults (ICD-10)	Mania in children and adolescents	ADHD
Flight of ideas or the subjective experience of thoughts racing	Flight of ideas if present is quite diagnostic. The child switches from one topic to another in a way that is impressive, unresponsive to redirection and frustrating. Younger children will have problems describing or confirming their thoughts racing. In severe cases, flight of ideas is obvious, speech is hard to follow, and it may show rhyming and echolalia.	Flight of ideas are not part of the core syndrome. Some very inattentive children may occasionally come up with comments that sound out of context, but they tend to be infrequent, and responsive to redirection by others.
Loss of normal social inhibitions, resulting in behaviour that is inappropriate to the circumstances	One of the most characteristic signs. The lack of inhibition of inappropriate behaviour is usually impressive. In severe cases the child can be sarcastic, threatening, and even assaultive.	Inappropriate behaviour has a more impulsive tone, unless oppositional behaviour has arisen. The discomfort of the child with the behaviour can be noticed, as well as his/her intent to control it in the face of great difficulties to do so.
Decreased need for sleep	Hard to report unless questioned, or if the parents are asked to observe the child during sleep. In severe cases, the child can report and/or deny any need to sleep.	Sleep difficulties are rarely prominent. In some hyperactive children, falling asleep can be difficult and is usually related to some degree of stimulation at bedtime.
Inflated self-esteem or grandiosity	If present this can be very helpful for the diagnosis. Content of grandiosity can be developmentally consistent. In severe cases grandiosity and even delusional grandiosity can be prominent.	It is not part of the core diagnosis. More often what is prominent is low self-esteem, especially in complicated cases with academic failure.

Distractibility or constant changes in activity or plans	It has a differentiating quality. The child seems keenly aware of his/her environment. At times it acquires an intrusive quality, as the child may comment on the interviewer's appearance, dress or reactions, usually in a joking or demeaning way.	It is a fundamental part of the core syndrome. It may be related to external or internal stimuli. Awareness of environment has a more fleeting quality. Although intrusiveness may be present, it seems less disturbing to those surrounding the child.
Behaviour that is foolhardy or reckless and whose risks the individual does not recognize, e.g., spending sprees, foolish enterprises, reckless driving	Reflects a grandiose sense of invulnerability. Patient may take risks at all levels, including sexually and financially. It may lead to problems with the law.	Although impulsive behaviour may appear reckless and lead to problems with authority figures, it is not common to see the serious foolhardy behaviours of the manic individual.
Marked sexual energy or sexual indiscretions	If present, especially in children brought up in very conservative homes and never subject to sexual abuse, may be almost pathognomonic. Sexual behaviour may take the form of profane expressions, overt sexual advances to other children or adults, or overt sexual acts such as masturbating in public.	Children may manifest some early interest in sex as an expression of impulsivity. However, the overt manifestations of inappropriate sexual behaviour seen in manic patients are uncommon.
No current psychoactive substance use	This is an important exclusion criterion. However, the clinician must take into account the fact that substance use is quite common in older manic adolescents and it may be difficult to differentiate a manic episode from the effect of drugs such as cocaine and other stimulants. Hospitalization and detoxification may be necessary to arrive at an accurate diagnosis in some cases.	Drug abuse is probably less frequent in this patient group. Careful observation and hospitalization may be necessary for differential diagnosis as well.
No organic mental disorder	No organic mental disorder.	No organic mental disorder.

the patient's behaviour since he/she will most probably have difficulties to provide the most useful information for an appropriate diagnosis to be made. This is most painfully obvious in the case of the manic patient.

When comparing the differential diagnostic criteria proposed here, one must take into account Geller and Luby's [6] emphasis on the need to evaluate children's affect in relationship with other historical features in the same way one evaluates the incongruity between the infectious elation of manic adult patients in the context of serious losses, such as the death of a loved one. This is a very important diagnostic clue, even though much needs to be done to develop accurate diagnostic methods for BD in children and adolescents.

REFERENCES

1. Werry J.S. (1996)   Brain and behavior. In *Child and Adolescent Psychiatry*, 2nd ed. (Ed. M. Lewis), pp. 86–96, Williams & Wilkins, Baltimore.
2. Kotrla K.J., Weinberger D.R. (2000)   Developmental neurobiology. In *Comprehensive Textbook of Psychiatry*, 7th ed. (Eds B.J. Sadock, V.A. Sadock), pp. 32–40, Lippincott, Williams, and Wilkins, Philadelphia.
3. Popper C.W. (1995)   Balancing knowledge and judgment: a clinician looks at new developments in child and adolescent psychopharmacology. *Child Adolesc. Psychiatr. Clin. North Am.*, **4**: 483–513.
4. Fristad M.A., Weller E.B., Weller R.A. (1992)   The Mania Rating Scale: can it be used in children? A preliminary report. *J. Am. Acad. Child Adolesc. Psychiatry*, **31**: 252–257.
5. Werry J.S., McClellan J.M., Chard L. (1991)   Childhood and adolescent schizophrenic, bipolar, and schizoaffective disorder: a clinical and outcome study. *J. Am. Acad. Child Adolesc. Psychiatry*, **30**: 457–465.
6. Geller B., Luby J. (1997)   Child and adolescent bipolar disorder: a review of the past 10 years. *J. Am. Acad. Child Adolesc. Psychiatry*, **36**: 1168–1176.

5.3
Emotion, Mood and Bipolar Disorder in Children

Ellen Leibenluft[1]

The thorough review compiled by Shulman *et al* details the gender and age differences that have been identified in the symptoms and treatment response of patients with bipolar disorder (BD). It is clear that we have

[1] *Unit on Affective Disorders, Pediatric and Developmental Neuropsychiatry Branch, National Institute of Mental Health, Building 10, Room 4N208, 10 Center Drive MSC 1255, Bethesda, MD 20892–1255, USA*

learned a good deal about gender effects in BD, although important questions remain, particularly about the impact of puberty and menopause on the illness, and about the management of BD during pregnancy and the postpartum. In the young and old, considerably more work needs to be done to understand age differences in the presentation and management of the illness. However, we can take heart from the increased research attention now being devoted to these topics.

While it has required a great deal of research effort to identify *what* gender and age effects exist in the presentation of BD, it is even more difficult to discover *why* these effects exist. To do so necessitates that we understand how brain function in male patients with BD differs from that of female patients, and how neural circuits function differently in children with BD than in older patients. Indeed, to do so requires that we first understand the pathophysiology of BD itself.

That latter goal has proven quite elusive—in all psychiatric illnesses, to be sure, but particularly in BD. Beyond some obvious and important impediments to research with patients with BD (ethical issues regarding studying medication-free patients; the "moving target" of mood state; difficulty differentiating biological traits from state-dependent changes), conceptual shortcomings hamper us. Within what theoretical framework can we place the psychobiological dysfunction occurring in patients with BD? The need for such a framework is most evident in the current state of neuroimaging research in mood disorders in general, and in BD in particular. While much progress has been made in defining the fronto–striatal–thalamic circuits mediating depressive symptoms [1], the field is hampered by a lack of appropriate neuroimaging paradigms. In other words, we are unclear as to what tasks we should ask patients with BD to perform in the scanner, in order to bring out differences between their pattern of brain activation and that of controls. The question is particularly important in the case of functional magnetic resonance imaging (fMRI) scans, which yield relative, not absolute, measures of brain activity and therefore require that one subtract activation measures obtained during a control task from those obtained during an experimental task. In essence, then, we are challenged to take what we know about the symptoms of BD, as manifest in a patient over days, weeks, and years, and to use that knowledge to devise a task—one that takes merely seconds to complete, but that will evoke meaningful differences between groups.

Put in other terms, the challenge is to identify *emotional* responses that distinguish patients with *mood* disorders from controls. The distinction between emotion and mood is an important one, although clinicians do not often focus on it. Definitions of emotion vary, but most theoreticians view emotion as an evoked response to a stimulus with motivational value, that is, a stimulus that the organism would want to approach or avoid [2].

The definition of mood has been more elusive than that of emotion, although again there is consensus that moods, in contrast to emotions, are more long-lasting and occur in response to pervasive and persistent environmental conditions, rather than to discrete events [3]. If we were to show an unpleasant picture to patients with depression and controls while obtaining fMRI data, we would learn whether the two groups, whom we know differ in *mood*, also differ in their *emotional* response to the stimulus.

Psychologists generally agree not only on the definition of emotion, but also on the idea that is it useful to categorize emotions in terms of their valence and the level of arousal that they evoke [4]. Thus, a positive valence emotional stimulus is one that the organism would want to approach (a person that one finds sexually attractive, or a bouquet of flowers), while a negative emotional stimulus is one that an organism would want to avoid (a charging tiger or a foul-smelling pool of muck). Arousal refers to the intensity of the evoked emotion; while both the flowers and the sexually attractive person evoke positive-valence emotion, the emotion evoked by the latter is usually at a higher level of arousal than that evoked by the former. And, just as we can characterize emotional states in terms of their arousal and valence, so can we categorize the mood states of BD: euphoric mania is a high-arousal, positive valence state; euthymia is a low-arousal, positive valence state; mixed mania and agitated depression are both high-arousal, negative valence states (thus accounting for the difficulty distinguishing them clinically); and retarded depression is a low-arousal, negative valence state. It is important to note that, while there are a number of psychiatric disorders characterized by negative valence states, pure mania is the *only* one that is positive valence.

This discussion of emotion, mood, arousal, and valence is particularly germane to the controversy surrounding the topic of early-onset BD and its clinical presentation. As Shulman *et al* note, youths with BD are thought to have shorter, more rapidly cycling mood states characterized by irritability rather than euphoria. In other words, *emotion* dysregulation may be a more prominent feature of the presentation of juvenile BD than *mood* dysregulation. The problem is that emotion dysregulation, in the form of irritability (i.e. increased responsiveness to negative emotional stimuli), is widespread among childhood psychiatric disorders. Irritability is a diagnostic criterion not only for mania, but for depression and oppositional defiant disorder, and frequently is associated with attention deficit hyperactivity disorder (ADHD) and pervasive developmental disorder [5]. Therefore, some researchers have reported that children with BD lack the mood state that is unique to the illness (euphoric mania) while exhibiting instead a very nonspecific mood state [6].

How, then, can a clinician make the diagnosis of BD in children? In our experience, as indeed in some published samples [7], children with BD *do* experience periodic episodes of euphoria, although they also experience a significant amount of irritability. In addition to euphoria, we have also found it helpful to focus on the other *cardinal* symptoms of BD, i.e. those that are not seen in other disorders. These include grandiosity, episodic *decreased need* for sleep (which is distinct from nonspecific insomnia), and increase in *goal-directed* activity. While these cardinal symptoms are specific to mania, other DSM-IV diagnostic criteria (subjective experience that thoughts are racing, flight of ideas, distractibility, and agitation) are seen in other disorders, most notably ADHD. Children who have no cardinal symptoms of BD may, in some instances, "squeak by" and technically meet DSM-IV criteria for the illness; however, in our research group we would find the diagnosis of BD in that case to be suspect. Such children are clearly ill, and may ultimately develop a course consistent with BD, but considerably more research is needed to determine whether they should be assigned the diagnosis or not.

In sum, our understanding of the phenomenology of BD, and of the effects of gender and age on it, can be enriched by a theoretical framework derived from studies of emotion in unaffected populations. Such a framework can aid us as we continue to reach beyond descriptions of what is, to explanations of why.

REFERENCES

1. Drevets W.C. (1998) Functional neuroimaging studies of depression: the anatomy of melancholia. *Annu. Rev. Med.*, **49**: 341–361.
2. Ekman P., Davidson R.J. (1994) *The Nature of Emotion: Fundamental Questions.* Oxford University Press, Oxford.
3. Morris W.N. The mood system. In *Well-Being: The Foundations of Hedonic Psychology* (Eds D. Kahneman, E. Diener, N. Schwarz), pp. 169–189, Russell Sage, New York.
4. Lang P.J., Bradley M.M., Cuthbert B.N. (1998) Emotion, motivation, and anxiety: brain mechanisms and psychophysiology. *Biol. Psychiatry*, **44**: 1248–1263.
5. American Psychiatric Association (2000) *Diagnostic and Statistical Manual of Mental Disorders (DSM-IV-TR).* American Psychiatric Association, Washington.
6. Wozniak J., Biederman J., Kiely K., Ablon J.S., Faraone S.V., Mundy E., Mennin D. (1995) Mania-like symptoms suggestive of childhood-onset bipolar disorder in clinically referred children. *J. Am. Acad. Child Adolesc. Psychiatry*, **34**: 867–876.
7. Geller B., Williams M., Zimerman B., Frazier J. Beringer L., Warner K.L. (1998) Prepubertal and early adolescent bipolarity differentiate from ADHD by manic symptoms, grandiose delusions, ultra-rapid or ultradian cycling. *J. Affect. Disord.*, **51**: 81–91.

5.4
Childhood Mania—Is it Bipolar Disorder?

Carrie M. Borchardt[1]

In their comprehensive review, Shulman *et al* point out that bipolar disorder frequently begins in youth, and is associated with significant morbidity and mortality. We, therefore, are interested in early identification and treatment to prevent complications. Recently there has been a substantial increase in the frequency of diagnosing children with bipolar disorder, and the use of pharmacotherapies (including mood stabilizers and atypical antipsychotics) to treat children with manic symptoms. While there is some good evidence to support continuity of adolescent mania into adulthood [1, 2], there is a lack of such evidence for preadolescents. A number of authors, including Shulman *et al*, have discussed this controversy of diagnosis [3, 4]. No doubt there are cases of children with mania who go on to have a typical bipolar disorder in adulthood. But it is also likely there are others who do not. Thus, bipolar children are likely a heterogeneous group. Clearly we have great need for good longitudinal studies which follow bipolar children into adulthood. Such studies would help to improve diagnostic precision and prediction.

Lack of diagnostic clarity contributes to several problems. First, it may lead to erroneous treatment. Second, how we define a disorder has major implications for research and research findings. For example, if the "disorder" we are studying turns out to be a different disorder than bipolar disorder, we may learn about the children studied but lack information about bipolar disorder in children. In the worst case scenario, the children studied are so heterogeneous we have difficulty interpreting the findings.

Currently, there are many more medication choices for the treatment of bipolar disorder than in years past. Atypical antipsychotic medications are frequently used in children for a range of problems (including mania), in part because the risk of tardive dyskinesia is less than with traditional antipsychotics. However, the long-term risks to children of the use of these medications have been inadequately studied. Potential long-term consequences of chronic use of atypical antipsychotics include tardive dyskinesia, weight gain, and diabetes.

Kurmra *et al* [5] presented data on 23 children and adolescents with schizophrenia, age 6–18, who were treated with olanzapine or clozapine. Over a six-week trial, the average weight gain was 3.4 ± 4.1 kg for subjects on olanzapine, and 5.0 ± 6.0 kg for subjects on clozapine. Clearly, if weight gain continues at that rate it would have serious consequences. Other studies have found similar troubling rates of weight gain for risperidone

_____

[1] *Division of Child and Adolescent Psychiatry, Box 95 Mayo, 420 Delaware Street, SE, Minneapolis, MN 55455, USA*

[6, 7]. There is a growing literature on the risk of diabetes mellitus in patients taking atypical antipsychotics. Henderson *et al* [8] studied 82 adult patients who were treated with clozapine over five years, and found increased risk for diabetes (36.6%) and weight gain. Surprisingly, diabetes risk was not linked to weight gain, which has been one of the hypothesized mechanisms. The risk to children and adolescents for diabetes due to atypical antipsychotics is unknown at this time. However, given the many potential years of exposure to the drugs, it is of great concern.

The widespread use of newer antidepressants in children raises other concerns. Reports in the literature show hyperactivity and irritability to be relatively common side effects of selective serotonin reuptake inhibitors in children, with rates of about 20% [9]. The dilemma is that this type of side effect is similar to manic symptoms, as well as attention-deficit hyperactivity disorder, which can again lead to diagnostic confusion. There are no studies of juveniles that help clarify whether this phenomenon is only a side effect or whether it represents bipolar disorder or a predisposition to bipolar disorder. This is similar to the controversy which erupted many years ago around tricyclic-induced mania.

Current diagnostic categorization treats childhood mania the same as adult mania and assumes it is part of a bipolar illness. Given the lack of knowledge about preadolescent mania, that may be premature. Perhaps our research and clinical work would be better served by having a separate category for preadolescent mania. This is similar to the approach that was taken for childhood anxiety disorders. Separate categories were maintained for childhood anxiety disorders in the earlier versions of the DSM. Research was conducted on the childhood disorders, and only after research showed continuity with the adult anxiety disorders, were the child and adult categories combined. Such an approach would promote study, and would lead to less diagnostic bias.

REFERENCES

1. Carlson G.A., Davenport Y.B., Jamison K. (1977)   A comparison of outcome in adolescent and late-onset bipolar manic-depressive illness. *Am. J. Psychiatry*, **134**: 919–922.
2. Goodwin F.K., Jamison K.R. (1990)   *Manic-Depressive Illness*. Oxford University Press, New York.
3. Biederman J. (1998)   Resolved: mania is mistaken for ADHD in prepubertal children. *J. Am. Acad. Child Adolesc. Psychiatry*, **37**: 1091–1093.
4. Klein R.G., Pine D.S., Klein D.F. (1998)   Resolved: mania is mistaken for ADHD in prepubertal children. *J. Am. Acad. Child Adolesc. Psychiatry*, **37**: 1093–1095.
5. Kumra S., Jacobsen L.K., Lenane M., Karp B.L., Frazier J.A., Smith A.K., Bedwell J., Lee P., Malanga C.J., Hamburger S. *et al* (1998)   Childhood-onset

schizophrenia: an open-label comparison of olanzapine and clozapine in children and adolescents. *J. Am. Acad. Child Adolesc. Psychiatry*, **37**: 1–9.

6. Nicolson R., Awad G., Sloman L. (1998) An open trial of risperidone in young autistic children. *J. Am. Acad. Child Adolesc. Psychiatry*, **37**: 372–376.

7. McDougle C.J., Holmes J.P., Bronson M.R., Anderson G.M., Volkmar F.R., Price L.A., Cohen D.J. (1997) Risperidone treatment of children and adolescents with pervasive developmental disorders: prospective open-label study. *J. Am. Acad. Child Adolesc. Psychiatry*, **36**: 685–693.

8. Henderson D.C., Cagliero E., Gray C., Nasrallah R.A., Hayden D.L., Schoenfeld D.A., Goff D.C. (2000) Clozapine, diabetes mellitus, weight gain, and lipid abnormalities: a five-year naturalistic study. *Am. J. Psychiatry*, **157**: 975–981.

9. Leonard H.L., March J., Rickler K.C., Allen A.J. (1997) Pharmacology of the selective serotonin reuptake inhibitors in children and adolescents. *J. Am. Acad. Child Adolesc. Psychiatry*, **36**: 725–815.

5.5
Bipolar Disorder in Children: Some Issues of Concern

Y.C. Janardhan Reddy and Shoba Srinath[1]

This extensive and timely review by Shulman and colleagues provides a useful perspective on the effect of gender and age on phenomenology and management of bipolar disorder. We consider here certain issues specific to bipolar disorder in children.

Bipolar disorder in the juvenile population is less well studied than in adults. There are several unresolved issues. Most important is the high rate of comorbidity with attention deficit hyperactivity disorder (ADHD). This had led some researchers to suggest that ADHD may be a marker of a very early onset bipolar disorder [1]. However, Indian studies do not report high rates of ADHD [2, 3]. Ascertainment bias and differing clinical characteristics of the samples seem to explain the disparity. While all the previous studies included referred clinical samples, often recruited from clinics well known for treating ADHD children, the Indian patients were largely self-referred and drug-naïve. Even a family study [4], which suggested that ADHD with bipolar disorder could be a familial subtype, suffered from similar ascertainment bias. Most of the data suggesting association between ADHD and juvenile bipolar disorder has come from the USA. Therefore, replication outside the USA and in representative samples is needed to resolve the controversy.

_____

[1] *Department of Psychiatry, National Institute of Mental Health and Neurosciences (NIMHANS), Bangalore 560029, India*

Another issue is the pathway to juvenile bipolarity. Akiskal *et al* [5] suggest that most children and adolescents with depressive disorder are pre-bipolar. Studies of depressed patients recruited from tertiary care centres support this possibility [6]. However, a recent follow-up study of adolescents with major depressive disorder in a community sample reported bipolarity in less than 1% of the sample [7]. A related issue is the relationship between temperamental predispositions and bipolarity. There is evidence to suggest that temperamental instability may be predisposing young depressives to develop bipolar II disorder [8]. However, the data on bipolar II disorder in juveniles is at present very limited, though the disorder is more prevalent than bipolar I disorder [9]. There is a need to study bipolar II disorder in the juvenile population and its relationship with temperamental instability and bipolar I disorder.

As noted in the review, the findings of course and outcome studies of the juvenile population differ greatly. The differences are striking when compared with the findings of the Indian study [2]. This study reported 100% recovery from index episodes, a high rate of relapse (67%), very low rates of comorbid conditions and suicide/suicide attempts, and absence of alcohol/substance abuse. Ninety percent of the relapses occurred within two years of recovery from the index episode. This finding provides justification to consider prophylaxis in juvenile bipolar disorder, even after only one episode.

An important aspect of the course in juvenile bipolar disorder is rapid cycling. A study by Geller *et al* [10] reported rapid cycling in 83% of their sample, with 75% of rapid cyclers having ultradian cycling. Interestingly, in the Indian samples, rapid cycling was observed in only 8 to 14% of the subjects [2, 3].

Clinical justification to use valproic acid in children and adolescents is based largely on its proven efficacy in adults. However, its safety in young females is yet to be established. In addition, it is associated with serious adverse effects such as hepatotoxicity and pancreatitis. Therefore, a safer alternative such as carbamazepine, a remarkably understudied drug, deserves proper evaluation in controlled trials. However, ethical problems are likely to arise in conducting any placebo-controlled trials involving severely ill bipolar children. Moreover, having a placebo arm has inherent difficulty in recruiting severely ill children and this may pose problems in detecting differences between active drugs and placebo. Therefore, employing placebo-controlled designs in children needs to be debated widely.

Overall, juvenile bipolarity is still largely understudied, with some early indications that the comorbidity patterns and course could be different in populations drawn from different cultural contexts. It is not clear whether these differences are the result of different ascertainment methods or true cross-cultural variations. A prospective follow-up of large samples is warranted to examine if these differences are truly cross-cultural, especially in the light of the finding that schizophrenia has a better prognosis in developing countries [11].

REFERENCES

1. Faraone S.V., Biederman J., Wozniac J., Mundy E., Menin D., O'Donnell D. (1997) Is comorbidity with ADHD a marker for juvenile-onset mania. *J. Am. Acad. Child Adolesc. Psychiatry.*, **36**: 1046–1055.
2. Srinath S., Reddy Y.C.J., Girimaji S.R., Seshadri S.P., Subbakrisjna D.K. (1998) A prospective study of bipolar disorder in children and adolescents from India. *Acta Psychiatr. Scand.*, **98**: 437–442.
3. Rajeev J., Somashekar B.S., Shashikiran M.G., Srinath S., Reddy Y.C.J., Girimaji S.C., Seshadri S.P. (1999) ADHD in childhood and adolescent bipolar disorder. Presented at the 5th Biennial Conference of the Indian Association for Child and Adolescent Mental Health, Bangalore, 18–20 November.
4. Faraone S.V., Biederman J., Menin D., Wozniac J., Spencer T. (1997) Attention-deficit hyperactivity disorder with bipolar disorder: a familial subtype? *Am. Acad. Child Adolesc. Psychiatry*, **36**: 1378–1387.
5. Akiskal H.S. (1995) Developmental pathways to bipolarity: are juvenile-onset depressions pre-bipolar? *J. Am. Acad. Child. Adolesc. Psychiatry*, **34**: 754–763.
6. Geller B., Luby J. (1997) Child and adolescent bipolar disorder: a review of the past 10 years. *J. Am. Acad. Child Adolesc. Psychiatry*, **36**: 1168–1176.
7. Lewinsohn P.M., Rhode P., Klein D.N., Seeley J.R. (1999) Natural course of adolescent major depressive disorder: I. Continuity into young adulthood. *J. Am. Acad. Child. Adolesc. Psychiatry.*, **38**: 56–63.
8. Akiskal H.S., Master J.D., Zeller P.J., Endicott J., Coryell W., Keller M., Warshaw M., Clayton P., Goodwin F. (1995) Switching from unipolar to bipolar II: an 11-year prospective study of clinical and temperamental predictors in 559 patients. *Arch. Gen. Psychiatry*, **52**: 114–123.
9. Lewinsohn P.M., Klein D.N., Seeley J.R. (1995) Bipolar disorders in a community sample of older adolescents: prevalence, phenomenology, comorbidity and course. *J. Am. Acad. Child Adolesc. Psychiatry.*, **34**: 454–463.
10. Geller B., Williams M., Zimerman B., Frazier J., Beringer L., Warner K.L. (1998) Prepubertal and early adolescent bipolarity differentiate from ADHD by manic symptoms; grandiose delusions; ultra-rapid or ultradian cycling. *J. Affect. Disord.*, **51**: 81–91.
11. Leff J., Sartorius N., Jablensky A., Korten A., Ernberg G. (1992) The International pilot study of schizophrenia: five-year follow-up findings. *Psychol. Med.*, **22**: 131–145.

5.6
Bipolar Disorder: The Need for Treatment Outcome Studies
Peter M. Lewinsohn[1]

Shulman *et al* present a very scholarly and comprehensive review of the empirical literature. It enables the reader to know the current state of the field and, importantly, where there are critical gaps in knowledge. For example, it is painfully clear that treatment outcome studies to evaluate the efficacy of treatments for bipolar disorder (BD) in children, adolescents, and older people are badly needed.

The coverage of the chapter is fairly complete, but there are some areas that deserve further attention. One of them is the importance of managing the suicidal behaviour of bipolar adolescents. One of the most firmly established facts in the literature is that adults with BD are at very high risk for suicidal behaviours, but knowledge about the suicide attempt and completion rates among adolescent bipolar patients is relatively sparse [1]. In our study with bipolar adolescents [2] we found that 72% had suicidal ideation and 44% had attempted suicide.

The controversy concerning possible differences in the phenomenology of child and adult BD and the fact that some [3] believe that the prevalence of mania in children may be substantial also might have been focused. The manifestations of childhood and adolescent mania and hypomania differ somewhat from those in adulthood. For example, the symptoms of grandiosity and excessive involvement in pleasurable activities can vary as a function of age and developmental level [4, 5]. In addition, juvenile BD is characterized by high rates of rapid cycling (e.g., > 4 cycles per year) and very high rates of comorbidity with attention deficit hyperactivity disorder (ADHD) [6] and conduct disorder [7]. In addition, prepubertal BD differs from adolescent BD in showing non-classical presentations such as dysphoric mania, irritability, aggressiveness, and the absence of clear-cut episodes which follow good premorbid adjustment. Juvenile BD appears to be a much more chronic condition that has a very early onset age [8]. These patients are severely impaired, showing a great deal of emotional lability and impulsivity. It is important to ascertain whether juvenile and classical forms of mania [9] are manifestations of the same disorder or not [8, 10, 11]. Identification of the psychosocial antecedents and consequences of prepubertal and adolescent BD need to be pursued by future research in order to facilitate development and evaluation of preventive and therapeutic interventions. For a review of this literature the reader is referred to a forthcoming book [12].

[1] *Oregon Research Institute, Eugene 97403–1983, USA*

Another gap in our knowledge involves the clear delineation of the psychosocial impairments that are associated with bipolar disorder and whether they persist after recovery. It is of considerable clinical importance to know whether bipolar patients who have recovered from the illness are able to return to their premorbid level of psychosocial functioning.

REFERENCES

1. Shaffer D. (1985) Depression, mania and suicidal acts. In *Child and Adolescent Psychiatry: Modern Approaches* (Eds M. Rutter, L. Hersov), pp. 689–719, Blackwell, Oxford.
2. Lewinsohn P.M., Klein D.N., Seeley J.R. (1995) Bipolar disorders in a community sample of older adolescents: prevalence, phenomenology, comorbidity, and course. *J. Am. Acad. Child Adolesc. Psychiatry*, **34**: 454–463.
3. Biederman J., Mick E., Faraone S.V., Spencer T., Wilens T.E., Wozniak J. (2000) Pediatric mania: a developmental subtype of bipolar disorder? *Biol. Psychiatry*, **48**: 458–466.
4. Bowring M.A., Kovacs M. (1992) Difficulties in diagnosing manic disorders among children and adolescents. *J. Am. Acad. Child Adolesc. Psychiatry*, **31**: 611–614.
5. Geller B., Luby J. (1997) Child and adolescent bipolar disorder. A review of the past 10 years. *J. Am. Acad. Child Adolesc. Psychiatry*, **36**: 1168–1176.
6. Geller B., Zimerman B., Williams M., Bolhofner K., Craney J.L., DelBello M.P., Soutullo C.A. (2000) Diagnostic characteristics of 93 cases of a prepubertal and early adolescent bipolar disorder phenotype by gender, puberty and comorbid ADHD. *J. Child Adolesc. Psychopharmacol.*, **10**: 157–164.
7. Biederman J., Faraone S.V., Hatch M., Mennin D., Taylor A., George P. (1997) Conduct disorder with and without mania in a referred sample of ADHD children. *J. Affect. Disord.*, **44**: 177–188.
8. Carlson G.A. (1995) Identifying prepubertal mania. *J. Am. Acad. Child Adolesc. Psychiatry*, **34**: 750–753.
9. Kraepelin E. (1921) *Manic-Depressive Insanity and Paranoia*. Livingstone, Edinburgh.
10. Biederman J. (1998) Resolved: mania is mistaken for ADHD in prepubertal children. *J. Am. Acad. Child Adolesc. Psychiatry*, **37**: 1091–1099.
11. Carlson G.A (1998) Mania and ADHD: Comorbidity or confusion. *J. Affect. Disord.*, **51**: 177–187.
12. Geller B., Delbello M. (Eds) (2002) *Child and Early Adolescent Bipolar Disorder*. Guilford, New York.

5.7

Juvenile Onset Bipolar Disorder: Longitudinal Studies Long Overdue

Jay N. Giedd[1]

Dr Shulman and colleagues have done a superb and scholarly job in reviewing the relevant literature regarding age and gender effects on the phenomenology and management of bipolar disorder. The most striking aspect of the review is not the details of the literature but the conspicuous paucity of paediatric studies. This is especially alarming given the large and increasing number of children and adolescents who are being treated with mood-stabilizing agents with little data to support or guide the use.

The reasons for the lack of pharmacological studies in children are myriad and include inherent difficulties in assessing outcome measures in subjects whose cognition and behaviour change rapidly in normal growth, the moving target of developmental physiology, issues of informed consent in minors, and protracted risk of litigation for pharmaceutical companies sponsoring the research.

Another issue that confounds paediatric bipolar research and treatment is diagnostic uncertainty, particularly the relationship between juvenile-onset bipolar disorder (BD) and attention deficit hyperactivity disorder (ADHD). Whether large numbers of children with BD are being misdiagnosed as ADHD is a raging topic in child psychiatry. The stakes of this debate are compounded by the fact that treatments for BD are generally ineffective for ADHD and treatments for ADHD are generally ineffective or may even induce mania in BD.

The clinical distinction between BD and ADHD is complicated by directly overlapping DSM-IV diagnostic criteria of talkativeness, distractibility, and psychomotor agitation. Other symptoms, although not identical in DSM-IV terminology, can be difficult to discern. For example, "decreased need for sleep" in BD can be confused with the sleep difficulties common in ADHD, "flight of ideas" in BD can be mistaken for "difficulty sustaining attention" in ADHD, and "excessive involvement in pleasurable activities that have a high potential for painful consequences" in BD may blur with "impulsivity" in ADHD. Both disorders frequently involve impairments in social and family relationships, school performance, and self-esteem. Also, both are highly comorbid with other disorders, such as learning disability, oppositional defiant disorder, or conduct disorder. ADHD is quite commonly diagnosed in juveniles with BD [1] although the reverse is not true—longitudinal studies of ADHD have generally not shown an increased incidence of BD [2].

[1] *Child Psychiatry Branch, National Institute of Mental Health, 10 Center Drive, MSC 1367, Bethesda, MD 20892, USA*

Despite this substantial overlap, there are some features that are fairly distinctive between these two disorders. For example, 52 of 60 BD children but only three of 60 ADHD children reported elevated mood and 51 BD versus four ADHD children reported grandiosity [3]. Also significantly more common in BD were decreased need for sleep, racing thoughts, and hypersexuality. A careful clinical history, usually involving the use of life charts to map the lifelong history of symptomatology, can often provide this important discriminatory data.

Family history may also be important in discriminating ADHD from BD. First-degree relatives of children with ADHD have higher rates of ADHD (but not BD), whereas first-degree relatives of children with combined BD and ADHD have higher incidences of both BD and ADHD [4].

In addition to ADHD, BD must be distinguished from normal development. The ability to modulate affect is a fairly advanced cerebral function. Children who exhibit displays of affect dysregulation may be doing so because the neurocircuitry subserving the ability to modulate affect is not yet mature, not because they have BD. This may explain why many children seem to "outgrow" the symptoms.

Another issue regarding juvenile-onset BD is whether the phenomenology is sufficiently different between children and adults to require separate diagnostic criteria. Geller and Luby, in a review of the juvenile-onset BD literature from 1987 to 1997, conclude that juvenile-onset BD is characterized by non-episodic, chronic, rapid-cycling, mixed manic states [5]. However, others argue that "discrete episodes" are the *sine qua non* of BD, pointing out that DSM-IV defines a manic episode as "A distinct period of abnormally and persistently elevated, expansive, and/or irritable mood. This represents a significant change in the patients' baseline mental status, and must last for at least one week (or any duration if hospitalization is necessary)." Longitudinal studies are needed to establish the continuity between the juvenile onset and adult form of BD. If continuity and age-dependent phenomenology can be firmly established, future generations of DSM should include a separate diagnostic entity of juvenile-onset BD.

Longitudinal paediatric studies are also desperately needed to assess the long-term benefits of early diagnosis and treatment and the effects of medication on the developing brain. Lacking well-controlled pharmacology data, clinicians working with children have had to extrapolate from adult studies to guide their medication management. Robust differences between the anatomy and physiology of adult and paediatric brains make these extrapolations perilous. Further evidence of this comes from data showing that tricyclic antidepressants are not as effective for childhood depression, despite high agreement that the disorder is continuous with the adult form [6].

In summary, despite the many inherent challenges, the need for well-controlled longitudinal studies of the phenomenology and pharmacology of juvenile-onset BD is paramount.

REFERENCES

1. Strober M., Morell W., Burroughs J., Lampert C. (1998) A family study of bipolar I disorder in adolescence: early onset of symptoms linked to increased familial loading and lithium resistance. *J. Affect. Disord.*, **15**: 255–268.
2. Gittleman R., Mannuzza S., Shenker R., Bonagura N. (1985) Hyperactive boys almost grown up. I: psychiatric status. *Arch. Gen. Psychiatry*, **42**: 937–947.
3. Geller B., Williams M., Zimmerman B. (1998) Prepubertal and early adolescent bipolarity differentiate from ADHD by manic symptoms, grandiose delusions, ultra-rapid or ultradian cycling. *J. Affect. Disord.*, **51**: 81–91.
4. Faraone S.V., Biederman J., Mennin D., Wozniak J., Spencer J. (1997) Attention-deficit/hyperactivity disorder with bipolar disorder: a familial subtype? *J. Am. Acad. Child. Adolesc. Psychiatry*, **36**: 1378–1387.
5. Geller B., Luby J. (1997) Child and adolescent bipolar disorder: a review of the past 10 years. *J. Am. Acad. Child Adolesc. Psychiatry*, **36**: 1168–1176.
6. Birmaher B., Dahl R.E., Perel J., Williamson D.E. (1999) Corticotropin-releasing hormone challenge in prepubertal major depression. *Biol. Psychiatry*, **39**: 267–277.

5.8
Development Issues in Bipolar Disorder: Comments, Controversies and Future Directions

Vivek Kusumakar[1]

Shulman *et al*, in their review of age and gender issues on phenomenology and management of bipolar disorder, have given the reader a most comprehensive view of the literature. The recurrent themes of discussion and debate about child and adolescent bipolar disorder include: Does bipolar disorder really onset in this age group? How common is it? How can one recognize bipolar disorder before there is threshold level mania? What are the overlaps and interfaces with attention deficit hyperactivity disorder (ADHD) and conduct disorder, alcohol and substance abuse, and borderline personality functioning? Are the clinical manifestations different from the classical adult onset variety of the disorder? Is there cognitive dysfunction and functional deficit in juvenile onset bipolar disorder? What are the effective treatments in this age group?

[1] *Department of Psychiatry, Dalhousie University, 5909 Veterans Memorial Lane, Halifax, Nova Scotia, Canada B3H 2E2*

Although much of the literature suggests that the age of onset of bipolar disorder is in the mid-20s, for those clinicians who work across the life cycle, it is evident that episodic anxiety, dysthymia and major depression often predate hypomania or mania by years. Egeland's seminal publication in 1987 [1] demonstrated that there is first impairment associated with affective symptoms at 15.5 years, first fulfilment of research diagnostic criteria for bipolar disorder with the manifestation of mania at 18.7 years, first treatment at 22.0 years and first hospitalization at 25.8 years. So, why is it that many studies continue to talk about bipolar disorder as a predominantly adult onset disorder, while North American literature abounds with adolescent and even preadolescent onset disorders? This could be because almost all studies have been retrospective in nature, and the age of the first manifestation of mania is taken to be that of first diagnosis, thus ignoring other affective symptoms that appear earlier. Clearly, clinicians and researchers who only consider bipolar type I disorder to be the "true illness" are apt to ignore bipolar type II and other forms of biphasic mood dysregulation. However, one must also consider that: bipolar disorder is a heterogeneous illness, with juvenile and adult onset variants; the age of onset of hypomania and mania has become earlier in successive generations due to genetic processes of anticipation; the increasing use of antidepressants, particularly in North America, in children and adolescents is unmasking the condition at a younger age.

At this point in scientific inquiry, the presence of anxiety and depressive syndromes in the presence of a history of bipolar disorder in a parent or sibling, psychotic symptoms as part of the depression, and pharmacologically induced hypomania or mania are all predictors of future bipolarity of illness. Yet the debate as to what is the most effective and least detrimental treatment for this phase of the condition remains unresolved. There are reports of the ineffectiveness of lithium or valproate in this phase. A recently reported 20-week randomized open study [2] of adolescents with major depression and with a parent or sibling with bipolar disorder treated with lamotrigine or sertraline demonstrated that lamotrigine is not only more likely to cause remission of depression but is also not associated with switching to mania or provoking accelerated and chaotic cycling of mood, as with sertraline. This begs the questions: should the use of antidepressants in this particular patient population be tempered? Should a mood stabilizer be the first-line treatment? Although a slow titration schedule with lamotrigine minimizes the risk of serious rash in the adolescent, pre-adolescents and all patients on concurrent valproate continue to have a higher risk of serious dermatological problems.

Offspring of bipolar type I, particularly lithium responder, parents tend to have a more episodic bipolar disorder, while the offspring of lithium non-responder parents present with significantly greater comorbidity and a more amorphous and less discrete clinical condition.

The wide variation in the reported prevalence rates of ADHD in juvenile bipolar disorder is intriguing. Canadian, Indian and US data are similar for all other types of comorbidity, except ADHD, which is reported to be over 50% in US studies and about 5% in Canadian studies, and 0% in an Indian study. Apart from the facetious comment that there is a greater risk of bipolar disorder comorbid with ADHD if you live in the USA, one must also consider that this might be an artefact of the overlapping diagnostic criteria for ADHD and mania. One cannot rule out that a subtype of ADHD may, in fact, demonstrate biphasic mood dysregulation at some point during the course of the illness.

Although clinicians often use dichotomous diagnostic thinking to come to a decision if an adolescent is suffering from a bipolar disorder or borderline personality functioning, the clinical realities are that: a) early childhood trauma and abuse are not uncommon in juvenile bipolar disorder, b) borderline personality functioning can be the interpersonal and behavioural manifestation of ultra rapid and ultradian biphasic mood cycling, and c) untreated or undertreated rapid cycling bipolar disorder during a critical stage of personality development can cause borderline personality functioning. Only carefully conducted prospective studies and well-designed case control studies can throw light on this issue.

There appears to be a consensus that chaotic and rapid biphasic mood cycling, particularly in bipolar type II disorder and likely with a female preponderance, is the hallmark of juvenile bipolar disorder. Mixed states and psychotic symptoms too are common. The 1970s' work of Strober and Carlson about the misdiagnosis of mania as schizophrenia holds good to this day.

Juvenile bipolar disorder is commonly associated with a turbulent course and with disabling sub-threshold symptoms even after a syndrome has been successfully treated. More recent work by Robertson and Kutcher [3] and MacMaster and Kusumakar [4] suggests that bipolar youth have problems in executive functioning not restricted to attentional problems. For example, functional magnetic resonance imaging (fMRI) studies suggest that prefrontal cortex functioning is impaired during the execution of mathematical tasks in bipolar and other mood disordered young people. These findings have major implications in treatment planning, which will have to include educational exercises to remobilize and reintegrate prefrontal cortex functioning, not simply the use of medication treatments.

The area of pharmacological treatment research is only in its infancy in juvenile bipolar disorder, as clearly reviewed by Shulman *et al*. A major challenge to any interpretation of effectiveness is the treatment non-adherence rates common in juvenile conditions. Clinicians and clinical services will be well advised to use the models of psychoeducation and collaborative management pioneered in juvenile diabetic clinics across the world.

REFERENCES

1. Egeland J.A., Blumenthal R.L., Nee J., Sharpe L., Endicott J. (1987) Reliability and relationship of various ages of onset criteria for major affective disorder. *J. Affect. Disord.*, **12**: 159–65.
2. Kusumakar V. (2000) Clinical usefulness of lamotrigine in bipolar disorder. *Int. J. Neuropsychopharmacol.*, **3**: (Suppl. 1): S22.
3. Bird D., Robertson H.A., Kutcher S.P. (1998) Mathematics deficits in bipolar youth. Presented at the American Psychiatric Association 131st Annual Meeting, Toronto, 30 May–4 June.
4. Khan S.C., MacMaster F.P., Schmidt M., Kusumakar V. (2001) Mathematical processing in mood disorders: an fMRI study. *Biol. Psychiatry*, **49**: 26S.

5.9

Suicide and Bipolar Disorder in Children and Adolescents

Raul R. Silva and Veronica Rojas[1]

Shulman *et al*'s review presents an interesting theoretical and academic framework for studying the significance of gender and age in the presentation and treatment of bipolar disorder (BD). In this commentary, we would like to examine and elaborate on one particular aspect, that is the issue of suicidality in BD, especially among children and adolescents.

In the United States alone, the estimated annual economic burden of BD is calculated at $45 billion. Suicide and lost income secondary to disability represents 80% of this figure [1]. The risk of suicide for patients with BD is higher than for those with other psychiatric and medical illnesses [2].

Sax *et al* [3] found that, in 88 consecutively admitted patients, those with onset of their affective illness before the age of 18 were significantly more suicidal than those with illness onset at older ages. Tondo *et al* [4] reported that younger patients in their sample of 310 BD subjects demonstrated higher risks of suicidal behaviour. Lewinsohn *et al* [5] found that suicide attempts are twice as common in adolescents with BD, when compared to adolescents with major depressive illness, and 44 times more common than in healthy controls.

Efforts have been made to further understand what features may increase suicidal risk in this population. Brent *et al* [6], in their psychological autopsy study, found that successful suicides were associated with mixed state presentations rather than manic states. Strakowski *et al* [7], in a study

[1] *Division of Child and Adolescent Psychiatry, New York University School of Medicine/Bellevue Hospital Center/ Child Study Center, 550 First Avenue, NB 21S6, New York, NY 10016, USA*

that included patients from the ages of 16 on, found that suicide attempt rates were higher in the group of BD patients with mixed versus manic presentation. They then analysed the role of severity of depression ratings in these patients and found that this factor was what most strongly predicted suicide attempts. They determined, in their sample of BD patients, that a rating score between 14 and 18 on the Hamilton Depression Scale correctly identified 90% of manic patients with a suicidal attempt.

Strober *et al* [8] identified that 20% of adolescents with BD attempt suicide within a five-year period. Tondo *et al* [4], in a sample of BD patients aged 12 years and older, found that more than 50% of serious suicide attempts occurred during the first five years of the illness. This is especially important since the elapsed time from first symptoms to starting medication was slightly over eight years in their investigation. Furthermore, in that study, suicide attempt rates were approximately 10 times greater prior to treatment and after stopping treatment with lithium when compared to the period of treatment with lithium. Tondo and Baldessarini [9] reported strikingly similar results on the protective effects of lithium against suicide. They examined 22 studies and found nearly a 7-fold decrease in annual rates of suicidal behaviour for patients on lithium maintenance treatment.

There are other elements that should be integrated in the conceptualization and assessment of suicidal behaviour. Mann *et al* [10] have postulated a stress-diathesis model to integrate the biologic factors and precipitants for suicidal behaviour. The biological factors include temperamental factors such as impulsiveness and aggression, altered brain functioning (such as altered serotonergic functioning), the use of illicit substances and alcohol, the existence of prolonged medical illness, and genetic or familial contributants. In this vein, it should be kept in mind that there is evidence that suicidal behaviour runs in families irrespective of psychiatric disorder [11]. Serious psychosocial stressors can include but are not limited to significant losses (of a friend, worldly possessions, or the death of a parent), or exposure to life-threatening circumstances such as physical or sexual abuse.

In conclusion, it should be borne in mind that children and adolescents with BD can present a significant suicidal risk. The characteristics of the studies mentioned above are factors that are important to sort out when evaluating a BD patient with suicidal potential. Factors such as age of illness onset, mixed BD presentations, significant depressive symptom manifestation, significant psychosocial or medical stressors, substance or alcohol abuse, the lack of proper treatment, and a family history of suicidal gestures or completion, can all increase the potential risk of these patients going on to seriously hurt themselves.

REFERENCES

1. Wyatt R.J., Henter I. (1995) An economic evaluation of manic-depressive illness. *Soc. Psychiatry Psychiatr. Epidemiol*, **30**: 213–219.
2. Jamison K.R. (2000) Suicide and bipolar disorder. *J. Clin. Psychiatry*, **61** (Suppl. 9): 47–51.
3. Sax K.W., Strakowski S.M., Keck P.E., McElroy S.L., West S.A., Bourne M.L., Larson E.R. (1997) Comparison of patients with early, typical and late-onset affective psychosis. *Am. J. Psychiatry*, **154**: 1299–1301.
4. Tondo L., Baldessarini R., Hennen J., Floris G., Silvetti F., Tohen M. (1998) Lithium treatment and risk of suicidal behavior in bipolar disorder patients. *J. Clin. Psychiatry*, **59**: 405–414.
5. Lewinsohn P.M., Klein D.N., Seeley J.R. (1995) Bipolar disorders in a community sample of older adolescents: prevalence, phenomenology, comorbidity, and course. *J. Am. Acad. Child Adolesc. Psychiatry*, **34**: 453–463.
6. Brent D.A., Perper J.A., Goldstein C.E., Kolko D.J., Allan M.J., Zelenak J.P. (1998) Risk factors for adolescent suicide: a comparison of adolescent victims and suicidal inpatients. *Arch. Gen. Psychiatry*, **145**: 35–40.
7. Strakowski S.M., McElroy S.L., Keck P.F., West S.A. (1996) Suicidality among patients with mixed and manic bipolar disorder. *Am. J. Psychiatry*, **153**: 674–676.
8. Strober M., Schmidt-Lackner S., Freeman R., Bower S., Lampert C., DeAntonio M. (1995) Recovery and relapse in adolescents with bipolar affective illness: a five-year naturalistic, prospective follow-up. *J. Am. Acad. Child Adolesc. Psychiatry*, **34**: 724–731.
9. Tondo L., Baldessarini R.J. (2000) Reduced suicide risk during lithium maintenance treatment. *J. Clin. Psychiatry*, **61** (Suppl. 9): 97–104.
10. Mann J.J., Waternaux C., Haas G.L., Malone K.M. (1999) Toward a clinical model of suicidal behavior in psychiatric patients. *Am. J. Psychiatry*, **156**: 181–189.
11. Brent D.A. (2000) Children of depressed mothers. *J. Am. Acad. Child Adolesc. Psychiatry*, **39**: 136–137.

5.10

Bipolar Children and Adolescents: A Latin American View

Edgard J. Belfort[1]

Reports in the scientific literature concerning childhood bipolar disorder are few and show several inconsistencies.

Shulman *et al*'s paper provides a useful overview of the epidemiology of this disorder, its impact on psychosocial functioning, the differences in its symptomatic expression with respect to bipolar disorder in the adult, its prognosis and comorbidities, and a guide to some of the treatment strategies presently available.

---

[1] *Venezuelan Central University, Avenida Libertador, Edificio Majestic, 6 Piso N. 64, Caracas, 1050 Venezuela*

The authors mention that an early age of onset of bipolar disorder is associated with greater psychosocial impairment. In Latin America, the complex interaction between adverse life events (poverty, malnutrition, adverse perinatal events, parental problems and the lack of a stable relationship with a parental figure during childhood, poor socioeconomic and educational status, lack of social support, physical illnesses, etc.) makes it even more difficult to evaluate the psychosocial implications of bipolar disorder in children and adolescents. Some clinical evidence suggests that a higher number of stressful life events is associated with the occurrence of emotional disorders in the child population [1]. It appears likely that genetic factors interact with environmental factors to influence the vulnerability of this population. In the absence of heritable risk factors, children appear to be less vulnerable to psychosocial adversity.

As reviewed in Shulman *et al*'s paper, the differences in the symptomatic expression of bipolar disorder in youth versus adults have not been consistently reported across studies. However, the existing data are sufficient to suggest that bipolar disorder with onset before the age of 18 years is essentially the same disorder as in adults. The same diagnostic criteria are used as for adults; youth may differ with regard to the developmental presentation of symptoms and comorbid psychiatric disorders.

Cross-cultural issues may influence the expression or interpretation of symptoms. In the Latin American context, the clinical experience has been consistent in finding that mixed mania is more frequent in the youth. The most common clinical aspects are psychomotor agitation, pressure of speech, somatic complaints, diminished concentration, distractibility, severe depressed mood and positive family history of bipolar disorder. As mentioned by Bowring and Kovacs [2], the changes noted in mood, psychomotor activity, and mental excitement are often markedly labile and erratic, rather than persistent. Thus, hallmark manic symptoms, such as grandiosity, psychomotor agitation, and reckless behaviour, must be differentiated from those of other more common childhood disorders, as well as from the normal childhood phenomena of boasting, imaginary play, overactivity, and youthful indiscretions. Although none of the individual elements of this cluster is invariably present, the syndrome occurs in many different clinical contexts.

A significant number of youth display comorbid attention deficit hyperactivity disorder (ADHD), conduct disorder and/or substance abuse [3]. Latin American children and adolescents with bipolar disorder show a similar comorbidity, which may further complicate the diagnosis of bipolar disorder in this age group. The presence of comorbid behavioural disorders and/or substance abuse negatively influences prognosis and treatment response [4].

To organize the clinical information using a life chart to characterize the course of illness, patterns of episodes, severity, and treatment response, according to each specific culture or locality, may be very helpful. Using such a longitudinal perspective to conceptualize the disorder helps with diagnostic accuracy.

REFERENCES

1. Backett M., Petros-Barzavian A. (1978)   El concepto de riesgo en la asistencia sanitaria. *Cuadernos de Salud Pública* 76, Organización Mundial de la Salud, Geneva.
2. Bowring M.A., Kovacs M. (1992)   Difficulties in diagnosing manic disorders in children and adolescents. *J. Am. Acad. Child Adolesc. Psychiatry*, **31**: 611–614.
3. Borchardt C.M., Bernstein G.A. (1995) Comorbid disorders in hospitalized bipolar adolescents compared with unipolar depressed adolescents. *Child Psychiatry Hum. Dev.*, **26**: 11–18.
4. Kovacs M., Pollock M. (1995), Bipolar disorder and comorbid conduct disorder in childhood and adolescence. *J. Am. Acad. Child Adolesc. Psychiatry*, **34**: 715–723.

5.11
Impact of Development on Diagnosis and Treatment of Bipolar Disorders
Elizabeth B. Weller[1]

Bipolar disorder (BD) is a severe and often chronic condition, which seriously disrupts the lives of children, adolescents and adults by the means of increased rates of suicide attempts and completion, poor academic performance, disturbed interpersonal relationships, increased rates of substance abuse, legal difficulties, and multiple hospitalizations [1, 2]. In spite of its potential to produce significant disability, BD in children has been poorly studied [3, 4].

To determine the direction of future research into childhood BD, it is important to review what is really known about BD in children. Shulman *et al*'s review addresses this need with current information about the impact of age and sex on the diagnosis and management of BD. The authors state that women may be more likely than men to be diagnosed with BD type II. Although the evidence on gender-specific prevalence of BD in children is limited, Carlson *et al* [5] suggest that young subjects with early-onset mania (before the age of 21) are more likely to be male (69.6% versus 26.6%), to have

[1] *Department of Child and Adolescent Psychiatry, Children's Hospital of Philadelphia, 34th and Civic Center Blvd., Philadelphia, PA 19104–4399, USA*

more complicated psychopathology (i.e., early onset of behaviour problems and substance abuse comorbidity, mixed episodes, and paranoid symptoms), to spend more time in the hospital overall, and to be less likely to remit completely over 24 months than subjects whose illness first emerges after age 30. This observation was also made by Costello, who suggests that early-onset BD is more common in males, especially in those with onset before 13 years [6].

In regard to the questions of prevalence of BD and the age of onset, Shulman et al cite Goodwin and Jamison [7], who reviewed 898 cases from 1977 to 1985 and estimated that 0.3% of patients had onset of illness before the age of 10. Our own study showed that mania was present in 22% of severely disturbed children (including definite, possible and probable manic children) [8].

Shulman et al also highlight the decline in psychosocial functioning, which is a significant problem in children with BD. Müller et al. [9] examined 80 family members of BD patients and found that they more often failed a grade (nine compared to one in the control group), obtained lower grades (38 compared to 23) and less often succeeded in their final examinations (15 compared to 38). Among the BD patients themselves 30% did not finish school. When an otherwise intelligent child is failing at school, mood disorder and substance abuse should be considered hand in hand with learning disabilities.

Antisocial behaviour in bipolar children is a cause of great concern. For example, Pliszka et al found 10 of 50 youths at an urban juvenile detention centre met criteria for mania, another 10 met criteria for major depressive disorder, and one met criteria for bipolar disorder, mixed type. The authors conclude that there is a high rate (42%) of affective disorders in juvenile offenders [10].

Suicide risk in youth, especially adolescents, with BD relative to children with other psychiatric illnesses is also a significant problem [11]. Eleven of 54 bipolar adolescents (20%) made suicide attempts that required medical attention during a five-year follow-up [2]. Comorbid substance abuse further increases a bipolar adolescent's risk for suicide [12].

Treatment of childhood BD is significantly understudied due to the paucity of controlled studies. The only completed double-blind, placebo-controlled study in this age group involved the use of lithium in adolescents with BD and comorbid substance use [13]. In this study there was decreased substance use on lithium. However, there were no comments on what happened to bipolarity symptoms. There are no contemporary controlled studies available to guide our therapeutic approach for the management of children with these very difficult, highly comorbid conditions. Thus, most clinicians use medications based on either their own clinical experience or on the results of studies in adults.

REFERENCES

1. Akiskal H.S., Downs J., Jordan P., Watson S., Daugherty D., Pruitt D.B. (1985) Affective disorders in referred children and younger siblings of manic-depressives. Mode of onset and prospective course. *Arch. Gen. Psychiatry*, **42**: 996–1003.

2. Strober M., Schmidt-Lackner S., Freeman R., Bower S., Lampert C., DeAntonio M. (1995) Recovery and relapse in adolescents with bipolar affective illness: a five-year naturalistic, prospective follow-up. *J. Am. Acad. Child Adolesc. Psychiatry*, **34**: 724–731.

3. Weller E.B., Weller R.A., Fristad M.A. (1995) Bipolar disorder in children: misdiagnosis, underdiagnosis, and future directions. *J. Am. Acad. Child Adolesc. Psychiatry*, **34**: 709–714.

4. Weller E. (2000) Bipolar children and adolescents: controversies in diagnosis and treatment. Presented at the American Psychiatric Association 153rd Annual Meeting, Chicago, 13–18 May.

5. Carlson G.A., Bromet E.J., Sievers S. (2000) Phenomenology and outcome of subjects with early- and adult-onset psychotic mania. *Am. J. Psychiatry*, **157**: 213–219.

6. Costello E.J. (1987) Child psychiatric disorders and their correlates: a primary care pediatric sample. *J. Am. Acad. Child Adolesc. Psychiatry*, **28**: 851–855.

7. Goodwin F., Jamison K. (1990) *Manic-Depressive Illness*. Oxford University Press, New York.

8. Weller R.A., Weller E.B., Tucker S.G., Fristad M.A. (1986) Mania in prepubertal children: has it been underdiagnosed? *J. Affect. Disord.*, **11**: 151–154.

9. Muller E., Schapowahl A., Seelander A. (1984) Catamnestic surveys on somato-psychosocial development in childhood and adolescence of patients with unipolar depressive and bipolar manic-depressive psychoses. *Psychiatr. Neurol. Med. Psychol.*, **36**: 480–488.

10. Pliszka S.R., Sherman J.O., Barrow M.V., Irick S. (2000) Affective disorder in juvenile offenders: a preliminary study. *Am. J. Psychiatry*, **157**: 130–132.

11. Brent D.A., Perper J.A., Moritz G., Allman C., Friend A., Roth C., Schweers J., Balach L., Baugher M. (1993) Psychiatric risk factors for adolescent suicide: a case-control study. *J. Am. Acad. Child Adolesc. Psychiatry*, **32**: 521–529.

12. Rich C.L., Young D., Fowler R.C. (1986) San Diego suicide study. I. Young vs. old subjects. *Arch. Gen. Psychiatry*, **43**: 577–582.

13. Geller B., Cooper T.B., Sun K., Zimerman B., Frazier J., Williams M., Heath J. (1998) Double-blind and placebo-controlled study of lithium for adolescent bipolar disorders with secondary substance dependency. *J. Am. Acad. Child Adolesc. Psychiatry*, **37**: 171–178.

5.12
Gender, Age and a Developmental Perspective in Mania
Gabrielle A. Carlson[1]

Shulman *et al.* have provided a thorough discussion of gender and age in bipolar disorder. I would like to examine three details more closely.

First, it is important to clarify whether one is considering lifetime rates of *bipolar disorder* obtained from a *community sample*, or current rates of *acute mania* obtained from a *clinical sample*. Community studies of adults with bipolar I disorder suggested an even distribution of gender (lifetime rates of 0.45% among men and 0.47% among women). The one-year incidence was 0.36% [1].

In the Oregon Adolescent Depression Project (OADP), Lewinsohn *et al* [2] reported bipolar rates of 0.95% (66.7% female) in 14–18 year olds. Rates and gender distribution have generally been interpreted as similar to adults. Reading the "fine print", however, reveals that only two teens (gender not reported) had lifetime rates of *mania*; the remainder reported lifetime hypomania with varying levels of *depression* severity (i.e., bipolar II disorder and cyclothymia). Basically, most subjects were depressed. The one-year mania incidence was 0.13%, significantly lower than in adults.

Since bipolar disorder often begins in adolescence and since a number of years may elapse before a person with bipolar disorder either seeks treatment or receives accurate diagnosis [3], we might speculate that young people with subsyndromal mania or major depression would be at high risk to develop full-blown mania. However, a follow-up of a subsample of the OADP subjects, conducted when they were 24 years old [4], revealed that only three additional patients (annual incidence 0.08%) had developed acute *mania* (another three had developed hypomania). Only one of these had progressed from earlier hypomania, and less than 1% of adolescents with major depression had switched to mania. Nor did subjects come from the 5.7% of teens felt to have subsyndromal mania. These findings suggest that extrapolation from community samples to clinical samples with bipolar disorder is not straightforward.

Although clinical samples and research designs reduce diagnostic problems, referral bias emerges. Gender ratios may depend on the kind of comorbidity selected by the clinical sample. Comparing hospitalized young adolescent (mean age 15) and adult manic patients (mean age 28), McElroy *et al* [5] found no difference in gender distribution (63% of adolescent, 55% of adult subjects were female). The young sample's mania was more "mixed"; few were substance abusing. The Suffolk County First Episode

———————————
[1] *Department of Child and Adolescent Psychiatry, State University of New York at Stony Brook, Putnam Hall-South Campus, Stony Brook, New York 11794–8790, USA*

Project, a community study of patients hospitalized with psychosis (including mania), reported clear age/gender differences at hospitalization in mania. Of manics hospitalized under age 20, only 33% were female; between ages 20–29, 47% were female; and those aged 30 and over were 69% female. The age/gender differences were significant ($X^2 = 8.317$, $p = 0.016$) [6 and unpublished data]. Mixed episodes were uncommon in this youth sample; rates of externalizing disorder and substance abuse were very common. Perhaps where externalizing comorbidities (and substance abuse) are more common, male gender will predominate. If those comorbidities are excluded, and if the scope of "bipolar disorder" is broadened to include subtypes in which depression is more prominent, females are better represented.

Finally, the conclusions drawn about "age of onset" depend on how onset is defined. Shulman *et al* noted the discrepancy between the comparatively poor outcome found for young bipolars in the above-mentioned Suffolk County Project and the similar long-term outcomes in adolescent vs. adult onset subjects admitted to Chestnut Lodge [3], a finding similar to that of Carlson *et al* [7] for a sample admitted to the National Institute of Mental Health. Differences between these studies are many. Most basically, the earlier studies only counted first *symptoms* of *any* mood problem, not first *hospitalization* for *acute mania*. Follow-up was also much longer. Though Carlson *et al* found poor two-year outcomes in the young-onset sample [6], outcomes in the two age groups had equalized by the four-year point, because the young sample had improved [8], a difference largely accounted for by their decreased substance abuse. This suggests that maturation as well as psychopathology may be interacting to affect outcome.

This re-examination hypothesizes that gender and outcome may depend on comorbidity and on age of onset of *mania*. A developmental perspective might add to our understanding of the interaction and its impact on outcome.

REFERENCES

1. Kessler R.C., Rubinow D.R., Holmes C., Abelson J.M., Shao S. (1997) The epidemiology of DSM III R bipolar I disorder in a general population survey. *Psychol. Med.*, **27**: 1079–1089.
2. Lewinsohn P.M., Klein D.N., Seeley J.R. (1995) Bipolar disorder in community sample of older adolescents: prevalence, phenomenology, comorbidity and course. *J. Am. Acad. Child Adolesc. Psychiatry*, **34**: 454–463.
3. McGlashan T.H. (1988) Adolescent vs adult onset of mania. *Am. J. Psychiatry*, **145**: 221–223.
4. Lewinsohn P.M., Klein D.N., Seeley J.R. (2000) Bipolar disorder during adolescence and young adulthood in a community sample. *Bipolar Disord.*, **2**: 281–293.

5. McElroy S.L., Strakowski S.M., West S.A., Keck P.E., Jr., McConville B.J. (1997) Phenomenology of adolescent and adult mania in hospitalized patients with bipolar disorder. *Am. J. Psychiatry*, **154**: 44–49.
6. Carlson G.A., Bromet E.J., Sievers S.B. (2000) Phenomenology and outcome of youth and adult onset subjects with psychotic mania. *Am. J. Psychiatry*, **157**: 213–219.
7. Carlson G.A., Davenport Y.B., Jamison K.R. (1977) A comparison of outcome in adolescent- and late-onset bipolar manic depressive illness. *Am. J. Psychiatry*, **134**: 919–922.
8. Carlson G.A., Bromet E.J., Lavelle J. (1999) Medication treatment in adolescents vs adults with psychotic mania. *J. Child Adolesc. Psychopharmacol.*, **9**: 221–231.

5.13
Gender and Age in Mixed States
Jean-François Allilaire[1]

Episodes occurring during the course of bipolar disorders which include symptoms of both mania and depression are referred to as mixed states.

Some investigators have reported that certain patient populations may be at higher risk than others of experiencing mixed episodes. Studies have repeatedly demonstrated that mixed episodes occur more commonly in female patients [1–3]. Adolescent mania has also been found more likely than adult mania to be mixed, with more frequently high rates of depressive features [4–7].

Mixed episodes have also been associated with a later age of onset, first treatment and first hospitalization compared with pure manic episodes. The first mixed episode has been shown to occur later (average age 39.2 years) in the course of illness than the patient's first depressive (average age 27.6 years) or manic (average age 30.6 years) episode. It has been also shown [3] that patients who experience mixed episodes are more likely than patients without mixed episodes to experience depressive episodes early in the course of illness. In a study by Dell'Osso *et al* [8] carried out on 108 female inpatients with bipolar disorders, 24.5% had a first episode which was mixed, 65.3% a depressive first episode, and 8.2% a manic first episode.

Contradictory data exist regarding whether or not bipolar patients with mixed episodes experience more episodes of illness than patients without mixed episodes. Suicidal ideation and attempts have been demonstrated to occur more frequently in the context of bipolar disorders with mixed versus pure manic episodes. Strakowski *et al* [9] found that 26% of patients with

[1] *Hôpital de la Salpêtrière, 47 bd. de L' Hôpital, Paris, F-75013, France*

mixed mania had suicidal ideation compared with 7% patients with pure manic episodes.

Higher rates of comorbid substance abuse have been found in bipolars with mixed states (46%) compared with bipolars without mixed episodes (20%) in the study by Himmelhoch et al [10].

Other clinical features associated with mixed episodes are a higher frequency of mood incongruent psychotic features and negative formal thought disorder and a lower frequency of positive formal thought disorder [11]. Longer hospital stays and stressors preceding the index episode have also been associated with mixed episodes.

Finally, the course of mixed states tends to be protracted, and antidepressants may induce exacerbation of excitatory symptoms and hyperlability.

The French EPIMAN study [12] showed that mixed mania defined crosssectionally by the simultaneous presence of at least two depressive symptoms represents a prevalent and clinically significant and distinct form of mania. Furthermore, subthreshold depressive admixtures with mania appear to represent the most common expression of dysphoric mania.

In terms of temperament, the EPIMAN study showed that men have more *pure manic episodes*, which may be due to the over-representation of hyperthymic temperament. On the other hand, the depressive temperament is over-represented in women and could explain the higher prevalence of mixed mania in women.

In conclusion, mixed states are frequent and differ with respect to gender and age distribution from other bipolar disorders. They require special attention concerning diagnosis and therapeutic management.

REFERENCES

1. Himmelhoch J.M., Garfinkel M.E. (1986) Mixed mania: diagnosis and treatment. *Psychopharmacol. Bull.*, **22**: 613–620.
2. McElroy S.L., Strakowski S.M., Keck P.E., Jr., Turgrul K.L., West S.A., Lonczak H.S. (1995) Differences and similarities in mixed and pure mania. *Compr. Psychiatry*, **36**: 187–194.
3. Nunn C.M.H. (1979) Mixed affective states and the natural history of manicdepressive psychosis. *Br. J. Psychiatry*, **134**: 153–160.
4. Himmelhoch J.M., Garfinkel M.E. (1986) Sources of lithium resistance in mixed mania. *Psychopharmacol. Bull.*, **22**: 613–620.
5. Horowitz H.H. (1977) Lithium and treatment of adolescent manic depressive illness. *Dis. Nerv. Syst.*, **38**: 480–483.
6. Krasa N.R., Tolbert H.A. (1994) Adolescent bipolar disorder: a nine-year experience. *J. Affect. Disord.*, **30**: 175–184.
7. West S.A., McElroy S.L., Strakowski S.M., Keck P.E., Jr., Mcconville B.J. (1995) Attention deficit hyperactivity disorder in adolescent mania. *Am. J. Psychiatry*, **152**: 271–273.

8. Dell'Osso L., Placidi G.F., Nassi R., Freer P., Cassano G.B., Akiskal H.S. (1991) The manic-depressive mixed state: familial, temperamental and psychopathologic characteristics in 108 female inpatients. *Eur. Arch. Psychiatry Clin. Neurosci.*, **240**: 234–239.
9. Strakowski S.M., McElroy S.L., Keck P.E., Jr. West S.A. (1996) Suicidality among patients with mixed and manic bipolar disorder. *Am. J. Psychiatry*, **153**: 674–676.
10. Himmelhoch J.M., Mulla D., Neil J.F., Detre T.P., Kupfer D.J. (1976) Incidence and significance of mixed affective states in a bipolar population. *Arch. Gen. Psychiatry*, **33**: 1062–1066.
11. Sax K.W., Strakowski S.M., McElroy S.L., Keck R.E., Jr., West S.A. (1995) Attention and formal thought disorder in mixed and pure mania. *Biol. Psychiatry*, **37**: 420–423.
12. Akiskal H.S., Hantouche E.G., Bourgeois M.L., Azorin J.-M., Sechter D., Allilaire J.-F., Lancrenon S., Fraud J.-P., Châtenet-Duchêne L. (1998) Gender, temperament, and the clinical picture in dysphoric mixed mania: findings from a French national study (EPIMAN). *J. Affect. Disord.*, **50**: 175–186.

5.14

Beyond Phenomenology: What are Mixed States and Do Children Really Develop Mania?

Guy Goodwin[1]

Gender and age are as neglected as the many aspects of bipolar disorder that remain under-investigated. The gender issues highlighted in Shulman *et al*'s review appropriately reflect our uncertainty about the status of depressive symptoms in bipolar disorder and in particular the evaluation of mixed states. The arbitrary definition of mixed states currently hinders rather than helps understanding. Furthermore, it is difficult to see how more detailed and sensitive instruments for assessing symptoms will ultimately resolve the more fundamental problems, because they simply, and inevitably, detect the target subsyndromal symptoms towards which they are directed. Fundamentally, the contradiction is that in bipolar disorder we expect mania and depression to occupy opposite poles and to be, in all respects, independent of each other. When they co-occur, this is puzzling; it implies either that mood can be in two places at once (and at its opposite poles) or the two poles have different neurological substrates and they can to some extent be expressed simultaneously. Either formulation is contradictory. The issue of how we progress from phenomenology to neuronal mechanisms is a fundamental challenge for the field at present. This particular

[1] *Department of Psychiatry, University of Oxford, Warneford Hospital, Oxford, OX3 7JX, United Kingdom*

gender debate simply sharpens a more general problem. It is a possibility that direct investigations of neuropsychological function or sleep may allow us to move on to some extent from phenomenology and also give us measures that are freer of bias and the preconceptions of observers.

As an example, our current work has shown that the manic phase of bipolar disorder is characterized by impaired performance across a range of tasks assessing executive, mnemonic and attentional functioning. However, two measures, verbal learning (the California Verbal Learning Test, CVLT) and sustained attention, are particularly potent indicators of the deficit in mania, correctly classifying 87% of manic subjects and 91% of subjects overall [1]. Additional tests do not contribute to the classification of manic subjects and therefore do not represent core markers of the manic state. In the euthymic state only performance on a measure of sustained attention was impaired after controlling for low levels of affective symptoms [2]. Thus, impaired sustained attention may represent a trait marker for bipolar disorder, related to vulnerability to the disorder at a structural and/or neurochemical level, while impaired memory function is a state marker sensitive to mood change. However, memory function is modulated by mood in diurnal depression in bipolars [3]. This poses an interesting question: is the memory impairment that appears intrinsic to depression present in mania because the manic state is inherently and always a mixed one or do mood elevation and depression have separate and independent capacities to cause memory impairment? The same question also arises for sleep architecture, which is similarly abnormal in mania and depression. The point is that a purely phenomenological question may actually have an answer rooted in neurobiology.

The problems relating to the impact of age on bipolar disorder are more fundamental. There remains a concern that the diagnosis of bipolar disorder in children occurs much more frequently in North America than it does in Europe. The explanation for this remains both uncertain and interesting. There are two perceptions at work here; one is that North American criteria for mood disorder in children are more inclusive (and therefore perhaps less reliable) than those employed in Europe. This certainly appears to be the case, for example, for attention deficit hyperactivity disorder (ADHD) in the same population. The fact that the two have an uncertain clinical interface adds to this impression for Europeans.

The other consideration relates to the bipolar/ADHD relationship, but is an independent reason for concern. It stems from the suggestion that the wide prescription of methylphenidate may serve to precipitate manic illness in vulnerable young people. Because the diagnosis of ADHD and the prescription of methylphenidate is so much more common in North America, this could explain a true increase in the frequency with which mania is described [4]. That this is at least contributory is suggested by the finding in

North American centres that the age at presentation of patients with bipolar disorder is earlier in those who have had previous exposure to methylphenidate than those who have not. The debate about childhood mood disorder is a critical one. Earlier diagnosis and effective treatment of bipolar disorder is a major challenge for patients and clinicians alike. The resolution of our present uncertainties seems to demand improvements that conventional clinical diagnosis are unlikely to be able to offer—improved sensitivity and specificity of diagnosis in young people. Whether really early intervention in high risk subjects is feasible or simply a misleading over-enthusiasm remains very uncertain.

Shulman *et al*'s review ends with a summary of what is described as "incomplete evidence" and "areas still open to research". One has to reflect that at this date none of the evidence is yet complete and no one would sensibly declare any area of research closed given our surprising ignorance of this important but neglected disease.

REFERENCES

1. Clark L., Iversen S.D., Goodwin G.M. (2001) Sustained attention deficit in bipolar disorder. *Br. J. Psychiatry* (in press).
2. Clark L., Iversen S.D., Goodwin G.M. (2001) A neuropsychological investigation of prefrontal cortex involvement in acute mania. *Am. J. Psychiatry* (in press).
3. Moffoot A.P.R., O'Carroll R.E., Bennie J., Carroll S., Dick H., Ebmeier K.P., Goodwin G.M. (1994) Diurnal variation of mood and neuropsychological function in major depression with melancholia. *J. Affect. Disord.*, 32: 257–269.
4. Reichert C.G., Nolen W.A., Wals M., Hillegers M.H.J. (2000) Bipolar disorder in children and adolescents: a clinical reality? *Acta Neuropsychiatrica*, 12: 132–135.

5.15
Late Life Depression and Mania

Carl Gerhard Gottfries[1]

Estimates of prevalence of late life depression vary widely according to the population studied, sample size, definition of depression and method of diagnosis. The prevalence of depression among people 65 years of age and older is usually estimated to 15% if all depressive disorders with clinically significant symptoms requiring intervention are included [1]. Major depressive disorders and bipolar affective disease occur somewhat less frequently

[1] *Institute of Clinical Neuroscience, Department of Psychiatry and Neurochemistry, SU/Molndal, Sweden*

among the elderly when compared to younger adults. There are few studies on the prevalence of mania in the elderly. Retrospective studies generally have found that the number of new cases of mania and the prevalence of mania in the population decrease, although there is evidence to contradict this belief [2]. The diagnosis of mania in the elderly is confounded by the overlap of manic symptoms with other syndromes that occur in the elderly, as dementia, confusional states, and delirium. Pure mania as a part of a bipolar disorder is rather rare. This may be the result of premature death of patients with bipolar disorders due to suicide or cardiovascular disease. It may, however, also reflect age-related differences in symptom presentation of both depression and mania in the elderly.

The symptomatology of late life depression is more heterogeneous than that of younger patients. The most common symptoms are somatic complaints, irritability, insomnia, fatigue, and comorbid anxiety. Compared to younger adults, elderly patients tend to somatize depressive symptoms. When mania is present, this is most often in the form of mixed mania with dysphoria and concomitant confusional states. Sometimes the syndrome is named disinhibition as uncontrolled emotional behaviour may dominate the picture.

Also the aetiology of late life depression is more heterogeneous than that of depression in younger adults. Women are more depressed than men are; the difference between the sexes, however, is less pronounced than in younger adults. Patients with a family history of depression are also more likely to be depressed than those with no family history of depression, but genetic factors seem to have less importance in old age depression.

In the elderly it is obvious that the ageing process and neurodegenerative disorders are important risk factors for syndromes of depression and mania. In patients with Alzheimer's dementia (AD) 25% also fulfil the criteria for major depressive disorders and in patients with vascular dementia (VAD) the frequency of depression is similarly high. In stroke patients the frequency of depression is almost 50% the year after the stroke attack. If not only depression but also behavioural and psychological symptoms in dementia (BPSD) are investigated, the frequency of these symptoms is around 85%. BPSD are often subdivided into subgroups. There are syndromes where overactivity is dominating, others where agitation and psychotic symptoms are dominating. Depression and insomnia are also frequent symptoms in BPSD. The prevalence of mania in demented patients is not well studied, and assumed to be low. However, if mixed mania, disinhibition syndromes and BPSD were investigated, the frequency of these syndromes might well be high.

As Shulman et al point out in their review, there is an association between cerebrovascular disease and bipolar disorders. Cognitive impairment is a prominent feature of old age mania. A clinical impression is that mania or disinhibition syndromes are more frequent in VAD and frontal lobe dementia (FLD) than in AD. In fact, both "vascular depression" and "vascular mania" are discussed [3]. Depression with onset in old age is associated with white matter lesion [4]. This may indicate that vascular disturbances may be present and these changes do not only cause cognitive impairment but also depression and BPSD.

In post-mortem human brain material from aged people and patients with AD and VAD, reduced levels of serotonin are reported [5]. This may well explain an increased risk for manic symptoms or disinhibited behaviour. However, white matter damage may also cause a disconnection between the frontal lobes and basal ganglia and brainstem, thus increasing the risk for disinhibited behaviour. This may also explain why patients with vascular depression appear to have more psychomotor retardation, greater lack of insight, and less agitation and guilt than elderly patients with early-onset depression without vascular risk factors.

The study of the one carbon metabolism has created interest lately. This metabolism is of importance for many metabolic processes in the body and in the brain. It is dependent on the access to folic acid, vitamin B12 and pyridoxine (vitamin B6). A marker for the one carbon metabolism is serum homocysteine, which increases if the metabolic process is disturbed. In elderly patients with depression, mania, cognitive impairment and elderly with heart-vessel disorders a disturbance of the one carbon metabolism has been observed [6–8]. Of still greater interest is that Coppen *et al.* [9] have shown that patients with affective disorders who are on long-term treatment with lithium have less morbidity if the treatment is combined with folic acid. Patients with low serum folate respond less favourably to treatment with selective serotonin reuptake inhibitors (SSRIs) and there is a correlation between the response to treatment with sertraline, an SSRI, and serum folate levels, although the levels are within the normal distribution [10]. A disturbed one carbon metabolism may thus be a common risk factor for depression, mania, cognitive impairment and vascular disorders in the elderly that should be considered in the treatment.

REFERENCES

1. Judd L.L., Kunovac J.L., Akiskal H.S., Rapaport M.H., Robertson P.F. (1994) Subsyndromal symptomatic depression: a new mood disorder? *J. Clin. Psychiatry*, **55**: 18–28.
2. McDonald W.M. (2000) Epidemiology, aetiology, and treatment of geriatric mania. *J. Clin. Psychiatry*, **61** (Suppl. 13): 3–11.
3. Alexopoulos G.S., Meyers B.S., Young R.C., Campbell S., Silbersweig D., Charlson M. (1997) "Vascular depression" hypothesis. *Arch. Gen. Psychiatry*, **54**: 915–922.

4. Krishnan K.R., Hays J.C., Blazer G.D. (1997) MRI-defined vascular depression. *Am. J. Psychiatry*, **154**: 497–501.
5. Gottfries C.G. (1990) Neurochemical aspects of ageing and diseases with cognitive impairment. *J. Neurosci. Res.*, **27**: 541–547.
6. Lehmann W., Gottfries C.G., Regland B. (1999) Identification of cognitive impairment in the elderly: homocysteine is an early marker. *Dement. Geriatr. Cogn. Disord.*, **10**: 12–20.
7. Diaz-Arrastia R. (1998) Hyperhomocysteinemia. *Arch. Neurol.*, **55**: 1407–1408.
8. Hasanah C.I., Khan U.A., Musalmah M., Razali S.M. (1997) Reduced red cell folate in mania. *J. Affect. Disord.*, **46**: 95–99.
9. Coppen A., Abou-Saleh M.T. (1982) Plasma folate and affective morbidity during long-term lithium therapy. *Br. J. Psychiatry*, **141**: 87–89.
10. Fava M., Borus J.S., Alpert J.E., Nirenberg A.A., Rosenbaum J.F., Bottiglieri T. (1997) Folate, B12 and homocysteine in major depressive disorder. *Am. J. Psychiatry*, **154**: 426–428.

6

The Economic and Social Burden of Bipolar Disorder: A Review

Joseph F. Goldberg[1, 2] and Carrie L. Ernst[3, 4]

[1] Department of Psychiatry, Weill Medical College of Cornell University, New York, NY, USA
[2] Bipolar Disorders Research Clinic, New York Presbyterian Hospital-Payne Whitney Clinic, New York, NY, USA
[3] Departments of Medicine and Psychiatry, Harvard Medical School, Boston, MA, USA
[4] Cambridge Hospital, Cambridge, MA, USA

INTRODUCTION

Despite remarkable advances in its detection, treatment, and management, bipolar illness remains a highly prevalent disorder of enormous cost to society, from an economic and social perspective as well as from the standpoint of morbidity and mortality. In 1996, the World Health Organization ranked bipolar disorder as one of the 10 leading worldwide causes of both temporary and permanent disability for individuals aged 15–45, exceeding the number of disability-adjusted life years (DALYs) associated with numerous other serious and chronic medical conditions such as human immunodeficiency virus (HIV) infection, diabetes mellitus, or asthma [1]. By the year 2020, it has been estimated that affective disorders will be second only to ischemic heart disease in DALY rank orderings [1]. Observational studies have found that psychosocial disability often extends far beyond the resolution of affective symptoms among bipolar as well as unipolar patients [2]. As noted in both cross-sectional and longitudinal findings from epidemiologic reports, functional disability for patients with severe mood disorders often persists after an index affective episode in ways that appear even more devastating than seen with many chronic medical conditions [3, 4].

This paper will review current information about the economic, occupational, and social disability attributed to bipolar illness, focusing on factors

Bipolar Disorder. Edited by Mario Maj, Hagop S. Akiskal, Juan José López-Ibor and Norman Sartorius.
© 2002 John Wiley & Sons Ltd.

relating both to the procurement of treatment as well as the interpersonal, familial and work-related implications of bipolar disorder and its likely complications. Issues involving healthcare and service utilization will be examined in relation to models of healthcare delivery, pharmacoeconomics, psychotherapy, and relapse prevention. Finally, evidence regarding the economic and social costs due to illness will be examined from the perspective of existing knowledge and future research directions.

To comprehend the financial and psychosocial impact of bipolar illness requires an appreciation for a number of illness domains, including: 1) its *epidemiology and diagnostic identification*; 2) its *treatment* (including the effect of misdiagnosis, delayed treatment initiation, appropriateness of treatment interventions, and pharmacoeconomics); 3) the costs and complications associated with *other psychiatric or medical conditions* (or related states such as pregnancy) as affected by comorbid bipolar illness; 4) its *occupational ramifications* (including worker absenteeism and lost productivity); 5) its *interpersonal dimensions* (including divorce or relationship discord, illness effects on child-rearing, and other family and social relationships); 6) the *domestic effects* of bipolar illness (involving implications for independent residential community dwellings vs. assisted-living needs or possible homelessness); 7) its *forensic consequences* (e.g., arrests, incarcerations, and harm to property and other individuals); and 8) *death*—due largely to suicide, but also to excess cardiovascular disease, accidents, and other reported sources of premature mortality [5]. Many of these dimensions are intermixed and merit consideration across varied contexts of the economic and social burden of illness.

A further component for understanding psychosocial illness burden involves differentiating the costs and liabilities associated with treated vs. untreated (or treatment-seeking vs. non-seeking) individuals, as well as the unknown characteristics of patients who remain unidentified or concealed within family or community settings. Less tangible or quantifiable aspects of the disease toll include diminished quality of life and satisfaction with the events of daily living [6, 7]. This phenomenon bears on reports that many bipolar patients experience subthreshold manic and/or depressive symptoms between periods of full manic or major depressive episodes [8], although subsyndromal psychopathology may not always be recognized as appreciably as distinct affective episodes.

ECONOMIC AND OCCUPATIONAL ILLNESS BURDEN

In 1990, the total annual prevalence-based cost in the United States associated with depression, including both unipolar and bipolar illness, was estimated as $44 billion [9]. This sum has been subdivided into direct costs (totaling approximately $7.6 billion/year, or 17% of total costs) and indirect expenses (about 83% of total costs, reflecting expenses due to worker absenteeism and diminished work productivity or lost wages, institutional costs, premature death, and family/caregiver burden). Direct expenses linked to affective disorders include nursing home (33%) and inpatient (26%) costs, crime (25%), substance abuse (8%), suicide (2%), medications (1%), shelters (1%), and research/training programme costs (1%) [9].

A different morbidity cost estimate for affective disorders, using a timing model with regression analysis based on data from 1985, determined that affective disorders comprised 21% of costs related to all forms of mental illness; a majority of expenses were accounted for by direct treatment costs (58.4%), while morbidity comprised 8.1% of costs and mortality constituted 28.9%; costs due to crime, diminished work productivity and caregiver services comprised 4.6% of costs [10].

Studying a more contemporary cohort, Begeley et al [11] developed an incidence-based model of cost estimates for bipolar patients with illness onset in 1998. Total lifetime costs in this group were estimated at $24 billion, with an average cost per case of $252 212. A marked financial difference was observed between patients with single manic episodes and a stable subsequent course (average cost $11 720) and those with more chronic, treatment-nonresponsive forms of illness (average cost $624 785). The $24 billion total cost for incident cases of bipolar illness reported by Begeley et al [11] contrasts with an approximately 200% greater cost among prevalent cases reported by Wyatt and Henter [9]. This disparity may reflect differences in the time until costs may actually be incurred, as well as the focus only on new cases beginning in 1998 (rather than existing plus new cases) described by Begeley [11].

Occupational disability remains extensive for many individuals with bipolar illness. For example, at six-month follow-up after an index manic episode, Dion et al [12] found that only 43% of bipolar patients were employed, while only 21% were functioning at expected levels, even though nearly 80% of the cohort was judged to be symptom-free or only mildly ill. Other authors have estimated that, in 1990, bipolar illness and depression collectively accounted for 289 million days of worker absenteeism [13]. Mintz et al [14] observed that the capacity to work may lag significantly after symptom remission from a depressive episode. Goldberg et al [15] found at both two- and five-year follow-ups that fewer than one-quarter of bipolar patients with affective relapses had steady work performance, and that affective relapse led to impaired work functioning more profoundly among bipolar than unipolar patients. Moreover, work-related problems may be more evident and more pervasive among individuals with either bipolar illness or schizophrenia than with any other psychiatric diagnoses [16].

Formal economic models have only partly begun to identify the relative indirect costs for individuals with treated vs. untreated bipolar illness, an effort of both clinical and economic importance in light of findings that only one-third of patients with bipolar disorder seek treatment [17]. Were this majority of untreated individuals to receive appropriate psychiatric care, it has been estimated that the overall economic burden associated with bipolar illness would be counterbalanced by an annual cost saving of $5.6 billion (attributable to offsetting indirect illness-related expenses [17]). When treatment is initiated near the onset of symptoms, the potential to forestall multiple relapses and related disease complications, such as substance abuse, would presumably generate even more dramatic cost savings.

Likely effects of treatment on indirect illness-related costs are illustrated by a survey of 500 patients with bipolar disorder conducted by the National Depressive and Manic-Depressive Association, which reported that after receiving effective treatment, patients were significantly less likely to commit minor crimes, experience financial difficulties, become divorced or encounter marital difficulties, injure themselves or others, gamble excessively, or abuse alcohol or drugs [18]. This portrait of the composite expense of bipolar disorder suggests that it is far more costly *not* to treat than to treat.

MISDIAGNOSIS AND ILLNESS DETECTION

Early detection through disease screening and public awareness has made a considerable impact on the prognosis, course, and costs related to numerous serious medical conditions. Programmes designed to enhance patients' abilities to recognize prodromal signs of affective relapse in bipolar disorder have demonstrated significant reductions in full relapses that require hospitalization [19]. Efforts to identify episodes before they become fully manifest are of particular importance, since at least one-quarter of euthymic bipolar patients show impaired insight and an inability to recognize affective prodromes [20]. Some authors have observed that the maximal benefits of lithium prophylaxis are most likely to occur when lithium is begun within the first five years of illness [21], and that lithium initiation after the passage of multiple episodes may be less efficacious both acutely [22] and prophylactically [23].

The likelihood with which mental health professionals diagnose bipolar illness has varied cross-culturally and internationally over the past several decades. In the 1970s, it became recognized that American psychiatrists were far more likely to diagnose schizophrenia than bipolar disorder as compared to their European counterparts [24]. This trend may have diminished in later years [25], although in recent assessments of community-based patients screened for affective disorders, substantial rates of under-diagnosis are still evident [26].

Ghaemi et al [27] observed that 40% of patients consecutively hospitalized for depression had a history of previously undiagnosed bipolar illness, with an average delay of 7.5 (SD = 9.8) years between receiving an initial diagnosis of unipolar depression and a rediagnosis of bipolar illness. Gold-berg et al [28] also found that among 74 young adult patients hospitalized for depression with no prior history of bipolar disorder, 45% met diagnostic criteria for mania or hypomania on one or more occasions over an ensuing 15-year follow-up period. Lag periods between illness onset and diagnosis have been reported for an average of 5–6 years in some studies (e.g., [29]), with increases proportional to age of onset [30, 31]. In the National Depres-sive and Manic-Depressive Association membership survey [18], approxi-mately one-third of respondents reported delays of more than 10 years from their initial symptom onset to receiving a diagnosis of bipolar disorder and initiation of treatment with a mood stabilizer.

The clinical significance of lag times in both the accurate diagnosis and initiation of treatment for bipolar disorder has become a subject of growing interest. From a psychosocial as well as economic standpoint, costs related to misdiagnosis and inaccurate treatments are difficult to estimate. Because antidepressants may induce manias or accelerate cycling patterns in at least 30–40% of bipolar patients [32], the possibility exists that prolonged expos-ure to antidepressants in bipolar patients who are misidentified as having unipolar depression may drastically destabilize a longitudinal symptom course and related functioning. Other factors, such as the abrupt versus gradual discontinuation of lithium, may directly worsen disease course by hastening relapse [33] or diminishing the likelihood of a favourable response upon rechallenge [34, 35]. Such iatrogenic effects of treatment, particularly early in the lifetime course of illness, may add to overall dis-ability and disease burden in ways that are difficult if at all possible to estimate.

SUICIDE, HOMICIDE AND FORENSIC ISSUES

Suicide accounts for a significant proportion of premature death among individuals with bipolar disorder [36]. It has been estimated that, on average, a 25-year-old woman with untreated bipolar disorder will lose nine years of life expectancy (due largely to suicide), although with appropriate treat-ment a 6.5-year increase in life expectancy may be recaptured [37]. Because suicide risk historically has been described as being particularly high during the first few years after the onset of affective symptoms [38–40], delays in accurate diagnosis and treatment could impact high-risk mortality periods

[41]. Once appropriate treatment is begun for bipolar disorder, current data suggest that lag times until initiation do not significantly diminish outcome [42]. Craig *et al* [43] also found no relation between the duration of untreated symptoms and two-year outcome among 119 psychotic first-admission bipolar patients, although the mean duration of untreated symptoms in that group was relatively brief (nine days). The impact of lithium and other treatments as affecting suicide risk are discussed below.

Forensic complications have been only partially addressed in considering the societal burden of bipolar illness. A review by Good [44] suggests that bipolar illness may exist in at least 10% of prison populations, yet its formal diagnosis is frequently either missed or ignored. The impact of comorbid substance abuse appears to be an important contributor to arrests for violent crime among men and women with severe affective disorders [45]. The extent to which costs involving the criminal justice system could be reduced via better detection and treatment of bipolar illness has not been fully estimated.

CHILDHOOD BIPOLAR DISORDER

Increasing attention has been paid in the literature to the recognition of bipolar illness that may develop during childhood [46], although its frequent non-prototypical features or comorbid presentation with other conditions (such as attention deficit hyperactivity disorder) hinder accurate and timely diagnoses. Little information is available on the psychosocial impact of juvenile-onset bipolar disorder with regard to school performance, social development, or longitudinal outcomes. However, data from the National Depressive and Manic-Depressive Association membership survey [18] point to a number of differences in psychosocial outcome following child/adolescent onset (before age 20, approximate $n = 295$) and adult onset (after age 20, approximate $n = 205$) bipolar disorder. Notably, child-adolescent onset bipolar disorder was more often associated with school dropout (55% of respondents), financial difficulties (70% of respondents), divorce or marital problems (73% of respondents), alcohol or drug abuse (52% of respondents), injuring self or others (46% of respondents), and committing minor crimes (36% of respondents). Receiving public assistance, being unemployed, or job firings did not differ among juvenile vs. adult onset bipolar patients, or among those with more highly recurrent vs. infrequent affective episodes.

PHARMACOECONOMICS AND PHARMACOTHERAPIES

Financial costs relating to treatment include not only the direct expense of medications and individual/institutional provider services but also expenses associated with treatment, including the need for adjunctive pharmacotherapies or antidotes to primary medication side effects, laboratory monitoring of medication blood levels and end-organ functioning, additional health service utilization (such as emergency department visits or medical/intensive care unit admissions due to medication toxicities or overdoses), and indirect cost estimates such as worker absenteeism, diminished productivity, and suicide.

The introduction of lithium in the United States has been credited with a dramatic reduction in both direct and indirect costs associated with bipolar illness. From 1970 to 1980, a $2.88 billion decrease was estimated due to lithium use in direct treatment costs (including prescription medications, laboratory monitoring, outpatient psychosocial treatments, and hospitalization) [47]. Relatedly, marked decreases in length of hospital stay within the United Kingdom have been observed in the pre- to post-lithium era, associated with an approximate $34 million saving in costs related solely to hospitalization [48, 49].

Several studies have compared relative treatment costs across distinct pharmacotherapies, although it warrants mention that much of the available contemporary data derive from research conducted under sponsorship by the pharmaceutical industry rather than government, private foundations, or other economically impartial agencies. Many studies also presuppose the exclusive or predominant use of psychotropic monotherapies (rather than combination drug therapies and/or concomitant psychotherapies), when in fact many if not most bipolar patients chronically receive two or more maintenance medications [50]. Data from Sajatovic *et al* [51] suggest that bipolar-manic patients who receive combinations of mood stabilizers may have hospitalizations of significantly longer duration than those on lithium or anticonvulsant monotherapy regimens (although clinicians' decisions to utilize monotherapies vs. combination drug therapies may be influenced by varied factors, such as differential severity of illness, treatment non-adherence, or side-effect tolerabilities). Potential outcome differences between treatment groups may be influenced by including special populations (e.g., bipolar I vs. bipolar II patients, those with or without substance abuse comorbidity, the presence or absence of rapid cycling) or other clinical, socioeconomic and demographic factors (e.g., high vs. low social supports, socioeconomic and current employment status), although such factors may not routinely be included or systematically accounted for in pharmacoeconomic analyses.

Keck *et al* [52] developed a pharmacoeconomic decision-analytic model of treatment for bipolar disorder over a one-year period, based on the use of either lithium carbonate or divalproex sodium as the primary mood stabilizer. One-year costs related to treatment of classic (pure), mixed, and rapid-cycling bipolar disorder with lithium were estimated as $31 426, $50 856 and \$49 078, respectively; corresponding costs with divalproex sodium were \$33 139, \$43 672, and \$42 792. A breakdown of component costs described initial hospitalization as comprising a major portion of annual costs (60% of total costs with lithium and 57% with divalproex sodium), followed by treatment costs related to relapses (mainly rehospitalization costs). Per-pill costs (numerically higher for divalproex sodium than lithium) were considered negligible. Relative cost savings with divalproex sodium for mixed or rapid-cycling mania were attributed in large part to an expected shorter length of hospital stay during the index manic episode.

Several limitations of the pharmacoeconomic model developed by Keck *et al* [52] have been described [53]. First, the relative lack of controlled data on differential maintenance pharmacotherapy makes uncertain the likely long-term outcome across different medication groups. In fact, the sole one-year maintenance comparison of lithium vs. divalproex sodium or placebo [54] failed to show any difference in relapse rates for mania with either active drug versus placebo, likely reflecting the enormous methodologic challenges for recruiting and retaining bipolar patients in long-term placebo-controlled studies. Such extrapolation from short-term outcome data limits the reliability of long-range outcome estimates. Second, the validity of assuming robust superiority of divalproex sodium over lithium for mixed states or rapid cycling—as suggested in recent reports [55, 56]—has been challenged by at least some treatment guidelines [57]. Basic assumptions about differential pharmacotherapy outcome in the pharmacoeconomic model may therefore be more tentative than was originally believed, particularly since clinical decisions to utilize combinations of mood stabilizers may be associated with longer durations of hospitalization [51]. Finally, length of hospital stay has been recognized as a highly variable parameter on which numerous nonclinical factors (e.g., economic, psychosocial) impinge. Because length-of-stay data used in this analysis were derived from a single source, their generalizability becomes further narrowed.

Frye *et al* [58] conducted a retrospective pilot review of hospital records for 78 bipolar inpatients receiving either lithium ($n = 52$), divalproex sodium ($n = 5$), carbamazepine ($n = 15$), or lithium plus carbamazepine ($n = 6$), and found that the average length of hospital stay was significantly shorter with divalproex sodium alone (10.2 ± 2.0 days) or with lithium plus carbamazepine (11.7 ± 2.1 days) than with lithium alone (17.6 ± 1.0 days) or carbamazepine alone (18.1 ± 3.0 days). In contrast, Goldberg *et al* [59] found no differences in mean hospital duration during routine treatment with lithium, divalproex sodium, carbamazepine, or combinations thereof, but did observe that the time necessary to achieve a therapeutic blood level of any one mood stabilizer was a significant correlate of clinical remission from acute mania during hospitalization. Specifically, for each week's delay to achieve a therapeutic blood level of lithium, divalproex sodium, or carbamazepine, the likelihood of remission prior to discharge decreased by 27%. From an economic as well as clinical perspective, this suggests that pharmacotherapies which can be optimized swiftly near the onset of an episode may lead to better outcomes than the same therapies under-dosed or used in too slow a dose escalation strategy. However, rapid dosage optimization may be less feasible with pharmacotherapies that have narrow therapeutic indices (such as lithium) or other significant toxicity potentials (such as severe, life-threatening dermatologic reactions with lamotrigine when rapidly dosed).

In a recent 12–week randomized comparison of divalproex sodium (orally loaded as 20 mg/kg) versus olanzapine (10 mg/day) monotherapy for acute mania, use of divalproex sodium ($n = 27$) was associated with an overall 12-week cost of $553 (SD = $325) as compared to $1109 (SD = $627) with olanzapine ($n = 26$) ($p = .003$) [60]. Much of the cost saving of divalproex sodium was primarily attributed to drug acquisition rather than related treatment expenses (e.g., laboratory monitoring, rehospitalization, emergency department visits, or other outpatient visits). However, relatively high dropout rates have been common during long-term randomized clinical trials (approximately 70% in either treatment arm in the study by Zajecka *et al* [60]), and a lack of data about subsequent outcomes for study dropouts further limits the practical significance of pharmacoeconomic estimates for clinicians.

Other pharmacoeconomic or treatment service studies have focused on bipolar subgroups such as geriatric populations. Conney and Kaston [61] retrospectively compared financial costs and clinical outcomes for 72 patients above age 54 with bipolar disorder and/or dementia in a Veterans Administration long-term skilled nursing care facility. Drug acquisition costs per patient-year were significantly lower with lithium ($15 for 600 mg daily) than divalproex sodium ($339 for 750 mg daily), although higher annual laboratory monitoring costs were associated with lithium ($278) than divalproex sodium ($53). Largely because of more adverse medication events and medical intensive care unit admissions, average net annual costs with lithium were $2875 higher than with divalproex sodium. Specific adverse events occurring more frequently during treatment with lithium than divalproex sodium included toxicity and/or dehydration (68% with lithium versus 7% with divalproex sodium), leukocytosis (25% with lithium versus 0% with divalproex sodium), whereas medical events more common with divalproex sodium than lithium included thrombocytopenia (10% versus 0%, respectively) and hepatotoxicity (7% versus 0%, respectively). Total mean costs related to treating mild-to-moderate morbidity (excluding intensive care unit costs) remained higher with lithium ($3472 per year) than divalproex sodium ($672 per year).

PSYCHOTHERAPY

The economic impact of psychotherapy for serious mental illnesses such as bipolar disorder remains difficult to estimate. Psychotherapy outcomes research has partly been hampered by the relatively few operationalized forms of psychotherapy specific to bipolar disorder [62]. Hence, the difficulty in separating the specific from nonspecific benefits of psychotherapy [63] limits the confidence with which one can ascribe an accurate cost benefit or liability to treatment effects. It is often assumed that patients who undertake a diagnosis-specific form of psychotherapy such as cognitive-behavioural therapy (CBT) or interpersonal psychotherapy (IPT) may have better clinical and psychosocial outcomes than those in other, less specific forms of psychotherapy where efficacy in bipolar disorder has not been demonstrated. Nevertheless, in a meta-analysis of 32 published outcome studies involving a variety of individual, group, family, or couples-based psychotherapies, Huxley et al [64] observed overall gains in objective measures of clinical stability and reduced hospitalizations across a range of psychotherapy modalities. At the same time, close clinical monitoring per se (without formal psychotherapy) has been linked with superior outcomes during pharmacotherapy for bipolar disorder [65]; surveillance may closely parallel medication adherence, and may account for much of the variability in outcome observed for patients who receive standard care within lithium clinics [66]. In this respect, the consistency of psychosocial support provided by a practitioner, grounded in an established therapeutic alliance, may contribute in large measure to relapse prevention and global improvement.

Gabbard et al [67], in a meta-analysis of 10 published studies involving randomized assignment to psychotherapy or clinical management in conjunction with standard pharmacotherapy, found significant overall cost savings attributable to psychotherapy for individuals with bipolar disorder as well as schizophrenia and borderline personality disorder. Much of the economic impact of psychotherapy was linked with reduced inpatient treatment and decreased work impairment, suggesting a benefit both for direct and indirect illness-related expenses.

TREATMENT NON-ADHERENCE

Non-adherence to medications or other treatments has been estimated to occur in over half of bipolar patients, and may be especially likely among those with comorbid substance abuse [68, 69], maladaptive personality traits [70], illness denial and poor coping skills [71], severity of mania during hospitalization [72] and the use of combinations of mood stabilizers [72]. Among bipolar patients with comorbid substance use disorders, medication adherence with few side effects may be greater among those taking valproate than lithium [73]. Substantial increases in both direct and indirect treatment costs for bipolar illness have been associated with medication noncompliance; for example, in a capitated healthcare setting, Durrenberger *et al* [74] estimate that every bipolar patient with poor treatment compliance consumes the equivalent healthcare share budgeted for 13 severely mentally ill treatment-compliant healthplan enrollees.

FAMILY AND CAREGIVER BURDEN

Marital conflict, separation and divorce are frequent occurrences among individuals with bipolar disorder, such that some studies report intact marital relationships in less than one-fifth of bipolar cohorts [2, 75]. Interpersonal problems with spouses or romantic partners have also been associated with elevated suicide risk in at least one bipolar cohort based in Taiwan [76].

Burdens on family members and caregivers for individuals with bipolar disorder are extensive (over 90% of caregivers report moderate or greater distress [77]) and may be more profound than occurs with either major depression alone [78] or schizophrenia [79]. Clinicians also have been shown to demonstrate a keener appreciation for the burden experienced by relatives of patients with schizophrenia than with bipolar disorder—particularly with regard to patients being delusional or displaying other positive symptoms, or showing lack of insight into the nature of their condition [79].

Factors related to severity of illness, number of episodes, and increasing age may especially be associated with severity of burden, while a less robust connection with family burden has been reported for occupation, education and family size [78]. Burden also appears greater for families in which comorbid substance abuse accompanies severe mental illness, accounted for by family members providing both increased time and financial support to patient-relatives (an average annual cost of $8489.21 for dual-diagnosis patients as compared to $3547.30 for adult children without chronic illness) [80]. Mean family expenditures for adult children with dual diagnosis psychopathology were particularly elevated for transportation, food and clothing, rent and utilities, and leisure activities [80].

Demographically, among families of severely mentally ill individuals in general, African American caregivers tend to report less subjective burden than do white family caregivers, independent of religious or other social factors [81]. The degree of caregiver burden perceived by the well siblings of severely mentally ill individuals appears directly linked to symptoms experienced by an affected sibling, and may also relate to perceptions by a well sibling that they possess some ability to control an ill sibling's behaviour [82]. Similarly, Perlick *et al* [77] found that family caregiver beliefs about bipolar disorder (e.g., illness awareness, perceptions of patient and family control) accounted for up to 28% of the variance associated with the severity of family burden, above and beyond the effects of a patient's clinical state and history.

These latter observations are consistent with findings by Miklowitz *et al* [83] that emotional overinvolvement by family members of bipolar patients may reflect one aspect of negative expressed emotion (EE), in turn heightening relapse risk. To that end, family-therapy based efforts to reduce EE levels may be of value not only as a means for improving medication compliance and individual patient outcomes, but also as an aid to reduce subjective caregiver burden aggravated by illness misperceptions.

Cross-culturally, severe mental illness in developing nations and Afro- or Afro-Caribbean countries is often related to culturally syntonic concepts about spiritual causation involving witchcraft and evil spells [84]. Family members not only bear the economic and care-giving ramifications of untreated psychopathology, but, moreover, are themselves often ostracized and isolated because of community-shared negative beliefs about spiritual meanings behind severe mental illness [84].

Spouses of bipolar patients have been shown to strongly favour the concept of genetic screening for bipolar illness were such technology to become available [85]. Survey data are mixed regarding family attitudes toward family planning and aborted pregnancies, were genetic markers to become available for anticipating eventual bipolar illness in a developing foetus. Some reports have found that most patients and spouses indicate they would not abort a developing foetus in such circumstances [85], while other studies suggest that nearly half of pregnant couples would terminate pregnancy if a foetus were thought definitely to develop bipolar illness, unless a "mild course" could be anticipated [86].

TREATMENT SETTINGS AND HEALTH INSURANCE PROGRAMMES

Several studies have compared aspects of treatment and service utilization for bipolar patients treated in prepaid or capitated health care programmes such as health maintenance organizations (HMOs) as compared to other clinical settings. Unutzer *et al* [87] found a treated prevalence of bipolar disorder of 0.42% in HMO enrollees, comprised mostly of women and younger individuals, the vast majority of whom (85%) were receiving treatment with at least one mood stabilizer. In addition, contrary to speculation that seriously mentally ill individuals become disenrolled from prepaid insurance programmes [88], the duration of HMO enrolment appears no shorter for bipolar patients than for nondiabetic HMO members, though somewhat shorter than for HMO members with diabetes mellitus [89]. At the same time, although bipolar patients treated within HMO settings appear to be high users of mental health services, their use of general medical services may be comparable to that of nonbipolar, nonpsychotic HMO members [89].

Laboratory monitoring of mood stabilizer blood levels or associated organ system effects (e.g., thyroid, renal functioning) has been shown to occur with substantially less frequency for Medicaid patients with bipolar disorder than would ordinarily be expected [90] based on treatment practice guidelines [91]. Conceivably, economic and clinical costs might secondarily elevate due to possible clinical deterioration resulting from subtherapeutic mood stabilizer use, or toxicities due to supratherapeutic medication use, or under-detection of secondary end-organ dysfunction (e.g., lithium-induced hypothyroidism or renal insufficiency, or glucose dysregulation induced by atypical antipsychotics). Actual adverse medical consequences due to laboratory under-monitoring were not documented in the report by Marcus *et al* [90], although elsewhere [92] regular blood monitoring of mood stabilizers has been associated with a 3–fold decreased likelihood of experiencing adverse drug events.

SERVICE UTILIZATION

In the United States and abroad, trends toward shortened inpatient hospitalizations for acute manic or depressive episodes have led to the development of intensive outpatient or day hospital programmes as alternatives to hospitalization. Although little prospective outcome data exist on the clinical and psychosocial impact of shortened lengths of stay, a recent retrospective study suggested that clinical status and treatment outcome at the time of discharge was not necessarily associated with greater illness severity status at discharge [93]. However, it remains an open question whether or not differences exist in subsequent outcome (e.g., return to work or independent community living, rates of suicide attempts) or service utilization (e.g., emergency room visits, rehospitalization) as a function of length of stay after a manic or major depressive episode. The availability and efficacy of alternatives to hospitalization (e.g., assisted outpatient treatment or partial hospital programmes) and/or community-based programmes such as intensive case management—which have been shown to reduce overall mental health service costs and reduce the frequency of inpatient care [94, 95]—would likely play an important role in such analyses.

Severely mentally ill individuals who receive integrated services through a centralized agency have been shown to have less hospitalization, better occupational functioning, less reliance on assisted living arrangements, diminished family/caregiver burden, and greater life satisfaction as compared to those receiving mental health services under ordinary conditions [96]. However, capitated costs for patients seen through integrated service agencies were significantly higher than for individuals seen in usual treatment settings [96]. The degree to which such increased direct costs may be offset by greater savings in indirect costs was not estimated.

Lack of health insurance for a substantial minority of United States citizens has been associated with increased economic costs both within medicine and psychiatry. Among uninsured patients, Simon and Unutzer [97] found that overall healthcare costs were significantly greater for those with bipolar illness than unipolar depression, diabetes mellitus, or general medical conditions. Moreover, bipolar illness accounted in this study for 90% of inpatient psychiatric costs and 40% of specialty mental health services, although parity of coverage for inpatient treatment was estimated to increase overall health expenditures by only 6%.

Among bipolar patients treated within the United States Department of Veterans Affairs, high rates of service utilization were associated with histories of childhood physical abuse, more than traditionally reported predictors of disease severity [98]. Thus, it is possible that developmental or other longitudinal factors that might contribute to coping skills or other psychosocial dimensions may be important contributors to mental health service use and economic outcome in bipolar patients.

Finally, with the emergence of a growing number of treatment algorithms and practice guidelines for the management of bipolar disorder [99], little is known, as yet, about the impact of guideline-based interventions versus treatment-as-usual on clinical and psychosocial outcomes as well as service utilization and related health economic parameters. Open trials suggest that guideline-based treatments may substantially increase antidepressant pharmacotherapy compliance among depressed patients in primary care medical settings [100], although it has not yet been determined whether such clinical outcomes produce economic savings that offset the costs associated with guideline development, teaching, and implementation.

SUMMARY

The morbidity, mortality, and economic consequences of bipolar disorder remain substantial, although much of its financial cost derives from indirect expenses related to undertreatment, misdiagnosis, and the vocational and other psychosocial ramifications of previous affective episodes. Advances in both pharmacotherapy and diagnosis-specific psychotherapies offer promise to lessen morbidity and thereby reduce the economic and social burden of disease. With regard to functional disability and treatment outcome of bipolar disorder, current pharmacoeconomic and other health care cost models vary in their methodologies and often either extrapolate from enriched patient samples or else draw conclusions based solely on expert opinion. Future studies that include more heterogeneous patient subtypes, followed in "effectiveness"- (rather than "efficacy"-) based models, are needed in order to develop better predictors of psychosocial burden, as well to inform practitioners and healthcare policy administrators about likely prognoses and outcomes under ordinary treatment conditions.

At present, the collective experience from clinical and research-based efforts suggests several areas in which knowledge about the psychosocial and economic burden of bipolar illness can be described with confidence. These may be summarized as follows.

Consistent Evidence

- Bipolar disorder remains a ubiquitous yet underrecognized and often misdiagnosed clinical phenomenon, one in which *inappropriate* treatments may worsen the overall course of illness, and for which delays in prompt detection may lead to increased morbidity and mortality, due to a high risk for suicide near illness onset.
- Psychosocial disability from bipolar disorder remains extensive and encompasses multiple domains, including work and social functioning, independent community living, family adjustment, premature mortality, and diminished quality of life.
- Comorbid substance abuse or other psychiatric diagnoses [101] and/or medical conditions [102] are highly prevalent in bipolar disorder and may contribute to diagnostic confusion as well as delayed introductions of appropriate treatments [103, 104].
- The development of newer pharmacotherapies as well as diagnosis-specific psychotherapies—combined with a more targeted use of existing treatments for specific bipolar subtypes—has begun to refine modern psychotherapeutics. The marked impact of lithium prophylaxis on reducing suicide risk stands as a major example of such enhanced outcome [105]. New therapeutic options are continually emerging for treatment-resistant forms of illness or as alternatives when standard drug side effects may be intolerable. The translation of such therapeutic strides into observable benefits (e.g., work and social adjustment, reintegration into community settings, and global life satisfaction) has become a growing focus of outcomes research.

- In the treatment of acute mania, the rapid initiation of divalproex [106], lithium [107] and possibly other therapeutic agents [108] may promote faster resolution of symptoms than more gradual dosing approaches. It is possible that swift interventions may help to diminish length of hospital stay [58] or altogether avert hospitalizations, and correspondingly reduce the direct and indirect costs associated with relapse.
- Shortened lengths of hospitalization and alternative community-based integrative treatments have become increasingly common for both the acute and long-term management of bipolar illness. Modern clinical practice has demanded an intense adaptation to this changing healthcare climate in order to manage severely ill bipolar patients. Clinicians often must balance issues of risk assessment and safety while at the same time accrue experience using new or complex pharmacotherapy regimens.
- Although economic costs of bipolar disorder are among the highest per capita mental health expenditures worldwide, these derive largely from indirect expenses related to underdiagnosis, undertreatment, and the psychosocial consequences of poorly controlled illness. Cost savings attributable to appropriate treatment far outweigh direct treatment expenses.

Incomplete Evidence

Alongside the above present-day circumstances, clinical and empirical evidence remains less conclusive in a number of areas, including the following:

- Pharmacoeconomic estimates of treatment costs remain imprecise. In the current literature, methodologies by which illness-related expenses are estimated vary, as existing studies utilize expert opinion summaries, insurance claims data, pharmacy registry surveys, and literature reviews without uniformity or systematic approaches [109, 110]. In addition, current long-range estimates are often derived either by extrapolation from short-term data or from individual treatment settings for which broad generalizations about outcome may be limited. Furthermore, many existing studies of the economic and social burden of bipolar disorder use data from epidemiologic surveys such as the Epidemiologic Catchment Area (ECA [111]) study or the National Comorbidity Survey (NCS [112]). Limitations of these databases include their exclusion of institutionalized patients or those over age 65, as well as their incorporation of patients from 1980–1985 (ECA) or 1990–1992 (NCS)—predating the contemporary use of newer pharmacotherapies, such as divalproex or other anticonvulsants (e.g., lamotrigine, topiramate, gabapentin) and atypical antipsychotics such as olanzapine, risperidone, quetiapine, and ziprasidone. Current data are mixed as to whether or not the chronic use of atypical antipsychotics is [113] or is not [114] generally associated with substantially better long-term outcomes in bipolar patients, although few systematic prospective studies exist in this area. Relatively high drop-out rates in virtually all long-term pharmacotherapy studies—perhaps an insurmountable obstacle when studying a condition so inherently unstable as bipolar illness—further limit pharmacoeconomic generalizability when drop-outs are not followed through to study completion. Finally, because inter-rater diagnostic agreement has shown substantial variability in epidemiologic studies (particularly for non-prototypical forms of bipolar illness such as bipolar II disorder, unipolar mania, and cyclothymia), it has been difficult to accurately estimate the psychosocial consequences of atypical forms of bipolarity.

- The criteria by which clinicians diagnose bipolar spectrum disorders have broadened considerably in recent years [117, 118], although debate has arisen about the validity of heterogeneous concepts of bipolar illness [119]. Estimates of the economic and social burden of bipolar disorder may vary widely when cyclothymic disorder, unipolar mania, or other atypical forms of possible bipolar disorder are subsumed alongside bipolar I illness. The degree to which bipolar II disorder differs from bipolar I illness with respect to functional impairment, treatment outcome, suicide risk, and other aspects of disability also remains an area in which little empirical data now exist.

- The rise of patient advocacy organizations and support groups both for patients and family members may provide important psychosocial resources for individuals affected by bipolar disorder, potentially helping to improve relationships within families, facilitate access to appropriate health care, and aid in the destigmatization of mental illness [120]. It is possible that such groups may aid in psychoeducation that could ultimately help patients to detect prodromal signs of relapse and possibly avert full affective episodes and rehospitalization. As described in earlier sections, organizations such as the National Depressive and Manic-Depressive Association in the United States have alerted patients as well as clinicians to issues regarding the misdiagnosis and inappropriate treatment of bipolar illness. Because it is difficult to estimate the likely socioeconomic impact of such groups in terms of helping to reduce direct and indirect illness costs, as well as quality of life, future studies might usefully incorporate their visibility and involvement in judging clinical outcomes.

- Treatment outcome and disability among special populations of bipolar patients—such as children, pregnant women, the elderly, and the medically ill—remain understudied. In the case of pregnancy, decisions to discontinue potentially teratogenic pharmacotherapies generally must be balanced against risks of affective relapse during pregnancy, and the potential for substantial post-partum morbidity when mood stabilizers are not resumed in the puerperium [121]. In geriatric mania, modified dosing schedules may yield better tolerability and less morbidity [122], although costs related to treatment outcomes, service utilization, side effects, and iatrogenic complications are not yet well documented in instances such as these.

Areas Still Open to Research

- It is essentially unknown whether, and when, and for which patients, combination drug therapies may produce better outcomes, fewer relapses, less disability, and diminished costs as compared to monotherapies. While profiles of good- versus poor-prognostic factors for lithium responsivity have become increasingly recognized [123], less is known about matching other drug treatments to illness subtypes or symptom constellations. Clinical, psychosocial, and economic outcomes have not been explored for deliberately sequenced treatments (i.e., specific iterative drug trials, or psychotherapy that is begun concomitant with medication adjustments versus subsequent to pharmacotherapy for acute episodes). Although combination drug therapy is common in the routine treatment of bipolar patients, further work is needed to determine when costs and outcomes are more favourable during specific monotherapies or specific combination therapies for given phases of illness.
- The clinical significance of lag times in the early detection and treatment of bipolar illness remains a subject of controversy. Further studies are needed to corroborate current impressions that lithium response may be poorer and suicide risk may be greater when lengthy delays transpire from the lifetime onset of illness to a first mood stabilizer treatment. Moreover, greater information is needed regarding the treatment outcome and illness costs related to bipolar disorder among children and adolescents. Begeley et al [11] estimated that 36% of incident cases of bipolar illness occur before age 14, yet controlled treatment studies of any kind in this age group are scarce or nonexistent. The clinical, social, and economic impact of surveillance screening for children at risk of bipolar parents has not yet been carefully evaluated, nor has the concept of introducing mood stabilizer pharmacotherapy either prophylactically in high-risk individuals or for prodromal features prior to a first manic or depressive episode. The possible over-use of antidepressants or psychostimulants [124] in this age group, potentially inducing kindling phenomena and adversely influencing subsequent illness course, also remains an area in which little information exists.
- Although efficacy-based studies provide a growing base in the literature from which clinicians can judge the utility of newer pharmacotherapies,

important differences may exist between treatment outcomes from controlled trials as opposed to routine practice conditions [125]. The increasing availability of research protocols for the treatment of bipolar disorder has led to a growing number of patients who enter randomized clinical trials [126]. At the same time, as larger numbers of newer possible drug therapies become popularized before their efficacy becomes established in large-scale controlled studies, it becomes difficult to estimate the effect on psychosocial outcome of relatively experimental or unproven new treatments (including herbal remedies and nutritional products not regulated for quality assurance).

- Amid increasingly stringent criteria for hospitalization under capitated or managed care health systems, outpatient programmes will likely treat greater numbers of severely ill individuals who previously would have received care in longer term inpatient settings. The impact of such "deinstitutionalization" on family and economic burden within the community cannot be fully estimated and represents a further area of future investigation.

- "Split" treatments between physician prescribers and nonmedical psychotherapists have gained in popularity within some healthcare systems, in part perhaps due to economic forces but also as the result of an increased presence of nonphysician mental health professionals who encounter patients with bipolar illness. There is unresolved debate as to when "split" treatments may be cost-effective, therapeutically advantageous, or frankly counterproductive in the treatment of depression and anxiety disorders [127, 128]. Virtually no data exist on this question in the treatment and outcome of bipolar illness.

- Finally, amid the growing number of treatment practice guidelines and evidence-based practice models within the literature, it remains to be demonstrated whether their implementation and adoption within large-scale health care settings will translate not only to improved quality of care, but also to cost savings [129]. Research projects such as the Texas Medication Algorithm Project (TMAP) for the treatment of bipolar disorder have begun to evaluate this question by comparing multi-year outcomes for bipolar patients who receive guideline-based treatment versus routine care [130]. As findings become available from empirical studies such as these, estimates of optimal treatment strategies alongside health economic issues will become less subject to sheer speculation.

ACKNOWLEDGEMENTS

Supported by research grants from the Theodore and Vada Stanley Foundation, the Nancy Pritzker Foundation, a NARSAD Young Investigator

Award, and by resources from a fund established in the New York Community Trust by DeWitt Wallace.

REFERENCES

1. Murray C.J.L., Lopez A.D. (1996) *The Global Burden of Disease: A Comprehensive Assessment of Mortality and Disability from Diseases, Injuries, and Risk Factors in 1990 and Projected to 2020.* Harvard University Press, Cambridge.
2. Coryell W., Scheftner W., Keller M., Endicott J., Maser J., Klerman G.L. (1993) The enduring psychosocial consequences of mania and depression. *Am. J. Psychiatry*, **150**: 720–727.
3. Wells K.B., Stewart A., Hays R.D., Burnam A., Rogers W., Daniels M., Berry S., Greenfield S., Ware J. (1989) The functioning and well-being of depressed patients: results from the Medical Outcomes Study. *JAMA*, **262**: 914–919.
4. Hays R.D., Wells K.B., Sherbourne C.D., Rogers W., Spritzer K. (1995) Functioning and well-being of patients with depression compared with chronic general medical illnesses. *Arch. Gen. Psychiatry*, **52**: 11–19.
5. Ahrens B., Müller-Oerlinghausen B., Schou M., Wolf T., Alda M., Grof P., Lenz G., Simhandl C., Thau K., Vestergaard P. *et al* (1995) Excess cardiovascular and suicide mortality of affective disorders. *J. Affect. Disord.*, **33**: 67–75.
6. Cooke R.G., Robb J.C., Young L.T., Joffe R.T. (1996) Well-being and functioning in patients with bipolar disorder assessed using the MOS 20-item short form (SF-20). *J. Affect. Disord.*, **39**: 93–97.
7. Atkinson M., Zibin S., Chuang H. (1997) Characterizing quality of life among patients with chronic mental illness: a critical examination of the self-report methodology. *Am. J. Psychiatry*, **154**: 99–105.
8. Keller M.B., Lavori P.W., Kane J.M., Gelenberg A.J., Rosenbaum J.F., Walzer E.A., Baker L.A. (1992) Subsyndromal symptoms in bipolar disorder. A comparison of standard and low serum levels of lithium. *Arch. Gen. Psychiatry*, **49**: 371–376.
9. Wyatt R.J., Henter I. (1995) An economic evaluation of manic-depressive illness: 1991. *Soc. Psychiatry Psychiatr. Epidemiol.*, **30**: 213–219.
10. Rice D.P., Miller L.S. (1995) The economic burden of affective disorders. *Br. J. Psychiatry*, **166** (Suppl. 27): 34–42.
11. Begeley C.E., Annegers J.F., Swann A.C., Lewis C., Coan S., Schnapp W.B., Bryant-Comstock L. (2001) The lifetime cost of bipolar disorder in the United States: An estimate based on incidence and course of illness. *Pharmacoeconomics*, **19** (5 Pt 1): 483–495.
12. Dion G.L., Tohen M., Anthony W.A., Waternaux C.S. (1988) Symptoms and functioning of patients with bipolar disorder six months after hospitalization. *Hosp. Commun. Psychiatry*, **39**: 652–657.
13. Greenberg P.E., Stiglin L.E., Finkelstein S.N., Berndt E.R. (1993) The economic burden of depression in 1990. *J. Clin. Psychiatry*, **54**: 405–418.
14. Mintz J., Mintz L.I., Arruda M.J., Hwang S.S. (1992) Treatments of depression and the functional capacity to work. *Arch. Gen. Psychiatry*, **49**: 761–768.
15. Goldberg J.F., Harrow M., Grossman L.S. (1995) Recurrent affective syndromes in bipolar and unipolar mood disorders at follow-up. *Br. J. Psychiatry*, **166**: 382–385.
16. Wold P.N., Rosenfield A.G., Dwight K. (1982) The relationship between work impairment and diagnosis. Schizophrenia and bipolar affective disorder impair

work performance more than other diagnostic entities. *Rhode Island Med. J.*, **65**: 161–164.

17. Prien R.F., Potter W.Z. (1990) NIMH workshop in treatment of bipolar disorder. *Psychopharmacol. Bull.*, **26**: 409–427.

18. Lish J.D., Dime-Meenan S., Whybrow P.C., Price R.A., Hirschfeld R.M.A. (1994) The National Depressive and Manic-depressive Association (DMDA) survey of bipolar members. *J. Affect. Disord.*, **31**: 281–294.

19. Perry A., Tarrier N., Mirriss R., McCarthy E., Limb K. (1999) Randomised controlled trial of efficacy of teaching patients with bipolar disorder to identify early symptoms of relapse and obtain treatment. *Br. Med. J.*, **318**: 149–153.

20. Lam D., Wong G. (1997) Prodromes, coping strategies, insights and social functioning in bipolar affective disorders. *Psychol. Med.*, **27**: 1091–1100.

21. Franchini L., Zanardi R., Smeraldi E., Gasperini M. (1999) Early onset of lithium prophylaxis as a predictor of good long-term outcome. *Eur. Arch. Psychiatry Clin. Neurosci.*, **249**: 227–230.

22. Swann A.C., Bowden C.L., Calabrese J.R., Dilsaver S.C., Morris S.S. (1999) Differential effect of number of previous episodes of affective disorder on response to lithium or divalproex in acute mania. *Am. J. Psychiatry*, **156**: 1264–1266.

23. Gelenberg A.J., Kane J.M., Keller M.B., Lavori P., Rosenbaum J.F., Cole K., Lavelle J. (1989) Comparison of standard and low serum levels of lithium for maintenance treatment of bipolar disorder. *N. Engl. J. Med.*, **321**: 1489–1493.

24. Cooper J.E., Kendell R.E., Gurland B.J., Sharpe L., Copeland J.R.M., Simon R. (1972) *Psychiatric Diagnosis in New York and London: A Comparative Study of Mental Hospital Admissions.* Maudsley Monograph No. 20, Oxford University Press, London.

25. Stoll A.L., Tohen M., Baldessarini R.J., Goodwin D.C., Stein S., Katz S., Geenens D., Swinson R.P., Goethe J.W., McGlashan T. (1995) Shifts in diagnostic frequencies of schizophrenia and major affective disorders at six North American psychiatric hospitals, 1972–1988. *Am. J. Psychiatry*, **152**: 299–300.

26. Hirschfeld R.M.A., Keller M.B., Panico S., Arons B.S., Barlow D., Davidoff F., Endicott J., Froom J., Goldstein M., Gorman J.M. *et al* (1997) Consensus statement: The National Depressive and Manic-Depressive Association consensus statement on the undertreatment of depression. *JAMA*, **277**: 333–340.

27. Ghaemi S.N., Boiman E.E., Goodwin F.K. (2000) Diagnosing bipolar disorder and the effect of antidepressants: a naturalistic study. *J. Clin. Psychiatry*, **61**: 804–808.

28. Goldberg J.F., Harrow M., Whiteside J.E. (2001) Risk for bipolar illness in patients initially hospitalized for unipolar depression. *Am. J. Psychiatry*, **158**: 1265–1270.

29. Kessler R.C. (1999) Treatment delays in bipolar disorders. *Am. J. Psychiatry*, **156**: 812.

30. Hilty D.M., Brady K.T., Hales R.E. (1999) A review of bipolar disorder among adults. *Psychiatr. Serv.*, **50**: 201–213.

31. Unutzer J., Simon G., Pabiniak C., Bond K., Katon W. (1998) The treated prevalence of bipolar disorder in a large staff-model HMO. *Psychiatr. Serv.*, **49**: 1072–1078.

32. Altshuler L.L., Post R.M., Leverich G.S., Mikalauskas K., Rosoff A., Ackerman L. (1995) Antidepressant-induced mania and cycle acceleration: a controversy revisited. *Am. J. Psychiatry*, **152**: 1130–1138.

33. Faedda G.L., Tondo L., Baldessarini R.J., Suppes T., Tohen M. (1993) Outcome after rapid versus gradual discontinuation of lithium treatment in bipolar disorders. *Arch. Gen. Psychiatry*, **50**: 448–455.

34. Post R.M., Leverich G.S., Altshuler L.L., Mikalauskas K. (1992) Lithium-discontinuation-induced refractoriness: preliminary observations. *Am. J. Psychiatry*, **149**: 1727–1729.
35. Tondo L., Baldessarini R.J., Floris G., Rudas N. (1997) Effectiveness of restarting lithium treatment after its discontinuation in bipolar I and bipolar II disorders. *Am. J. Psychiatry*, **154**: 548–550.
36. Goodwin F.K., Jamison K.R. (1990) *Manic-Depressive Illness*. Oxford University Press, New York.
37. United States Department of Health, Education and Welfare (1979) *Medical Practice Project: A State of the Science Report for the Office of the Assistant Secretary for the US Department of Health, Education and Welfare*. Policy Research, Baltimore.
38. Guze S.B., Robins E. (1970) Suicide and primary affective disorders. *Br. J. Psychiatry*, **117**: 437–438.
39. Tsuang M.T., Woolson R.F. (1977) Mortality in patients with schizophrenia, mania, depression and surgical conditions. *Br. J. Psychiatry*, **130**: 162–166.
40. Johnson G.F., Hunt G. (1979) Suicidal behavior in bipolar manic-depressive patients and their families. *Compr. Psychiatry*, **20**: 159–164.
41. Baldessarini R.J., Tondo L., Hennen J. (1999) Treatment delays in bipolar disorders. *Am. J. Psychiatry*, **156**: 811.
42. Johnstone E.C., Owens D.G., Crow T.J., Davis J.M. (1999) Does a four-week delay in the introduction of medication alter the course of functional psychosis? *J. Psychopharmacol.*, **13**: 238–244.
43. Craig T.J., Bromet E.J., Fennig S., Tanenberg-Karant M., Lavelle J., Galambos N. (2000) Is there an association between duration of untreated psychosis and 24-month clinical outcome in a first-admission series? *Am. J. Psychiatry*, **157**: 60–66.
44. Good M.I. (1979) Primary affective disorder, aggression, and criminality. *Arch. Gen. Psychiatry*, **35**: 954–960.
45. Brennan P.A., Mednick S.A., Hodgins S. (2000) Major mental disorders and criminal violence in a Danish birth cohort. *Arch. Gen. Psychiatry*, **57**: 494–500.
46. Sanchez L., Hagino O., Weller E., Weller R. (1999) Bipolarity in children. *Psychiatr. Clin. North Am.*, **22**: 629–648.
47. Reifman A., Wyatt R.D. (1980) Lithium: a brake in the rising cost of mental illness. *Arch. Gen. Psychiatry*, **37**: 385–388.
48. Morrison D.P., McCreadie R.G. (1985) The impact of lithium in South-West Scotland: II. A longitudinal study. *Br. J. Psychiatry*, **146**: 74–77.
49. McCreadie R.G. (1987) The economics of lithium therapy. In *Depression and Mania: Modern Lithium Therapy*, (Ed. F.N. Johnson), pp. 257–259, IRL Press, Oxford.
50. Frye M.A., Ketter T.A., Leverich G.S., Huggins T., Lantz C., Denicoff K.D., Post R.M. (2000) The increasing use of polypharmacotherapy for refractory mood disorders: 22 years of study. *J. Clin. Psychiatry*, **61**: 9–15.
51. Sajatovic M., Gerhart C., Semple W. (1997) Association between mood-stabilizing medication and mental health resource use in the management of acute mania. *Psychiatr. Serv.*, **48**: 1037–1041.
52. Keck P.E. Jr., Nabulsi A.A., Taylor J.L., Henke C.J., Chmiel J.J., Stanton S.P., Bennett J.A. (1996) A pharmacoeconomic model of divalproex versus lithium in the acute and prophylactic treatment of bipolar I disorder. *J. Clin. Psychiatry*, **57**: 213–222.
53. Dardennes R.M., Even C. (1997) Is divalproex a cost-effective alternative in the acute and prophylactic treatment of bipolar I disorder? *J. Clin. Psychiatry*, **58**: 495–496.

54. Bowden C.L., Calabrese J.R., McElroy S.L., Gyulai L., Wassef A., Petty F., Pope H.G. Jr., Chou J.C., Keck P.E. Jr., Rhodes L.J. *et al* (2000) A randomized, placebo-controlled 12-month trial of divalproex and lithium in treatment of outpatients with bipolar I disorder. Divalproex Maintenance Study Group. *Arch. Gen. Psychiatry*, **57**: 481–489.

55. Freeman T.W., Clothier J.L., Pazzaglia P., Lesem M.D., Swann A.C. (1992). A double-blind comparison of valproate and lithium in the treatment of acute mania. *Am. J. Psychiatry*, **149**: 108–111.

56. Swann A.C., Bowden C.L., Morris D., Calabrese J.R., Petty F., Small J., Dilsaver S.C., Davis J.M. (1997) Depression during mania. Treatment response to lithium or divalproex. *Arch. Gen. Psychiatry*, **54**: 37–42.

57. Bauer M.S., Callahan A.M., Jampala C., Petty F., Sajatovic M., Schaefer V., Wittlin B., Powell B.J. (1999) Clinical practice guidelines for bipolar disorder from the Department of Veterans Affairs. *J. Clin. Psychiatry*, **60**: 9–21.

58. Frye M.A., Altshuler L.L., Szuba M.P., Finch N.N., Mintz J. (1996) The relationship between antimanic agent for treatment of classic or dysphoric mania and length of hospital stay. *J. Clin. Psychiatry*, **57**: 17–21.

59. Goldberg J.F., Garno J.L., Leon A.C., Kocsis J.H., Portera L. (1998) Rapid titration of mood stabilizers predicts remission from mixed or pure mania in bipolar disorder. *J. Clin. Psychiatry*, **59**: 151–158.

60. Zajecka J., Weisler R., Sommerville K.W. (2000) Divalproex sodium versus olanzapine for the treatment of mania in bipolar disorder. Presented at the 39th Annual Meeting of the American College of Neuropsychopharmacology, San Juan, Puerto Rico, December 10–14.

61. Conney J., Kaston B. (1999) Pharmacoeconomic and health outcome comparison of lithium and divalproex in a VA geriatric nursing home population: influence of drug-related morbidity on total cost of treatment. *Am. J. Managed Care*, **5**: 197–204.

62. Craighead W.E., Miklowitz D.J. (2000) Psychosocial interventions for bipolar disorder. *J. Clin. Psychiatry*, **51** (Suppl. 13): 58–64.

63. Strupp H.H., Hadley S.W. (1979) Specific versus nonspecific factors in psychotherapy: a controlled study of outcome. *Arch. Gen. Psychiatry*, **36**: 1125–1136.

64. Huxley N.A., Parikh S.V., Baldessarini R.J. (2000) Effectiveness of psychosocial treatments in bipolar disorder: state of the evidence. *Harvard Rev. Psychiatry*, **8**: 126–140.

65. Masterson G., Warner M., Roxburgh B. (1988) Supervising lithium—A comparison of a lithium clinic, psychiatric outpatient clinic and general practice. *Br. J. Psychiatry*, **152**: 535–538.

66. Maj M., Pirozzi R., Magliano L., Bartoli L. (1998) Long-term outcome of lithium prophylaxis in bipolar disorder: a 5-year prospective study of 402 patients at a lithium clinic. *Am. J. Psychiatry*, **155**: 30–35.

67. Gabbard G.O., Lazar S.G., Hornberger J., Spiegel D. (1997) The economic impact of psychotherapy: a review. *Am. J. Psychiatry*, **154**: 147–155.

68. Keck P.E. Jr., McElroy S.L., Strakowski S.M., Bourne M.L., West S.A. (1997) Compliance with maintenance treatment in bipolar disorder. *Psychopharmacol. Bull.*, **33**: 87–91.

69. Goldberg J.F., Garno J.L., Leon A.C., Kocsis J.H., Portera L. (1999) A history of substance abuse complicates remission from acute mania in bipolar disorder. *J. Clin. Psychiatry*, **60**: 733–740.

70. Colom F., Vieta E., Martinez A., Reinares M., Benabarre A., Gasto C. (2000) Clinical factors associated with treatment noncompliance in euthymic bipolar patients. *J. Clin. Psychiatry*, **61**: 549–555.

71. Greenhouse W.J., Meyer B., Johnson S.L. (2000) Coping and medication adherence in bipolar disorder. *J. Affect. Disord.*, **59**: 237–241.

72. Keck P.E. Jr., McElroy S.L., Strakowski S.M., Stanton S.P., Kizer D.L., Balistreri T.M., Bennett J.A., Tugrul K.C., West S.A. (1996) Factors associated with pharmacologic noncompliance in patients with mania. *J. Clin. Psychiatry*, **57**: 292–297.

73. Weiss R.D., Greenfield S.F., Najavits L.M., Soto J.A., Wyner D., Tohen M., Griffin M.L. (1998) Medication compliance among patients with bipolar disorder and substance use disorder. *J. Clin. Psychiatry*, **59**: 172–174.

74. Durrenberger S., Rogers T., Walker R., de Leon J. (1999) Economic grand rounds: the high costs of care for four patients with mania who were not compliant with treatment. *Psychiatr. Serv.*, **50**: 1539–1542.

75. Gitlin M.J., Swendsen J., Heller T.L., Hammen C. (1995) Relapse and impairment in bipolar disorder. *Am. J. Psychiatry*, **152**: 1638–1640.

76. Tsai S.Y., Lee J.C., Chen C.C. (1999) Characteristics and psychosocial problems of patients with bipolar disorder at high risk for suicide attempt. *J. Affect. Disord.*, **52**: 145–152.

77. Perlick D., Clarkin J.F., Sirey J., Raue P., Greenfield S., Struening E., Rosenheck R. (1999) Burden experienced by care-givers of persons with bipolar affective disorder. *Br. J. Psychiatry*, **175**: 56–62.

78. Chakrabarti S., Kulhara P., Verma S.K. (1992) Extent and determinants of burden among families of patients with affective disorders. *Acta Psychiatr. Scand.*, **86**: 247–252.

79. Mueser K.T., Webb C., Pfeiffer M., Gladis M., Levinson D.F. (1996) Family burden of schizophrenia and bipolar disorder: perceptions of relatives and professionals. *Psychiatr. Serv.*, **47**: 507–511.

80. Clark R.E. (1994) Family costs associated with severe mental illness and substance abuse. *Hosp. Commun. Psychiatry*, **45**: 808–813.

81. Stueve A., Vine P., Struening E.L. (1997) Perceived burden among caregivers of adults with serious mental illness: comparison of black, Hispanic, and white families. *Am. J. Orthopsychiatry*, **67**: 199–209.

82. Greenberg J.S., Kim H.W., Greenley J.R. (1997) Factors associated with subjective burden in siblings of adults with severe mental illness. *Am. J. Orthopsychiatry*, **67**: 231–241.

83. Miklowitz D.J., Simoneau T.L., George E.L., Richards J.A., Kalbag A., Sachs-Ericsson N., Suddath R. (2000) Family-focused treatment of bipolar disorder: 1-year effects of a psychoeducational program in conjunction with pharmacotherapy. *Biol. Psychiatry*, **48**: 582–592.

84. Patel V., Musara T., Butau T., Maramba P., Fuyane S. (1995) Concepts of mental illness and medical pluralism in Harare. *Psychol. Med.*, **25**: 485–493.

85. Trippitelli C.L., Jamison K.R., Folstein M.F., Bartko J.J., dePaulo J.R. (1998) Pilot study on patients' and spouses' attitudes toward potential genetic testing for bipolar disorder. *Am. J. Psychiatry*, **155**: 899–904.

86. Smith L.B., Sapers B., Reus V.I., Freimer N.B. (1996) Attitudes towards bipolar disorder and predictive genetic testing among patients and providers. *J. Med. Genet.*, **33**: 544–549.

87. Unutzer J., Simon G., Pabinak C., Bond K., Katon W. (1998) The treated prevalence of bipolar disorder in a large staff-model HMO. *Psychiatr. Serv.*, **49**: 1072–1078.

88. Sharfstein S.S. (1994) Capitation versus decapitation in mental health care. *Hosp. Commun. Psychiatry*, **45**: 1065.
89. McFarland B.H., Johnson R.E., Hornbrook M.C. (1996) Enrollment duration, service use, and costs of care for severely mentally ill members of a health maintenance organization. *Arch. Gen. Psychiatry*, **53**: 938–944.
90. Marcus S.C., Olfson M., Pincus H.A., Zarin D.A., Kupfer D.J. (1999) Therapeutic drug monitoring of mood stabilizers in Medicaid patients with bipolar disorder. *Am. J. Psychiatry*, **156**: 1014–1018.
91. Frances A., Docherty J.P., Kahn D.A. (1996) The Expert Consensus Guideline Series: treatment of bipolar disorder. *J. Clin. Psychiatry*, **57** (Suppl. 12A): 1–88.
92. Ried L.D., Horn J.R., McKenna D.A. (1990) Therapeutic drug monitoring reduces toxic drug reactions: a meta-analysis. *Ther. Drug Monit.*, **12**: 72–78.
93. Thomas M.R., Kassner C.T., Fryer G.E., Giese A.A., Rosenberg S.A., Dubovsky S.L. (1997) Impact of shorter lengths of stay on status at discharge in bipolar mania. *Ann. Clin. Psychiatry*, **9**: 139–143.
94. Quinlivan R., Hough R., Crowell A., Beach C., Hofstetter R., Kenworthy K. (1995) Service utilization and costs of care for severely mentally ill clients in an intensive case management program. *Psychiatr. Serv.*, **46**: 365–371.
95. Rakfeldt J., Tebes J.K., Steiner J., Walker P.L., Davidson L., Sledge W.H. (1997) Normalizing acute care: a day hospital/crisis residence alternative to inpatient hospitalization. *J. Nerv. Ment. Dis.*, **185**: 46–52.
96. Chandler D., Meisel J., Hu T.W., McGowen M., Madison K. (1996) Client outcomes in a three-year controlled study of an integrated service agency model. *Psychiatr. Serv.*, **47**: 1337–1343.
97. Simon G.E., Unutzer J. (1999) Health care utilization and costs among patients treated for bipolar disorder in an uninsured population. *Psychiatr. Serv.*, **50**: 1303–1308.
98. Bauer M.S., Shea N., McBride L., Gavin C. (1997) Predictors of service utilization with bipolar disorder: A prospective study. *J. Affect. Disord.*, **44**: 159–168.
99. Goldberg J.F. (2000) Treatment guidelines: current and future management of bipolar disorder. *J. Clin. Psychiatry*, **61** (Suppl. 13): 12–18.
100. Katon W., von Korff M., Lin E., Walker E., Simon G.E., Bush T., Robinson P., Russo J. (1995) Collaborative management to achieve treatment guidelines. Impact on depression in primary care. *JAMA*, **273**: 1026–1031.
101. McElroy S.L., Altshuler L.L., Suppes T., Keck P.E. Jr., Frye M.A., Denicoff K.D., Nolen W.A., Kupka R.W., Leverich G.S., Rochussen J.R. *et al* (2001) Axis I psychiatric comorbidity and its relationship to historical illness variables in 288 patients with bipolar disorder. *Am. J. Psychiatry*, **158**: 420–426.
102. Strakowski S.M., McElroy S.L., Keck P.E. Jr., West S.A. (1994) The co-occurrence of mania with medical and other psychiatric disorders. *Int. J. Psychiatry Med.*, **24**: 305–328.
103. Ananth J., Vandewater S., Kamal M., Brodsky A., Gamal R., Miller M. (1989) Missed diagnosis of substance abuse in psychiatric patients. *Hosp. Commun. Psychiatry*, **40**: 297–299.
104. Lehman A.F., Myers C.P., Corty E. (1989) Assessment and classification of patients with psychiatric and substance abuse syndromes. *Hosp. Commun. Psychiatry*, **40**: 1019–1025.
105. Tondo L., Baldessarini R.J. (2000) Reduced suicide risk during lithium maintenance treatment. *J. Clin. Psychiatry*, **61** (Suppl. 9): 97–104.
106. Keck P.E. Jr., McElroy S.L., Tugrul K.C., Bennett J.A. (1993) Valproate oral loading in the treatment of acute mania. *J. Clin. Psychiatry*, **45**: 305–308.

107. Keck P.E. Jr., Strakowski S.M., Hawkins J.M., Dunayevich E., Tugrul K.C., Bennett J.A., McElroy S.L. (2001) A pilot study of rapid Lithobid administration in the treatment of acute mania. *Bipolar Disord.*, **3**: 68–72.

108. Goldberg J.F., Garno J.L., Leon A.C., Kocsis J.H., Portera L. (1998) Rapid titration of mood stabilizers predicts remission from mixed or pure mania. *J. Clin. Psychiatry*, **59**: 151–158.

109. Hodgson T.A., Meiners M.R. (1982) Cost-of-illness methodology: a guide to current practices and procedures. *Milbank Quarterly*, **60**: 429–462.

110. Hodgson T.A. (1994) Costs of illness in cost-effectiveness analysis: a review of the methodology. *PharmacoEconomics*, **6**: 536–552.

111. Regier D.A., Myers J.K., Kramer M., Robins L.N., Blazer D.G., Hough R.L., Eaton W.W., Locke B.Z. (1984) The NIMH Epidemiologic Catchment Area program. Historical context, major objectives, and study population characteristics. *Arch. Gen. Psychiatry*, **41**: 934–941.

112. Kessler R.C., McGonagle K.A., Zhao S., Nelson C.B., Hughes M., Eshelman S., Wittchen H.U., Kendler K.S. (1994) Lifetime and 12-month prevalence of DSM-III-R psychiatric disorders in the United States: results from the National Comorbidity Survey. *Arch. Gen. Psychiatry*, **51**: 8–19.

113. Vieta E., Martinez G., Fernandez A., Gasto C. (1999) Risperidone treatment of bipolar disorder: findings of a 6-month open-label study in Spain. Presented at the 152nd Annual Meeting of the American Psychiatric Association, San Diego, May 15–20.

114. Zarate C.A. Jr., Tohen M. (2000) Antipsychotic drug treatment in first-episode mania: a 6-month longitudinal study. *J. Clin. Psychiatry*, **61**: 33–38.

115. Tohen M.F., Jacobs T.G., Meyers T.M., Risser R.C., Keeter E.L., Breier P.D. (2000) Efficacy of olanzapine combined with mood stabilizers in the treatment of bipolar disorder. Presented at the 153rd Annual Meeting of the American Psychiatric Association, Chicago, May 13–18.

116. Müller-Oerlinghausen B., Retzow A., Henn F.A., Giedke H., Walden J. (2000) Valproate as an adjunct to neuroleptic medication for the treatment of acute episodes of mania: a prospective, randomized, double-blind, placebo-controlled, multicenter study. *J. Clin. Psychopharmacol.*, **20**: 195–203.

117. Akiskal H.S., Pinto O. (1999) The evolving bipolar spectrum: prototypes I, II, III and IV. *Psychiatr. Clin. North Am.*, **22**: 517–534.

118. Angst J. (1998) The emerging epidemiology of hypomania and bipolar II disorder. *J. Affect. Disord.*, **50**: 143–151.

119. Baldessarini R.J. (2000) A plea for the integrity of the bipolar concept. *Bipolar Disord.*, **2**: 3–7.

120. Heller T., Roccoforte J.A., Hsieh K., Cook J.A., Pickett S.A. (1997) Benefits of support groups for families of adults with severe mental illness. *Am. J. Orthopsychiatry*, **67**: 187–198.

121. Viguera A.C., Nonacs R., Cohen L.S., Tondo L., Murray A., Baldessarini R.J. (2000) Risk of recurrence of bipolar disorder in pregnant and nonpregnant women after discontinuing lithium maintenance. *Am. J. Psychiatry*, **157**: 179–184.

122. Goldberg J.F., Sacks M.H., Kocsis J.H. (2000) Low-dose lithium augmentation of divalproex in geriatric mania. *J. Clin. Psychiatry*, **61**: 304.

123. Goldberg J.F. (2000) Treatment of bipolar disorders. *Psychiatr. Clin. N. Am. Ann. Drug Therapy*, **7**: 115–149.

124. DelBello M.P., Soutullo C.A., Henricks W., Niemeier R.T., McElroy S.L., Strakowski S.M. (2001) Prior stimulant treatment in adolescents with bipolar disorder: association with age at onset. *Bipolar Disord.*, **3**: 53–57.

125. Stahl S.M. (2001)   Does evidence from clinical trials in psychopharmacology apply in clinical practice? *J. Clin. Psychiatry*, **62**: 6–7.
126. Robinson D.S., Rickels K. (2000)   Concerns about clinical drug trials. *J. Clin. Psychopharmacol.*, **20**: 593–596.
127. Goldman W., McCulloch J., Cuffel B., Zarin D.A., Suarez A., Burns B.J. (1998)   Outpatient utilization patterns of integrated and split psychotherapy and pharmacotherapy for depression. *Psychiatr. Serv.*, **49**: 477–482.
128. Dewan M. (2000)   Are psychiatrists cost-effective? An analysis of integrated versus split treatment. *Am. J. Psychiatry*, **156**: 324–326.
129. Drake R.E., Goldman H.H., Leff H.S., Lehman A.F., Dixon L., Mueser K.T., Torrey W.C. (2001)   Implementing evidence-based practices in routine mental health service settings. *Psychiatr. Serv.*, **52**: 179–182.
130. Shon S.P., Crimson M.L., Toprac M.G., Trivedi M., Miller A.L., Suppes T., Rush A.J. (1999)   Mental health care from the public perspective: the Texas Medication Algorithm Project. *J. Clin. Psychiatry*, **60** (Suppl. 3): 16–20.

Commentaries

6.1
What is the True Cost of Bipolar Disorder?
Paul E. Keck, Jr[1]

Much has been and should be made of the findings of *The Global Burden of Disease* project which revealed that major psychiatric disorders accounted for five of the 10 most common causes of disability worldwide in 1990 [1]. Without improved treatment access, adherence and advances, these disorders were projected to remain causes of profound disability well into this century. Among these illnesses, bipolar disorder was ranked as the sixth leading cause. This clearly is bad news. Goldberg and Ernst have compiled their scholarly and encyclopaedic review of the economic and social burden of bipolar disorder from the available studies conducted in this area to date. Notably, they conclude their review with an important call to arms for new research in desperately understudied areas.

Epidemiology. Bipolar disorder is a recurrent severe psychiatric disorder that usually begins in late adolescence and early adulthood. Thus, it is commonly a lifelong malady. Epidemiological studies conducted around the globe yield remarkably similar lifetime prevalence rates of approximately 1% for bipolar I disorder [2]. Recent surveys suggest that when bipolar II disorder and cyclothymic disorder are included, the lifetime prevalence rates of bipolar disorders may exceed 3% [3]. This potent combination of common prevalence, lifelong duration, morbidity associated with mood episodes and subsyndromal symptoms between episodes, and lag in functional recovery behind syndromal and symptomatic recovery contributes to disability from bipolar disorder [4]. This illness is also associated with a significant risk of suicide. Fortunately bipolar disorder is a highly treatable illness and the economic costs of untreated illness far outweigh those associated with treatment.

Economic and occupational illness burden. Occupational function is a common casualty of bipolar disorder. In a recent survey of patients with bipolar disorder conducted by the US National Depressive and Manic-Depressive Association (NDMDA), more than 80% of respondents stated

[1] *Department of Psychiatry, University of Cincinnati College of Medicine, 231 Albert Sabin Way, ML 559, Cincinnati, OH 45267–0559, USA*

that bipolar disorder detracted from their ability to perform at work and 79% indicated that their illness had foreshortened their career goals [5]. Nearly 40% reported that they had stopped working outside the home due to their illness. The economic impact study of Begeley *et al* uncovered an important difference in lifetime costs between those patients who had only one manic episode and a stable course (average lifetime cost $11 720 in 1998 dollars) and those with chronic, treatment-nonresponsive manifestations of the illness ($624 785) [6]. In other words, the cost of multiple episodes and a chronic course of illness was a staggering 53 times higher than for individuals with limited episodes and protracted periods of euthymia. These direct cost estimates do not capture the enormous collateral damage or indirect costs of bipolar disorder, such as divorce, bankruptcy, criminal violence, caretaker morbidity, injuries and accidents, gambling and other impulse control disorders, and the devastating sequelae of comorbid alcoholism and substance use disorders.

Misdiagnosis and illness detection. The stark contrast in the cost of well-managed and treatment-responsive illness versus chronic, recurrent, treatment-resistant illness described above underscores the need for early detection and treatment interventions. Unfortunately, even recent data indicate that an average of approximately 10 years lapse between illness onset and accurate diagnosis for patients with bipolar disorder [6, 7]. These delays in diagnosis and treatment can wreck havoc on people's lives and lead to violence and suicide. In the US, there has been no national public education effort about bipolar disorder similar to that deployed for depression in the 1990s. The NDMDA has been one of few organizations to take on this important role. Improved public understanding and awareness of the signs and symptoms of bipolar disorder are extremely important factors in getting patients to treatment early and preventing the costs in human suffering associated with untreated illness and treatment refractoriness associated with multiple episodes.

Increased public awareness needs to be coupled with improved diagnostic precision and vigilance by mental health professionals. The recent NDMDA survey found that bipolar disorder was not accurately diagnosed in 69% of patients upon initial presentation to a psychiatrist for treatment [5]. A diagnosis of bipolar disorder can be difficult to establish when patients present for treatment of depressive episodes because of the frequent comorbidity of other psychiatric disorders (e.g., alcohol and substance use disorders, anxiety, impulse control and eating disorders). Obtaining a history of hypomanic or manic symptoms can be difficult due to under-reporting, lack of recognition or simply not asking. Recently, the first diagnostic screening tool for bipolar disorder, the Mood Disorders Questionnaire (MDQ) developed jointly by the NDMDA and the National

Alliance for the Mentally Ill (NAMI), was published and represents an important step in rigorously including an assessment for bipolar features in patients presenting for psychiatric treatment [8].

Childhood bipolar disorder. Early recognition, diagnosis and treatment begin with improved understanding of the manifestations and prodromal symptoms of bipolar disorder in children and adolescents. Only 20 years ago, psychodynamic theories posited that mood disorders *per se* could not present in childhood. Much enlightenment has ensued since then, but clinical research in the phenomenology and treatment of bipolar disorder in children and adolescents is still in its infancy. Early intervention initiatives such as those sponsored by the Stanley Foundation should help to identify children at risk and improve preventative strategies [7].

Forensic issues. Perhaps the most scandalously ignored consequence of untreated bipolar disorder is violence and other behaviour resulting in criminal convictions. Conservative estimates place the prevalence of bipolar disorder in correctional facilities at least at 10% [9]. The few available data suggest that these individuals often are not diagnosed and poorly treated or untreated. Many prison formularies are restricted to older, less expensive medications. Effective integration of state mental health and correctional services is so rare as to be remarkable when a pilot model is established.

Pharmacoeconomics and pharmacotherapies. Goldberg and Ernst correctly point out that nearly all major pharmacological treatment advances for patients with bipolar disorder resulted from clinical trials sponsored by pharmaceutical companies "rather than government, private foundations, or other economically impartial agencies". The neglect of treatment research by the latter sources of research support is beginning to be addressed. The Stanley Foundation currently funds more treatment research in bipolar disorder annually than the US National Institute of Mental Health (NIMH). The NIMH is sponsoring a much-needed long-term treatment effectiveness multi-site trial, the STEP-BD initiative. However, greater funding dedicated to treatment research is sorely needed.

Goldberg and Ernst point out that medications or medication dosing strategies that can rapidly achieve symptom remission in patients with acute affective episodes might bring the dual rewards of promptly alleviating human suffering and saving substantial treatment costs. This is an aspect of psychopharmacology that has recently been studied. Rapid loading studies of lithium [10] and divalproex [11], and a rapid titration trial of ziprasidone [12], as well as naturalistic data support the notion that "pharmacotherapies which can be optimized swiftly near the onset of an episode may lead to better outcomes than the same therapies under-dosed or used in too slow a dose escalation strategy".

A number of new medications (e.g., new antiepileptics and atypical anti-psychotics) offer promise as potential treatments for aspects of bipolar disorder. In addition to important questions about the comparative efficacy and safety of these agents, inevitable pharmacoeconomic questions will also arise. These will be important in not only justifying their use, but also in making them accessible to patients with bipolar disorder globally. Better techniques for measuring treatment costs are needed, in representative clinical settings, using multiple treatment paradigms (e.g., monotherapy or combination therapy) to fully understand the impact of and improve on these interventions.

REFERENCES

1. Murray C.J.L., Lopez A.D. (1996)   *The Global Burden of Disease*. Harvard School of Public Health, Cambridge.
2. Weissman M.M., Bland R.C., Canino G.J., Faravelli C., Greenwald S., Hwu H.G., Joyce P.R., Karam E.G., Lee C.K., Lellough J. *et al* (1996). Cross-national epidemiology of major depression and bipolar disorder. *JAMA*, **276**: 293–299.
3. Akiskal H.S., Maser J.D., Zeller P.J., Endicott J., Coryell W., Keller M., Warshaw M., Clayton P., Goodwin F. (1995)   Switching from "unipolar" to bipolar II: an 11 year prospective study of clinical and temperamental predictors in 559 patients. *Arch. Gen. Psychiatry*, **52**: 114–123.
4. Keck P.E., McElroy S.L., Strakowski S.M., West S.A., Sax K.W., Hawkins J.M., Bourne M.L., Haggard P. (1998)   Twelve-month outcome of bipolar patients following hospitalization for a manic or mixed episode. *Am. J. Psychiatry*, **155**: 646–652.
5. Lewis L.L. (2001)   Patient perceptions of bipolar illness: results of a national survey. Presented at the 154th Annual Meeting of the American Psychiatric Association, New Orleans, 5–9 May.
6. Begeley C.E., Annegers J.F., Swann A.C., Lewis C., Coan S., Schnapp W.B., Bryant-Comstock L. (2001)   The lifetime cost of bipolar disorder in the United States: an estimate based on incidence and course of illness. *Pharmacoeconomics* **19** (5 Pt 1): 483-495, 2001.
7. Post R.M. (2001)   Update on Stanley Foundation programs in bipolar disorder. Presented at the Fourth International Conference on Bipolar Disorder, Pittsburgh, June 14–16.
8. Hirschfeld R.M.A., Williams J.B.W., Spitzer R.L., Calabrese J.R., Flynn L., Keck P.E., Jr., McElroy S.L., Lewis L., Post R.M., Russell J.M. *et al* (2000)   Development and validation of a screening instrument for bipolar spectrum disorder: the Mood Disorder Questionnaire. *Am. J. Psychiatry*, **157**: 1873–1875.
9. Good M.I. (1979)   Primary affective disorder, aggression, and criminality. *Arch. Gen. Psychiatry*, **35**: 954–960.
10. Keck P.E., Jr., Strakowski S.M., Hawkins J.M., Dunayevich E., Tugrul K.C., Bennett J.A., McElroy S.L. (2001)   A pilot study of rapid lithium administration in the treatment of acute mania. *Bipolar Disord.*, **3**: 68–72.
11. Hirschfeld R.M.A., Allen M.H., McEvoy J., Keck P.E., Jr., Russell J. (1999)   Safety and tolerability of oral loading divalproex sodium in acutely manic bipolar patients. *J. Clin. Psychiatry*, **60**: 815–818.

12. Keck P.E., Jr., Ice K.N., and the Ziprasidone Study Group (2000). A double-blind, placebo-controlled trial of ziprasidone in the treatment of acute mania. Presented at the 53rd Annual Meeting of the American Psychiatric Association, Chicago, 14–17 May.

6.2

Reducing the Social and Economic Burden of Bipolar Disorder

Jürgen Unützer[1]

Goldberg and Ernst provide a comprehensive overview of the tremendous social and economic burden associated with bipolar affective disorder. Most of the studies reviewed involve adults with bipolar disorder who live in community settings in the United States and receive treatment in specialty mental health facilities. Less seems to be known about the impact of bipolar disorder in other settings of care, in other countries, in children, adolescents, older adults, or institutionalized persons.

While bipolar disorder is less common than unipolar depression, it is more common than many clinicians suspect and often missed or misdiagnosed for years before a diagnosis is made. Compared to unipolar major depression, most treatment for bipolar disorder occurs not in primary care but in the mental health care sector. However, there may be important opportunities to identify the disorder in settings outside of mental health such as primary care, schools, and correctional institutions.

Goldberg and Ernst go beyond epidemiology and disease burden to discuss the availability and potential impact of current treatments on the burden associated with bipolar disorder. Their review suggests that good treatments are available and that such treatments, if properly used, should be associated with a substantial reduction in the disease burden associated with bipolar disorder. This is, however, hard to prove, and there is little evidence of such reductions on a population level. There is a substantial literature to suggest that residual symptoms and persistent social, family, and occupational dysfunction are common, even in treated bipolar patients [1–5].

There is a substantial gap between the efficacy of treatments for bipolar disorder in carefully conducted research studies and the effectiveness of treatments for bipolar patients in the real world [6], but we know little about the factors responsible for this gap. Goldberg and Ernst discuss the lack of adherence to treatments that may be associated with poor outcomes for as many as 50% of treated patients [7–10]. In addition to nonadherence to

[1] *Center for Health Services Research, Neuropsychiatric Institute, University of California at Los Angeles, 10920 Wilshire Boulevard, Suite 300, Los Angeles, CA 90024, USA*

medications, there is insufficient continuity in the treatment of bipolar individuals even in organized systems of care [11–12]. Much research remains to be done to help us understand patient, provider, practice, and policy barriers to the effective use of evidence-based treatments for bipolar disorder.

Goldberg and Ernst point out that much of the recent literature on the cost-effectiveness of treatments for bipolar disorder comes from pharmacoeconomic modelling exercises sponsored by pharmaceutical companies. Such studies have a number of limitations, including selection bias and assumptions about patient and provider behaviour that may not be representative of the real world. For example, most studies of treatment efficacy exclude patients with significant comorbid medical, alcohol, or substance use disorders, all common problems for bipolar patients in the real world. Pharmacoeconomic studies tend to focus on the choice of specific antimanic agents as the key independent variable, even though medications only account for a portion of the overall treatment costs and patients in the real world frequently switch from one agent to another or take combinations of psychotropic drugs.

Similar limitations may apply to the usefulness of treatment algorithms for bipolar disorder. Many algorithms are based on efficacy studies of selected subjects who are initiating one monotherapy versus another. Such algorithms may provide only limited guidance for the many patients who are on guideline-level doses of one or two mood stabilizers and an antidepressant and who continue to experience subthreshold hypomanic and depressive symptoms that substantially impair their functioning.

In recent years, a number of disease management models have been developed to improve care for real-world samples of patients with depression [13–14] and other chronic illnesses [15]. We should try to adapt such models of chronic illness care to meet the special challenges in the care of bipolar disorder. Much work remains to be done to determine the optimal combination of public policies, public health and community interventions, clinical programmes of care involving both patients and significant others, and specific pharmacologic and psychosocial treatments that are needed in order to reduce the tremendous economic and social burden associated with bipolar disorder.

REFERENCES

1. Maj M. (2000) The impact of lithium prophylaxis on the course of bipolar disorder: a review of the research evidence. *Bipolar Disord.*, **2**: 93–101.
2. Kulhara P., Basu D., Mattoo S.K., Sharan P., Chopra R. (1999) Lithium prophylaxis of recurrent bipolar affective disorder: long-term outcome and its psychological correlates. *J. Affect. Disord.*, **54**: 87–96.

3. Harrow M., Goldberg J.F., Grossman L.S., Meltzer H.Y. (1990) Outcome in manic disorders. A naturalistic follow-up study. *Arch. Gen. Psychiatry*, **47**: 665–671.
4. Gitlin M.J., Swendsen J., Heller T.L., Hammen C. (1996) Relapse and impairment in bipolar disorder. *Am. J. Psychiatry*, **152**: 1635–1640.
5. Keck P.E., Jr., McElroy S.L., Strakowski S.M., West S.A., Sax K.W., Hawkins J.M., Bourne M.L., Haggard P. (1998) 12–month outcome of patients with bipolar disorder following hospitalization for a manic or mixed episode. *Am. J. Psychiatry*, **155**: 646–652.
6. Guscott R., Taylor L. (1994) Lithium prophylaxis in recurrent affective illness. Efficacy, effectiveness, and efficiency. *Br. J. Psychiatry*, **164**: 741–746.
7. Gitlin M.J., Cochran S.D., Jamison K.R. (1990) Maintenance lithium treatment: side effects and compliance. *J. Clin. Psychiatry*, **50**: 127–131.
8. Lee S., Wing Y.K., Wong K.C. (1992) Knowledge and compliance towards lithium therapy among Chinese psychiatric patients in Hong Kong. *Aust. N.Z. J. Psychiatry*, **26**: 444–449.
9. Keck P.E., Jr., McElroy S.L., Strakowski S.M., Stanton S.P., Kizer D.L., Balisteri T.M., Bennett J.A., Tugrul K.C., West S.A. (1996) Factors associated with pharmacologic noncompliance in patients with mania. *J. Clin. Psychiatry*, **57**: 292–297.
10. Schumann C., Lenz G., Berghofer A., Müller-Oerlinghausen B. (1999) Nonadherence with long-term lithium prophylaxis: a 6–year naturalistic follow-up study of affectively ill patients. *Psychiatry Res.*, **89**: 247–257.
11. Johnson R.E., McFarland B.H. (1996) Lithium use and discontinuation in a health maintenance organization. *Am. J. Psychiatry*, **153**: 993–1000.
12. Unützer J., Simon G.E., Pabiniak C., Bond K., Katon W. (2000) The use of administrative data to assess quality of care for bipolar disorder in a large staff model HMO. *Gen. Hosp. Psychiatry*, **22**: 1–10.
13. Katon W.J., Von Korff M., Lin E.H.B., Unützer J., Simon G., Walker G.E., Ludman E., Bush T. (1997) Population-based care of depression: effective disease management strategies to decrease prevalence. *Gen. Hosp. Psychiatry*, **19**: 169–178.
14. Wells K.B., Sherbourne C., Schoenbaum M., Duan N., Meredith L., Unützer J., Miranda J., Carney M.F., Rubenstein L.V. (2000) Impact of disseminating quality improvement programs for depression in managed primary care: a randomized controlled trial. *JAMA*, **283**: 212–220.
15. Von Korff M., Gruman J., Schaefer J., Curry S.J., Wagner E.H. (1997) Collaborative management of chronic illness. *Ann. Intern. Med.*, **127**: 1097–1102.

6.3
Why We Care About the Economic and Social Burden of Bipolar Disorder
Gregory E. Simon[1]

Our interest in the economic and social burden of bipolar disorder is not primarily motivated by scientific curiosity. Instead, we hope to use data on the burden of illness to influence public policy and identify priority areas for clinical and quality improvement.

[1] *Center for Health Studies, Group Health Cooperative, 1730 Minor Ave. #1600, Seattle, WA, USA*

Continued discrimination against those with mental disorders depends on a series of prejudicial assumptions. The first is that mental disorders have relatively minor consequences compared to general medical conditions. The second is that adverse consequences of mental disorders are relatively fixed, with little potential for improvement. The third is that psychiatric treatments are relatively ineffective—and therefore a poor investment of societal resources.

Regarding the first of these assumptions, Goldberg and Ernst clearly describe the large economic and social burden associated with bipolar disorder. Costs to the health care system include modest increases in use of general medical services and a large burden of inpatient psychiatric costs and costs due to substance use disorders—both of which might be reduced by more appropriate treatment. Social costs include decreased work participation, increased work absenteeism, lost productivity due to suicide, costs associated with crime and the criminal justice system. Major elements of burden that are difficult to express in monetary units include decreased educational attainment, marital instability, and family burden. Unfortunately, few of the data available allow direct comparison of the burden associated with bipolar disorder to that associated with general medical conditions. In contrast, research on unipolar depression has long focused on such explicit comparisons. Evidence that the burden of depression equals or exceeds that of medical conditions traditionally viewed as more "serious" [1, 2] has been an important tool in the struggle for more equitable treatment of depressive disorders.

Regarding the second of these assumptions, fewer data are available regarding the "economic and social" prognosis of bipolar disorder. Addressing this question will require data on synchrony of change (i.e., is improvement in mood symptoms associated with improvement in various measures of burden?) rather than cross-sectional association (i.e., comparison of people with bipolar disorder to control or comparison samples without). Nearly all of the studies reviewed by Goldberg and Ernst were cross-sectional in design. One exception is the National Depressive and Manic-Depressive Association survey [3] showing marked improvements in psychosocial function following initiation of treatment.

Regarding the third assumption, available data are insufficient to support strong conclusions regarding the effects of treatment for bipolar disorder on health services utilization, functional impairment/disability, and family burden. Demonstrating the effects of treatment (on either clinical or economic outcomes) requires data from true experiments or randomized trials. Abundant experimental evidence supports the clinical efficacy of specific pharmacotherapy, and emerging evidence supports the efficacy of specific psychosocial treatments. Traditional clinical trials, however, have rarely evaluated reduction in economic or social burden as an outcome of treatment. One notable exception is Gelenberg's comparison of more and less intensive lithium treatment [4] demonstrating improved psychosocial function among those receiving more intensive pharmacotherapy. Goldberg and Ernst use data from observational studies to argue that improved treatment (either expanding access to treatment or increasing quality among those now treated) could lead to substantial economic gains. While it is likely that this argument will be proven correct, it is also unlikely that evidence currently available is strong enough to change policy. Research on the effectiveness and cost-effectiveness of treatments for unipolar depression is several years ahead of similar research on treatments for bipolar disorder. In the area of unipolar depression, recent randomized trials have demonstrated that improved depression treatment improves daily functioning [5], increases work productivity [6, 7], and can be considered cost-effective when compared to generally accepted medical treatments [8, 9]. We can hope that the next generation of effectiveness trials for bipolar disorder will produce similar evidence.

The second motivation for our interest in the economic and social burden of bipolar disorder is our interest in improving the quality of current clinical care. Two questions are relevant here. The first concerns the identification of priority populations for care improvement efforts. The second concerns the differential effects of specific treatments on measures of economic and social burden.

Regarding the first question, data on burden of illness can help to identify clinical populations in which expanded access to treatment or improved quality of treatment might produce the greatest societal benefit. While clinical research and decision making often focus on symptom reduction, symptoms alone may not be an adequate measure of the impact of a disorder or the effects of treatment. From the perspective of patients and families, restoration of function may actually be a more important goal than symptom change. One example of burden-of-illness research helping to establish clinical priorities is the impact of research on impairment associated with residual symptoms of mood disorders. Studies demonstrating the impact of persistent subthreshold mood symptoms [10, 11] have helped to re-orient clinicians toward complete remission (rather than modest improvement) as the goal of mood disorder treatment.

Regarding the second question (comparisons of economic outcomes for alternative treatments), Goldberg and Ernst review recent data regarding alternative mood stabilizers. Most of the studies reviewed were retrospective analyses of existing records data or decision-analytic models. Such designs do not support strong enough conclusions to warrant significant changes in practice or policy. The single randomized comparison (of divalproex vs. olanzapine for acute mania) [12] is difficult to interpret given high drop-out rates in both groups. Valid economic comparisons of alternative treatments will require representative samples, random assignment of treatment, high follow-up rates, and sufficient sample sizes to permit cost comparisons.

REFERENCES

1. Wells K., Stewart A., Hays R., Burnam M., Rogers W., Daniels M., Berry S., Greenfield S., Ware J. (1989) The functioning and well-being of depressed patients: results from the Medical Outcome Study. *JAMA*, **262**: 914–919.
2. Wells K., Golding J., Burnam M.A. (1988) Psychiatric disorder and limitations in physical functioning in a sample of the Los Angeles general population. *Am. J. Psychiatry*, **145**: 712–717.
3. Lish J., Dime-Meenan S., Whybrow P., Price R., Hirschfeld R. (1994) The National Depressive and Manic-Depressive Association (DMDA) survey of bipolar members. *J. Affect. Disord.*, **31**: 281–294.
4. Solomon D., Ristow R., Keller M., Kane J., Gelenberg A., Rosenbaum J., Warshaw M. (1996) Serum lithium levels and psychosocial function in patients with bipolar I disorder. *Am. J. Psychiatry*, **153**: 1301–1307.
5. Coulehan J., Schulberg H., Block M., Madonia M., Rodriguez E. (1997) Treating depressed primary care patients improves their physical, mental, and social functioning. *Arch. Intern. Med.*, **157**: 1113–1120.
6. Mintz J., Mintz L.I., Arruda M.J., Hwang S.S. (1992) Treatments of depression and the functional capacity to work. *Arch. Gen. Psychiatry*, **49**: 761–768.
7. Wells K., Sherbourne C., Schoenbaum M., Duan N., Meredith L., Unützer J., Miranda J., Carney M., Rubenstein L. (2000) Impact of disseminating quality improvement programs for depression in managed primary care: a randomized controlled trial. *JAMA*, **283**: 212–230.
8. Simon G., Katon W., von Korff M., Unützer J., Lin E., Walker E., Bush T., Rutter C., Ludman E. (2001) Cost-effectiveness of a Collaborative Care program for primary care patients with persistent depression. *Am. J. Psychiatry* (in press).
9. Simon G., Manning W., Katzelnick D., Perarson S., Henk H., Helstad C. (2001) Cost-effectiveness of systematic depression treatment for high utilizers of general medical care. *Arch. Gen. Psychiatry*, **58**: 181–187.
10. Coryell W., Scheftner W., Keller M., Endicott J., Maser J., Klerman G.L. (1993) The enduring psychosocial consequences of mania and depression. *Am. J. Psychiatry*, **150**: 720–727.
11. Judd L., Akiskal H., Zeller P., Paulus M., Leon A., Maser J., Endicott J., Coryell W., Kunovac J., Mueller T. *et al* (2000) Psychosocial disability during the long-term course of unipolar major depressive disorder. *Arch. Gen. Psychiatry*, **57**: 375–380.
12. Zajecka J., Weisler R., Sommerville K. (2000) Divalproex sodium versus olanzapine for the treatment of mania in bipolar disorder. Presented at the 39th Annual Meeting of the American College of Neuropsychopharmacology, San Juan, December 10–14.

6.4

The Importance of Boundaries and Comorbidities on Morbidity and Mortality: An Urgent Case for Early and Continuous Treatment

Paula J. Clayton[1]

Mania is derived from a Greek word meaning "to be mad" and the description of such patients dates back to Greek times. If we assume that names are

[1] *University of Minnesota School of Medicine, 231 Paseo de la Tierra, Santa Fe, New Mexico 87506, USA*

given to illnesses in an attempt to organize clinical information, then we can also assume that the occurrence and recognition of manic patients was apparent to clinicians throughout history. When we defined mania and stressed the psychotic symptoms, we were calling attention to an illness with features similar to schizophrenia, but that had an episodic course [1]. This was further elaborated in the textbook that followed [2]. Although the illness is now easily recognized, we are still struggling to define its boundaries. And the boundaries fix not only the prevalence, but also the burden of the illness. Goldberg and Ernst recognize this conflict and try to discuss the burden of the illness in regard to symptoms (pure versus mixed mania, bipolar I and II, psychotic versus nonpsychotic, mania that includes schizoaffective mania, etc.), to age (childhood versus adolescence versus adult), to comorbidity and to select study populations. If we expand the boundaries as we now seem to want to do, then the World Health Organisation disability projections, as quoted by Goldberg and Ernst, will only be greater. But even with the more conservative definitions, the illness, worldwide, is one of the 10 leading causes of temporary and permanent disability. Premature death also occurs. Recent data by Angst *et al* corroborates this [3]. In a 34–38 year follow-up of hospitalized mood disordered patients, they reported that bipolar patients, compared to appropriate controls, have increased death rates from all causes except cancer, but that it is particularly striking for suicide, accidents/intoxications, cardiovascular disorders and all vascular diseases. The most startling finding, however, was that even though the investigators had no influence on the treatment, if the bipolars were treated, most commonly with lithium in combination with antidepressants and/or neuroleptics, but also with lithium alone, neuroleptics plus antidepressants or a monotherapy of neuroleptics or antidepressants, the mortality was significantly lowered. This emphasizes the importance of treatment on outcome, both in regards to morbidity and mortality.

Goldberg and Ernst have provided a thorough and comprehensive review of the ramifications of the illness ranging from the actual cost of treating the illness compared to the cost of missing the diagnosis, applying inappropriate treatments, slow treatments and no treatment. They include the effect each has on outcomes other than symptom remission, such as ability to go to school, to form relationships, to marry, to work, to stay out of trouble and to have the liberty to enjoy life.

Their emphasis on prompt detection and rapid treatment particularly deserves reinforcement. Recently, Keck and his colleagues reviewed articles dealing with pharmacological loading in the treatment of acute mania [4]. They subsequently published a pilot study of rapid lithium administration [5]. The use of neuroleptics and antidepressants in the treatment of bipolar patients also should be stressed.

Since this is a lifelong illness, Goldberg and Ernst's review of psychological treatments calls attention to the crucial need for consistency in the treatment of these patients. Although it is essential for psychiatrists and other mental health workers in training to see and treat these patients, it is probably not in the best interest of these patients, almost more than any other psychiatric patients, to have different physicians or other caretakers every six to 12 months. Although we now have clozapine clinics due to the need of blood monitoring for schizophrenic patients, the old "lithium clinics" for the most part have disappeared and many universities do not even have mood disorder clinics. Whether this makes a difference, of course, is a researchable question.

In their discussion of future research, Goldberg and Ernst acknowledge that an understudied area is the problem of comorbid disease, especially substance abuse. Even without research, it is clear that drug use and abuse influence the morbidity and mortality of the illness. But because the drug use may start as early as the bipolar illness itself, it will have to be investigated by following adolescents in treatment with pure substance abuse, with pure depression and with either episodes of mania or bipolar illness, prospectively. The unclear relationship particularly between alcohol use and cocaine use in these patients needs to be studied. Frequently, the alcohol use is de-emphasized and neglected in the ongoing treatment, yet it may inaugurate episodes of cocaine use and even, by itself, contribute to the morbidity and mortality. These patients, when manic, are extremely intrusive. With drugs, they may become offensive. In the collaborative study of affective disorders, the first patient in the St Louis centre follow-up to die was a manic patient who got in a fight in a bar and was killed during the encounter. Only very detailed monitoring of bipolar patients will answer these questions. Clearly, along with the sophisticated genetic research, there is still a need for straightforward clinical research.

REFERENCES

1. Clayton P.J., Pitts F.N., Winokur G. (1965) Affective disorder. IV. Mania. *Compr. Psychiatry*, **6**: 313–322.
2. Winokur G., Clayton P.J., Reich T. (1969) *Manic-Depressive Illness*. Mosby, St. Louis.
3. Angst F., Stassen H.H., Clayton P.J., Angst J. (2001) Mortality of patients with mood disorders: follow-up over 34 to 38 years. *J. Affect. Disord.* (in press).
4. Keck P.E., McElroy S.L., Bennett J.A. (2000) Pharmacologic loading in the treatment of acute mania. *Bipolar Disord.*, **2**: 42–46.
5. Keck P.E., Strakowski, S.M., Hawkins J.M., Dunayevich E., Tugrul K.C., Bennett J.A., McElroy S.L. (2001) A pilot study of rapid lithium administration in the treatment of acute mania. *Bipolar Disord.*, **3**: 68–72.

6.5
Beyond Pharmacotherapy: The Difficult Lives of Bipolar Individuals

Michael J. Gitlin[1]

Over the last 30 years, treatment approaches in psychiatry in general and bipolar disorder specifically have been dominated by biological thinking, leading to the quest for increasingly effective pharmacotherapies. Given this emphasis, outcome studies focused on measuring symptoms and relapse rates. The effect of bipolar disorder on the lives of those we treated seemed almost irrelevant in our quest for a magic bullet to eradicate the disorder. In the last few years, however, the limitations of this important, understandable but narrow view became evident. Even as the range of pharmacotherapies multiplied, naturalistic studies of bipolar populations showed continued morbidity and marked functional impairment in treated populations [1]. Additionally, economic considerations, both for treatment and to society, became increasingly important. It is timely, therefore, for Goldberg and Ernst to comprehensively produce a broader analysis of bipolar disorder, focusing on its cost—both financial and psychosocial—to individuals, to families and to society. A corollary of this view is the consideration of therapeutic approaches for bipolar individuals that target other than directly diminishing symptoms, such as enhancing occupational and social function.

One of the enormous difficulties in providing pharmacotherapy as the only treatment modality (and a partial explanation for the less than optimal results of treatment in community samples of bipolar disorder) is the difficulty in eliciting adequate treatment adherence that would allow for a medication's efficacy. The recent maintenance treatment study of bipolar disorder by Bowden *et al* exemplifies this issue [2]. Among those ($n = 372$) who were recovered from an acute manic episode (already selected for enhanced compliance) and were randomized to one of three treatments, 29% dropped out of the study because of a mood episode whereas 40% discontinued treatment for other reasons. Thus, in a setting in which patients were followed more closely than is typical in the community, patients are more likely to drop out of treatment than to relapse. Without further attention to compliance issues for bipolar patients, even the best pharmacotherapies will be relatively ineffective, thereby adding substantially to both direct costs and to greater morbidity and indirect costs of the disorder.

Although reviewed more extensively in Chapter 4 of this book, psychotherapies—or, more broadly stated, psychosocial approaches—are central to addressing some of the problems described by Goldberg and Ernst.

───────────

[1] *Department of Psychiatry, University of California at Los Angeles, 300 UCLA Medical Plaza, Suite 2200, Los Angeles, CA 90095, USA*

Goals of these approaches include treatment adherence, diminishing the family stressors so common in families of bipolar individuals, recognizing the prodromal signs of mania, maintaining the kinds of lifestyles (e.g., regular sleep patterns) that minimize the likelihood of manic episodes, and helping patients re-enter the workplace in a manner that maximizes the chances for success. As noted in the chapter, integrated treatment of this type is associated with fewer hospitalizations and better psychosocial outcome, but also higher direct costs. Whether these increased directs are offset by savings in indirect costs is unclear. Yet, even if direct costs were documented to be offset by savings in fewer missed days of work, greater productivity at work, less need for government financial assistance and so forth, linking the two is problematic. Saving money in one pot will not necessarily translate into transferring that money into another pot which is guarded by different pot-keepers with different priorities. Integrated services must be matched by integrated book-keeping for optimal progress.

Goldberg and Ernst review the studies that document the functional disability of bipolar patients. Of equal interest is the evidence of a disparity between syndromal and functional outcome in these patients, i.e. bipolar individuals get better from episodes according to symptom rating scales, yet their lives—as measured by occupational or psychosocial ratings—do not improve in concert [3]. The reasons for this disparity are still unclear. Possibilities acting individually or in concert include: the effect of subsyndromal symptoms, neurocognitive deficits, the toxic effects of the poor social support common to bipolar individuals, and demoralization associated with fear of relapse. Studies examining the role of these factors in explaining the poorer level of functional vs. syndromal outcome in bipolar individuals will help target appropriate interventions to combat these negative prognostic factors.

As we attempt to disentangle the multiple causes for the psychosocial dysfunction associated with bipolar disorder, another fruitful area to consider is the potential differential effects of manic vs. depressive symptoms. Some studies have suggested that depressive symptoms—both as part of a major depression but also at a subsyndromal level—may be more associated with functional disruption, but the data are far from clear. It is also possible that the effects of depressive symptoms on occupational dysfunction might be mediated by neurocognitive deficits [4].

Finally, virtually all studies in the areas of occupational and psychosocial dysfunction in bipolar disorder have examined those with bipolar I disorder. Yet, some recent data have suggested that bipolar II disorder, in which the manic states are by definition less severe but the depressions of at least equal severity compared to bipolar I disorder, may be more common [5]. If so, then comparing bipolar I vs. bipolar II patients may allow us to better understand the relative effects of mania vs. depression on functional outcome.

REFERENCES

1. Gitlin M.J., Swendsen J., Heller T.L., Hammen C. (1995) Relapse and impairment in bipolar disorder. *Am. J. Psychiatry*, **152**: 1638–1640.
2. Bowden C.L., Calabrese J.R., McElroy S.L., Gyulai L., Wassef A., Petty F., Pope H.G., Jr., Chou J. C.-Y., Keck P.E., Rhodes L.J. *et al* (2000) A randomized, placebo-controlled 12-month trial of divalproex and lithium in treatment of outpatients with bipolar I disorder. *Arch. Gen. Psychiatry*, **57**: 481–489.
3. Dion G.L., Tohen M., Anthony W.A., Waternaux C.S. (1988) Symptoms and functioning of patients with bipolar disorder six months after hospitalization. *Hosp. Commun. Psychiatry*, **39**: 652–657.
4. Van Gorp W.G., Altshuler L., Theverge D.C., Wilkins J., Dixon W. (1998) Cognitive impairment in euthymic bipolar patients with and without prior alcohol dependence: a preliminary study. *Arch. Gen. Psychiatry*, **55**: 41–46.
5. Angst J. (1998) The emerging epidemiology of hypomania and bipolar II disorder. *J. Affect. Disord.*, **50**: 143–151.

6.6
Bipolar Disorder: How High the Cost?

Gordon Parker[1]

Goldberg and Ernst's review informs us how little we truly know about the economic and social consequences of bipolar disorder, much due to the many variables confounding analyses and interpretation of many of the key studies.

In the last decade we have come to appreciate that bipolar disorder is not quite the pristine episodic condition presented in many textbooks. The archetypal patient is no longer the individual who develops a "high" as a manic defence to some stress and whose mood cycles up and down for several weeks before long quiescent periods of euthymia and normal functioning. We now recognize that bipolar disorder can emerge in adolescence or early adulthood; that it is often preceded by protean *forme fruste* perturbations in childhood; that inter-episode periods of normal mood and functioning are probably not the norm; and that both the swings and their consequences expose the individual to a range of adverse outcomes.

Estimates of the prevalence and consequences of bipolar disorder are clearly influenced by a range of factors, with detection and definition being key confounders of analysis and interpretation. As noted, a significant percentage of those with bipolar disorder have the condition for more than a decade before coming to notice, with cost estimates rarely encompassing its early expression. The elasticity of the diagnostic application of bipolar II

[1] *School of Psychiatry, Prince of Wales Hospital, Randwick 2031, Australia*

disorder ensures many false positives, and, as a category, requires redrawing or abandonment. The changes in health care delivery over the last decade alone have influenced direct costs (especially hospitalization) enormously. Thus, our capacity to compare studies across decades and across health care systems is limited in terms of determining economic burden. Unique amongst psychiatric disorders, bipolar disorder comes, like having a spouse with expensive tastes, with a hyperspend guarantee. It must be the only disorder where a credit cardectomy may be part of the management armamentarium. How do we price such costs?

Yet not all the impact of bipolar disorder is negative. When mood is mildly elevated, its contribution to creativity may be a distinct advantage, as described decades ago by Jonathan Logan (the Broadway producer of *South Pacific*). Most enjoy their "highs" and it is often only following remission (when behaviours and indiscretions are remembered, and the bills start coming in) that negative components are conceded. While there are great dangers in romanticizing bipolar disorder, we do need to consider its overrepresentation in creative people and, as summarized by Kay Jamison [1], the "importance of moods in igniting thought, changing perceptions, creating chaos, forcing order upon that chaos, and enabling transformation". How do such parameters get costed?

Retrospective judgements of the overall effects and benefits vary, almost certainly more influenced by the impact and severity of the depressive episodes rather than the highs. The comedian Spike Milligan [2] observed: "I cannot reassure myself that it has been worthwhile. . . . I do not hold with this romantic view . . . As far as I am concerned it is without a redeeming feature." By contrast, the Australian writer Penelope Rowe [3] stated "I can 'thank' my illness for shaving off some prickly edges and giving me greater tolerance (although I wish there had been an easier way!)." Again, the American psychiatrist and bipolar researcher Kay Jamison [4] stated that, if given a choice about having manic-depressive illness, she would so choose ("Even when I have been most psychotic—delusional, hallucinated, frenzied—I have been aware of finding new corners in my mind and heart"). How then do we apply standard cost-benefit analyses to such a disorder which, like having children, can be variably exhilarating and a burden?

Cost estimates for unipolar depression comprise both costs of the "depression" and of a range of embedded predisposing factors (e.g., personality style, socio-economic deprivation). The contribution of the latter to unipolar depression is substantive, but difficult to disentangle from the costs of the depressed mood state alone. By contrast, few such factors are over-represented in those who develop bipolar disorder. Over-represented psychopathology is more likely to be a consequence rather than an antecedent of bipolar disorder. To the extent that bipolar disorder is the more "pristine" disorder, certain analytic strategies seem favoured. Particularly, comparison of bipolar subjects and matched general community samples, as well as comparison of treated and untreated bipolar individuals. Goldberg and Ernst provide illuminative data from such studies but their relative rarity suggests that findings remain guesstimates.

In addition to further quantitative studies pursuing such analyses, bipolar disorder invites more qualitative and ethnographic analyses, particularly pursuing personal costs. To the extent that the word "disorder" implies gloom or doom, here we have a gloom and boom condition. While highs have certain negative (and even dangerous) consequences, and generally respond well to medication, there are individuals who do achieve some benefit from such mood states and who can boom without busting. We need then to respect quite differing expressions of the condition in any costing analyses, and move beyond a current focus on quantitative studies.

REFERENCES

1. Jamison K.R. (1993)   *Touched with Fire*. Free Press, New York.
2. Jamison K.R. (1995)   *An Unquiet Mind*. Vintage Books, New York.
3. Milligan S., Clare A. (1994).   *Depression and How to Survive It*. Arrow Books, London.
4. Rowe P. (1999).   Van Gogh and lithium. Creativity and bipolar disorder: perspective of a writer. *Austr. N.Z. J. Psychiatry*, **33** (Suppl.): S117–S119.

6.7
Reducing the Impact of Bipolar Disorder: A Developmental Perspective

Melissa P. DelBello[1]

The devastating impact of bipolar disorder on individuals, families, and our society had become apparent with recent investigations of the phenomenology, neurobiology, treatment and outcome of adults with this illness. Goldberg and Ernst's comprehensive review of the economic and social effects of bipolar disorder provides a useful perspective of future research directions that are necessary to reduce these functional and financial deficits. There are several issues relevant to the field of child and adolescent psychiatry that are worth emphasizing, since primary and secondary prevention of bipolar disorder will ultimately be the responsibility of this specialty.

[1] *Department of Psychiatry, University of Cincinnati College of Medicine, 231 Bethesda Ave., P.O. Box 559, Cincinnati, OH 45267, USA*

In a retrospective survey, 59% of adult bipolar members of the National Depressive and Manic-Depressive Association reported the onset of their symptoms during childhood or adolescence [1]. Furthermore, in this study, child and adolescent onset bipolar disorder was associated with increased social morbidity, which was diminished by effective treatment. This survey highlights the imperative need for studies involving bipolar children and adolescents. Targeted early intervention strategies for children and adolescents at familial risk for developing bipolar disorder will be successful only after the phenomenology and biology of, and effective treatments for, paediatric bipolar disorder are better understood.

There are several ongoing preliminary investigations assessing the effectiveness of mood stabilizers in children at familial risk for bipolar disorder who exhibit subsyndromal affective symptoms. While these studies are important, given the lack of controlled data regarding effective treatments for paediatric bipolar disorder and the paucity of longitudinal studies of children and adolescents with familial risk for developing bipolar disorder, they may be premature. Moreover, as Goldberg and Ernst appropriately point out, the impact of early screening and treatment has yet to be systematically studied.

During the past five years, several reports have clarified the age-specific phenotypic manifestations of bipolar disorder in children and adolescents [2–5]. These studies consistently demonstrate that paediatric bipolar disorder commonly presents with comorbid attention deficit hyperactivity disorder (ADHD), conduct, and substance use disorders, is associated with poor outcome and high relapse and school drop-out rates, and often requires polypharmacologic intervention. Recently, the first study to assess the psychosocial impact of paediatric bipolar disorder described that bipolar children exhibit significant impairment in child–parent and child–peer interactions and social skills compared with ADHD children and healthy controls [6].

Despite these recent advances, there are still many areas that need further exploration prior to the development of prevention and early intervention programmes. For example, outcome studies of children with major depression revealed that those who experience recurrence of major depression during follow-up have higher rates of major depression in first-degree relatives [7]. It remains unclear whether this is also the case for children with bipolar disorder. Furthermore, children and adolescents with bipolar disorder are likely to have significant financial and psychosocial consequences, since many of the factors which largely contribute to the economic and social burden of bipolar disorder, such as the presence of comorbidity, polypharmacy, high relapse rates and psychosocial impairment, are present. However, there are no published cost-estimate studies and little is known about the long-term outcome of children who are diagnosed with bipolar disorder. Another area which deserves further attention is the utility of psychoeducation and early intervention substance use programmes aimed at bipolar adolescents, since data suggest that subsequent to the onset of *adolescent* bipolar disorder there is a significant risk for developing a substance use disorder [4, 8]. Additionally, neurobiological investigations are necessary to further validate and characterize the phenotypic variability of paediatric bipolar disorder. Prospective longitudinal outcome and biological studies of bipolar children and adolescents into adulthood are also needed to determine the psychosocial and neurobiological developmental trajectories associated with paediatric bipolar disorder, to identify neurobiological predictors of illness course and treatment response, and to clarify whether paediatric bipolar disorder is a distinct entity or a developmental variant of adult bipolar disorder.

It is difficult to develop early-intervention strategies when treatment efficacy data in children are scarce. There has been only one placebo-controlled study of a mood stabilizer in children and adolescents with bipolar disorder [7]. Furthermore, the effects of stimulants and antidepressants on children and adolescents with and at risk for developing bipolar disorder are not completely understood. As Goldberg and Ernst describe, clinical experience and several recent studies suggest that exposure to stimulants or antidepressants may hasten the onset of and exacerbate the course of bipolar disorder in children [9, 10]. Future prospective investigations of the effects of stimulants and antidepressants on illness course of children at familial risk for developing bipolar disorder are necessary.

Bipolar offspring studies are useful in that they permit characterization of a population with a high genetic loading, identification of phenomenological and neurobiological predictors of psychopathology and prodromes, and eventually, development of early detection and intervention strategies. Several investigations suggest that children and adolescents who have at least one parent with bipolar disorder have an increased risk for developing affective disorders in addition to a wide range of other psychopathology [11]. However, most bipolar offspring studies are not longitudinal and, therefore, are unable to assess stability of diagnoses, outcome of unaffected offspring, and environmental and neurobiological predictors of and risk factors for the development of bipolar disorder. Additionally, further characterization of the neurobiology and phenomenology of paediatric bipolar disorder is essential to enable identification of prodromal, subsyndromal, and syndromal manifestations and neurodevelopmental antecedents of bipolar disorder in "high-risk" youth. Therefore, only after research accomplishments advance our understanding of paediatric bipolar disorder will we be able to develop useful and effective early intervention programmes aimed at reducing the economic and social disabilities associated with bipolar disorder.

REFERENCES

1. Lish J.D., Dime-Meenan S., Whybrow P.C., Price R.A., Hirschfeld R.M. (1994) The National Depressive and Manic-depressive Association (DMDA) survey of bipolar members. *J. Affect. Disord.*, **31**: 281–294.
2. Geller B., Zimerman B., Williams M., Bolhofner K., Craney J.L., DelBello M.P., Soutullo C.A. (2000) Diagnostic characteristics of 93 cases of a prepubertal and early adolescent bipolar disorder phenotype by gender, puberty and comorbid attention deficit hyperactivity disorder. *J. Child Adolesc. Psychopharmacol.*, **10**: 157–164.
3. Geller B., Craney J.L., Bolhofner K., DelBello M.P., Williams M., Zimerman B. (2001) One-year recovery and relapse rates of children with a prepubertal and early adolescent bipolar phenotype. *Am. J. Psychiatry*, **58**: 303–305.
4. Wilens T.E., Biederman J., Milstein R.B., Wozniak J., Hahesy A.L., Spencer T.J. (1999) Risk for substance use disorders in youth with child- and adolescent-onset bipolar disorder. *J. Am. Acad. Child Adolesc. Psychiatry*, **38**: 680–685.
5. Wozniak J., Biederman J., Kiely K., Ablon J.S., Faraone S.V., Mundy E., Mennin D. (1995) Mania-like symptoms suggestive of childhood-onset bipolar disorder in clinically referred children. *J. Am. Acad. Child Adolesc. Psychiatry*, **34**: 867–876.
6. Geller B., Bolhofner K., Craney J.L., Williams M., DelBello M.P., Gundersen K. (2000) Psychosocial functioning in a prepubertal and early adolescent bipolar phenotype. *J. Am. Acad. Child Adolesc. Psychiatry*, **39**: 1543–1548.
7. Weissman M.M., Wolk S., Wickramaratne P., Goldstein R.B., Adams P., Greenwald S., Ryan N.D., Dahl R.E., Steinberg D. (1999) Children with prepubertal-onset major depressive disorder and anxiety grown up. *Arch. Gen. Psychiatry*, **56**: 794–801.
8. Geller B., Cooper T.B., Sun K., Zimerman B., Frazier J., Williams M., Heath J. (1998) Double-blind and placebo-controlled study of lithium for adolescent bipolar disorders with secondary substance dependency. *J. Am. Acad. Child Adolesc. Psychiatry*, **37**: 171–178.
9. DelBello M.P., Soutullo C.A., Hendricks W., Niemeier R.T., McElroy S.L., Strakowski S.M. (2001) Prior stimulant treatment in adolescents with bipolar disorder: association with age at onset. *Bipolar Disord.*, **3**: 53–57.
10. El-Mallakh R.S., Cicero D., Holman J., Robertson J. (2001) Antidepressant exposure in children diagnosed with bipolar disorder. *Bipolar Disord.*, **3** (Suppl. 1): 35.
11. DelBello M.P., Geller B. (2001) Review of studies of child and adolescents offspring of bipolar parents. *Bipolar Disord.* (in press).

6.8
Stress, Relapse and Disability in Bipolar Disorder
Joyce E. Whiteside[1]

The extent of disability, family disruption and fatality associated with bipolar disorder truly makes it one of the most financially impacting

[1] 145 East 26th Street, Suite 3C, New York, NY 10010, USA

illnesses affecting mankind. Goldberg and Ernst describe the economic impact of bipolar illness not only in direct costs, but also in the hard to define indirect costs of social impact.

As they report, there is a large body of research suggesting psychosocial disability may be profound among bipolar patients even after affective symptoms remit [1] and poor psychosocial functioning is highly prevalent among these patients. For example, Miklowitz and Frank [2] show that "for the 6 months after an acute manic or depressive episode, 57% of patients cannot maintain employment, and only 21% work at their expected level of employment even when they are relatively symptom free and maintained on standard drug regimes". An inability to regain pre-illness functioning can act as a vicious cycle for the bipolar patient, increasing financial and family pressure, which in turn may affect the probability of relapse.

The interplay between disruptive family history and poor coping strategies may set up a malicious cycle of depressive episodes and stressful events. Regardless of origin, these psychological events could lead to biological results. Researchers have suggested that stressful conditions or dysregulated stress reactions may alter neurochemical activity or neurohormonal functioning, respectively [3].

Ellicott et al [4] examined the importance of stress in affective episodes in a population of bipolar patients with similar conclusions. The research indicated that genetic and biological components are important in the etiology of manic-depressive illness, but they cannot entirely explain the variance in the magnitude or length between episodes. They found a greater likelihood of recurrent episodes in patients with high levels of stress compared with those with low to no stress. Though their research controlled for medication compliance, stress may lead patients to poor medication compliance, which in turn could lead to an increase in symptoms. They concluded: "psychological and medical interventions might need to be increased at times of stress". Their findings also suggest that while high levels of stress may lead to an exacerbation of illness, stressful life circumstances are not in themselves likely to be direct causes of affective episodes; rather, an individual's reaction to stress may be a mitigating factor.

This is supported by later observations by Swendsen et al [5], who found that psychiatric history, age of onset, or number of prior episodes did not predict relapse in bipolar patients, but personality variables did, such as introversion and obsessionality. They concluded that "psychological factors appeared to moderate the association between stress and relapse". In a prospective study, Hunt et al [6] examined the relationship between significant social stressors and affective relapse among 57 bipolar I patients during the course of two years. The findings suggest that while there is no clear causal relationship between life events and relapse, there is a significant increase in life stressors in the month prior to relapse. However, with the cyclical nature of bipolar disorder, it is difficult to separate in time those events preceding an affective relapse and those stressors that are symptoms of the illness. This is especially difficult with manic episodes.

Silverstone and Romans-Clarkson's review of the literature [7] suggests that many if not most patients (28–99%) who have an initial episode will relapse and of those most relapse three or more times. They conclude that psychosocial and environmental stressors play a greater role in the initial episodes than in successive relapses. Post [8] supports these findings indicating the onset of the illness, regardless of the state (i.e. manic or depressed), is more strongly correlated with a major psychosocial stressor than successive mood episodes. In addition, his research explores the neurobiology underlying the disorder "indicating how electrical and chemical stimulation and psychosocial stressors affect gene expression, thus present [ing] a way in which acute events can have long lasting effects on the subsequent reactivity of the organism".

Through a complex model in which psychosocial stresses may lead to a selective activation sequence of gene transcription, Post hypothesizes that significant life stress which precipitates a first mood episode may directly alter gene expression. This, in turn, affects neurotransmission, allowing future episodes to evolve spontaneously. A study of occupational functioning among 130 bipolar and unipolar patients and their relatives [9] supports Post's view: while previous research has demonstrated the detrimental effects of bipolar illness on occupational functioning, the "relationships between bipolar disorder and social adjustment are complex and cannot be conceived of simply in terms of negative consequences".

Related to this perspective, it has been reported [3] that suicide attempts in bipolar patients were often linked to stressful life events, but that such life stresses were more often than not the consequence of self-damaging behaviours acted out by patients themselves. As Goldberg and Ernst describe, suicide is the most frequent cause of premature death among bipolar patients. This illustrates the importance of monitoring a patient's stressors in order to increase medication compliance, decrease cycling and improve life expectancy.

REFERENCES

1. Gitlin M.J., Hammen C. (1999) Syndromal and psychosocial outcome in bipolar disorder: a complex and circular relationship. In *Bipolar Disorders: Clinical Course and Outcome* (Eds J.F. Goldberg, M. Harrow), American Psychiatric Press, Washington.
2. Miklowitz D.J., Frank E. (1999) New psychotherapies for bipolar disorder. In *Bipolar Disorders: Clinical Course and Outcome* (Eds J.F. Goldberg, M. Harrow), American Psychiatric Press, Washington.

3. Hammen C., Davila J., Brown G., Ellicott A., Gitlin M. (1992)   Psychiatric history and stress: predictors of severity of unipolar depression. J. Abnorm. Psychol., **101**: 45–52.
4. Ellicott A., Hammen C., Gitlin M., Brown G., Jamison K. (1990)   Life events and the course of bipolar disorder. Am. J. Psychiatry, **147**: 1194–1198.
5. Swendsen J., Hammen C., Heller T., Gitlin M. (1995)   Correlates of stress re-activity in patients with bipolar disorder. Am. J. Psychiatry, **152**: 795–797.
6. Hunt N., Bruce-Jones W., Silverstone T. (1992)   Life events and relapse in bipo-lar affective disorder. J. Affect. Disord., **25**: 13–20.
7. Silverstone T., Romans-Clarkson S. (1989)   Bipolar affective disorder: causes and prevention of relapse. Br. J. Psychiatry, **154**: 321–335.
8. Post R.M. (1992)   Transduction of psychosocial stress into the neurobiology of recurrent affective disorder. Am. J. Psychiatry, **49**: 999–1010.
9. Verdoux H., Bourgeois M. (1995)   Social class in unipolar and bipolar probands and relatives. J. Affect. Disord., **33**: 181–187.

6.9
Broadening the Perspective on Bipolar Disorder Outcome

James H. Kocsis[1]

Goldberg and Ernst have contributed a thorough and incisive review of the enormous economic and psychosocial burden associated with bipolar disorder diagnoses. Unfortunately this field is beset with even more daunting methodologic challenges than traditional research in areas such as treatment efficacy and clinical outcomes. While it is obvious to clinicians, patients and family members that bipolar illness remains difficult to treat and is associated with enormous economic and social consequences, very little is certain concerning the impact of treatment, in particular the effects of long-term treatment on either the illness itself or its associated consequences [1].

Ironically, some of the lack of clarity stems from recent advances in diagnosis and therapeutics. Our best information on the long-term course and consequences of treatment derives from studies of the use of the oldest of the modern mood stabilizers, lithium, in typical patients with bipolar I illness [2–5]. In recent years, the importance of a wider spectrum of bipolar subtypes has been recognized, e.g., bipolar II, rapid-cycling bipolar and atypical bipolar. The evolving use of a variety of new antiepileptic agents and novel atypical antipsychotic drugs as mood stabilizers has greatly broadened our therapeutic options. Many years of systematic follow-up research will be required to fill the information gap concerning the usefulness and importance of each of these treatments applied to the various

[1] *Department of Psychiatry, Weill-Cornell Medical College, New York Hospital, 525 East 68th St., New York, NY 10021, USA*

subtypes of bipolar illness. Such studies will need to address not only the reduction and prevention of bipolar symptoms and episodes, but also the effects of treatment on the broader psychosocial and economic burdens associated with these disorders. As Goldberg and Ernst emphasize, additional research attention needs to be given to "real-world" clinical diagnosis and treatment to achieve a true measure of the impact of new advances in nosology and drug development on the bipolar population.

In the United States, the National Institute of Mental Health has recognized these issues as an important priority of the mental health research agenda. Among the new initiatives of the Institute has been the Systematic Treatment Enhancement Program for Bipolar Disorder (STEP-BP), which is a systematic, multisite follow-up of a large cohort of bipolar patients over a five-year period. Many of the newer therapeutic options, including psychotherapy, will be delivered based on clinically driven algorithms. A broad range of outcomes, including psychosocial and cost-effectiveness measures, will be assessed. The results will inform us about the effectiveness, the psychosocial consequences and the costs of the treatments delivered. This effort is a "step" in the right direction. Much remains to be done.

REFERENCES

1. Bowden C.L., Calabrese J.R., McElroy S.L., Gyulai L., Wassef A., Petty F., Pope H.G. Jr., Chou J.C., Keck P.E. Jr., Rhodes L.J. *et al* (2000) A randomized, placebo-controlled 12-month trial of divalproex and lithium in treatment of outpatients with bipolar I disorder. Divalproex Maintenance Study Group. *Arch. Gen. Psychiatry*, **57**: 481–489.
2. Reifman A., Wyatt R.D. (1980) Lithium: a brake in the rising cost of mental illness. *Arch. Gen. Psychiatry*, **37**: 385–388.
3. Morrison D.P., McCreadie R.G. (1985) The impact of lithium in South-West Scotland: II. A longitudinal study. *Br. J. Psychiatry*, **146**: 74–77.
4. McCreadie R.G. (1987) The economics of lithium therapy. In *Depression and Mania: Modern Lithium Therapy* (Ed. F.N. Johnson), pp. 257–259, IRL Press, Oxford.
5. Tondo L., Baldessarini R.J. (2000) Reduced suicide risk during lithium maintenance treatment. *J. Clin. Psychiatry*, **61** (Suppl. 9): 97–104.

6.10
The Current Economic Picture of Bipolar Disorder: Your Money or Your Life!

J. Raymond DePaulo[1]

Goldberg and Ernst have provided an integrated picture of the economics and treatment effectiveness research in bipolar disorders. My comments are purposefully provocative and will reflect my experience as both an ageing American clinician and an advocate for and sometimes practitioner in the etiological research of affective disorders.

The authors' tracking of the research on bipolar disorder from global epidemiology, to the bedside, and back again (via the home, community, and societal institutions) is elegant. I am quite familiar with the research covered, but it would not have occurred to me to connect the economy/ social impact research (such as the WHO study) with treatment effectiveness research (e.g. guidelines-based psychopharmacology).

I have championed the Global Burden of Disease studies as validating the importance of major psychiatric syndromes. The studies show that psychiatric disorders make up five of the top 10 causes of disability worldwide in 1990 [1]. I have argued that the appropriate responses to these findings would be to treat them and to "cover them", like any other mysterious medical syndromes, and to increase substantially the commitment to basic etiological as well as clinical research on bipolar disorder (as well as the other four conditions listed).

To synopsize my argument in the light of Goldberg and Ernst's essay, I will risk creating a "straw man in order to knock it down", as I highlight the need for greater emphasis on etiologic research in bipolar disorder. First, let me give a few reasons why I do not usually connect the Global Impact Research with treatment effectiveness research: both lines of research are in their infancy in psychiatry and we should expect conflicting results from serious investigators for several years before anchor points are accepted. As an example, what is the somatic equivalent impairment for a three-month episode of uncomplicated major depression? Or, is lamotrigine an antidepressant or is it a specific treatment for bipolar II illness? In addition, I have a general concern about the value that will come from the current effectiveness trials based on treatment guidelines. This research may be premature, not just new. Why? The research, as highlighted in the essay, is limited in its scope. It fits into an American view of treatment that is not widely shared around the world. Americans tend to value the anticonvulsant medications and "diagnosis specific" psychotherapies in ways that our

[1] Department of Psychiatry and Behavioral Sciences, Johns Hopkins Medical Institutions, 600 N. Wolfe Street, Baltimore, MD 21287–7381, USA

European, Asian, and Australian colleagues do not, so that the research has narrow generalizability. I predict that over time, we Americans will think more like the rest of the world does about bipolar disorder management— not the reverse.

Finally, at a more fundamental level, I do not see how we can achieve treatment guidelines that have any durability over time without greater knowledge of the brain mechanisms (genetic, pharmacological, and structural) involved in bipolar disorder and the critical mechanisms of therapeutic action of our treatments. It would be like developing guidelines for diabetes management before we knew about glucose, insulin, and their relationship. This is not to say that we will not get some value from the guidelines-based research. We will undoubtedly learn a lot—including much that will surprise us, I believe. But we will not, in my judgement, create widely useful or durable treatment guidelines for treating bipolar disorder. We need to match the new funds going into treatment research (from governmental and foundation sources) with new funds to support basic genetic, brain imaging, and basic pharmacological research which will provide us with insight into the pathogenesis of bipolar disorder, in the way it has done for Alzheimer's disease [2]. This will provide us with improving diagnostic methods and rational treatment targets over decades to come and will provide the anchors needed for better treatment studies.

REFERENCES

1. Lopez A.D., Murray C.C. (1998) The global burden of disease, 1990–2020. *Nature Med.*, **4**: 1241–1243.
2. Selkoe D.J. (2001) Alzheimer's disease: genes, proteins, and therapy. *Physiol. Rev.*, **81**: 741–766.

6.11
The Economic and Social Burden of Affective Disorders: Unmet and Growing Needs

Daniel Souery[1]

Until the last few years, it has been suggested that no more than 1% of the general population has bipolar disorder. The recent literature on the lifetime prevalence of the bipolar spectrum suggests higher prevalence rates of up to

[1] *Department of Psychiatry, University Clinics of Brussels, Erasme Hospital, 808 Route de Lennik, 1070 Brussels, Belgium*

6.5%. The Zurich cohort study [1] identified a prevalence rate up to age 35 of 5.5% of DSM-IV hypomania/mania. The significant increase in prevalence rates from previous studies may be explained by softer and subthreshold clinical forms of bipolar disorder such as bipolar II, depression followed by antidepressant-associated hypomania, brief hypomania (recurrent and lasting 1–3 days). Despite being among the most prevalent psychiatric conditions in the community, these manifestations of the clinical spectrum of bipolarity remain under-recognized and often misdiagnosed.

Goldberg and Ernst, in their review, go far beyond the classical observations on epidemiology and morbidity and offer a comprehensive dissection of the different components involved in the economic and social burden of bipolar disorder. The Global Burden of Disease study mentioned in the review [2] provides a remarkable way to capture both the mortality effects and the disabling consequences of mood disorders using one single indicator (the Disability-Adjusted Life Year or DALY). This approach revealed the "unseen burden" of psychiatric disorders such as depression and bipolar disorders, almost invisible to public health.

Despite the development of new pharmacotherapies and treatment guidelines, the consequences of under-recognition, misdiagnosis, inappropriate treatments and psychosocial disabilities remain impressive. The results we actually achieve with available pharmacologic and psychotherapic treatments fall far short of what is achievable.

In Europe, very few existing studies address these issues. The lifetime prevalence of depression has been recently studied in a large European community survey [3], the Depression Research in European Society (DEPRES). In this survey, 78 463 persons within a demographically representative sample were interviewed using a standardized diagnostic instrument compatible with DSM-IV diagnostic criteria (Mini-International Neuropsychiatric Interview, MINI). A total of 13 359 of the 78 463 adults who participated in screening interviews across six countries were identified as suffering from depression, a six-month prevalence of 17%. Major depression accounted for 6.9% of the cases of depression, and minor depression for 1.8%. Depressive symptoms were responsible for substantial work and social impairment in both major and minor depression. A significant proportion of sufferers from depression (43%) failed to seek treatment for their depressive symptoms. Sufferers from major depression imposed the greatest demand on healthcare resources, making almost three times as many visits to their family doctor as non-sufferers (4.4 vs. 1.5 visits over six months). More than two-thirds of depressed subjects (69%) were not prescribed any treatment and, when drug therapy was prescribed (31%), only 25% of these subjects were given antidepressant drugs. The number of days of work lost due to illness increased with the severity of depression. Major depression had most impact on productive work, with sufferers losing four times as many working days over six months as non-sufferers. The results of the DEPRES survey confirm the burden imposed on the individual sufferer in terms of impaired quality of life and on society in terms of healthcare utilization and lost productivity.

Continuing medical education and the development of systematic quality management projects may help to improve the situation. Several factors are decisive for achieving an optimal quality of care and an optimal outcome. At the level of clinical practice, these are related to medical decisions, treatment habits, cost-benefit profile, patient compliance. Quality of care in psychiatry is often reflected by subjective aspects such as quality of life, psychosocial functioning or satisfaction with treatment. Objective measures include among others severity of symptoms, relapse rate, side effect rate, number of hospitalizations, and treatment response. The parallel monitoring of these aspects is difficult in daily practice and in the long term can only be achieved through quality measurement systems. This kind of system facilitates the collection of patient data for use in hospitals or across a country and may improve the quality of care in reducing relapse rates, increasing compliance and reducing direct and indirect costs.

It appears that, although successfully practised in other medical disciplines, quality management programmes are not largely accepted in psychiatry [4]. Much more money and manpower should be invested in such initiatives. There is therefore a requirement to demonstrate that investment is needed in such directions, and generate evidence on affordable and cost-effective management and prevention strategies.

REFERENCES

1. Angst J. (1998)   The emerging epidemiology of hypomania and bipolar II disorder. *J. Affect. Disord.*, **50**: 143–151.
2. Murray C.J.L., Lopez A.D. (1996)   *The Global Burden of Disease: A Comprehensive Assessment of Mortality and Disability from Diseases, Injuries, and Risk Factors in 1990 and Projected to 2020.* Harvard University Press, Cambridge.
3. Lepine J.P., Gastpar M., Mendlewicz J., Tylee A. (1997)   Depression in the community: the first pan-European study DEPRES (Depression Research in European Society). *Int. Clin. Psychopharmacol.*, **12**: 19–29.
4. Kissling W. (2001)   Who is interested in quality of everyday psychiatric care? *Int. Clin. Psychopharmacol.*, **16** (Suppl. 3): S1–S4.

6.12
Difficulties in Evaluating the Economics of Bipolar Disorder in Developing Countries

Ahmed Okasha[1]

We are indebted to Goldberg and Ernst for their seminal review about the economic and social burden of bipolar disorder in spite of the scarcity of the literature on this subject.

The economics of mental disorders is rarely estimated in developing countries, because the resources needed for such studies are unavailable in low-income countries. The studies done on bipolar disorder are scarce even in developed countries. However, they can be a paradigm for cost estimates of mental disorders in developing countries.

In a recent study, Angst [1] reported that, while 13 epidemiologic studies since 1980 had persistently found a low lifetime prevalence of mania (0.0–1.7%), the application of DSM-IV criteria by trained clinical psychologists produced a prevalence for mania and hypomania of 5.5% by age 35. A broadening of diagnostic criteria to include other aspects of the bipolar spectrum (hypomania, cyclothymia, and bipolar disorder not otherwise specified) in six studies since 1978 yields a prevalence ranging between 3.0 and 8.8%.

This high prevalence suggests that bipolar disorder is a general health problem with significant social and economic sequelae, a fact of which policy makers should be aware.

The economic burden of treatment of bipolar disorder is poorly understood. A recent study [2] discussed the direct cost of care for bipolar disorder in an employer claims database representing the healthcare experience of approximately 1.6 million covered lives. The study examined the estimated cost of care including expenditures for hospitalization, hospital outpatient services, outpatient medications, psychiatric day/night facilities, nursing home facilities, office visits, laboratory tests, substance abuse treatment, and other services. The prevalence of bipolar disorder in the population was 5.5 patients per 1000 eligible members. These patients incurred significant annual expenditures, totalling $13 402 in 1995, $11 856 in 1996, and $11 146 in 1997. These expenditures were comparable to the costs of treatment for schizophrenia in the same population during this period. Annual costs for outpatient use of mood stabilizers and antipsychotic medications increased by $168 (42%) over the study interval, totalling $568 in 1997. However, other costs of care for these patients decreased by $2424 (i.e., more than 80%) during the same period.

_____

[1] *Institute of Psychiatry, Ain Shams University, 3 Shawarby Street, Kasr El Nil, Cairo, Egypt*

In 1990, the total annual prevalence-based cost associated with depression, including both unipolar and bipolar illness, was estimated as $44 billion in the United States [3]. This sum has been subdivided into direct costs (totaling approximately $7.6 billion/year, or 17% of total costs) and indirect expenses (about 83% of total costs). Direct expenses related to affective disorders include nursing home (33%) and inpatient costs (26%), crime (25%), substance abuse (8%), suicide (2%), medications (1%), shelters (1%), and research/ training programme costs (1%). In developing countries, because of lack of quality services and underpayment of mental health professionals, the cost of medications, especially the novel ones, reaches 20–25% of the total cost.

To my knowledge, the only research on economics of bipolar disorder in developing countries was delivered by Okasha and Ramy [4]. Sixty manic inpatients, whose diagnosis had been confirmed by the SCID-IV on case records and whose severity had been assessed using the Bech–Rafaelsen Mania Scale, were divided into two groups according to whether or not they received electroconvulsive therapy (ECT) in addition to pharmacotherapy consisting of antipsychotics, lithium and/or anticonvulsants. Both the duration of hospital stay and the total treatment cost were significantly higher for non-ECT patients than for ECT patients (duration: 37.13 days versus 19.02 days; cost: $1904 versus $1097). This means that giving ECT will reduce the cost and the duration of hospitalization by about 50%. For the last 30 years I have been teaching that ECT is the best treatment for acute mania, but only recently the American Psychiatric Association included ECT as the first choice of management in its guidelines.

An ongoing study on ECT maintenance for resistant and relapsing bipolar patients is giving encouraging results in Egypt. This is a policy recommended for low-income countries with limited resources.

Goldberg et al [5] found at both two- and five-year follow-ups that fewer than one-quarter of bipolar patients with affective relapses had steady work performance, and that affective relapse led to impaired work functioning more profoundly among bipolar than unipolar patients. At least one-quarter of euthymic bipolar patients show impaired insight and an inability to recognize affective prodromes.

In recent years, much progress has been made in the diagnosis and treatment of schizophrenia and depression. Bipolar disorder, however, remains frequently misunderstood, leading to inconsistent diagnosis and treatment. Bipolar disorder is underdiagnosed and under-recognized and frequently misdiagnosed as unipolar major depressive disorder, which can increase the burden of the disorder. Antidepressants are probably overused and mood stabilizers underused. Reasons for underdiagnosis include: a) patients' impaired insight into mania, b) failure to involve family members in the diagnostic process, c) inadequate understanding by clinicians of manic symptoms.

Psychosocial disability from bipolar disorder remains extensive and encompasses multiple domains, including work and social functioning, independent community living, family adjustment, premature mortality, and diminished quality of life. Comorbid substance abuse or other psychiatric diagnoses [6] and/or medical conditions [7] are highly prevalent in bipolar disorder.

Further research is required in low-income countries with limited resources on the economics of mental disorder.

REFERENCES

1. Angst J. (1998)   The emerging epidemiology of hypomania and bipolar II disorder. *J. Affect. Disord.* **50**: 143–151.
2. Johnstone M.B., Loosbrock D.L., Stockwell Morris L., Gibson P.J., Barber B.L, Lichtenstein M., Henderson S., Dulisse B.K. (2001)   Estimated costs of treatment for bipolar affective disorder in a large employer database. Health Outcomes Evaluation Group, United States Medical Division, Eli Lilly and Company.
3. Wyatt R.J., Henter I. (1995)   An economic evaluation of manic-depressive illness: 1991. *Soc. Psychiatry Psychiatr. Epidemiol.*, **30**: 213–219.
4. Okasha T., Ramy H. (2000)   Using electroconvulsive therapy (ECT) in the treatment of manic episodes: economic aspects. Presented at the Meeting on Mental Health Economics in Arab and Sub-Saharan Countries, Cairo, October 10–12.
5. Goldberg J.F., Harrow M., Grossman L.S. (1995)   Recurrent affective syndromes in bipolar and unipolar mood disorders at follow-up. *Br. J. Psychiatry*, **166**: 382–385.
6. McElroy S.L., Altshuler L.L., Suppes T., Keck P.E. Jr., Frye M.A., Denicoff K.D., Nolen W.A., Kupka R.W., Leverich G.S., Rochussen J.R. *et al* (2001)   Axis I psychiatric comorbidity and its relationship to historical illness variables in 288 patients with bipolar disorder. *Am. J. Psychiatry*, **158**: 420–426.
7. Strakowski S.M., McElroy S.L., Keck P.E. Jr., West S.A. (1994)   The co-occurrence of mania with medical and other psychiatric disorders. *Int. J. Psychiatry Med.*, **24**: 305–328.

6.13

The Present Role of Advocacy Organizations in the Long-Term Management of the Bipolar Patient

Paolo Lucio Morselli[1]

In the present situation, where all over Europe psychiatric care is being transferred from institutions to the community, access to care and adher-

[1] *Fondazione IDEA and GAMIAN Europe, Via Statuto 8, 20121 Milano, Italy*

ence to treatment are far from being satisfactory [1–3]. Patient-driven advocacy organizations may play an important role in the long-term management of persons with mental disorders, for the reduction of the present burden that afflicts not only the patients but also their family and the community as well. More specifically, they may play an important role in helping to reintegrate into a more active and productive life those who suffered from mood and/or anxiety disorders. This is particularly true for those suffering from bipolar disorders, in whom the lingering effects of the disease may be very long lasting and relapses are more frequent than in other mood disorders. The interventions of patient-driven advocacy associations may also help in reducing the indirect costs related to the disorders [4].

At present, in Europe, these interventions are oriented along two main lines: a) information and education of the patient, his/her family and the general population; b) direct intervention and support through self-help groups favouring increase of the individual self-esteem and improvement of social adjustment, hence permitting a more rapid reintegration and a better quality of life.

A recent survey carried out among members of Fondazione IDEA, an advocacy association based in Italy, indicated that, out of 1130 patients who suffered from mood disorders (25% bipolar) 3–5 years before and were free of symptoms at the moment of the survey, lingering effects of the disease and impaired social functioning were present in 35% of the cases, despite their apparent return to working or professional activities and social interactions. The most severely impaired items were those referring to the "relationship with the other" or "capability to communicate with the other", both at the workplace and within the family. Furthermore, about 20% of the respondents reported they felt "stigmatized" both within the family and at the workplace or socially. As generally known, a poor or reduced social adjustment is associated with a poor quality of life and a higher risk of relapses [5].

Self-support groups do act specifically on this aspect. By improving the patient's ability to communicate, to express his/her ideas, by allowing him/her to realize that many others have suffered from the same disease, by permitting increased knowledge and understanding of the disease and its treatment, self-support groups gradually transform the sufferer from a passive executor of the physician's instructions, that are only partially understood, to a person that assumes an active role. Furthermore, those who participate actively in self-support groups discover that their suggestions and comments may be useful and important for the "others". All this leads to an increased self-esteem and to a better quality of life. Stigmatization is no longer feared and the future appears brighter.

"Relatives-oriented" self-support groups do also make it possible to reduce the burden on family members. In fact, relatives' improved knowledge and education about the disease and the way they should behave with respect to the sufferer lead to a better understanding of the situation of the sufferer, making it less conflicting. Furthermore, in case of relapses, relatives may become able to identify the prodromes of an episode, with a consequent earlier intervention by mental health workers.

Today patient-driven advocacy organizations also have an important role in the information and education of the general population. Despite tremendous advances of neuroscience and neuropsychopharmacology, despite an increased understanding of various brain disorders, mental illnesses still remain a "taboo" for a large part of the general population and, unfortunately, also for a part of the medical profession. Bipolar disorder is still too often labelled as "manic-depressive psychosis", where the term "psychosis" is linked to the concept of "incurable disease" and the term manic is associated with very negative connotations. This creates the stigma, that hits not only the patient but his/her family too. In the above-mentioned survey among 1020 relatives (not suffering from mood disorders), 20% declared they felt to be or were stigmatized because of having within the family a person suffering from mood disorder.

Relatives and family members may have an important role in the follow-up of the bipolar patient, but they know very little about the disease, are not prepared to manage the patient, and are not informed on the meaning of emerging manic symptoms. They can only be witnesses of the strange changes of their beloved and are powerless against the devastating march of the disorder.

Because of the above, the general population should be better educated and informed about bipolar disorder. They should know that bipolar disorder is not a "divine malediction" nor an "untreatable disease", but it is a chronic, biological, curable disorder that, if not treated, may lead to a serious impairment of the social role of the individual and of his/her family, and in 15% of cases to suicide.

Patient-driven advocacy organizations do the best they can, but a more integrated effort should be implemented with the help of governmental structures and scientific societies. The voice of mental illness advocacy organizations should be listened to more attentively, and these organizations should be allowed to participate in the decisions on mental health policy programmes. An integrated approach, based on an active co-operation between patients, families, psychiatrists, primary care physicians and governmental agencies, would hopefully lead to the necessary changes in the organization and availability of psychiatric services and consequently to a reduced burden of the disorder.

REFERENCES

1. Christiana J.M., Gilman S.E., Guardino M., Mickelson K., Morselli P.L., Olofson M., Kessler R.C. (2000) Duration between onset and time of obtaining initial treatment among people with anxiety and mood disorders: an international survey of members of mental health patient advocacy groups. *Psychol. Med.*, **30**: 693–703.
2. Wang P.S., Gilman S.E., Guardino M., Christiana J.M., Morselli P.L., Mickelson K., Kessler R.C. (2000) Initiation and adherence to treatment for mental disorders. Examination of patient advocate group members in 11 countries. *Med. Care*, **38**: 926–936.
3. Morselli P.L. (1999) What the patients tell us: report on the GAMIAN international survey with specific reference to the Italian data. In *Manage or Perish* (Eds J. Guimon, N. Sartorius), pp. 475–488, Kluwer, New York.
4. Morselli P.L. (2000) Present and future role of mental illness advocacy associations in the management of the mentally ill: realities, needs and hopes at the edge of the third millennium. *Bipolar Disord.*, **2**: 294–300.
5. Hirschfeld R.M.A., Montgomery S.A., Keller M. B., Kasper S., Schatzberg A.F., Möller H.J., Healy D., Baldwin D., Humble M., Versiani M. *et al* (2000) Social functioning in depression: a review. *J. Clin. Psychiatry*, **61**: 268–275.

Index

Acknowledgements

The Editors would like to thank Drs Paola Bucci, Umberto Volpe and Andrea Dell'Acqua, of the Department of Psychiatry of the University of Naples, for their help in the processing of manuscripts.

The publication has been supported by an unrestricted educational grant from Sanofi-Synthelabo, which is hereby gratefully acknowledged.